HEALTH PROMOTION AND DISEASE PREVENTION IN CLINICAL PRACTICE

SECOND EDITION

HEALTH PROMOTION AND DISEASE PREVENTION IN CLINICAL PRACTICE

SECOND EDITION

STEVEN H. WOOLF, MD, MPH

Professor
Departments of Family Medicine, Epidemiology and Community Health
Virginia Commonwealth University
Richmond, Virginia

STEVEN JONAS, MD, MPH

Professor
Department of Preventive Medicine
Graduate Program in Public Health
School of Medicine
Stony Brook University
Stony Brook, New York

EVONNE KAPLAN-LISS, MD, MPH

Assistant Professor
Department of Preventive Medicine
Graduate Program in Public Health
Department of Pediatrics, and School of Journalism
Stony Brook University
Stony Brook, New York

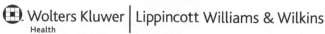 Wolters Kluwer | Lippincott Williams & Wilkins
Health

Philadelphia · Baltimore · New York · London
Buenos Aires · Hong Kong · Sydney · Tokyo

Acquisitions Editor: Sonya Seigafuse
Managing Editor: Nancy Winter
Project Manager: Fran Gunning
Senior Manufacturing Manager: Ben Rivera
Marketing Manager: Kimberly Schonberger
Design Coordinator: Terry Mallon
Compositor: Laserwords Private Limited, Chennai, India

© 2008 by LIPPINCOTT WILLIAMS & WILKINS, a Wolters Kluwer business

530 Walnut Street
Philadelphia, PA 19106 USA
LWW.com

Printed in the USA

Library of Congress Cataloging-in-Publication Data

Health promotion and disease prevention in clinical practice / [edited by] Steven H. Woolf, Steven Jonas, Evonne Kaplan-Liss—2nd ed.

   p. ; cm.

  Includes bibliographical references and index.

  ISBN-13: 978-0-7817-7599-1

  1. Health promotion. 2. Medicine, Preventive. 3. Clinical health psychology. I. Woolf, Steven H. II. Jonas, Steven. III. Kaplan-Liss, Evonne.

  [DNLM: 1. Health Promotion—United States. 2. Preventive Health Services—United States. 3. Preventive Medicine—United States. WA 110 H4345 2008]

RA427.8.H4923 2008

613—dc22

2007031954

10 9 8 7 6 5 4 3

We dedicate this book to Carol, Chezna, and Ron, whose love and support make all things possible, and to all those who have devoted themselves to the promotion and practice of healthy living. We also dedicate this book to our children: to Sarah, Rebecca, and Elizabeth; to Jacob, Lillian and grandson Nathan, and Mark; and to Joshua and Jacob. For what we advocate in this book is ultimately for their generation, and for those that follow, in the hope that lives in the future will enjoy ever greater health and quality of life.

FOREWORD

J. Michael McGinnis

From the time that the elements of medicine and health were first recorded, prevention has provided a philosophical and conceptual cornerstone. Some 2500 years ago, Hippocrates penned into the physician's solemn oath a pledge to help keep patients from harm, and used *On Air, Waters, and Places* to elaborate in detail on the physician's obligation to learn and understand the strong influence of external influences on sickness and disease.

Prevention also provided the foundation for the major leaps in life expectancy experienced in the last century. Declines in mortality rates and in the infectious diseases that claimed the lives of young and old occurred because of public health advances such as improved sanitation, housing, nutrition and an expanding body of knowledge about the role of pathogens and other modifiable causes of disease, such as cigarette smoking.

Concepts and science to the contrary, the overwhelming focus of medical practice has been on treatment and confronting the problems at hand, rather than attending to future prospects. In recent years, however, with growing recognition of the tools available for clinicians to make a difference in preventing disease—through immunizations, through targeted disease screening, and through behavioral counseling—modern medicine has increasingly embraced prevention as an integral component of routine patient care. Even now, however, the clinician's time for these activities is generally displaced by competing demands, notably the predominant attention to the more urgent—and more lucrative—needs to treat acute illness, injuries, and chronic diseases.

This relative disadvantage has put preventive medicine in the position of having to make a stronger case for itself, often on an uneven playing field in which its interventions must meet standards of proven benefit and cost-effectiveness that society does not expect of diagnostic tests, medications, and surgeries for patients with extant disease. Perhaps by shouldering this added burden of proof, the prevention science community adopted a pioneering role in the evolution of the quality improvement movement and in the critical appraisal of scientific evidence of effectiveness.

Two decades ago, medical practice guidelines in most specialties were based largely on expert opinion, and notions about "evidence-based medicine" were in their infancy. Archie Cochrane, David Eddy, and other early writers about the movement were urging a more systematic approach to developing guidelines based on evidence, but few groups had developed a methodology for doing so. Into this void stepped two government task forces, one in Canada and a task force established subsequently in the United States, intent on developing rigorous methods to evaluate the effectiveness of clinical preventive services. The rules of evidence and grading system for recommendations promulgated by the Canadian Task Force on the Periodic Health Examination and the U.S. Preventive Services Task Force inspired guideline development efforts in other clinical specialties and in public health, catalyzing the evolution of the evidence-based medicine movement.

We now understand, however, that evidence of effectiveness and the promulgation of practice guidelines are not enough to ensure the delivery of quality health care, in preventive medicine or any other clinical domain. Three other prerequisites exist: First, clinicians and systems of care need appropriate tools and approaches to deliver the services properly. Second, systems must be redesigned in a manner that will maximize efficiency in making the services available to all patients in need. Third, the health care system must reflect economic and professional incentives and standards to assure their delivery.

Herein lays the importance of the contribution of *Health Promotion and Disease Prevention in Clinical Practice*: it tells us in practical and very specific terms how to deliver quality preventive care. Assembled, edited, and authored by pioneers in the modern-day science and practice of preventive medicine, its pages offer detailed guidance on how to help patients adopt healthy lifestyles, perform recommended screening tests and immunizations, and modify practice systems to ensure quality in their delivery. Guidelines on these topics exist elsewhere, but the details of how to implement them fill the pages of this book, along with guidance to tables, websites, and other resources where readers can obtain even more information.

The signature feature of this book is its focus on modifiable risk factors—for example, smoking, diet, physical activity—the leading causes of death in the United States. The first third of the book is devoted to helping clinicians learn how to identify these risk factors and to counsel patients on the difficult work of changing their lifestyle. The authors understand the importance of these risk factors in changing the trajectory of disease in the industrialized world, and as practitioners themselves they provide readers a clear and practical map for how to incorporate these weighty issues into the busy cadence of patient care. They miss few details, including chapters on such relevant topics as practice redesign, electronic medical records, and reimbursement issues.

The first edition of this book, issued in 1996, was itself a major contribution. Clinicians were quick to recognize its usefulness to their practices and clinics, and it soon became required reading in medical and nursing schools, residency programs, and allied health training programs. As

Former Surgeon General C. Everett Koop, MD, ScD wrote in the foreword of the first edition, "[t]his single reference brings together in one place the essential information that practitioners need in the office and at the bedside to provide high-quality preventive care." The same remains true of the second edition, which retains the best elements of the first—readers will recognize the same structure and philosophy—but the book now includes updated information about the latest options for preventive care and current guidelines, statistics, and contact information for additional resources. A new chapter on preventive care for children and adolescents gives due emphasis to this very important population.

The shape of preventive medicine in our children's generation will be fundamentally shaped and enhanced by emerging insights, unfolding in current research, that are helping us to better understand the interactions between behavioral, social, environmental, and genetic factors as determinants of the course of human diseases. Advances in genetics and information technology will permit more efficient targeting of preventive interventions and technologies to those patients most likely to benefit. Patients' risk for disease will be more predictable and precise, allowing clinicians to give tailored advice about which interventions are necessary and which will not outweigh their risks. Over time, it seems likely that today's distinctions between prevention and treatment will become evermore blurred.

As we move forward toward that future, this useful book will serve as an important tool to refocus the priorities of health care on the interventions that matter most in improving our prospects, and those of our children, for better health and wellbeing. The pages that follow prepare us for the care tomorrow that will transform our futures. The editors and authors of *Health Promotion and Disease Prevention in Clinical Practice* have delivered a resource essential to all who are the stewards of the present and architects of the future for health care in the nation.

PREFACE

This book is intended for physicians, nurses, nurse practitioners, physician assistants, psychologists, clinical social workers, dietitians, and other clinicians and trainees who provide clinical preventive services as part of primary care. *Clinical preventive services* include counseling about personal health behaviors, screening tests for the early detection of risk factors and disease, immunizations, and chemoprophylactic regimens that are offered to patients before they develop clinical evidence of disease. These health maintenance interventions represent an important part of the daily activities of most clinicians, epecially family physicians, pediatricians, general internists, nurse practitioners, physicians' assistants, and other health professionals who practice primary care medicine.

For many years, major professional groups have issued guidelines on the periodic health examination and on specific clinical preventive services that should be offered to patients as part of ongoing personal health care. Groups such as the U.S. Preventive Services Task Force (USPSTF) have summarized existing scientific evidence in support of clinical preventive services. Although these recommendations have helped define which preventive services should be offered to patients, they provide limited information about how the preventive maneuvers should be performed. The guidelines indicate, for example, how often women should receive a Pap test but do not explain how to obtain the specimen properly. Clinicians are advised to discuss tobacco use, exercise, and sexual practices, but the recommendations generally provide little information about how to counsel patients about these personal health behaviors.

It was to fill this void that this book was published in its first edition in 1996. Since then, the first edition has been widely used by clinicians, educators, and health systems to study the "how-to" of preventive medicine. This new edition proudly carries forward that mission but has been enhanced by the deep expertise of its contributors, who have filled the chapters with more current concepts, clinical guidance, data, and resource lists.

The purpose of this book remains the same as in the first edition: It provides clinicians with practical information about how to perform clinical preventive services. The book is organized in the same sequence as the clinical encounter. The chapters in Section I explain how to gather information in the history, physical, and laboratory examination to evaluate the risk profile of the individual patient and to screen for early-stage disease. The chapters in Section II explain what to do with that information: how to talk to patients about specific health behaviors such as smoking or physical inactivity, how to immunize patients, and how to work up abnormal results from screening tests. The chapters in Section III offer practical suggestions about how to implement these recommendations in the office and in other health care settings: how to organize office and clinic systems to deliver preventive services; the use of computers, health maintenance schedules, and reminder systems; and the larger policy concerns surrounding the delivery of preventive care.

The focus of this book on risk factors rather than target conditions is intentional. Most chapter titles address personal health behaviors (e.g., smoking, nutrition) rather than the prevention of specific disorders or disease categories (e.g., prevention of cancer or coronary artery disease). This emphasis on risk factors is important for three reasons.

First, unlike the care of symptomatic patients, for whom the "problem" requiring attention is a disease or symptom complex, the problems in preventive care are risk factors for disease (e.g., physical inactivity, susceptibility to infectious diseases), or the preclinical stages of a disease (e.g., asymptomatic cervical dysplasia, abnormal screening mammogram). Although clinicians and patients may share the broad goal of "preventing heart disease," the practical means to that end, with which they contend on a daily basis, are modifying dietary fat intake, serum lipids, physical activity, and blood pressure.

Second, individual risk factors often affect more than one disease category. For example, smoking, which increases the risk of atherosclerosis, cancer, and other conditions, cannot be discussed exclusively under the label of one disease or another.

A third reason for emphasizing risk factors is that they provide the basis for designing a tailored health maintenance plan for the individual patient, rather than performing a standard battery of clinical preventive services. The adolescent who smokes cigarettes and has multiple sexual partners may require a different set of interventions than the adolescent who avoids these behaviors but is overweight and hypertensive. For the clinician, personal health behaviors assume the same role in the development of a treatment plan for preventive care as do presenting complaints for the management of a symptomatic patient. Just as abdominal pain triggers a series of focused questions, examination techniques, and laboratory tests to establish a diagnosis and prevent complications, a history that identifies health behaviors and other risk factors for disease should initiate a focused clinical approach tailored to the risk factors and the disorders with which they are associated.

This book is designed to help in that task. It is organized to provide guidance to the clinician on how to collect risk factor information in the history, physical, and laboratory examination; how to help patients modify risk factors; and how to use risk factor information to structure decisions about follow-up testing, treatment, and immunizations. The recommendations in this book generally conform to those of evidence-based groups, such as the USPSTF. Wherever appropriate, the recommendations of the USPSTF, government agencies, medical specialty societies, and private groups (e.g., American Cancer Society) are summarized.

The book is not designed to "sell" clinicians on the idea of practicing health promotion and disease prevention. Its emphasis on providing clinicians with practical information on how to provide preventive services leaves little space for discussing the scientific rationale for the recommendations or for citing relevant individual studies. Many references in the book are to publications that provide clinical practice guidelines and not to original research. An understanding of the scientific background for preventive care recommendations is, however, essential for the well-informed clinician. Detailed descriptions of the supporting evidence for clinical preventive services are available in systematic reviews published by groups such as the USPSTF. References to these reviews are often cited in individual chapters.

In the United States, many, if not most, clinical preventive services are provided by physicians. Primary care physicians, in particular, engage regularly in the practice of health promotion and disease prevention and are the principal target audience for this book. Medical terminology and concepts familiar to physicians are therefore often used without further explanation. Nonetheless, the editors have, wherever appropriate, intentionally used the word "clinician" rather than "physician" to speak directly to non-physician health professionals who also provide clinical preventive services. Non-physician health professionals are often more skilled in educating and counseling patients about specific prevention issues and can devote more time to these efforts than can many physicians. In many practice settings, these clinicians work collaboratively with physicians in a team approach to deliver preventive care. In some geographic regions of this country, including many rural areas, nurses, nurse practitioners, physician assistants, and other health professionals are the only primary care providers and have lead responsibility for the delivery of clinical preventive services.

Preventive services for pregnant women are not discussed in this book, in part because space limitations preclude an adequate discussion of the details of clinical implementation. Nonetheless, most chapters in Section II provide information of direct relevance to pregnant women, especially those who smoke tobacco, use alcohol or other drugs, or engage in other health behaviors that threaten the health of both mother and fetus. Guidelines on nutrition during pregnancy are provided. The chapters in this book do not, however, deal in detail with the special factors that clinicians should consider when selecting screening tests and immunizations during pregnancy. Preventive services that are unique to pregnancy (e.g., screening for neural tube defects with amniocentesis or prenatal ultrasound) are not discussed. Recommendations on these topics are available in guidelines issued by the USPSTF, the American College of Obstetricians and Gynecologists, and other groups.

This book is not intended as a substitute for other medical textbooks. It is oriented toward preventive care and does not emphasize discussions of the treatment of existing disease. For example, discussions of cancer screening describe how to detect early-stage disease and do not provide detailed guidance on staging, chemotherapy, and other treatment measures once the cancer is detected. The range of conditions reviewed in this book is broad and includes many diseases for which new data and research findings are published regularly. The contents of this book are current as of 2007. Readers in subsequent years are encouraged to update the information by reviewing recent journal articles and publications that discuss current advances and new recommendations.

This book is targeted at clinicians in the United States; listings of epidemiologic data and the official recommendations of major groups generally refer to this country. This exclusion is made only for practical purposes; information from other countries is too extensive to include in one book. Moreover, health promotion and disease prevention priorities differ considerably in other countries, especially in developing nations, where many of the costly preventive technologies discussed in this book are of less importance than basic public health and social services. Similarly, limited resources and special priorities influence the practice of preventive medicine in clinics in the United States that are located in disadvantaged communities and neighborhoods, where many of our uninsured population live. By selecting elements of this book that are appropriate for their specific practice setting, it is hoped that primary care clinicians will find this publication useful in enhancing the quality of preventive care and the overall health status of their patients.

Steven H. Woolf, MD, MPH
Steven Jonas, MD, MPH
Evonne Kaplan-Liss, MD, MPH

CONTRIBUTORS

Randall T. Brown, MD
Assistant Professor
Department of Family Medicine
School of Medicine
University of Wisconsin, Madison
Madison, Wisconsin

Karen T. Feisullin, MD
Director of Women's Health,
Community Health Services;
Clinical staff
Department of Women's Health
Hartford Hospital
Hartford, Connecticut

Laura E. Ferguson, MD
Associate Professor of Pediatrics
Department of Pediatrics
University of Texas Houston Medical School;
Medical Director, Well Baby Nursery
Department of Pediatrics
Lyndon B. Johnson General Hospital
Houston, Texas

Michael F. Fleming, MD, MPH
Professor
Department of Family Medicine
University of Wisconsin, Madison;
Member
Institute of Medicine, National Academy
of Sciences
Madison, Wisconsin

Daniel E. Ford, MD, MPH
Professor and Vice Dean of Clinical Investigation
Department of Medicine, Psychiatry,
and Behavioral Sciences
Johns Hopkins School of Medicine
Baltimore, Maryland

Paul S. Frame, MD
Clinical Professor
Department of Family Medicine
University of Rochester School of Medicine
and Dentistry
Rochester, New York;
Chief of Family Medicine
Noyes Memorial Hospital
Dansville, New York

Russell E. Glasgow, PhD
Senior Scientist
Institute for Health Research
Center for Health Dissemination
and Implementation
Kaiser Permanente Colorado
Denver, Colorado

Michael G. Goldstein
Associate Director
Clinical Education and Research
Institute for Healthcare Communication
New Haven, Connecticut

Janelle Guirguis-Blake, MD
Clinical Assistant Professor
Department of Family Medicine
University of Washington
Tacoma Family Medicine Residency Program;
Clinical Faculty
Department of Family Medicine
Tacoma General Hospital
Tacoma, Washington

Russell Harris, MD, MPH
Professor
Department of Medicine
University of North Carolina
Chapel Hill, North Carolina

John M. Hickner, MD, MSc
Professor and Vice Chair
Department of Family Medicine
The University of Chicago Pritzker School
of Medicine
Chicago, Illinois

Steven Jonas, MD, MPH
Professor
Department of Preventive Medicine
Graduate Program in Public Health
School of Medicine, Stony Brook University
Stony Brook, New York

Linda S. Kinsinger, MD, MPH
Chief Consultant/Director
National Center for Health Promotion
and Disease Prevention
Office of Patient Care Services
Veterans Health Administration
Durham, North Carolina

Evonne Kaplan-Liss
Assistant Professor
Department of Preventive Medicine
Graduate Program in Public Health
Department of Pediatrics, and School
of Journalism
Stony Brook University
Stony Brook, New York

Charles M. Kodner
Associate Professor
Department of Family and Geriatric Medicine
University of Louisville
Louisville, Kentucky

Alex H. Krist, MD, MPH
Assistant Professor
Department of Family Medicine
Virginia Commonwealth University
Fairfax Family Practice Center Residency
Program
Fairfax, Virginia

Robert S. Lawrence, MD
Professor of Environmental Health Sciences,
Health Policy, and International Health
Director, Center for a Livable Future
Johns Hopkins Bloomberg School of Public
Health
Baltimore, Maryland

Terence McCormally, MD
Clinical Assistant Professor
Department of Family Medicine
Virginia Commonwealth University
Fairfax Family Practice Center Residency
Program
Fairfax, Virginia

J. Michael McGinnis, MD, MPP
Senior Scholar, Institute of Medicine
National Academy of Sciences;
Former Assistant Surgeon General and Deputy
Assistant Secretary through four
Administrations (1977–1995);
Founder, U.S. Preventive Services Task Force
Washington, DC

Virginia A. Moyer, MD, MPH
Professor
Department of Pediatrics
Baylor College of Medicine;
Section Head
Academic General Pediatrics
Texas Children's Hospital
Houston, Texas

Heidi D. Nelson, MD, MPH
Professor
Department of Medical Informatics and Clinical
Epidemiology and Department of Medicine
Oregon Health and Science University;
Medical Director
Women and Children's Program and Research
Center
Providence Health and Services
Portland, Oregon

Betsy Nicoletti, MS
Private Consultant
Medical Practice Consulting, LLC
Springfield, Vermont

J. Marc Overhage, MD, PhD
Professor of Medicine
Department of Medicine, Medical Informatics
Indiana University School of Medicine;
Attending Physician
Department of Medicine
Wishard Memorial Hospital
Indianapolis, Indiana

Kevin Patrick, MD, MS
Professor
Department of Family and Preventive Medicine
University of California, San Diego
La Jolla, California

Michael Pignone, MD, MPH
Chief
Division of General Internal Medicine
University of North Carolina-Chapter Hill
Chapel Hill, North Carolina

Stephen F. Rothemich, MD, MS
Associate Professor
Department of Family Medicine
Virginia Commonwealth University
Richmond, Virginia

Kavitha Bhat Schelbert, MD, MS
Assistant Professor
Department of Family Medicine
Georgetown University
Washington, DC

Roger A. Shewmake, PhD, LN
Professor and Director, Section of Nutrition
Department of Family Medicine
University of South Dakota School of Medicine;
Director, Nutrition Program
Sioux Falls Family Practice Residency
Sioux Falls, South Dakota

Leif I. Solberg, MD
Senior Investigator and Director of Care
*   Improvement Research*
HealthPartners Research Foundation
Minneapolis, Minnesota

Carolyn L. Westhoff, MD, MSc
Professor
Department of Obstetrics and Gynecology,
*   Epidemiology, Population and Family Health*
Columbia University;
Attending Physician
Department of Obstetrics and Gynecology
New York Presbyterian Hospital
New York, New York

Robert M. Wolfe, MD, FAAFP
Associate Professor
Department of Family Medicine
Northwestern University Feinberg School
*   of Medicine*
Chicago, Illinois;
Attending Physician
Department of Family Medicine
Evanston Northwestern Healthcare
Evanston, Illinois

Steven H. Woolf, MD, MPH
Professor
Departments of Family Medicine, Epidemiology
*   and Community Health*
Virginia Commonwealth University
Richmond, Virginia

CONTENTS

III Putting Prevention Recommendations into Practice

INTRODUCTION

Steven H. Woolf, Steven Jonas, Robert S. Lawrence
and Evonne Kaplan-Liss

Health promotion and disease prevention[a] have an inherent logic: It has always seemed more sensible to prevent the occurrence of diseases, or to stop them early in their natural history, than to delay treatment until the process of pathogenesis has. resulted in irreversible damage to body tissues, organ systems, and physiologic processes. Clinicians know too well how ineffective medical and surgical interventions can become at this late stage in the process, when controlling symptoms and forestalling progression, rather than curing the disease itself, are often all that can be offered to patients.

Yet millions of Americans suffer from chronic diseases, such as heart disease, cancer, renal failure, stroke, chronic obstructive pulmonary disease, and diabetes. The burden of suffering has forced the health care system to invest heavily in caring for complications from these conditions, rather than in preventing the disease processes that caused them. On any given day in America, health care for end-stage diseases dominates the activities of physicians, hospitals, emergency departments, and nursing homes.

The dominance of late-stage interventions in medicine is a major factor in producing the high cost of health care delivery in this country. The United States spends more on health care than does any other nation; in 2005, it spent $2 trillion (16% of its gross domestic product) (3). The most expensive, high-technology elements of American medicine are consumed in providing intensive care for late-stage conditions. Treatments in the last year of life account for 25% of all Medicare expenditures, and approximately 40% of this expense is incurred in the last month of life (4,5). In contrast, prevention accounts for only 2–3% of health care expenditures in the United States (6,7), lying in the shadow of the sophisticated diagnostic and therapeutic technologies that dominate medicine.

[a] *Health promotion* is defined as "any combination of educational, organizational, economic, and environmental supports for behavior and conditions of living conducive to health." (1) Modifying personal health behaviors to reduce the risk of disease and injury is often described as health promotion. *Disease prevention* encompasses primary, secondary, and tertiary prevention. "*Primary preventive* measures are those provided to individuals to prevent the onset of a target condition (e.g., routine immunization of healthy children), whereas *secondary preventive* measures identify and treat asymptomatic persons who have already developed risk factors or preclinical disease but in whom the disease itself has not become clinically apparent. Obtaining a Pap smear to detect cervical dysplasia before the development of cancer and screening for high blood pressure are forms of secondary prevention. Preventive measures that are part of the treatment and management of persons with clinical illnesses ... are usually considered *tertiary prevention*."(2).

Three important trends make it likely that the prevalence and costs of chronic diseases will worsen over the coming years. The "baby boom" generation began to reach 60 years of age in 2006, and as it ages further it will dramatically swell the ranks of older adults. The number of seniors in the United States is expected to double from 36 million in 2003 to 72 million in 2030 (8). Second, as advances in medical care improve life expectancies and lengthen life spans, the prevalence of chronic diseases will increase. Already, almost half of Americans have one or more chronic illnesses, and the number is expected to grow by 29% from 133 million in 2005 to 171 million in 2030 (9). Third, the costs of medical care for those chronic diseases are climbing rapidly. Three diseases—cardiovascular disease, cancer, and stroke—already account for $600 billion per year in spending (10). It is a safe prediction that the convergence of these three trends will result in a higher prevalence of chronic diseases and that health care costs to treat the complications of those diseases will climb. Economic pressures from rising costs are already substantial for major employers, and the trends just mentioned portend a growing threat to corporate America and to the solvency of the Medicare program.

The obesity epidemic (11) complicates matters further. As of 2004, two out of three Americans were overweight or obese (12). The chronic diseases that threaten the viability of the health care system are causally linked to obesity and are therefore likely to grow even more prevalent as obesity rates climb. Obesity accounted for 27% of the rise in per capita health care spending between 1987 and 2001 (13). If current obesity trends continue, it is estimated that obesity will increase future Medicare beneficiary spending by 34% (14).

The rising prevalence of pediatric obesity is further cause for concern. Between 1999 and 2004, the prevalence of overweight among children aged 2–19 years increased from 14 to 17% (12). Obesity is expected to overtake smoking as the leading cause of death and to give today's children a shorter life expectancy than their parents (15), not to mention its psychosocial consequences. The next generation will also experience an escalation in obesity-related chronic illnesses—the prevalence of diabetes in children is already increasing—for which the current health care system is unprepared.

With this surge in disease looming on the horizon, prevention offers individuals, the health care community, and society at large a more rational strategy for dealing with disease and promoting health than the current model of deferring treatment until illness develops, often with little success. The logic behind prevention is obvious. It is far more effective to prevent the occurrence of heart disease by controlling cardiac risk factors (e.g., avoiding tobacco use, increasing physical activity) or preventing childhood obesity than it is to attempt, years later, to restore the function of stenosed coronary arteries or ischemically damaged myocardium. It is better to administer a vaccine to a healthy infant than to care for the child who subsequently develops poliomyelitis. It is more rational to screen for and treat asymptomatic persons with high blood pressure than, years later, to provide hemodialysis therapy to patients with hypertensive renal failure or rehabilitative services to victims of stroke. Benjamin Franklin understood this principle well when he popularized the maxim: "An ounce of prevention is worth a pound of cure" (16).

Despite this logic, the critical role of health promotion and disease prevention was not well recognized as a priority area of national health policy until the early 1970s. At that time, a seminal Canadian document, the Lalonde Report, presented a new model that raised awareness about the importance of an integrated health promotion policy for improving the health status of the population as a whole (17). The Lalonde Report signaled the transformation of health promotion from the preceding "wellness" movement, a succession of vitamin and stress-reduction fads with little supporting scientific evidence, to a well-recognized epidemiologic and clinical science linking behavioral risk factors to specific disease outcomes. The incorporation of these principles into national health policy was formalized in the United States in 1979–1980, when the federal government published *Healthy People: The Surgeon General's Report on Health Promotion and Disease Prevention* (18) and *Promoting Health/Preventing Disease: Objectives for the Nation* (19), setting specific goals to be achieved by 1990. By the time that new objectives for the year 2010 (*Healthy People 2010*) were released in 2000 (20), health promotion and disease prevention had become a well-accepted component of national health policy. Health promotion policy has now diffused to the regional and local level, where initiatives to promote wellness and preventive care are common priorities of local governments, health care institutions, insurance plans, employers, and retailers.

THE CURRENT SCOPE OF HEALTH PROMOTION AND DISEASE PREVENTION

Society can practice health promotion and disease prevention through several channels: (a) controlling communicable diseases, (b) protecting the environment, (c) modifying personal behaviors that affect health, and (d) preventing, or reducing the severity of, noncommunicable and chronic disabling conditions (21). The last century has witnessed achievements in health promotion and disease prevention in each of these areas. Through improved public sanitation, housing, immunization programs, and nutrition, infectious diseases that were the leading causes of death and disability in the United States at the beginning of the 20th century have now become uncommon. Poliomyelitis, for example, caused paralysis and death in hundreds of thousands of Americans before the polio vaccine was introduced in 1954 and the incidence of the disease began a steady decline; since 1991, no new cases of disease caused by wild-type polio virus have been reported in the Western hemisphere. Government and industry have worked to improve the cleanliness of air, water, and soil and to increase the safety of products and transportation services, thereby reducing the incidence of infectious diseases, environmental and occupational illnesses, and injuries. Between 1970 and 1997, total emissions of the six principal air pollutants decreased by 31% (20). Greater attention is now being given to threats to the safety of the food supply arising from the industrialization of agriculture and the globalization of food systems.

Personal health consciousness has been integrated into daily American life. Joggers and power walkers became common sights on residential streets in the 1970s. Concerns about nutrition and the importance of lifestyle in preventing infection with human immunodeficiency virus (HIV) grew in the 1980s. Now, other examples of health promotion have become evident in society: print and television advertisements feature messages about healthy, low-fat products and physical fitness; motorists routinely fasten their seat belts; children are protected by car safety seats and bicycle helmets; no-smoking policies have been adopted by local and state governments, employers, airlines, restaurants, and other public facilities; and celebrities, advertisers, and public service announcements encourage cancer screening, safe sex, and avoiding drug and alcohol abuse and drunk driving. The personal health behaviors of Americans have changed. Since 1964, the proportion of Americans who smoke cigarettes has fallen from 40 to 21% (22,23). Currently, approximately 11% of adults consume the recommended amount of fruits and vegetables, and 30% exercise regularly (23,24). Americans have become more conscientious about cancer screening. Between 1988 and 1993, the proportion of women older than 50 years who received a recent mammogram more than doubled (22); by 2003, 75% of women aged 40 years and older reported having received a recent mammogram (23).

These changes have been accompanied by favorable trends in the incidence of death and disability in the United States. Between 1950 and 2003, age-adjusted death rates for Americans decreased from 1,446:100,000 to 833:100,000, and life expectancy at birth increased from 68 to 78 years. Between 1950 and 2003, infant mortality rates fell from 30:1,000 to 7:1,000 live births (23). Between 1980 and 2003, age-adjusted death rates decreased significantly for heart disease (44% reduction), cerebrovascular disease (44% reduction), and cancer (9% reduction) (23). Behavioral risk factor modification accounts for a large proportion of these reductions. Heart disease mortality fell dramatically between 1970 and 2000; reductions in risk factors (e.g., smoking, lipids) contributed more to this trend (by a median ratio of 1.3:1) than did medical care (25). Similarly, reduced stroke mortality is believed to be due to early detection and treatment of hypertension. Age-adjusted mortality for lung cancer, following a more than sixfold increase between

1940 and 1982, has been decreasing since 1991, due largely to decreased tobacco use (26,27).

These achievements aside, far too many Americans continue to suffer from diseases and injuries that are largely preventable. The health status of the population is far lower than it should be, primarily because the full benefits of health promotion and disease prevention have yet to be realized. Heart disease remains the leading cause of death in the United States, killing almost 700,000 Americans annually (23). In 2003 in the United States, there were more than 550,000 deaths from cancer, 150,000 deaths from stroke, 120,000 deaths from chronic lower respiratory disease, and thousands more from other chronic diseases (23). Approximately one-third of such deaths are potentially preventable, caused by a short list of modifiable risk factors (tobacco use, unhealthy diet, physical inactivity, and problem drinking) (28). Mortality from motor vehicle injuries (approximately 40,000 deaths each year) could be reduced in half if seat belt use was maximized and drinking and driving were curtailed (29). Fully 38,000 deaths each year are caused by firearms (30), a situation that prudent handgun policies could remedy. Approximately 40,000 persons are diagnosed each year with acquired immunodeficiency syndrome (AIDS) (23). HIV infection is almost completely preventable by altering sexual practices and exposure to infected blood products. In 2004, more than 10% of all live births occurred among mothers aged 19 years or younger, and 8% of newborns were of low birth weight (23).

The incidence, morbidity, and mortality of certain diseases are disproportionately higher among disadvantaged and minority populations. The life expectancy of a black infant at birth is approximately 5 years less than that of a white infant, and the infant death rate is more than double that of whites (23). Among African Americans, age-adjusted death rates for ischemic heart disease and cancer are 21–24% higher than those for whites, and stroke mortality rates are 45% higher (23). Similar disparities are reported for other minorities, such as Hispanics, Native Americans, and Asians and Pacific Islanders, who suffer from increased rates of diabetes, HIV infection, overweight, tuberculosis, and other conditions. As summarized in Table 1, data on the receipt of clinical preventive services consistently report disproportionate gaps in preventive care among minorities and disadvantaged populations.

The reasons for the inadequacies in the availability and use of health promotion and disease prevention services are multifactorial. Strategies available to society for preventing diseases are limited by logistic, political, financial, religious, and philosophic obstacles. Regulations to protect the safety of the environment place economic and administrative burdens on private industry and governmental agencies. Vaccines and screening services are costly to society and often unavailable to persons with limited access to health

TABLE 1   Receipt of Preventive Services by Persons in the United States

Preventive Services	Proportion of Eligible Persons in the United States Who Had Received the Preventive Service, 2006 (%)
Children (aged 19–35 mo)	
Immunizations	
DTP (4 or more doses)	85
Polio (3 or more doses)	92
MMR (1 dose)	92
Hib (3 or more doses)	94
HBV (3 or more doses)	93
Combined series	82
Adults (aged 18 yr and older)	
Cholesterol (checked in last 5 yr)	73
Low-income[a] Americans	64
African Americans	74
Hispanic Americans	53
Colonoscopy or sigmoidoscopy screening (ever)	57
Low-income[a] Americans	50
African Americans	53
Hispanic Americans	44
Women (aged 40 yr and older) who have received a mammogram in the last 2 yr	77
Low-income[a] women	65
African Americans	80
Hispanic Americans	76
Pneumococcal vaccine (once at 65 yr or older)	67
Low-income[a] Americans	67
African Americans	47
Hispanic Americans	45

TABLE 1   *(Continued)*

Preventive Services	Proportion of Eligible Persons in the United States Who Had Received the Preventive Service, 2006 (%)
Influenza vaccine (last 12 mo at 65 yr or older)	70
Low-income[a] Americans	62
African Americans	49
Hispanic Americans	57

National Center for Health Statistics. *Health, United States, 2006 with chartbook on trends in the health of Americans.* Hyattsville: Accessed at http://www.cdc.gov/nchs/data/hus/hus06.pdf; Behavioral Risk Factor Surveillance System, Prevalence Data, http://apps.nccd.cdc.gov/brfss/index.asp. 2006.
DTP = diphtheria-tetanus-pertussis vaccine; MMR = measles-mumps-rubella vaccine; Hib = *Haemophilus influenzae* type b vaccine; HBV = hepatitis B vaccine; Td, tetanus-diphtheria booster.
[a] Low income less than or equal to $15,000 per year.

care. The biologic efficacy of vaccines and antibiotics to control infectious diseases is threatened by the emergence of new organisms, antibiotic-resistant strains, and vaccine failure. Perhaps the most effective means of promoting health, convincing individuals to change personal behaviors, cannot succeed if individuals lack the motivation or resources to change behavior. To change behavior voluntarily is difficult because unhealthy behaviors are often enjoyable or deeply ingrained in lifestyle and culture. Unhealthy foods, tobacco, and alcohol products are actively promoted by advertisers. Forcing changes in behavior, such as requiring motorcyclists to wear helmets, poses philosophic, ethical, political, and legal problems and generally conflicts with American preferences for individual freedom.

HEALTH PROMOTION AND DISEASE PREVENTION IN CLINICAL PRACTICE

It is in this context of societal efforts that this book explores the role of clinicians in promoting health and preventing disease. As noted in the Preface, this book is targeted to the full spectrum of *clinicians*—not just to physicians—and takes great care to use that term because nurses, nurse practitioners, physician assistants, dentists, psychologists, clinical social workers, pharmacists, dietitians, and other clinicians all play vital roles in promoting health. The limitations of clinicians in this effort, however, are as immediately apparent as their capabilities. Clinicians cannot ensure the cleanliness of water and food supplies, cannot redesign motor vehicles to improve safety, cannot redesign the built environment to facilitate outdoor physical activity, and cannot control the behavior of their patients.

Nonetheless, the potential capabilities of clinicians in promoting health are substantial. Clinicians, perhaps better than anyone, know the consequences of allowing conditions to progress to their final stages and the futility of offering treatments late in the natural history of disease. Clinicians are therefore among the most persuasive advocates of health promotion. Clinicians also have special access to the population; approximately 84% of Americans have contact with a physician each year, averaging more than three office visits per year (23). Patients value the advice of doctors and other clinicians. Studies suggest that patients' decisions to stop smoking, undergo a mammogram, or have their child immunized are often traceable to the encouragement of their doctor. The clinician is essential to the delivery of many preventive services (e.g., Pap smears, screening colonoscopy, and prescription medication to help with smoking cessation).

Clinicians have therefore always tried to emphasize preventive services in clinical practice. Pediatricians and family physicians, for example, have, for decades, prioritized health promotion and disease prevention issues during well-baby and well-child visits. Nurse practitioners, nurses, physicians' assistants, and other clinicians have emphasized nutrition, exercise, and other aspects of wellness. Much of the prenatal care provided by obstetricians, family physicians, and nurse midwives is dominated by prevention topics. Many specialists also engage in preventive care. Cardiologists devote much of their time to encouraging patients to modify cardiac risk factors, gastroenterologists screen for colorectal cancer, dermatologists encourage the prevention and early detection of skin cancer, ophthalmologists and optometrists screen for glaucoma, and so on.

Most clinicians, however, do fall short in providing the preventive services that are recommended for their patients. A widely cited study estimated that Americans receive only 55% of recommended preventive services (31). Studies have consistently found that patients routinely receive checkups without being questioned about personal health behaviors or receiving other recommended clinical preventive services (32). In 2004, only 69% of smokers in commercial health plans reported receiving some advice to quit, and only 37% and 38%, respectively, went on to receive counseling about cessation strategies or medications (33). Table 1 documents the extent to which Americans have not received recommended clinical preventive services. Nearly half of Americans older than 50 years have not undergone colonoscopy or sigmoidoscopy for colorectal cancer screening (34). One out of three adults 65 years and older has not received a pneumococcal vaccination (34).

BARRIERS TO THE DELIVERY OF CLINICAL PREVENTIVE SERVICES

There are many reasons for inadequate attention to preventive services in the clinical setting. A fundamental barrier is that clinicians may lack motivation to practice prevention, for several perceived reasons. First, health promotion and disease prevention activities are often less "interesting" than curative medicine. Talking to healthy patients about personal behaviors is thought to provide less intellectual stimulation and to offer fewer dramatic clinical challenges than contending with full-blown diseases.[b] Discussing low-fat diets, performing Pap smears, and injecting vaccines offer less professional excitement and remuneration than performing crash resuscitations, transluminal angioplasty, laser surgery, joint reconstruction, and other high-technology medical procedures. The latter provide an opportunity to apply more fully the advanced scientific knowledge acquired during clinical training and from keeping abreast of current research. The scientific principles and practice of preventive medicine, by comparison, receive relatively little emphasis in most training curricula and seem less captivating to many clinicians. Among those graduates who are interested in preventive care, the deficit in training creates a problematic gap in knowledge, skills, and motivation—all of which influence a clinician's sense of self-efficacy.

A second disincentive to providing clinical preventive services is skepticism about their effectiveness. Uncertainty about the ability of screening tests, counseling, and immunizations to reduce morbidity and mortality has been a longstanding obstacle to preventive care for many years. It was this skepticism that prompted the U.S. Public Health Service to establish the U.S. Preventive Services Task Force (USPSTF) in 1984. The USPSTF, modeling its approach after that of the Canadian Task Force on the Periodic Health Examination[c] (35), carefully examined the evidence for more than 200 clinical preventive services. Although it found that many preventive services lacked sufficient evidence to reach conclusions about their effectiveness or ineffectiveness, it was able to identify a core package of clinical preventive services for which there was compelling evidence of significant health benefits (2). The USPSTF findings have been regularly updated over two decades (36) and have been reinforced by other expert panels and medical

[b]The inaccuracy of these perceptions often does not become apparent until one begins to practice health promotion and disease prevention as part of daily patient care. As any primary care clinician can attest, helping patients to adopt a healthier lifestyle and to detect disease at an early stage can be among the most challenging and gratifying aspects of medicine.
[c]The Canadian Task Force on the Periodic Health Examination, which was later renamed the Canadian Task Force on Preventive Health Care, continued to issue updated recommendations until 2005. At this writing its funding is tenuous, however, and it is not currently operational. Readers should consult the website of the Canadian Task Force on Preventive Health Care (http://www.ctfphc.org/) for updates on its status and a complete list of its recommendations.

groups. Together, the findings of these groups provide a strong scientific argument for emphasizing these measures in daily patient care.

A third, more practical, disincentive for clinicians interested in providing preventive services is uncertainty about exactly what to do: which preventive services to provide, how often, and on which patients. The USPSTF and other expert panels, government agencies, medical specialty societies, and private groups have responded to this need by issuing practice guidelines that specify the proper indications for a variety of clinical preventive services (see Table 2). Although there is some disagreement among professional organizations about the appropriateness of certain screening tests, there is a growing consensus around a core package of clinical preventive services of proven effectiveness that should be offered to patients (see Appendix A at the end of this book).

The strength of the consensus around effective preventive care has not been fully appreciated because of highly publicized controversies about relatively narrow areas of disagreement (e.g., screening for prostate cancer). Unfortunately, these marginal debates have distracted clinicians from the many important recommendations about which there is little disagreement. For the busy clinician, the areas of consensus provide more than enough work, without even taking on the controversial elements of preventive care. Ensuring the delivery of the core package of clinical preventive services that is supported by all expert groups (e.g., ensuring that all patients who smoke receive counseling, that persons age 50 and older are screened for colorectal cancer, that childhood immunizations are up-to-date) presents, by itself, a formidable challenge for most busy clinicians. If this alone could be achieved, many of the deficiencies in the current practice of preventive medicine would be remedied.

Which specific clinical preventive services should be provided? The recommended clinical preventive services for patients in specific age- and risk groups have been specified by the USPSTF and other groups (Table 2). The USPSTF recommendations are summarized in Appendix A of this book, and the scientific evidence on which the recommendations are based is documented in detail in USPSTF publications and in systematic literature reviews posted on its website (http://www.ahrq.gov/clinic/uspstfix.htm). The details of *how* to perform the recommended clinical preventive services are the principal focus of this book. As noted in the Preface, Section I describes how to collect risk factor information during the history, physical, and laboratory examination. Section II presents the ways and means of using that information to help patients modify risk factors and to determine appropriate follow-up tests, treatments, immunizations, and counseling. Section III addresses implementation systems, which are necessary to achieve comprehensiveness and efficiency in providing complete, high-quality preventive care to all patients.

TABLE 2 Examples of Groups Issuing Practice
Recommendations on Clinical Preventive Services

Groups	Clinical Preventive Services Topic Areas
Federal Agencies	
Agency for Healthcare Research and Quality *http://www.ahrq.gov/*	Clinical practice guidelines on selected clinical preventive services. See U.S. Preventive Services Task Force (below)
Centers for Disease Control and Prevention *http://www.cdc.gov/*	Recommendations on immunizations and screening tests for infectious diseases and selected chronic diseases. National Immunization Program (http://www.cdc .gov/nip/default.htm). See Advisory Committee on Immunization Practices (below)
Advisory Committee on Immunization Practices *http://www.cdc.gov/nip/ ACIP/default.htm*	Immunization guidelines developed under the auspices of the Centers for Disease Control and Prevention, usually with endorsement by the American Academy of Pediatrics, American Academy of Family Physicians, and/or American College of Physicians
National Institutes of Health *http://www.nih.gov/*	Recommendations on screening and follow-up for high blood cholesterol and dietary guidelines, developed by the National Cholesterol Education Program and Adult Treatment Panel (ATC) (http://www.nhlbi .nih.gov/guidelines/cholesterol/index.htm); screening and follow-up for high blood pressure and lifestyle interventions, developed by the National High Blood Pressure Education Program and the Joint National Committee (JNC) (http://www.nhlbi.nih.gov/ guidelines/hypertension/index.htm); recommendations on obesity prevention and treatment (http://www.nhlbi.nih.gov/ guidelines/obesity/ob_home.htm)

(continued)

TABLE 2 *(Continued)*

Groups	Clinical Preventive Services Topic Areas
Specialty Societies	
American Academy of Pediatrics *http://www.aap.org/*	Recommendations regarding screening tests, anticipatory guidance, health promotion, and immunizations for children and adolescents developed by committees in specific topic areas (http://aappolicy.aappublications.org/practice_guidelines/index.dtl); immunization guidelines developed as part of the Advisory Committee on Immunization Practices (see above), including *Report of the Committee on Infectious Diseases* ("Red Book") at http://aapredbook.aappublications.org/
American Academy of Family Physicians *http://www.aafp.org*	Recommended clinical preventive services during the periodic health examination (http://www.aafp.org/online/en/home/clinical/exam.html) and immunization guidelines (http://www.aafp.org/online/en/home/clinical/immunizationres.html)
American College of Obstetricians and Gynecologists *http://acog.org/*	Recommendations on selected screening, counseling, immunizations, and chemoprophylaxis during prenatal and well-woman care
American College of Physicians *http://www.acponline.org/*	Recommendations on screening tests and chemoprophylaxis (http://www.acponline.org/clinical/guidelines/?hp); immunization guidelines developed as part of the Advisory Committee on Immunization Practices (see above)
Independent Panels	
U.S. Preventive Services Task Force *http://www.ahrq.gov/clinic/uspstfix.htm*	Recommendations on more than 200 screening, counseling, immunization, and chemoprophylactic interventions, including *Guide to Clinical Preventive Services* (http://www.ahrq.gov/clinic/pocketgd.htm)

TABLE 2   *(Continued)*

Groups	Clinical Preventive Services Topic Areas
Private Advocacy Groups	
American Cancer Society *http://www.cancer.org*	Recommendations on cancer screening and lifestyle change to reduce risk factors for cancer
American Heart Association/American College of Cardiology *http://www .americanheart.org*	Recommendations on screening tests for heart disease and cardiac risk factors, nutrition, and other cardiac risk factor modification

This list is not exhaustive. Many other government agencies, specialty societies, and private organizations publish recommendations on specific types of clinical preventive services. Most organizations have resources on related topics as well as websites and materials for patients and consumers. Many of these resources are listed in subsequent chapters of this book.

Unfortunately, even the well-motivated clinician encounters many additional barriers related to delivering clinical preventive services. Practice organization and health care systems often present obstacles in busy clinical settings. Chief among these are lack of time, especially for counseling; lack of self-confidence in professional skills to provide preventive care, often due to inadequate emphasis on prevention during clinical training; and simply forgetting about prevention in the midst of other clinical responsibilities. Many patients see their clinicians only when sick, when neither the patient nor clinician may be inclined to deal with prevention issues. Physician reimbursement for clinical preventive services has, for many years, been inadequate under traditional indemnity (fee-for-service) health insurance plans. Support for prevention increased when managed care predominated as the insurance model in the 1990s, but current reimbursement schemes give clinicians weak incentives to invest time in counseling patients about lifestyle change or about the tradeoffs associated with screening tests.

Other barriers to preventive care involve patients: People find it difficult to change their health habits, and those in need of clinical services often do not receive them because they are disinterested, fearful, or lack access to health care. Approximately 16% of Americans, or approximately 47 million persons, currently lack health insurance (23).

Recent years have witnessed efforts by government agencies, medical organizations, and health care delivery systems to address many of these implementation barriers. Government agencies, medical specialty societies, and medical journals have worked to disseminate clinical preventive services recommendations to clinicians through their websites and through Internet-based interactive tools, journal articles, conferences, and organizational publications aimed at preventive care. A national campaign launched in 1994, "Put Prevention into Practice," was the forerunner of many subsequent efforts to provide clinicians with implementation tools for providing preventive services in the primary care setting. Computerized reminder systems have been designed to help clinicians remember which preventive services are indicated. Public education campaigns have used print and broadcast advertisements and programs, magazine articles, and other media (e.g., online services) to encourage Americans to visit their doctor to obtain screening tests, immunizations, and other recommended preventive services.

Problems with patient access to, and clinician reimbursement for, clinical preventive services have also received attention from policy makers. *Healthy People 2000* (37), the national health objectives laid out in 1990, made access to clinical preventive services an explicit priority for the country. Since then, national health care reform discussions have increasingly emphasized the need for Americans to have access to a minimum benefits package of effective clinical preventive services. Health insurers, employers, and the Medicare program have widened coverage of clinical preventive services as part of their efforts to control the rising costs of health care. Preventive services are popular with consumers, and many plans compete for patient enrollment by advertising their respective preventive services packages. The performance review criteria used by organizations that evaluate the quality of health care (e.g., the National Committee for Quality Assurance, quality improvement organizations [QIOs] for Medicare, and the National Quality Foundation) emphasize preventive services delivery as a cornerstone for judging the quality of care provided to patients.

The emphasis on the clinical setting as a venue for preventive care has been accompanied by the growing recognition of the importance of population-based efforts and community programs in health promotion and disease prevention. Legislation, product redesign, initiatives by school districts and employers, and neighborhood campaigns can often accomplish more to prevent disease than the efforts of individual clinicians. A counterpart to the USPSTF—the Task Force on Community Preventive Services—has been working since the 1990s to identify evidence-based strategies outside the clinical setting that are effective and actionable (38). The greatest promise lies in leveraging the power of both venues through partnerships between clinicians and such community programs. For example, more effective smoking cessation counseling can occur when primary care clinicians augment efforts in the office by referring smokers to proactive telephone counseling provided by quit lines. Success in addressing obesity requires the collective efforts of families, retailers, and school systems to facilitate behavior change and collaborations between clinicians and community resources (e.g., commercial weight loss programs) to deliver intensive weight loss counseling.

THE IMPORTANCE OF PATIENT EDUCATION AND COUNSELING IN PREVENTIVE MEDICINE

The clinical preventive services that clinicians should provide are classified by the USPSTF as: (a) counseling interventions, (b) screening tests, (c) immunizations, and (d) chemoprophylaxis. *Counseling interventions* refer to efforts to educate patients about the consequences of personal health behaviors (e.g., smoking, diet, physical inactivity, substance abuse, sexual practices, and injury prevention) and to work in a collaborative manner on strategies for risk factor modification. *Screening tests* are special tests or standardized examination procedures for the early detection of preclinical conditions (e.g., cervical dysplasia) or risk factors (e.g., elevated serum cholesterol) in asymptomatic persons. *Immunizations* include the use of vaccines and immunoglobulins to prevent infectious diseases. *Chemoprophylaxis* refers to the use of drugs, nutritional and mineral supplements, or other natural substances by asymptomatic persons to prevent future disease.

This book gives special emphasis to counseling patients about risk factors. Modifying personal health behaviors is probably the most effective way for patients to prevent disease. According to one analysis, a 45-year-old female smoker is 23 times more likely to avoid a premature death by stopping smoking than by getting a screening mammogram (39). Despite the relative superiority of health behavior change over testing as a strategy to prevent disease, the former is more challenging, and a typical patient is more likely to see the latter emphasized in clinical practice. As in other areas of medicine, preventive care is dominated by procedures and testing. Patients seeking preventive care are more likely to undergo a rectal examination or cholesterol test than to be asked whether they smoke, what they eat, or whether they exercise.

To some extent, the disaffection with counseling is due to factors already mentioned, such as lack of time, inadequate reimbursement, deficient skills, and skepticism about effectiveness. More broadly, however, the emphasis on testing is a generic phenomenon in medicine, owing to medicolegal concerns about the risks of not ordering tests, test-ordering habits acquired during clinical training, fascination with high technology, a poor appreciation of the potential harms of testing, intellectual curiosity about test results, and patient demand (40). Patients feel that their doctor is more competent and that they are receiving better care if they undergo extensive testing, regardless of the effectiveness of the tests. In one national survey, 87% of adults indicated that routine cancer screening is "almost always a good idea;" 73% said that they would prefer to receive a total-body computed tomographic scan instead of receiving $1,000 in cash (41).

There are, however, additional reasons for the reluctance of clinicians to emphasize personal health behaviors and other risk factors during patient assessment. First, clinicians are accustomed to dealing with the here and now. Clinical training and the pragmatic realities of patient care encourage attention to current problems and not to risk factors for future disease. Their distant and uncertain impact in the future gives health behaviors the perception of being less serious than "real" pathology in the present, in part because of the universal human tendency to discount future events. Such perceptions often conflict with the facts. A patient's discomfort from reflux esophagitis, for example, may *seem* more important than a discussion of health behaviors. But if the patient smokes cigarettes, failure to have this discussion will allow the patient's most likely cause of death (heart disease) to escape attention at a time in life when it might be preventable. In the final analysis, dyspepsia is less important than death, and yet in practice it may receive more attention.

A second reason for the tendency of clinicians to emphasize testing over talking is the perception that screening tests are more effective than counseling. Once again, this perception is often erroneous. The extensive review of the literature performed by the USPSTF determined that, although routine screening can lower mortality for selected conditions (e.g., breast, cervical, and colorectal cancer, hypertension), routine screening for most other diseases appears to have little or no effect on health outcomes (36). In contrast, unhealthy personal behaviors are the leading causes of death in the United States; fully 38% of all deaths are caused by smoking, physical inactivity, poor diet, and problem drinking (11). In 2000 in the United States, there were 435,000 deaths attributable to tobacco use, 400,000 deaths from unhealthy eating habits and physical inactivity, 85,000 deaths from alcohol use, 29,000 deaths from firearms, and 20,000 deaths attributable to sexual practices (11). Given the magnitude of these effects, even if a clinician has only modest success in convincing patients to change behavior, the effort is far more likely to prevent disease than administering tests.

The general ineffectiveness of screening tests stands to reason. If one considers the time line of the natural history of disease (see Fig. 1), it becomes apparent that screening tests cannot detect a disorder until the disease process has produced a measurable pathophysiologic abnormality, even if it is asymptomatic. Treatment interventions at this stage are often of limited effectiveness because the pathophysiologic process has often advanced to the point of producing irreversible disease. Personal health behaviors that cause disease, on the other hand, play a key etiologic role much earlier on the time line. Modifying such behaviors early in the natural history can prevent (or, in some

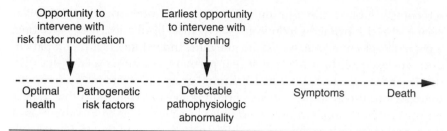

Figure 1 • "Time line" for pathogenesis of preventable disease, which begins with modifiable risk factors that, over time, can lead to pathophysiologic abnormalities. Once these abnormalities develop, screening tests may be able to detect the problem before the patient develops symptoms but not until the disease process has progressed to the point of producing a detectable pathophysiologic disorder. Through modification of personal health behaviors, the patient can intervene much earlier in the process and is therefore more likely to be effective.

cases, reverse [42]) progression of the disease many years before it would be detectable by physical examination or screening tests. Attention to these causes of disease and injury can accomplish real prevention, whereas the inherent nature of screening requires one to wait for the disease process to begin.

PRINCIPLES OF EXCELLENCE AND QUALITY IN PREVENTIVE MEDICINE

Basic to the practice of good preventive medicine, as to the practice of all medicine, is taking a thorough history. The clinician cannot determine which preventive services are indicated for a particular patient without first considering the patient's risk factors. It is self-evident that the clinician cannot recognize the need to advise a patient to stop smoking without first inquiring whether he or she smokes. The need to advise an adolescent about sexual practices will not become apparent until the clinician determines whether the teen is sexually active. The need to begin colorectal screening at an earlier age because of hereditary polyposis will not become apparent unless the clinician inquires about the family history. A diagnostic approach to risk factors is of as much importance in designing a plan for prevention as is a diagnostic approach in determining how to treat symptomatic patients. Proposing a uniform ("one size fits all") health maintenance plan for all patients is as inappropriate as suggesting a single treatment plan for all patients with chest pain. The history, physical, and laboratory examination must be used to construct an individual risk profile. Only then can one determine which preventive services are indicated and which deserve priority.

The risk factors identified in the evaluation should be treated as real problems, recorded on the patient's "problem list" along with diseases, physical findings, and symptoms. Unhealthy personal behaviors, inadequate screening, and overdue immunizations represent problems that require as clear and as determined a follow-up plan as atrial fibrillation, rectal bleeding, a palpable spleen, or a new systolic murmur. Indeed, the fact that a patient does not exercise, has multiple sexual partners, consumes a high-fat diet, drinks and drives, or has not had a mammogram in 5 years may represent a more serious threat to the patient's health than most conditions that appear on conventional problem lists. Certainly they require as much attention if the patient is to reduce the risk of adding new diseases to the problem list in future years. The bulk of this book (see Section II) is devoted to advising the clinician on how to address risk factors once they are identified.

Preventive medicine cannot be practiced properly without a seamless integration with other aspects of health care. Providing preventive services in isolation from the patient's primary health care often limits their effectiveness. Appropriate counseling about personal health behaviors, such as advising safe exercise levels, requires an awareness of the patient's past history and coexisting medical problems. Screening tests performed in isolation from the primary care clinician (e.g., screening at community health fairs) can leave the patient without a means for acting on the results. Clinicians who prescribe preventive therapics (e.g., who start antihypertensive medications on a patient noted to have high blood pressure) without consulting the primary care clinician may be unaware of other medications and medical problems that need to be considered and may duplicate or complicate efforts undertaken by the primary care clinician. The same concern applies to comprehensive testing programs offered to corporate executives by "boutique" practices and to freestanding imaging centers in shopping malls that promote computed tomography scanning and ultrasonographic testing to the general public. The overuse of tests by such enterprises produces a large proportion of false-positive results and may give those with negative tests a false sense of security that makes them less attentive to modifying health habits. Such testing programs are often poorly equipped to counsel patients appropriately, either to put the results in context, to communicate the findings to their primary care clinician, or to make other appropriate referrals.

This book is therefore targeted at primary care clinicians, who are most knowledgeable about the patient's complete medical history, have the skills to diagnose and manage the broad array of clinical problems that arise in health promotion and disease prevention, and have a relationship with the patient that facilitates continuity in the health maintenance program. The primary care clinician is best suited to coordinate the patient's referrals to specialists, ensuring that patients receive necessary expert care in categorical areas without allowing other problems to "fall through the cracks."

Clinicians who are not primary care providers, such as specialists (e.g., cardiologists, ophthalmologists), emergency department clinicians, and hospital nurses, should also provide preventive services. It is important, however, that their focused contribution to the patient's preventive care be integrated into a comprehensive health maintenance plan under the coordination of the primary care clinician. A dermatologist who performs a skin cancer screening examination, a gastroenterologist who performs a screening colonoscopy, or an emergency department nurse who administers a vaccination, for example, should notify the primary care clinician about the services delivered and should forward copies of their findings to be included in the patient's primary care medical record.

Discussions in this book about patient education and counseling emphasize a shared decision-making model and a respectful style of discourse between clinicians and patients. This approach differs from the old-fashioned paternalistic counseling style in which the doctor "tells the patient what to do." The philosophy espoused in this book is that patients are entitled to make informed decisions about how they live their lives and about their health care. Clinicians have a professional responsibility to ensure that patients' decisions are based on complete and accurate health information but do not have a right to force the outcome of decisions. Once they have given the patient the necessary information about benefits and harms, they must respect the patient's preferences, even if the patient decides against doing what the clinician recommends. An authoritarian approach to promoting personal behavior change is rarely effective. Instead, this book encourages a collaborative model for decision making, which permits the clinician and patient to work together to determine the best choice for that individual. The book speaks of choices, not "orders;" patient initiative, not "compliance;" and partnership, not "prescription."

Although this trend in patient empowerment in decision making is occurring throughout medicine, it is especially appropriate in the practice of preventive health care. In health promotion, the "locus of control" lies more with the patient than with the clinician. In curative medicine, the clinician can often perform a procedure to solve the patient's problem (e.g., by placing a cast, removing an infected gallbladder, or suturing a laceration). In health promotion, only the patient can solve the problem. Stopping smoking, changing eating habits, increasing physical activity, and other changes in lifestyle are under the control of the patient and occur outside of the doctor's office or clinic. The clinician can, and should, provide information about the health risks associated with the behavior, encourage change, and suggest strategies for doing so, but the ultimate determinant of whether change occurs is the patient and not the clinician. The patient's feelings and attitudes about these health issues therefore require the full attention and respect of the clinician. (The clinician can also collaborate with public health colleagues to advocate changes in environmental factors, such as advertising for unhealthy foods, which interfere with even the most highly motivated patient's ability to practice health-promoting behaviors.)

This book's emphasis on patient education is reflected in the "Resources—Patient Education Materials" section at the end of most chapters, which include a list of organizations, government agencies, and federal clearinghouses that provide useful websites, brochures, counseling services, and other information resources. Characteristic of the current "information age" and the growth of medical consumerism, the scope of health information available to patients and the technologies for obtaining it are expanding rapidly. This information can supplement and reinforce the counseling provided by the clinician and can help the patient frame new questions, as well as identify the resources for answering them. It is the clinician's responsibility to ensure that patients are aware of these information resources and how to obtain them. Of all the services that clinicians can provide in the practice of health promotion and disease prevention, information is certainly the most valuable.

Finally, excellence in the practice of health promotion requires a holistic approach to understanding "health." The biomedical paradigm that dominates modern medicine has a tendency to be reductionist, to measure health in terms of blood test results, radiographic findings, and electrocardiographic changes. Clearly, health is more than the absence of disease, and it comprises more than the discrete biophysical entities that we are currently capable of measuring. Our understanding of the interconnections between the mind and body is steadily improving. It seems clear that health is influenced not only by biophysical factors but also by emotional and spiritual life, family dynamics and relationships, work satisfaction, income, food security, educational status, personal achievements, and social support.

Busy clinicians can easily overlook these issues, especially if these problems are not perceived as "medical" concerns. Failure to consider the broader context of health can limit or undermine the clinician's efforts to help patients. A clinician who is preoccupied with a patient's "noncompliance" in getting a mammogram, without considering her personal life and the barriers she faces, may never discover that depression over her husband's death has diminished her interest in living longer. An overweight inner city youth concerned about basic survival and gang-related shootings will be helped little by a clinician preoccupied with weight management as a singular focus. Clinicians benefit from taking the time to consider these issues. By learning more about their patients' lives, clinicians can enjoy fuller and more satisfying relationships with their patients and their families. Their suggested strategies for behavior change are more likely to be relevant to their patients' living conditions and, accordingly, are more likely to achieve results. Defining health objectives more broadly gives clinicians the gratification of knowing that their efforts are directed toward goals that are meaningful to their patients and that relate directly to the overall quality of their lives.

References

1. Green LW. Prevention and health education. In: Last JM, Wallace RB, eds. *Maxcy-Rosenau-Last. Public health and preventive medicine*, 13th ed. Norwalk: Appleton & Lange, 1992:787–802.

2. U.S. Preventive Services Task Force. *Guide to clinical preventive services*, 2nd ed. Baltimore: Williams & Wilkins, 1996.

3. Catlin A, Cowan C, Heffler S, et al. National health spending in 2005: the slowdown continues. *Health Aff (Millwood)* 2007;26:142–153.

4. Hogan C, Lynn J, Gabel J, et al. *Medicare beneficiaries' costs and use of care in the last year of life*. Medicare Payment Advisory Commission, Report No. 00–1. Washington, DC: Medicare Payment Advisory Commission, May 2000.

5. Lubitz JD, Riley GF. Trends in Medicare payments in the last year of life. *N Engl J Med* 1993;328:1092–1096.

6. U.S. Centers for Disease Control and Prevention. Estimated national spending on prevention—United States, 1988. *MMWR* 1992;41:529–531.

7. Satcher D. The prevention challenge and opportunity. *Health Aff* 2006;25:1009–1011.

8. He W, Sengupta M, Velkoff VA, et al. U.S. Census Bureau. *Current population reports, P23–209, 65+ in the United States: 2005*. Washington, DC: U.S. Government Printing Office, 2005.

9. Horvath J. *Chronic conditions in the U.S.: implications for service delivery and financing*. Rockville: Agency for Healthcare Research and Quality, http://www.ahrq.gov/news/ulp/hicosttele/sess2/horvathstxt.htm. Accessed 2007.

10. Eyre H, Kahn R, Robertson RM. ACS/ADA/AHA Collaborative Writing Committee. Preventing cancer, cardiovascular disease, and diabetes: a common agenda for the American Cancer Society, the American Diabetes Association, and the American Heart Association. *CA Cancer J Clin* 2004;54:190–207.

11. Mokdad AH, Bowman BA, Ford ES, et al. The continuing epidemics of obesity and diabetes in the United States. *JAMA* 2001;286:1195–1200.

12. Ogden CL, Carroll MD, Curtin LR, et al. Prevalence of overweight and obesity in the United States, 1999–2004. *JAMA* 2006;295:1549–1555.

13. Thorpe KE, Howard DH. The rise in spending among Medicare beneficiaries: the role of chronic disease prevalence and changes in treatment intensity. *Health Aff* 2006;25(5):w378–w388.

14. Lakdawalla DN, Goldman DP, Shang B. The health and cost consequences of obesity among the future elderly. *Health Aff* 2005;24(Suppl 2):W5R30–W5R41.

15. Olshansky SJ, Passaro DJ, Hershow RC, et al. A potential decline in life expectancy in the United States in the 21st century. *N Engl J Med* 2005;352:1138–1145.

16. Independence Hall Association. *The quotable Franklin*. Philadelphia: Independence Hall Association, at http://www.ushistory.org/franklin/quotable/quote67.htm. Accessed 2007.

17. Lalonde M. *A new perspective on the health of Canadians*. Ottawa: Information Canada, 1974.

18. U.S. Department of Health, Education, and Welfare. *Healthy people: the Surgeon General's report on health promotion and disease prevention*. HEW Publication No. 79–55071. Washington, DC: U.S. Department of Health, Education, and Welfare, 1979.

19. U.S. Department of Health and Human Services. *Promoting health/preventing disease: objectives for the nation.* Washington, DC: U.S. Department of Health and Human Services, 1990.

20. U.S. Department of Health and Human Services. *Healthy People 2010: Understanding and Improving Health.* 2nd ed. Washington, DC: U.S. Government Printing Office, November 2000.

21. Last JM, Wallace RB, eds. *Maxcy-Rosenau-Last public health and preventive medicine*, 13th ed. Norwalk: Appleton & Lange, 1992.

22. McGinnis JM, Lee PR. *Healthy people 2000 at mid decade. JAMA* 1995;273:1123–1129.

23. National Center for Health Statistics. *Health, United States, 2006 with chartbook on trends in the health of Americans.* Hyattsville, MD: National Center for Health Statistics. Accessed at http://www.cdc.gov/nchs/data/hus/hus06.pdf. 2006.

24. Casagrande SS, Wang Y, Anderson C, et al. Have Americans increased their fruit and vegetable intake? The trends between 1988 and 2002. *Am J Prev Med* 2007;32:257–263.

25. Woolf SH. The big answer: rediscovering prevention at a time of crisis in health care. *Harvard Health Policy Rev* 2006;7:5–20.

26. Garfinkel L, Silverberg E. Lung cancer and smoking trends in the United States over the past 25 years. *CA Cancer J Clin* 1991;41:137–145.

27. National Cancer Institute. *SEER cancer statistics review, 1975–2004.* Rockville: National Cancer Institute, http://seer.cancer.gov/csr/1975_2004/sections.html. Accessed 2007.

28. Mokdad AH, Marks JS, Stroup DF, et al. Actual causes of death in the United States, 2000. *JAMA* 2004;291:1238–1245.

29. Dinh-Zarr TB, Sleet DA, Shults RA, et al. Task Force on Community Preventive Services. Reviews of evidence regarding interventions to increase the use of safety belts. *Am J Prev Med* 2001;21(4 Suppl):48–65.

30. Miniño AM, Anderson RN, Fingerhut LA, et al. *Deaths: injuries, 2002.* National vital statistics reports, vol 54, no. 10. Hyattsville: National Center for Health Statistics, 2006.

31. McGlynn EA, Asch SM, Adams J, et al. The quality of health care delivered to adults in the United States. *N Engl J Med* 2003;348:2635–2645.

32. Cifuentes M, Fernald DH, Green LA, et al. Prescription for health: changing primary care practice to foster healthy behaviors. *Ann Fam Med* 2005;3(Suppl 2):S4–11.

33. National Committee for Quality Assurance. *The state of health care quality: 2005. Industry trends and analysis.* Washington, DC: National Committee for Quality Assurance, 2005.

34. National Center for Chronic Disease Prevention and Health Promotion. *Behavioral risk factor surveillance system, prevalence data.* http://apps.nccd.cdc.gov/brfss/index.asp. Accessed 2007.

35. Canadian Task Force on the Periodic Health Examination. *The Canadian guide to clinical preventive health care.* Ottawa: Canada Communication Group, 1994.

36. U.S. Preventive Services Task Force. *The guide to clinical preventive services, 2006. Recommendations of the U.S. Preventive Services Task Force.* Rockville: Agency for Healthcare Research and Quality, http://www.ahrq.gov/clinic/pocketgd.pdf. 2006.

37. U.S. Public Health Service. *Healthy people 2000: national health promotion and disease prevention objectives.* Publication (PHS) 91–50212. Washington, DC: U.S. Department of Health and Human Services, 1991.

38. Zaza S, Briss PA, Harris KW, eds. *The guide to community preventive services: what works to promote health? Task Force on Community Preventive Services*. Oxford University Press, 2005.
39. Woolf SH. The need for perspective in evidence-based medicine. *JAMA* 1999;282: 2358–2365.
40. Woolf SH, Kamerow DB. Testing for uncommon conditions: the heroic search for positive test results. *Arch Intern Med* 1990;150:2451–2458.
41. Schwartz LM, Woloshin S, Fowler FJ Jr, et al. Enthusiasm for cancer screening in the United States. *JAMA* 2004;291:71–78.
42. Ornish D, Scherwitz LW, Billings JH, et al. Intensive lifestyle changes for reversal of coronary heart disease. *JAMA* 1998;280:2001–2007.

Gathering Information

CHAPTER 1

Principles of Risk Assessment

Steven H. Woolf

Case 1: *A 21-year-old male college student was brought to the emergency department following a motor vehicle accident. He was the unbelted driver of an automobile involved in a high-speed collision. The patient was ejected from the vehicle on impact and thrown 50 yd, sustaining fatal head injuries. The deceased patient's blood alcohol concentration was 0.24%. Past medical history revealed that he had been seen for acute gastritis at the student health center on three occasions in the last year. The records revealed no discussion of his alcohol use, which had been a problem since high school, or his regular practice of driving without using a seat belt.*

Case 2: *A 52-year-old woman presented to a gastroenterologist with a 3-month history of progressive left lower quadrant abdominal pain, weight loss, and fatigue. In the last few days she had noted bloody stool. A colonoscopic examination with biopsy revealed an obstructing adenocarcinoma of the sigmoid colon. The patient underwent a partial colectomy and colostomy placement. Past medical history was noteworthy for ulcerative colitis, which was diagnosed when the patient was 24 years old but which had not required extensive medical care. The patient's previous clinical encounters had been limited to preventive visits to her gynecologist, who had never discussed her ulcerative colitis and had not recommended periodic colonoscopy or sigmoidoscopy.*

Case 3: *A 49-year-old corporate executive was brought to the emergency department 45 minutes after clutching his chest and collapsing during a business meeting. The electrocardiogram revealed 3-mm ST-segment depression in the anterior leads. Shortly thereafter the patient developed ventricular fibrillation and could not be resuscitated. Postmortem examination revealed a blood cholesterol level of 356 mg/dL and large stenotic plaques in the left main and anterior descending coronary arteries. Family members indicated that the patient had been gaining weight and smoking more heavily in recent years but was otherwise healthy. His siblings were also considered to be healthy, but two sisters were being treated for elevated serum lipid levels. The patient's father and uncle had also died at a young age from unanticipated heart attacks. The patient visited a physician* *only three times as an adult, primarily for treatment of joint injuries received during unsuccessful attempts at jogging. The physician's notes addressed the joint injuries but did not discuss the patient's tobacco use, family history, eating habits, or physical inactivity. No prior record of the patient's lipid levels could be found in the chart.*

Case 4: *A 20-month-old girl was admitted to the hospital with a 1-day history of fever, headache, and increasing lethargy. Physical examination was suggestive of meningitis, and culture of the cerebrospinal fluid demonstrated the presence of* Haemophilus influenza *type b. After completion of intravenous antibiotic therapy, the patient was discharged from the hospital but was noted to have permanent hearing impairment. Review of the family physician's records revealed that the patient had received appropriate immunizations until 9 months of age, but subsequent appointments for well-child examinations were canceled by the parents for unexplained reasons and therefore the* Haemophilus *vaccination series was never completed. The patient's mother did see the family physician on two occasions for treatment of facial lacerations, but the child's immunization status and the conditions at home were not discussed. Six months later, a telephone call from a neighbor prompted an evaluation by the local child protective services agency, which revealed that both the child and mother were regular victims of beatings by the father.*

What these unfortunate cases have in common is clear to the reader: each patient suffered or died from conditions that were potentially preventable earlier in life. Diseases (e.g., coronary artery disease, colon cancer), injuries (e.g., motor vehicle accidents, physical abuse), and infections (e.g., meningitis) were preceded months, years, and decades earlier by the presence of risk factors or preclinical disease states that were amenable to prevention but that escaped detection and intervention.

Unfortunately, prevention failures of this magnitude are neither exceptional nor uncommon in the United States. Each day, many thousands of Americans undergo treatment for conditions that could have been prevented earlier in their lives if the underlying causal risk factors had been identified. The failure to detect and treat those risk factors while patients are otherwise healthy often culminates years later in the need for aggressive medical interventions (e.g., chemotherapy, surgery, dialysis) and in chronic impairment (pain, paralysis, mental illness, disability, death). Such personally, socially, and financially costly consequences can be prevented through relatively simple interventions such as modifying harmful health behaviors (e.g., smoking), immunizations, and screening for early detection of disease before it becomes clinically apparent. The reality that so many Americans do not take these steps, despite being under the care of a clinician, has created a growing concern among both professionals and the public.

Americans receive only half of recommended clinical preventive services (1). Preventive care in the United States is inadequate for many reasons, including limited access to health services, patient noncompliance, and costs. In many cases, however, the failure to receive preventive care is attributable to the failure of clinicians to include risk assessment in their routine care of asymptomatic and healthy patients. The purpose of this chapter is to review the importance of clinical risk assessment and the theoretic principles that underlie the related activities discussed in this book. See Chapters 2–4 for details on how to perform risk assessment as part of the history, physical examination, and laboratory testing.

THE PLACE OF PREVENTION IN ILLNESS VISITS

In this book, the terms *asymptomatic* and *healthy* are not meant to describe patients without complaints; only a few patients visit their doctor without complaints for the sole purpose of obtaining preventive checkups. Rather, the terms refer to the absence of signs or symptoms of *target conditions*. For example, the executive who was seen on three occasions for joint injuries was "symptomatic" in the usual sense of the term—he had acute joint pain—but he was asymptomatic with respect to the target condition of coronary artery disease.

This, in fact, is the usual context of preventive care: the detection of risk factors in patients who are asymptomatic with respect to target conditions often occurs during clinical encounters that have been scheduled by the patient to address other, more immediate problems. For example, a patient schedules an appointment to deal with sinusitis, but is found to be physically inactive and returns home with *both* an exercise and antibiotic prescription. A patient presents with a vaginal yeast infection but is noted to have not had a Papanicolaou smear for 5 years. A preschool boy with inadequate well-child care is rushed to the emergency department for treatment of acute otitis media and receives his second measles-mumps-rubella vaccination before being discharged.

See Chapter 20 for further discussion of the advantages and disadvantages of delivering preventive care opportunistically during such illness visits, as opposed to during well-person examinations dedicated to prevention.

WHAT IS RISK ASSESSMENT?

Risk assessment in the clinical setting refers to the collection of information about risk factors during the history, physical, and laboratory examination.[a] *Risk factors* are personal characteristics, physiologic parameters, symptoms, or preclinical disease states that increase the likelihood that an individual has or will develop a particular disease. Examples of personal characteristics that can increase risk are personal health behaviors (e.g., smoking), family history, genotype, environmental exposures, and occupation. Examples of physiologic risk factors, which can be determined by measurement, include laboratory test results (e.g., serum lipid levels), anthropomorphic measurements (e.g., body mass index), and other laboratory information (e.g., audiometry results). Similarly, symptoms and past or present disease states may also increase a patient's likelihood of developing a related disease.

Chapters 2, 3, and 4 discuss how to perform risk assessment during the history, physical, and laboratory examination, respectively. Section II of this book discusses what to do with the findings.

Risk assessment should not be regarded as a unique clinical activity, separate from routine patient care. It is, after all, a well-established component of the thorough history, physical, and laboratory examination taught throughout clinical training. Personal characteristics that increase health risk, such as smoking and family history, are commonly addressed in the social and family history sections of the history. Preclinical disease states are sought in a careful physical examination. Physiologic risk factors are often detected in conventional laboratory tests. Yet many clinicians perform incomplete risk assessments when evaluating healthy patients for preventive care.

THE IMPORTANCE OF RISK ASSESSMENT

Why do clinicians not conduct complete risk assessments? Why, for example, did the businessman's physician not investigate his family history and cardiac risk factors? In some cases, the oversights are due to *lack of knowledge* and the clinician's unfamiliarity with current guidelines. The gynecologist may not have remembered that ulcerative colitis is a risk factor for colon cancer and that periodic endoscopic surveillance may be necessary. In other instances, the oversight is due to *lack of time*. The physician in a busy student health center may have lacked the time to ask about the patient's drinking habits or seat belt use. In some cases, the oversight is due to *distraction* by the patient's current

---

[a]Population-based risk assessment, such as the measurement of environmental and other health risks facing society (e.g., pandemics, bioterrorism), is not discussed here.

complaints. The family physician's concentration on suturing the mother's facial lacerations may have made him less attentive to the source of her injuries or her daughter's missed appointments. Sometimes the oversight is *attitudinal,* due to a lack of appreciation of the clinical importance of prevention. Problem drinking, seat belt use, unsuccessful attempts at regular exercise, unhealthy eating habits, and missed appointments may all have seemed unimportant at the time, and the serious consequences of overlooking them may have been inapparent. Finally, *inadequate reimbursement* by insurers lessens the enthusiasm of some clinicians to devote large portions of office visits to preventive care.

An important reason for incomplete risk assessments is the reluctance of clinicians to believe that preventive interventions are worthwhile. Many do not appreciate the linkage between the quality of preventive care provided and the thoroughness of risk assessment, despite its obviously logical basis—clinicians cannot provide patients with rational advice on health maintenance or intervene with early-stage disease without first identifying the risk factors and disease states that most deserve their attention. A standardized "prevention package" for all patients is rarely appropriate, effective, or well received. The prevention priorities for a 55-year-old smoker with a family history of premature heart disease obviously differ from those of the health-conscious young athlete, the drug-using, depressed adolescent who talks of suicide, or the elderly nursing home patient. If the clinician is to have a meaningful and effective impact on the patient's risk of future disease, the prevention message must be tailored to the risk profile of that individual.

Risk assessment is also necessary for the rational ordering of screening tests. For many years, physicians administered a standard battery of laboratory tests as part of annual checkups, such as screening blood counts and chemistries, urinalyses, chest radiographs, and electrocardiograms. Many clinicians continue this practice now. One problem with this approach, aside from its enormous cost, is that it generates large numbers of false-positive results (see Chapters 4 and 19). This, in turn, leads to a so-called screening cascade of what in fact are unnecessary diagnostic workups and treatment interventions.

Because these adverse effects are less likely when screening is targeted to patients with specific risk factors (in whom the pretest probability and positive predictive value are increased), expert panels, such as the U.S. Preventive Services Task Force (USPSTF) (2), have recommended that clinicians avoid routine test batteries and instead order selected screening tests based on the patient's individual risk profile. This recommendation obviously requires the clinician to first identify the patient's risk factors. It also reinforces the need for clinicians to return to the time-honored tradition of careful history taking and to limit the currently common overreliance on laboratory testing.

THE BASIS OF INCOMPLETE RISK ASSESSMENT BY CLINICIANS: THE ILLNESS-BASED VERSUS THE RISK FACTOR–BASED THOUGHT PROCESSES

The tendency of clinicians to perform incomplete risk assessments may result from using the wrong thought process when evaluating patients. The commonly used clinical thought process when evaluating symptomatic patients identifies the chief complaint(s) as the primary problem(s) and has as its objective the clarification of the diagnosis and treatment plan. This *illness-based thought process* is, appropriately, oriented to the present and not the future. In such patients, risk assessment—the collection of risk factor information in the history, physical, and laboratory examination—is performed to explain the patient's *current* symptoms and signs. In this context assessment of *future* risk plays a relatively minor role. Experienced clinicians know that the history of present illness and physical examination findings are usually all that are needed to make the diagnosis. Although risk factor information can occasionally enhance diagnostic accuracy, most clinicians discover over time that their diagnostic accuracy is rarely compromised by an incomplete social, family, or occupational history. Clinicians accustomed to caring for symptomatic patients are therefore not driven to thorough questioning about risk factors.

In preventive medicine, risk assessment has a different purpose, because the patient has not yet developed clinical evidence of the target conditions. Therefore, a different *risk factor–oriented thought process* is necessary. The patients' risk factors—not their current complaints—come to be viewed as the primary problem. In contrast to their relatively minor role in evaluating current symptoms, risk factors constitute the primary problem in preventive care. Therefore, risk assessment becomes the essential starting point for addressing the scope of the problem. What should follow in the thought process is a problem-oriented examination of how to modify the identified risks.

A patient with the risk factors of tobacco use, prior exposure to tuberculosis, and susceptibility to influenza requires a special program of smoking cessation counseling, tuberculin skin testing, and influenza vaccination. A patient with the risk factors of multiple sexual partners, injection drug use, and a history of dysplastic nevi requires a special program of sexual practices and substance abuse counseling, screening for malignant melanoma, and vaccination against hepatitis B. These interventions will not be carried out if the clinician does not first establish the risk factor "problem list" through risk assessment.

Clinicians are more accustomed to the thought process used for symptomatic patients than to the thought process used for preventive care. Their tendency to use the customary illness-based thought process in preventive care probably accounts for the frequency of incomplete risk assessments. To further illustrate the consequences of this mismatch, let us return to the example of a clinician accustomed to the illness-based thought process who enters the examination room of the previously mentioned patient with sinusitis. Because the illness-based thought process defines current complaints as the primary problem, the clinician immediately identifies purulent rhinorrhea and maxillary tenderness as the primary matter at hand. With additional physical examination findings to confirm the diagnosis, there is little reason to pursue risk assessment. For a patient with obvious sinusitis, why should the clinician obtain a social, family, or occupational history? The only risk factors to which the illness-based thought process might direct the clinician are those related to sinusitis. The patient would be sent home with an antibiotic prescription, but without a discussion of the need to engage in regular exercise.

High-quality preventive care requires the clinician to adopt a risk factor–oriented thought process that is independent of the evaluation of current complaints. Once the current complaints have been addressed, the next step is to switch to a risk factor–oriented thought process, which begins a comprehensive search for unrecognized risk factors. In a systematic process that takes less than a few minutes to complete, the clinician supplements the sinusitis history with information about the risk factors discussed in Chapter 2 and checks whether the patient is up-to-date on the recommended physical examination and laboratory screening procedures discussed in Chapters 3 and 4. (Reminders produced by electronic health records or other office systems discussed in Chapters 21 and 22 can speed this process and make it routine.) In this example, questions drawn from Chapter 2 would call attention to the patient's physical inactivity and would prompt a discussion of regular exercise or arrangements for a return visit devoted to this topic.

The risk factors identified through this process vary among patients. Each patient's risk factor "problem list" constitutes an *individual risk profile*. It provides global information on the patient's overall risk for developing future disease, as well as a framework for tailoring the health maintenance plan to the patient's particular needs. For example, consider a patient who makes an appointment with a physician to obtain a bone density measurement. Rather than simplistically responding to this request, the physician performs a brief but thorough risk assessment to review the individual's risk profile. This reveals that the patient has multiple risk factors for other diseases, including a family history of premature coronary artery disease and a personal history of smoking, hypertension, overweight, and hypercholesterolemia. This "big picture" perspective enables the physician and patient to review the complete list of risk factors and to work together to "triage" the priorities. They first agree that the cardiac risk factors pose a greater threat to future health than does osteoporosis, defer the bone density measurement, and use the remaining time to devise a plan for cardiac risk factor modification. It is rarely appropriate or possible to address all risk factors at once. Health maintenance planning involves collaborative work with the patient: setting priorities by determining which problems the patient is willing and able to address first and agreeing on a follow-up plan for addressing other risk factors. See Chapter 5 for further details about this process.

SETTING REASONABLE LIMITS AND PRIORITIES IN RISK ASSESSMENT

There are at least hundreds of personal characteristics, physiologic parameters, environmental exposures, symptoms, and preclinical disease states that can increase an individual's risk for future disease. Practical and scientific reasons make it implausible for clinicians to screen for all risk factors during risk assessments. The most important practical constraint is lack of time; a typical office visit can accommodate a discussion of no more than two or three risk factors. Moreover, for many risk factors, there is insufficient scientific evidence that they pose *significant* risks or that attempts to modify them are effective in improving health. At its best, devoting time to these unproved measures may be useless. At its worst, this practice can divert the clinician and patient away from more important risk factors that deserve their attention. Thirty eight percent of deaths in the United States are attributable to three behaviors: smoking, diet, and physical activity (3).

How, then, should the clinician select the factors to address in risk assessment? These are the key questions to ask: (a) How serious is the target condition? (b) How common is the risk factor? (c) What is the magnitude of risk associated with the risk factor? (d) How accurately can the risk factor be detected? (e) What is the evidence that potential interventions improve health outcomes? (f) How does this information compare with other health priorities? Similar questions are pertinent in setting reasonable limits for almost every topic in this book.

How Serious Is the Target Condition?

Risk factors for a trivial health problem may not deserve attention. The burden of suffering from the target condition is best judged by its frequency and severity. Frequency is typically measured in terms of incidence or prevalence. *Incidence* is the proportion of the population that acquires the condition in a given period of time. *Prevalence* is the proportion of the population that has the condition at any given time. A variety of outcome measures are used to estimate the severity of a health condition. Traditional measures include morbidity, mortality, and survival rates, but health services research has encouraged the use of more meaningful measures of quality of life, functional status, and overall well-being. In terms of mortality,

TABLE 1.1   Leading Causes of Death in the United States

Rank	Cause of Death	Number of Deaths, 2002	Age-Adjusted Death Rate (per 100,000)	Percentage of Total Deaths
1	Heart disease	696,947	240.8	28.5
2	Malignant neoplasms	557,271	193.5	22.8
3	Cerebrovascular diseases	162,672	56.2	6.7
4	Chronic lower respiratory diseases-	124,816	43.5	5.1
5	Unintentional injuries	106,742	36.9	4.3
6	Diabetes mellitus	73,249	25.4	3.0
7	Influenza and pneumonia	65,681	22.6	2.7

Adapted from National Center for Health Statistics. *Health, United States, 2005 with chartbook on trends in the health of Americans*. Hyattsville: National Center for Health Statistics, http://www.cdc.gov/nchs/data/hus/hus05.pdf#summary. 2005.

a convenient ranking of the importance of diseases is the leading causes of death, which can be determined for the general population (see Table 1.1) or stratified by specific risk groups. Table 1.2 lists the leading causes of death for specific age-groups.

How Common Is the Risk Factor?

A risk factor that is extremely uncommon may not be worthy of routine screening, and some risk factors that are extremely common may be weak predictors of future disease. Like target conditions, the frequency of the presence of a risk factor in the population is generally measured by prevalence and incidence rates and may vary considerably in different segments of the population.

What Is the Magnitude of Risk Associated with the Risk Factor?

The magnitude of risk conferred by a risk factor can be defined in terms of relative or absolute risk. *Relative risk* is the ratio between the risk of disease among persons with the risk factor and the risk among those without the risk factor. A relative risk of 2.0 suggests that persons with the risk factor are twice as likely to develop the disease as persons without the risk factor.

TABLE 1.2 Leading Causes of Death, United States, by Age-group, 2002

1–4 Years	5–14 Years
Unintentional injuries	Unintentional injuries
Congenital malformations, deformations, and chromosomal abnormalities	Malignant neoplasms
Homicide	Congenital malformations, deformations, and chromosomal abnormalities
Malignant neoplasms	Homicide
Heart diseases	Suicide
Influenza and pneumonia	Heart diseases
Septicemia	Chronic lower respiratory diseases
Chronic lower respiratory diseases	Septicemia
Conditions originating in perinatal period	Cerebrovascular diseases
In situ, benign, and other neoplasms	Influenza and pneumonia
15–24 Years	**25–44 Years**
Unintentional injuries	Unintentional injuries
Homicide	Malignant neoplasms
Suicide	Heart diseases
Malignant neoplasms	Suicide
Heart diseases	Homicide
Congenital malformations, deformations, and chromosomal abnormalities	HIV disease
Chronic lower respiratory diseases	Chronic liver disease and cirrhosis
HIV disease	Cerebrovascular diseases
Diabetes mellitus	Diabetes mellitus
Cerebrovascular diseases	Influenza and pneumonia

TABLE 1.2 *(Continued)*

45–64 Years	65 Years and Older
Malignant neoplasms	Heart diseases
Heart diseases	Malignant neoplasms
Unintentional injuries	Cerebrovascular diseases
Cerebrovascular diseases	Chronic lower respiratory diseases
Diabetes mellitus	Influenza and pneumonia
Chronic lower respiratory diseases	Alzheimer's disease
Chronic liver disease and cirrhosis	Diabetes mellitus
Suicide	Nephritis, nephrotic syndrome, nephrosis
HIV disease	Unintentional injuries
Septicemia	Septicemia

Adapted from National Center for Health Statistics. *Health, United States, 2005 with chartbook on trends in the health of Americans.* Hyattsville: National Center for Health Statistics, http://www.cdc.gov/nchs/data/hus/hus05.pdf#summary. 2005.
HIV = human immunodeficiency virus.

Such ratios, which are often used in both the medical literature and lay media to emphasize (and sensationalize) the magnitude of risk, can be misleading if not accompanied by information about the *absolute risk,* the actual proportion of persons with the risk factor who will develop the disease.

To clarify the distinction, consider hypothetical risk factors A and B. Risk factor A is a risk factor for disease A, risk factor B is a risk factor for disease B, and both diseases are fatal. The relative risk of risk factors A and B are 2.0 and 1.1, respectively. Readers of the medical literature and lay media are likely to conclude at first glance that risk factor A is almost twice as dangerous as risk factor B. The missing information is the absolute risk. Suppose the absolute risk for persons with risk factor A is 1:50,000, whereas the risk is 1:100,000 for persons without risk factor A. Therefore, although it is true that the relative risk is 2.0 (1:50,000 is twice the risk of 1:100,000), the patient's absolute risk of developing disease A is increased by only 0.001% (1:100,000 subtracted from 1:50,000) by having risk factor A. Put differently, 99.998% of persons with risk factor A will not develop the disease.

Next consider the situation for risk factor B, which has a lower relative risk (1.1) than risk factor A (2.0). Suppose, however, that the absolute risk for disease B is 1:10 (0.1) among persons with this risk factor and 1:11 (0.0909) for persons without this risk factor. Therefore, although it is true that the relative risk associated with risk factor B is 1.1 (0.1/0.0909), it increases the absolute risk for disease B by 0.9% (0.1–0.0909). Recall that the absolute risk for disease A was increased 0.001% by risk factor A. Therefore, although the relative risk of risk factor B (1.1) is approximately half that of risk factor A (2.0), the absolute risk data tell us that persons with risk factor B are 900 times (0.9/0.001) more likely to develop disease B than are persons with risk factor A to develop disease A. (Note that, even with this higher risk, 90% of persons with risk factor B will not develop the disease.)

Absolute risk helps to clarify the distinction between risk factors and real disease, a common source of confusion among both clinicians and the public. Once the relation between a risk factor and a disease is established and public education campaigns are launched to raise awareness of the risk factor, there is a tendency for both clinicians and patients to feel that a disease has been discovered when they detect a risk factor. Both patients and clinicians often need reminders and reassurance that heightened risk—whether from an increase in high-density lipoproteins, C-reactive peptide, prediabetes, or prehypertension—warrants attention but is not tantamount to disease.

Unfortunately, it is all too common for the public, policymakers, and clinicians to overlook these details when they make arguments for or against health-promoting interventions. For example, based on the information given in the preceding text, is it appropriate for a newspaper headline to claim that risk factor A or B is a more serious problem? The answer is that neither relative nor absolute risk data provide sufficient information to answer the question. The analysis is incomplete without considering the *population-attributable risk,* the proportion of the population affected. Suppose that 1 million Americans have risk factor A, but only 1,000 have risk factor B. Reducing the absolute risk of disease A by 0.001% will save 1,000 (1 million × 0.001%) lives, whereas reducing the absolute risk of disease B by 0.9% will save only 9 (1,000 × 0.9%) lives. Therefore, whether in the government or clinic, the importance of a risk factor requires consideration of relative, absolute, and population-attributable risk.

How Accurately Can the Risk Factor Be Detected?

Even if the target condition and risk factor are serious, efforts to detect risk factors may be ineffective or harmful if the screening test is inaccurate. Inaccurate screening tests can produce *false-positive* results, which suggest incorrectly the presence of the risk factor, or *false-negative* results, which suggest incorrectly the absence of the risk factor. False-positive results can generate unnecessary anxiety, follow-up testing, and treatment. False-negative results can lead to delays in the detection and treatment of the risk factor. The accuracy of a screening test is measured in terms of *sensitivity, specificity,* and *predictive value.* In general, a screening test is more likely to produce false-positive results if the risk factor is uncommon in the population. See Chapter 4 for definitions of these terms and for further discussion of these concepts.

What Is the Evidence that Potential Interventions Improve Health Outcomes?

Even if the risk factor and target condition are important and the available screening tests are accurate, there is little point in screening if there is inadequate evidence that available interventions improve outcomes. The best evidence to this effect are intervention studies demonstrating that patients who undergo risk factor modification achieve better health outcomes than those without the intervention. More often, however, all that is available is epidemiologic evidence suggesting that the presence of the risk factor is causally associated with the disease. In such cases, proponents of risk factor modification may use this evidence of causality to infer that modifying the risk factor will be effective in reducing the incidence of the disease.

Unfortunately, such assumptions are not always valid. For example, there is considerable evidence of an association between dietary fat and cancer, but prospective trials have not convincingly demonstrated that lowering dietary fat intake reduces the incidence of cancer. In exceptional cases, the effectiveness of risk factor modification can be inferred from the strength and consistency of the evidence. For example, there has never been a controlled intervention study demonstrating that smoking cessation reduces the incidence of cancer. The performance of such a study is highly unlikely for both ethical and legal reasons. The enormous strength and consistency of the causal evidence and the lower rates of disease in persons who stop smoking are considered adequate evidence, even without a controlled trial, to infer that such measures are effective.

How Does This Information Compare with Other Health Priorities?

Individual risk factors and diseases do not exist in a vacuum. In deciding whether to devote limited time and energy to a particular risk factor or health problem, the conscientious clinician must also consider its relative importance in relation to the other risk factors and health problems that also require attention. Advising patients about dietary fiber intake may be important, but is it more important than using the same time to discuss dietary fat consumption, tobacco use, the need for breast cancer screening, or blood pressure monitoring? Advocates of prostate cancer screening may emphasize that almost 30,000 Americans die each year from this disease but, by examining the data in Table 1.1, the clinician can put these numbers in perspective as they relate to other serious diseases the patient and clinician must consider.

SETTING PRIORITIES

Fortunately for the clinician, the risk factors and screening tests that usually deserve attention in the clinical encounter have already been identified by several expert panels, which have devoted years of research to examining the above issues. The USPSTF (2) is an independent panel established by the federal government in 1984 to develop evidence-based recommendations on which preventive services to include in the periodic health examination. The USPSTF recommendations are summarized in Appendix A at the end of this book. Some clinicians prioritize the services to which the task force gives an "A" or "B" recommendation, indicating strong evidence of net health benefit. Comprehensive preventive care recommendations have also been issued by medical specialty societies, and more specific recommendations on screening tests, immunizations, and health behaviors have been issued by government agencies, medical groups, and private organizations (4). These recommendations form the basis for the risk factor evaluations and screening tests discussed in Chapters 2–4.

Tools have been developed for clinicians to quickly determine which preventive services are recommended for an individual patient. For example, the Agency for Healthcare Research and Quality (AHRQ) has created a software program that can be used online or downloaded to a personal digital assistant (PDA) and uses clinical information inputted by the clinician to identify the services recommended by the USPSTF for an individual with that history (see http://epss.ahrq.gov/PDA/index.jsp).

For most primary care practices, however, the complete list of preventive services recommended by these programs is too extensive to offer in a single office visit or even a routine health maintenance examination. A widely cited estimate is that it would take 7.8 hours/day for most clinicians to deliver all of the preventive services recommended by the USPSTF (5). Choices must be made. As discussed further in Chapter 20, practices must often focus on ensuring the delivery of a subset of the preventive services that they consider most important.

Assistance in deciding which preventive services are most important is provided in the 2006 report of the National Commission on Prevention Priorities (6), which ranked preventive services based on their relative clinical effectiveness and cost-effectiveness (see Table 1.3). Clinicians should consult these rankings when setting priorities and establishing protocols for their own practices, considering the local contextual issues discussed in Chapter 20 (e.g., patient population needs, agreement from colleagues). Moreover, as discussed earlier, the most important preventive services for individual patients are likely to differ based on personal risk profiles.

TABLE 1.3 Rankings of Clinical Preventive Services by National Commission on Prevention Priorities

Preventive Service	Clinically Preventable Burden	Cost-Effectiveness
Aspirin chemoprophylaxis	5	5
Childhood immunization series	5	5
Tobacco use screening and brief intervention	5	5
Colorectal cancer screening	4	4
Hypertension screening	5	3
Influenza immunization	4	4
Pneumococcal immunization	3	5
Problem drinking screening and brief counseling	4	4
Vision screening for adults	3	5
Cervical cancer screening	4	3
Cholesterol screening	5	2
Breast cancer screening	4	2
Chlamydia screening	2	4
Calcium chemoprophylaxis	3	3
Vision screening for children	2	4
Folic acid chemoprophylaxis	2	3
Obesity screening	3	2
Depression screening	3	1
Hearing screening	2	2
Injury prevention counseling	1	3

(continued)

TABLE 1.3 *(Continued)*

Preventive Service	Clinically Preventable Burden	Cost-Effectiveness
Osteoporosis screening	2	2
Cholesterol screening in high risk young adults	1	1
Diabetes screening	1	1
Diet counseling	1	1
Tetanus-diphtheria booster	1	1

How to interpret the scores

Score	Clinically Preventable Burden (QALYs Saved)	Cost-Effectiveness (Dollars/QALY Gained)
5	≥360,000	Cost saving
4	185,000–360,000	0–14,000
3	40,000–185,000	14,000–35,000
2	15,000–40,000	35,000–165,000
1	<15,000	165,000–450,000

Adapted from: Maciosek MV, Coffield AB, Edwards NM, et al. Priorities among effective clinical preventive services: results of a systematic review and analysis. *Am J Prev Med* 2006;31:52–61.
QALY = quality adjusted life year.
Services that produce the most health benefits received the highest clinically preventable burden (CPB) score of 5. Services that are most cost effective received the highest cost-effectiveness (CE) score of 5.

TOOLS TO HELP INDIVIDUALIZE RISK ASSESSMENT

A variety of tools are available to help clinicians compile and analyze information about patients' risk factors. For generations it has been customary for patients to provide such information on forms completed when they register at practices and, less consistently, for this database to be updated over time. Health risk appraisals—introduced in the 1970s to collect risk data from patients and generate epidemiologically based, personalized risk projections—are still in use by some practices. See Chapter 2 for further discussion of the role of questionnaires about risk factors and health history.

The emergence of electronic health records has introduced a more systematic means for organizing and maintaining information about individual risk factors. As discussed further in Chapters 21 and 22, electronic health records can be programmed to generate prompts and reminders to alert clinicians when attention to risk factors (e.g., counseling) or to overdue preventive services is warranted. Interoperable electronic databases also enable risk factor data to be shared between practices, hospitals, and other institutions and to be updated as changes occur.

Beginning with the use of handheld minirecords and health passports in the 1980s, patients have assumed an active role in keeping track of their personal health information and, increasingly, are using interactive websites and software for self-management of their health. They use their computers and handheld devices to obtain health information from websites and to maintain personal health records—the consumer counterpart to the electronic health record maintained by clinicians. Interactive websites and software products on which patients store past medical history and risk factor data can be programmed to advise patients about unhealthy behaviors (e.g., physical inactivity, smoking) and preventive services recommended for individuals with their risk profile. They can print out summaries and prompts for patients to bring to their doctor, and some systems can, with the patient's permission, interface directly with electronic health records to transfer patient-entered data directly into the practice database and to review results of laboratory tests.

Finally, clinicians must often rely on specific risk calculation tools to determine whether some preventive services are indicated. For example, body mass index calculators, which can be accessed at websites or stored on PDAs, help clinicians quickly determine whether patients are overweight or obese and require counseling about weight management (see Chapters 3 and 17). Decisions about the chemoprevention of coronary artery disease and treatment of elevated serum lipids are often guided by the Framingham risk equation (see Chapters 15 and 18), which can be calculated for individual patients using the guide in Figure 1.1 or by using handheld or online software tools. Similarly, the appropriateness of medications to prevent breast cancer, such as tamoxifen and raloxifene, are influenced by the 5-year risk of breast cancer, which can be calculated using the Gail model (see Chapter 15). Online calculation tools are listed at the end of this chapter, and further details about their application in decisions about chemoprevention are provided in Chapter 15.

APPLYING THE PRINCIPLES OF RISK ASSESSMENT IN PRACTICE

Applying the principles of risk assessment requires more than implementing guidelines and using risk assessment tools, although these are helpful. Each day, clinicians have the opportunity to incorporate the principles discussed in this chapter when counseling patients and when setting policy in their practice. When counseling patients about the meaning of risk factors, the conscientious clinician will provide information about both relative and absolute risk, allowing the patient to make a more informed decision about

To calculate 10 year risk of CHD

Age	M	F
20–34	–9	–7
35–39	–4	–3
40–44	0	0
45–49	3	3
50–54	6	6
55–59	8	8
60–64	10	10
65–69	11	12
70–74	12	14
75–79	13	16
Points		

Total Cholesterol	Age 20–39		Age 40–49		Age 50–59		Age 60–69		Age 70–79	
	M	F	M	F	M	F	M	F	M	F
<160	0	0	0	0	0	0	0	0	0	0
160–199	4	4	3	3	2	2	1	1	0	1
200–239	7	8	5	6	3	4	1	2	0	1
240–279	9	11	6	8	4	5	2	3	1	2
>280	11	13	8	10	5	7	3	4	1	2
Points										

HDL	Points
>60	–1
50–59	0
40–49	1
<40	2
Points	

Systolic BP	If untreated		If treated	
	M	F	M	F
<120	0	0	0	0
120–129	0	1	1	3
130–139	1	2	2	4
140–159	1	3	2	5
>160	2	4	3	6
Points				

Smoking	Age 20–39		Age 40–49		Age 50–59		Age 60–69		Age 70–79	
	M	F	M	F	M	F	M	F	M	F
Non smoker	0	0	0	0	0	0	0	0	0	0
Smoker	8	9	5	7	3	4	1	2	1	1
Points										

Points: Age ___ + Total Cholesterol ___ + HDL ___ + Systemic BP ___ + Smoking ___ =

Men 10 year risk of coronary heart disease in the next 10 years

Points	<0	0	1	2	3	4	5	6	7	8	9	10	11	12	13	14	15	16	17
Risk %	<1%	1	1	1	1	2	2	3	4	5	6	8	10	12	16	20	25	>30%	

Women 10 year risk of coronary heart disease in the next 10 years

Points	<9	9	10	11	12	13	14	15	16	17	18	19	20	21	22	23	24	>24
Risk %	<1%	1	1	1	1	2	2	3	4	5	6	8	11	14	17	22	27	>30%

Figure 1.1 • Calculation of a patient's Framingham risk score. Risk factors included in the Framingham-based calculation of 10-year coronary artery disease risk are age, total cholesterol, high-density lipoprotein (HDL) cholesterol, systolic blood pressure, treatment for hypertension, and smoking status. Points are assigned for each risk factor according to the tables, and the sum of points is used in the gender specific tables to determine the 10-year risk to develop coronary heart disease. The cholesterol and HDL cholesterol values should be the average of at least two measurements. The systolic blood pressure should be the current blood pressure, but the need for antihypertensive therapy is an additional risk factor. CHD, coronary heart disease; BP, blood pressure. (Adapted from: National Cholesterol Education Program. *Detection, evaluation, and treatment of high blood cholesterol in adults (adult treatment panel III)*. Available at: http://www.nhlbi.nih.gov/guidelines/cholesterol/atp3_rpt.htm. Last reviewed January, 2006.)

the importance or unimportance of the risk factor and limiting unnecessary anxiety. For example, providing only relative risk information to patients with risk factor A—telling them that they are twice as likely to develop a fatal disease than persons without the risk factor—is more likely to generate anxiety than if the absolute risk is also described. Patients who realize that their absolute risk of disease is only 0.002% will put this information in proper perspective and will be less likely to abandon more important health concerns to address this risk factor. Also, the realization that 99.998% of persons with risk factor A will not develop disease will also help them avoid the pitfall of confusing risk factors with disease.

The principles of risk assessment can also be applied when developing policy for one's practice. Although national guidelines are available to define important health priorities, local practice conditions or the emergence of new information following publication of the guidelines may prompt the need to supplement or modify recommendations for local practice. For example, organizations disagree about the appropriateness of routine screening for diabetes in the general population. However, clinicians caring for Native Americans, in whom the prevalence of diabetes is high among certain tribes, might need to examine whether a different policy is indicated in their practice. Local news reports may heighten a community's concern over a particular risk factor (e.g., exposure to hazardous emissions), a health problem (e.g., avian influenza), or a bioterrorist incident, which may exert pressure on clinicians to screen for this condition. Finally, the medical literature may provide new information about the importance of a risk factor or the availability of a new screening test before national expert panels have had an opportunity to publish recommendations.

In each of these cases, the clinician should use the principles discussed in this chapter to determine the relative importance of the risk factor and its relation to other established health priorities. How serious is the target condition? How common is the risk factor? What is the magnitude of risk associated with the risk factor? How accurately can the risk factor be detected? What is the evidence that potential interventions improve health outcomes? How does this information compare with other health priorities?

Clinicians should also examine the source of articles advocating increased clinical attention to a particular risk factor. As noted in the preceding text, such recommendations often originate from individuals, medical organizations, or government agencies that have a specialized interest in the topic. If an individual's research or an organization's mission is devoted to the eradication of a particular disease or risk factor, it may advocate full attention to this problem without first considering the effect of its recommendations on other serious health problems outside its focus of concern. Clinicians, who have the responsibility to address all of the patient's health needs, must be careful to use independent judgment before adding such topics to their risk assessment protocol. See Chapter 6 for a helpful list of questions to consider in making such choices.

CONCLUSION

What follows in Chapters 2–4 are the details of how to perform risk assessment during the history, physical, and laboratory examination. Section II of this book contains chapters devoted to the risk factors that clinicians are most likely to encounter during risk assessments. These chapters are designed to provide the clinician with detailed information about what to do when a particular risk factor is discovered, including further questions for completing the risk assessment, screening tests for related disorders, counseling, and treatment. These efforts are paramount if the clinician is to have a meaningful impact on helping patients to reduce their risk of developing diseases in later life.

RESOURCES — PATIENT EDUCATION MATERIALS

Harvard Center for Risk Analysis
Risk Quiz
http://www.hcra.harvard.edu/quiz.html#risks

National Cancer Institute. Cancer Risk
Understanding the Puzzle
http://understandingrisk.cancer.gov/

SUGGESTED READINGS

AHRQ Electronic Preventive Services Selector
http://epss.ahrq.gov/PDA/index.jsp

Online Risk Calculation Tools

Body Mass Index

National Heart, Lung, and Blood Institute
Calculate Your Body Mass Index
http://www.nhlbisupport.com/bmi/(downloadable format for Palm Os and PocketPC2003 devices at http://hp2010.nhlbihin.net/bmi_palm.htm).

Coronary Artery Disease (Framingham Risk) Calculator

The Framingham Risk Equation is often used to estimate the patient's 10-year risk of cardiovascular events, using an appropriate risk calculator. The estimate for a specific patient can be obtained from Figure 1.1 or can be calculated automatically using online tools. See National Heart, Lung, and Blood Institute *Risk Assessment Tool for Estimating 10-year Risk of Developing Hard CHD (Myocardial Infarction and Coronary Death)* at http://hp2010.nhlbihin.net/atpiii/calculator.asp?usertype=prof.

Breast Cancer Risk Calculator

The Gail model is an assessment tool that calculates a woman's risk of developing breast cancer over the next 5 years and over her lifetime. See National Cancer Institute *Breast Cancer Risk Assessment Tool* at http://www.cancer.gov/bcrisktool/.

References

1. McGlynn EA, Asch SM, Adams J, et al. The quality of health care delivered to adults in the United States. *N Engl J Med* 2003;348:2635–2645.
2. U.S. Preventive Services Task Force. *Guide to clinical preventive services*. Available at http://www.ahrq.gov/clinic/pocketgd.htm. 2006.
3. Mokdad AH, Marks JS, Stroup DF, et al. Actual causes of death in the United States, 2000. *JAMA* 2004;291:1238–1245.
4. American Academy of Family Physicians Recommendations for Clinical Preventive Services. Available at http://www.aafp.org/online/en/home/clinical/exam.html.2007.
5. Yarnall KS, Pollak KI, Ostbye T, et al. Primary care: is there enough time for prevention? *Am J Pub Health* 2003;93:635–641.
6. Maciosek MV, Coffield AB, Edwards NM, et al. Priorities among effective clinical preventive services: results of a systematic review and analysis. *Am J Prev Med* 2006;31:52–61.

CHAPTER 2

The History: What to Ask About

Alex H. Krist, Janelle Guirguis-Blake, and Steven H. Woolf

INTRODUCTION

Most of the leading causes of death and disability in the United States are caused by only a small number of risk factors (1). The primary task of health promotion and disease prevention in clinical practice is to identify modifiable risk factors during the history, physical, and laboratory examination and to minimize the impact of these factors by recommending preventive interventions. Ultimately, the goal is to improve the patient's quality and years of healthy life. Preventive interventions include the modification of personal health-related behaviors (e.g., sedentary lifestyle), early detection of disease (e.g., cervical dysplasia), immunizations, and chemoprophylaxis.

This chapter discusses how clinicians should approach collecting risk factor information while obtaining a history from their patients. Two types of questions are used to collect a preventive history. *Primary screening questions* are those that determine whether more detailed, *exploratory questions* are necessary. The chapter assumes that the patient is asymptomatic, i.e., lacking signs or symptoms of the target condition. Patients who have already developed the target condition will often require different risk assessment questions. An example of a primary screening question is, *"Do you smoke?"* More detailed questions such as *"At what age did you start smoking"* or *"How many packs do you smoke each day?"* are examples of exploratory questions and will be addressed in the chapters in Section II.

This chapter offers examples of potential *primary screening* questions that should be asked during history taking. Chapters 3 and 4 discuss how to obtain further evidence of risk factor exposure during the physical and laboratory examination, respectively. The chapters in Section II of this book address specific risk factors and the appropriate exploratory questions and techniques that should be used for learning more about these risk factors. Section II also addresses the interventions that should be recommended once a risk factor is identified.

A prevention history is not the same as a conventional medical history. The conventional history that is taken when evaluating symptomatic patients includes questions about chief complaints, history of present illness, past medical and surgical history, current medications, drug allergies, and a review of systems; all of which relate to the *current* situation. This chapter focuses on how to question patients about *past and present* risk factors for *future* disease or injury, with the hopes of intervening and preventing their occurrence or minimizing their impact. As noted in Chapter 1, in the evaluation of current complaints the questions that relate to future risks are generally not stressed. Clinicians often consider this information to be less relevant than establishing a diagnosis for a current complaint. Instead, many clinicians reserve detailed questions about modifiable risk factors for special visits, separate from acute care or disease management visits, such as when they first meet a patient or when a patient presents for a periodic health examination (PHE) (i.e., "annual physical," preventive checkup) (see Chapter 20 for further discussion of this topic).

General Approach to the Prevention History

Clinicians can use a wide range of information sources to collect a prevention history, including the patient, family, friends, caregivers, outpatient records, and hospital records, as well as prior laboratory, radiographic, and procedure results. Preferably before entering the room, the clinician should briefly review the patient's medical record to determine which risk factors have been discussed at previous visits, to recall the patient's previous successful or unsuccessful attempts at risk factor modification, and to determine which risk factors and clinical preventive services deserve attention at the current visit. A preventive care "problem list" or reminder notes, displayed prominently in paper-based or electronic medical records (see Chapters 21 and 22), will obviously facilitate doing such a review. In fact, having to rifle through a multipaged medical record to compile a current risk factor list diminishes the likelihood that such a task will be undertaken. If the patient has already successfully modified a risk factor (e.g., smoking cessation), the clinician will want to offer positive reinforcement during the current visit and to verify that the patient has not relapsed. Other risk factors and outstanding preventive services that have not been addressed should then be identified, and, working with the patient, the clinician should determine which deserve attention in the current interview.

Patients may be psychologically unprepared for a detailed discussion of their lifestyle, especially at a visit other than a scheduled preventive checkup. When risk assessment questions are introduced, patients (or parents of young patients) may be surprised by the sudden change of subject or may be disturbed or offended by the personal nature of the questions. Transition statements serve an important function in laying the groundwork for such questions:

"Well, Mrs. Jones, I'm glad you've agreed to see Dr. Smith for an opinion on having gallbladder surgery. It will be good to get that resolved. You know,

sometimes we can get so preoccupied with a specific medical problem—such as your gallbladder—that we lose sight of other important health matters. I'd like to run through a short list of questions to make sure we aren't overlooking something important that also needs our attention. Is that alright with you?"

"So, Mr. White, I anticipate that your back pain will ease up if you follow the plan that we discussed, but I want you to let me know next week if it still bothers you. By the way, there are some personal health matters we haven't discussed in the past that, although they have nothing to do with your back, might someday affect your health in other ways. I'd hate for something important to fall through the cracks. For example, you once mentioned that you had been dating several people. As you know, there can be important health implications to sexual activity. I wonder if you might be willing to discuss how many sexual partners you have had in the last year."

"Mrs. Jackson, I think your daughter's ear infection will respond well to the antibiotic I'm prescribing today. I'd like to see her again in a few weeks to reexamine her ear. Before you leave, though, I want to ask you a few questions about Tracy, double-check her shot record, and go over some conditions at home that might affect her risk of future illness or injuries. Is that all right?"

During both the introductory statement and the question period, the clinician should monitor the patient's emotional reactions. The patient's comments, vocal quality (tone, pitch, tempo), and nonverbal communication may signal discomfort, impatience, or a reluctance to discuss certain lifestyle issues. Recognizing these reactions and sharing the observations with the patient through reflection (e.g., *"You seem uncomfortable talking about this."*) are important for several reasons. First, if patients do not bring these emotions to the surface, they may suppress them or develop feelings of resentment or anger toward the clinician. Second, open discussion of the emotions and their validation by the clinician can often reduce patient anxiety. Third, although some patients use their discomfort or impatience as an excuse for changing the subject, the clinician's open acknowledgment of their feelings gives many patients the strength to return to the topic in greater detail. Often these patients will "open up" with disclosures that would not have been mentioned if the clinician were less empathic.

The clinician should also monitor the patient's choice of words, which may disclose important information about risk factors. Clues are often deeply imbedded in dialogue about other problems. The clinician may obtain more information by carefully listening to these subtle comments than from the patient's answers to routine screening questions:

"The chest pains seem to occur after meals, although lately I've wondered whether it's because of the way my life is going. Anyway, I tried antacids . . ."

"Doctor, you know it's got to be bad for me to come in—I haven't been to a doctor in years—I hate all those tests—but I just can't stand this shoulder pain anymore."

"I didn't start the baby on the medicine yet because I needed John to pick it up for me. He's been on a short string lately and I'm afraid to push him, with the way he gets. Now the baby has a fever and pulls on her ears ..."

"No, my stomach pain isn't any worse after fatty meals. Lately, with my schedule, I've been getting a daily dose of French fries and greasy food, but that has never brought on the pain. It's only when I don't eat ..."

"I doubt the headaches are due to the birth control pills. I stopped taking those things two months ago. My boyfriend thinks I've got migraines, which do run in our family ..."

TECHNIQUES FOR TAKING THE PREVENTION HISTORY

Collecting a prevention-focused history requires a unique set of history-taking skills that includes the *integration* of a range of topics into an encounter, *prioritization* of essential topics for discussion and an *appropriately timed and systematic* approach.

Integration

Sick visits comprise most patient encounters at the office, clinic, emergency department, hospital, or nursing home. Therefore, if risk assessments and preventive interventions are omitted from sick visits and offered only during well visits, then only a small percentage of patients will benefit from preventive care. As Chapter 20 discusses further, many clinicians therefore attempt to incorporate preventive medicine into routine illness visits. Acute care and disease management visits often pose a greater challenge for integrating a prevention history, however, because patients and clinicians frequently have a predefined problem-focused agenda. The most appropriate means for integrating a prevention history into a clinical encounter will vary from clinician to clinician, patient to patient, and encounter to encounter. Primary screening questions can be an effective and simple means for a clinician to introduce a prevention topic during a sick visit. By systematically administering health risk assessments before the encounter (see Chapter 21), practices can set the tone that prevention will routinely be addressed. Additionally, patients themselves frequently give cues to potential prevention needs through their chief complaint or history.

Aside from sick visits, visits by new patients and PHEs provide additional and often more conducive opportunities to address prevention. Visits by new patients represent a unique opportunity to get to know a patient. History taking commonly extends beyond the presenting problem and naturally includes topics such as the patient's occupation and health behaviors. The PHE is, by design, centered on prevention. Therefore, the issue is not how to integrate the taking of a prevention history into the visit, but rather how to ensure that all appropriate topics are addressed when such a history is obtained.

Prioritization

It is obviously unrealistic for clinicians to address all risk factors during a short patient visit. Prioritization is essential (see Chapter 1 for general information about how to prioritize risk factors and other preventive services, and see Chapter 20 for guidance on how priorities should be tailored by individual practices). The average primary care office visit lasts 17 minutes (2), and most of that time must be devoted to the patient's chief complaints. Investing more than a few minutes in risk assessment is rarely feasible. These minutes do provide enough time, however, to ask a few primary screening questions. A clinician can leverage small amounts of time for maximum health benefit by selecting questions about risk factors that could potentially yield the greatest health benefit for a patient or that a patient is mostly likely to act upon. Given that tobacco use is the leading cause of death in the United States (1), clinicians who have time for only one question should probably ask the most valuable primary screening question: *"Do you smoke?"* The same question should be asked of parents regarding their children or adolescents (refer to Chapter 9 for further details).

Timing

- **Identifying risk factors.** When is the right time during a sick visit to ask questions about risk factors? Inserting the questions into the history obtained for the presenting problem is one approach. Another is to first address the presenting problem and, at the conclusion of the visit, to bring up the matter of the patient's risk factors. Both models are illustrated in the subsequent text for a hypothetical patient who has visited the clinician for a chief complaint of flu-like symptoms:

  During the History

  Clinician: *". . . So, to summarize, you've had a fever since Friday, and for the past two days you've had muscle aches, a sore throat, and fatigue. I want to examine you but, before I do, let me ask you a question that also relates to your health. Do you smoke?"*

  At the End of the Clinical Encounter

  Clinician: *". . . and remember to drink plenty of fluids. Call me if you feel that you are getting worse or if you notice new symptoms. Before you* *leave, I want to address an unrelated issue that also affects your health. How much exercise do you get?"*

- **Giving advice and counseling.** Another timing issue is when during the encounter to advise and counsel a patient. Clinicians may be tempted to counsel a patient about an unhealthy behavior during the questioning period, when the patient first mentions it. Compared to waiting until the end of the encounter, this has the advantage of limiting the possibility of forgetting to address the health behavior later and being faced with the challenge of delivering multiple counseling messages on a range of topics. It is a potential pitfall, however, to provide counseling before collecting the entire history. It can diminish the impact of the counseling message if patients feel that the clinician has not heard their entire story. Further, the clinician may neglect other important information, obtained later in the encounter that would alter advice or could be used as further motivation when counseling the patient.

  This book includes separate chapters on the history, physical examination, and screening tests. However, during an encounter these tasks will often be appropriately undertaken together. Specific findings on physical examination should prompt further risk assessment questions (such as asking about alcohol consumption in much greater depth if a patient is found to have hepatomegaly). Additionally, many elements of the physical examination do not require silence, allowing an opportunity to ask primary screening questions during inspection and palpation. Caution is warranted in determining which questions are appropriate during portions of the examination. Some questions might make patients uncomfortable, and clinicians should monitor nonverbal cues as they perform the physical examination.

- **Using windows of opportunity.** During a problem-focused visit, whether for a new problem or chronic disease management, opportunities may arise in which clinicians can address prevention. These opportunities can serve as tools for both prioritizing and integrating the prevention history into the encounter. They allow for natural transitions in conversation from the presenting problem to a prevention topic, and can create a "teachable moment." Teachable moments will often occur when a patient's problem is caused or exacerbated by a modifiable risk factor. Through improved health behaviors, a patient may not only be able to significantly ameliorate the presenting problem, but may also secure a better health future. One example of a teachable moment is a smoker who presents with a community-acquired pneumonia. By asking about smoking status and then providing brief counseling, the patient may recognize how his behaviors have contributed to his illness, increasing his receptivity to smoking cessation and providing him with further reasons to quit.

- **Longitudinal history taking.** Clinicians should not view the prevention history as an isolated event. Not only do risk factors and health behaviors change over time but also clinicians lack the time to effectively address all of the questions listed in this chapter during a single visit. Patients lack the capacity to act on all potential interventions. Taking advantage of a longitudinal relationship between a clinician and patient can allow for the more effective delivery of preventive care across a patient's lifespan. Establishing a system to track which preventive questions have been asked, which primary screening questions deserve follow-up, and which modifiable risk factors need to be addressed, is necessary to allow for longitudinal preventive care. Coupling such tracking systems with reminders (as discussed in Chapters 21 and 22) can assist clinicians in remembering to address timely prevention topics and to reinforce past discussions at future encounters. Clinicians should schedule a return visit dedicated to addressing those risk factors that cannot be covered in the current visit. The latter may be the best option for patients who only visit the clinician sporadically for illness visits.

Systematic Approach

Despite the best intentions, many clinicians overlook important risk factors, even when they are attempting to be complete. A systematic approach to asking about risk factors can help ensure a complete prevention history. Many such strategies exist and can be used alone or in conjunction with one another. Some examples of systematic approaches, which are covered in greater detail in Chapter 21, include health risk assessments, regular questionnaires such as intake forms, flow sheets, checklists, electronic medical record prompts, team-based delivery of care, and information collection performed as part of the "vital sign" process performed by nursing staff.

Another option is for clinicians to regularly use an organized verbal script to collect a prevention history. This is more time consuming for clinicians and may result in missing some questions. However, the approach allows for patient-specific individualization of the history taking. Additionally, a team approach can be adopted, utilizing several members of the office staff to collect elements of the prevention history at designated stages of the intake process (see "vital sign" procedure on page 31) and to even initiate the delivery of counseling interventions and referrals (3). Such a team approach takes the burden off of the individual clinician, allows for duplication of history collection (increasing the likelihood of completeness), increases office staff satisfaction, and ultimately improves patients' health status.

WHAT TO ASK ABOUT

This section provides sample language for screening questions but the clinician, who can identify the optimal communication strategy for his or her patient, best determines the wording in clinical practice. Moreover, for most risk factors, research has not yet determined the "correct" wording for such questions nor tested their sensitivity and specificity. (See discussion of Screening Questionnaires on pages 45–46.) The wording that clinicians use when asking risk factor questions should reflect their practice style and their relationship with the patient. The questions also need to be sensitive to the patient's age, educational background, primary language, culture, and health belief model. Because questions about risk factors often address sensitive aspects of personal behavior, the clinician should avoid judgmental or directive questions, or those that will put most patients on the defensive. Patients who are asked *"You aren't homosexual, are you?"* or *"I assume that you don't drink and drive"* may be reluctant to answer honestly. Similarly, facial expressions (e.g., raised eyebrows) and other nonverbal communications that suggest the clinician's disapproval are inappropriate.

Table 2.1 gives examples of the type of primary screening questions that clinicians should employ on a routine basis to begin constructing an individual's risk profile. In the subsequent text we discuss the major topics in some detail. These questions address a fundamental set of risk factors: health behaviors (tobacco use, physical activity, dietary intake, sexual practices, alcohol and other drug use, injury prevention, exposure to ultraviolet light, dental hygiene); mental health and functional status; risk factors from past medical and family history; occupational and environmental exposures; travel history; and the status of recommended screening tests, immunizations, and chemoprophylaxis. Questions for pediatric patients need to be tailored to the patient's age to determine the content of the question and whether the patient or parents should be asked. While general principles are discussed here, see Chapter 17 for details about the pediatric and adolescent examinations.

Health Behaviors
TOBACCO USE

Sample primary screening question: *"Do you smoke cigarettes or use other types of tobacco?"*

Exploratory Questions and Follow-up
If there is only one risk factor that a clinician can address in a clinical encounter, it should be tobacco use. One means to ensure that smoking status is assessed at every clinical encounter is to include smoking status as a "vital sign" routinely collected at the same time as other vital signs (see Chapter 9).

TABLE 2.1 Sample Primary Screening Questions about Key Risk Factors

Note: See text for complete wording of questions. Different questions are indicated for patients in specific age or risk groups and for parents of infants and small children.

Do you smoke cigarettes or use other types of tobacco?

How much exercise do you get?

What foods have you eaten in the last 24 hr?

Do you have sex with men, women, or both? How many partners do you have now, and how many were there in the past? Are you interested in getting pregnant, or are you using some form of birth control?

Do you drink alcohol? Have you ever used cocaine or other drugs?

Do you always fasten your seat belt when you are in a car? Do you ever drive after drinking, or ride with a driver who has been drinking?

Do you protect yourself from the sun when you are outdoors?

How often do you brush your teeth and how often do you floss? When did you last visit the dentist?

How are your spirits these days?

Have you ever been told that you had heart trouble, cancer, diabetes or a serious infectious disease?

Is there a family history of heart trouble, cancer, or diabetes?

What sort of work do (did) you do?

Have you ever been in other countries, or are you planning a trip to one?

When was your last —————————————— ?
(recommended screening test)

When was your last —————————————— ?
(recommended immunization)

Are you taking daily aspirin?

Tobacco use accounts for 435,000 deaths each year in the United States (1). All adults, adolescents, and, occasionally, older children should be asked whether they smoke or use smokeless tobacco. If they do not currently use tobacco, the clinician should inquire whether they used tobacco previously and, if so, when they quit. Exposure to environmental smoke (at home or at work) should also be addressed. Because patients who stop smoking often relapse, tobacco use should be readdressed periodically throughout the clinician's relationship with the patient. The topic also needs to be revisited regularly with children and adolescents, who are always at risk of starting to smoke or use smokeless tobacco for the first time.

PHYSICAL ACTIVITY

Sample primary screening question: *"How much exercise do you get?"*

Exploratory Questions and Follow-up

Physical inactivity, an important risk factor for coronary artery disease, hypertension, obesity, and other chronic conditions, should be addressed with adults (including the elderly) as well as with children and adolescents (see Chapter 6). Depending upon their age such questions may need to be directed to the parents. Both the clinician and patient should have a clear understanding of what they mean by the term *exercise*. *"Well, doc, what I mean by 'exercise' is that I have to take several walks through the factory each day to inspect production lines. I also have a flight of stairs at my apartment."* At a minimum, further questions should explore the intensity, frequency, and duration of physical activity.

DIETARY INTAKE

Sample primary screening questions: *"Tell me about your typical diet. How many servings of fruits and vegetables do you eat in a typical day? Do you typically try to avoid fatty foods?"*

Exploratory Questions and Follow-up

The range of nutritional issues that can be addressed by the clinician is broad, including dietary intake of calories, saturated fat, *trans* fats, cholesterol, carbohydrates, fruits and vegetables, sodium, iron, calcium, and vitamins (see Chapter 7). Clinicians cannot offer meaningful counseling about these nutrients without first performing a dietary assessment of the foods that the patient typically eats. It is difficult to ask a single primary screening question that identifies all patients in need of counseling, and a *complete* dietary assessment for each food category is usually beyond the scope of a single visit (and may well be beyond the competency of the given clinician). However, of all the nutrients and foods in the patient's diet, those that most affect the patient's future health are total calories, fat, and fruits and vegetables (see Chapter 7). At a minimum, clinicians with limited time should consider exploring these topics. Further questions can explore consumption of meat, fried food, and fast foods as well as the general frequency of food consumption, meal skipping habits, and portion sizes. In patients with poor dietary habits, exploring their barriers for eating healthier foods and reviewing improvement strategies that they have tried in the past can help to guide clinicians with the counseling that follows.

Infants and Children

Nutritional questions are essential during well-baby and well-child examinations. However, primary screening questions about nutrition should also be considered during other visits, especially if compliance with recommendations made during well-child examinations is not anticipated or poor feeding practices are suspected. The most important nutritional priorities during childhood are to ensure that the diet is appropriate for healthful growth and development and that intake of dietary fats and sweets is limited. Chapter 7 provides further details on nutritional guidelines for infants and children.

Older Adults

In addition to the nutritional issues that confront all adults, older adults face the added risks of nutritional deficiencies and malnutrition. They can also experience potentially harmful interactions between their dietary practices and their medical conditions and medications. Clinicians should assess whether the patient suffers from impaired functional status and whether this impairment may be caused by nutritional deficiencies. Impaired functional status can further exacerbate poor dietary intake by creating barriers to obtaining and preparing healthy foods. One specific nutritional deficiency to recognize in older adults is inadequate calcium intake, which results in an increased risk for osteoporosis and subsequent fractures (see Chapter 7).

SEXUAL PRACTICES

Sample primary screening questions: *"Do you have sex with men, women, or both? How many partners do you have now, and how many did you have in the past? Are you interested in getting pregnant, or are you using some form of birth control? How do you protect yourself against sexually transmitted infections?"*

Exploratory Questions and Follow-up

The U.S. Preventive Services Task Force (USPSTF) recommends screening for several sexually transmitted infections in populations at risk for acquiring the infection, such as human immunodeficiency virus (HIV), syphilis, gonorrhea, and Chlamydia (see Chapters 11 and 12). This requires clinicians to take an appropriate sexual history on all adolescent and adult patients to ascertain each patient's risk. Clinicians must, of course, be exceedingly careful and sensitive in asking such questions and may want to develop their own approaches and preferred language. The information is important, however, for identifying high-risk individuals who could benefit from further laboratory screening or specific counseling. Owing to the sensitive nature of this topic, clinicians often need to introduce questions about sexual behavior by explaining its relevance to their health; see Chapter 12 for suggested language. This introduction is especially important if the patient is being seen for an unrelated health problem. Clinicians also frequently need to overcome their own discomfort with discussing sexual behavior. Even in urban practices with many high-risk patients, less than 40% of physicians obtain a sexual history from their patients (4).

Depending on the patient's answers to screening questions about sexual practices, further questions are often necessary regarding the use of condoms, birth control methods, duration of current sexual relationships, current or prior sexual practices (e.g., anal or oral sex, association between alcohol or drug use and sexual activity, prostitution), and sexual contact with partners who used injection drugs, had multiple partners, or had known sexually transmitted infections. The sexual history may reveal evidence of dysfunctional relationships (e.g., *"I don't need birth control because we hardly make love anymore," "Don't tell my wife, but I've been with other women in the past year"*). Such findings deserve further exploration for psychosocial reasons.

Adolescents

Surveys suggest that more than half the number of students in grades 9 to 12 report having had sexual intercourse (5). The usual discomfort that patients experience when asked about sexual behavior is magnified further for adolescents, who are often reluctant to admit to sexual activity or are afraid that the information they provide to the clinician will not be kept confidential. A commonly used approach is to begin by normalizing and depersonalizing the practice (e.g., *"A lot of high school students are having sex these days"*) and assuring the patient of confidentiality before asking the first question about sexual habits, such as *"Have you ever had sex?"* Some clinicians ease into the subject by first inquiring about peers (*"How about your friends?"*) and showing a nonjudgmental demeanor as the patient describes the sexual activity of his or her friends. Many adolescents then become comfortable enough to discuss their own sexual histories. See Chapter 17 for further details.

ALCOHOL AND OTHER DRUG USE

Sample primary screening questions: *"Do you drink alcohol? Have you ever used any drugs such as marijuana or cocaine?"*

Exploratory Questions and Follow-up

The USPSTF, Institute of Medicine, American Academy of Pediatrics, and other groups recommend screening all adult and adolescent patients for evidence of alcohol dependence, problem drinking, or excessive alcohol consumption (see Chapter 10). Patients who report drinking alcohol should be asked about the quantity and frequency of their consumption as well as whether drinking has resulted in any adverse effects on their life (such as causing trouble with work or relationships). However, patients' self-reports of their alcohol use may not provide accurate information to identify problem drinking. The reported sensitivity of historic inquiry about alcohol use is only 10–50%. Similarly, patients with a current or past history of illicit drug use may be even more reluctant to discuss the subject because of its legal implications. Clinicians must often rely on clues in the patient's responses and to other aspects of the medical history and lifestyle to detect a problem. For example, the answer, *"I just drink socially,"* requires further exploration.

Commonly used alcohol abuse questionnaires, such as the CAGE and Alcohol Use Disorders Identification Test (AUDIT) instruments or the Michigan Alcoholism Screening Test (MAST) (see Chapter 10 for further details), can provide a nonthreatening approach for patients to honestly report alcohol habits. Long-term continuity relationships between primary clinicians and patients can also foster trust over time by creating a safe environment for patients to accurately describe their alcohol and drug use. Patients with a history of drug use or sexually transmitted infections should be asked specifically about past or present injection drug use. Patients who use either alcohol or other drugs should be asked about driving while intoxicated and about binge drinking.

Adolescents

As with sexual behavior, adolescents may be reluctant to admit to alcohol or other drug use for fear of disapproval or disclosure to parents, teachers, or the legal authorities. Nonetheless, because, for example, intoxication accounts for approximately half of adolescent deaths in motor vehicle crashes, and because substance abuse often begins at this age, broaching this subject with teens is especially important. Again, it is often useful to first depersonalize the practice (e.g., *"A lot of high school students drink or use drugs these days"*), assure confidentiality, inquire about peers (*"How about your friends?"*), and then ask about the patient's habits (*"Have you ever used drugs?"*). See the discussion of respecting confidentiality with adolescents under "Patient Privacy" on pages 43–44.

INJURY PREVENTION PRACTICES

Sample primary screening questions: *"Do you always fasten your seat belt when you are in a car? Do you ever drive after drinking, or ride with a driver who has been drinking?"*

> *For parents of infants and small children:* "Is your child always secured in a safety seat when you or others transport him (her) in the car?"
> *For parents of older children:* "Does your child fasten his (her) seat belt whenever he (she) is transported in a car?"

Exploratory Questions and Follow-up

Many clinicians believe that a patient's driving habits are not a clinical concern, and yet motor vehicle accidents account for approximately 50,000 deaths and

5 million injuries each year in the United States. They are the leading cause of injury-related deaths among persons younger than 45 years (1). Clinician inquiry can further validate and support safe driving practices.

Older Adults
Falls are a common cause of injury in older adults, especially among those older than 75 years, in whom falls are the leading cause of injury-related deaths (due largely to the complications of hip fractures and head trauma). The clinician should ask the patient, family members, or caregivers whether the home has been inspected for fall hazards. A sample screening question is, *"Have you gone through the house to look for bad lighting; things that could cause you to trip or slip on the floor, steps, rugs, or bathtub; or sharp corners or hard floors that could hurt you if you fell?"* The clinician should also review the patient's medications, which may increase the risk of falls.

EXPOSURE TO ULTRAVIOLET LIGHT

Sample primary screening question: *"Do you protect yourself (your child) from the sun when you are outdoors?"*

Exploratory Questions and Follow-up
Further questions could explore a patient's cumulative sun exposure, history of severe or frequent sunburns, activities (e.g., occupation, weekend hobbies, or visiting tanning salons) associated with increased sun exposure, methods used to avoid sun exposure (avoidance of midday sun or use of protective clothing), and use of sunscreen.

Excess exposure to the ultraviolet radiation of sunlight carries a significantly increased risk of all types of skin cancer. Reducing exposure to ultraviolet rays through avoidance of midday sun or the use of protective clothing can help to prevent skin cancer. Additionally, use of sunscreen can prevent the development of squamous and basal cell skin cancers. Whether sunscreen prevents melanoma is less clear. If individuals who use sunscreen are more likely to increase the time they spend in the sun, melanoma risks could be increased, unless other preventive measures (e.g., sitting in the shade, protective clothing) are observed. Whereas avoidance of ultraviolet radiation can decrease the risk of skin cancer, there is insufficient evidence to demonstrate that clinician counseling changes patients' skin exposure behaviors (6).

DENTAL HYGIENE PRACTICES

Sample primary screening questions: *"How often do you brush your teeth? How often do you floss? When did you last visit the dentist?"*

For parents: "How often does your child brush his (her) teeth? When was he (she) last taken to the dentist? Does your child drink adequately fluoridated water? If not, is your child receiving fluoride supplements to prevent tooth decay?"

Exploratory Questions and Follow-up
Further exploratory questions could include "Are you having any problems with your mouth, throat, or teeth? Do your gums bleed when you brush or floss? Do you have trouble chewing your food? Do you have any questions about your oral health?"

In general, patients should be encouraged to see their dentist at least once every 12 months. Patients may need prompt referral for inflamed or bleeding gums, decayed or loose teeth, or lesions suggestive of oral cancer. Patients should also be encouraged to avoid the risk factors for poor oral health—which include smoking, chewing tobacco, and consuming refined sugars (e.g., sodas)—and to minimize the risks of dental injuries. Parents of infants should be asked about baby bottle-feeding practices, and clinicians should inquire about fluoride intake to determine if supplementation is necessary (see Chapter 17). The USPSTF endorses fluoride supplementation for those children 6 months of age and older whose primary water source is inadequately fluoridated but found insufficient evidence for primary care clinicians to conduct routine pediatric screening for dental disease. The USPSTF has not recently reviewed evidence for adult dental care (6).

Mental Health and Functional Status

Sample primary screening question (Mental Health): *"How are your spirits these days?"*

Sample primary screening question (Functional Status and Development):

> *For parents:* "What has your child learned to do recently?"
> *For older adults:* "Are you having any trouble taking care of things at home, such as getting your meals or cleaning ?"

Exploratory Questions and Follow-up
See Chapters 13 and 17.

Mental Health
The scope of potential problems and complications that fall under this category is broad, ranging from poor self-esteem, depression, and abuse (as victim or perpetrator), to violence and suicidal behavior. A single primary screening question is often inadequate to detect these problems. Therefore, in order to detect a problem, the clinician must be alert to clues in the patient's behavior, affect, family dynamics, and physical examination findings, not only during the risk assessment visit but also throughout the relationship with the patient. Patients who have recently experienced an important loss (e.g., death, divorce, loss of job) are at increased risk of depression. If there

is evidence of depression, the patient should be asked whether he or she has had suicidal or homicidal ideation (e.g., *"Have you ever thought of hurting yourself or others?"*). Commonly used screening instruments for depression include the Zung Self-Rating Depression Scale, Center for Epidemiological Studies Depression Scale, the Beck Depression Inventory, and the Patient Health Questionnaire (see Chapter 13).

The clinician must also remain alert for signs of interpersonal conflict, domestic violence, or other risk factors for intentional injuries (e.g., child abuse, spouse abuse, sexual violence, homicide). Because patients and family members often display their "best behavior" during clinical encounters, the clinician must be able to see past this presentation to unmask signs of escalating tensions in a relationship, an individual's inability to resolve conflicts nonviolently, or the physical findings of abuse or neglect. A patient or family member's grimace, shrug, or hesitation in answering a screening question, such as, *"How are things at home?"* or their responses to open-ended questions, such as *"What are the good things and bad things about your relationship?"* are often the clinician's best clues in detecting an important problem at home. In responding to such questions, patients may give clues to their possible misuse of alcohol or other drugs or to the presence of other codependent behaviors. Although unproved, acting on these findings by arranging for psychotherapy, marital counseling, substance abuse treatment, or social services may improve family dynamics and the emotional well-being of its members. In more advanced cases, these interventions may prevent physical illnesses and injuries, emotional morbidity from abuse or neglect, unwanted pregnancies, family dysfunction, unintentional firearm injuries, and even homicide.

Functional Status
Functional status refers broadly to an individual's ability to perform age-appropriate tasks of self-care and self-fulfillment. In childhood, this is often affected by abnormal physical or mental growth and development. Childhood development is covered in Chapter 17 and is therefore not discussed further in this chapter. In old age, functional status can be impaired by both physical and mental illness. The consequences affect other health-related behaviors, such as nutrition patterns and injury avoidance.

When examining older adults, clinicians should remain alert for evidence of difficulty in performing the activities of daily living. Screening for cognitive impairment is more difficult, because undertaking a lengthy mental status examination is often impractical in the brief clinical encounter and may lack accuracy or effectiveness as a screening test. The clinician must often seek readily obtainable clues in the patient's speech, ability to understand medical instructions, behavior in the office, and statements made about home or living conditions. Additionally, if the clinician thinks that a patient may be cognitively impaired, the patient can be asked to complete the Mini-Mental State Examination (MMSE), a screening instrument that provides a general measure of basic cognitive functions (see Chapter 13).

Obtaining the Presence of Risk Factors from the Past Medical History

Sample primary screening question: *"Have you ever been told that you had heart trouble, cancer, diabetes, or a serious infectious disease?"*

EXPLORATORY QUESTIONS AND FOLLOW-UP

Beginning with an open-ended question and progressing to questions about specific conditions can be an effective means to elicit a comprehensive prevention-focused past medical history. However, there are other sources for obtaining such information. Prior health records may be more efficient and effective than direct questioning to acquire an understanding of a patient's past medical history. Whether obtained from direct questioning or the medical record, the past medical history can provide critical information for determining whether patients fall within risk groups requiring special screening tests, immunizations, or other preventive services (see Chapters 3, 4, 18, and 19 for details). The medical history form that patients usually complete before their first interview will often be very helpful in focusing the discussion (see "Screening Questionnaires" on pages 45–46 and further discussion in Chapter 21).

Learning about Risk Factors from the Family History

Sample primary screening question: *"Do you have a family history of heart trouble, cancer, or diabetes?"*

EXPLORATORY QUESTIONS AND FOLLOW-UP

A thorough conventional family history can cover a wide range of topics and conditions. However, from a prevention standpoint coronary artery disease, cerebrovascular accidents, cancers (colorectal, breast, ovarian, prostate, and skin), and diabetes represent potentially inherited conditions that place patients in risk groups requiring screening tests specified for high-risk populations or at an earlier age than routinely recommended for the general population (see Chapters 3 and 4). In particular, clinicians should inquire whether these conditions occurred in first degree relatives, or in multiple family members, or if family members with the condition had an early age of disease onset. Although time consuming to complete, the family history can provide a comprehensive look at the patient's entire medical pedigree. A family history questionnaire (such as https://familyhistory.hhs.gov/) that a patient completes before the encounter can facilitate this process.

Occupational and Environmental Exposures

Sample primary screening questions: *"What sort of work do (did) you do? Does (did) your job or other activities expose you to loud noise, the sun, harmful chemicals, radiation, or other hazardous materials?"*

> *For parents:* "Where do you live, how old is your home, and what is the source of your drinking water?"
>
> *For older adults:* "Where do you live? Who do you live with? Who is available to assist you if needed?"

EXPLORATORY QUESTIONS AND FOLLOW-UP

A thorough occupational or environmental history requires more detailed questions about risks of occupational illnesses and injuries than can be addressed in this book. The earlier questions are intended to screen for selected exposures that place patients in risk groups requiring routine screening tests and immunizations (see Chapters 3, 4, and 18). For example, skin and hearing screening may be warranted for patients with occupational or recreational exposure to excessive sunlight or noise, respectively. Health care workers are at increased risk of being exposed to or transmitting tuberculosis, hepatitis B, HIV, and other harmful organisms (e.g., rubella). Questions for determining a worker's need for occupational screening tests (e.g., air sampling, pulmonary function testing), however, are addressed in standard occupational medicine and environmental health texts.

Questions about living conditions can also provide important environmental risk information for tailoring the patient's health maintenance plan. Crowded or unsanitary living conditions, for example, increase the risk of tuberculosis, influenza, and other pathogens. Determining that a patient lives in a homeless shelter, correctional institution, nursing home, or migrant worker camp suggests the need for tuberculosis screening (see Chapter 4). A number of environmental factors are potentially relevant to children, some of which have already been addressed (e.g., passive exposure to environmental tobacco smoke). Characteristics of the home, such as its age (dwellings constructed before 1960 often contain lead-based paint) and the presence or absence of fluoride in the water supply, have special relevance to a child's risk of developing disease. The Centers for Disease Control and Prevention has developed a website detailing each state's policies with respect to lead screening as well as questions to identify which children need screening (7). For older adults, clinicians should determine the patient's living environment (e.g., private home, assisted living facility, or nursing home) and what support systems exist to help patients with their needs.

Travel History

Sample primary screening question: *"Have you (or your child) ever been in other countries, or are you planning a trip to one?"*

EXPLORATORY QUESTIONS AND FOLLOW-UP

The risk of certain target conditions (e.g., hemoglobinopathies) or of exposure to infectious diseases (e.g., tuberculosis, hepatitis, HIV infection) is increased for immigrants from certain countries in Asia, the Pacific Islands, Africa, Central and South America, and the Mediterranean (see Chapters 3, 4, and 16). Patients traveling to developing countries or other regions in which malaria and other preventable infectious diseases are endemic require certain immunizations and chemoprophylaxis before their departure (see Chapter 16).

Clinical Preventive Services

The clinician should ask patients (or the parents of infants and children) whether they have received appropriate clinical preventive services— screening tests, immunizations, and chemoprevention regimens—that are recommended for their age and risk profile. Clarifying the risk group requires not only determining when the patient last received the service but also understanding the patient's risk for disease and the results of prior screening tests. Medical records, and flow sheets or screen prompts that summarize pertinent data, may be particularly helpful in gathering this information. Appendix A of this book lists the key screening tests that are indicated for average risk adults. See Chapters 3, 4, 15, and 16 for further details on when screening tests, immunizations, and chemoprevention regimens are indicated for particular patients and see Chapters 21 and 22 for further details on the role of flow sheets and reminder tools to track delivery of these services.

SPECIAL CONSIDERATIONS

Infants, Children, and Adolescents

See Chapter 17.

Older Adults

Obtaining accurate risk factor information from some older adults can be difficult for both organic and attitudinal reasons. Organic barriers in the elderly include the patient's difficulty in understanding questions or providing coherent answers, due to hearing loss, cognitive impairment, or other medical factors. Clinicians often need to accommodate these limitations through special measures, such as speaking more slowly in a loud, low voice; clearly writing the questions on paper; or obtaining the information from caregivers. Attitudinal barriers include the patient's hesitation to identify a risk factor as a problem because of a belief that it is a natural consequence of aging (e.g., hearing loss), it is something that should not be complained about (e.g., depression), it is too late in life to benefit from risk factor modification (e.g., smoking cessation after decades of tobacco use), or it will result in the loss of freedoms (e.g., the ability to drive or live independently). Clinicians often need to spend time with the patient to correct misconceptions, educate them about healthy aging, encourage open discussion, and foster a trusting and collaborative relationship.

Patient Privacy

Asking about risk factors with other individuals in the room is generally inappropriate for several reasons. First, taking a history under these conditions violates patient confidentiality. Second, the presence of other individuals often makes patients uncomfortable and reluctant to discuss personal behaviors. The patient may give inaccurate or incomplete information, such as denying or minimizing their involvement with behaviors that might be judged negatively by others (e.g., the adolescent who denies sexual activity or substance abuse when the parents are present). Third, if the visit includes a physical examination, the visitors must leave the room anyway to respect the patient's privacy.

On the other hand, family members, caregivers, or friends who accompany patients can often provide important information about risk factors that may not be volunteered by the patient. For example, a teenage patient denies tobacco use, but the mother tells the clinician that she routinely sees a cigarette package in his shirt pocket. A wife complains about her husband's drinking problem although he denies such behavior. The children of an older adult, who denies problems at home, inform the clinician that they have witnessed frequent episodes of disorientation and memory loss. It is therefore useful, in the appropriate setting, to ask individuals who have accompanied a patient whether they have any health concerns that they would like to discuss. They should then be asked to leave the room.

Most individuals accompanying patients, once given an opportunity to express their concerns, are quite agreeable to leaving the examination room. Some parents of adolescents or older children may be surprised by or resistant to the request, in part because this practice was unnecessary when their children were younger, but a brief explanation will usually suffice to ease their anxieties. Some sample language may include, "*I always make sure to give my teenage patients a chance to ask questions.*" Or "*I routinely ask parents to step out of the room for a few minutes so that we can talk.*" Each clinician will develop and each patient encounter will dictate an individualized approach to interviewing patients and caretakers. A commonly used sequence is to interview everyone present, then interview the patient alone, conduct an examination, review the assessment and plan with only the patient, and summarize the encounter with everyone present, of course taking care to omit from that discussion any matters that any of the participants asked to be kept confidential. This can allow an opportunity for everyone to contribute to the history and the plan of action while maintaining patient privacy and providing the patient an opportunity to limit what will be shared with others. The adamant refusal of family members to leave the examination room or a tendency to dominate the interview should raise the clinician's index of suspicion that there are issues of abuse, neglect, or other problems that they do not want disclosed.

Interview Problems and Strategies

Silence, which frequently makes both clinicians and patients uncomfortable, is nevertheless often helpful in collecting risk factor information. Patients may introduce silence themselves, pausing after mentioning a risk factor to collect their thoughts or to marshal the courage to bring up a difficult topic. Rather than breaking the silence with another question, clinicians who wait for the patient to break the silence are often rewarded with additional information. *"No, I don't use any drugs, and I hardly touch alcohol . . .* (silence introduced by patient) *. . . Did I ever tell you, doctor, that I was once in a rehab program? I was using crack and heroin back then . . ."* Even if the patient does not introduce silence, the clinician may intentionally pause to see how the patient fills the silence. *"Things at home are fine, I guess . . .* (silence introduced by clinician) *. . . I do wish things were better between my husband and the kids, though . . ."*

Resistance is often manifested by a patient's hesitation in answering questions, vagueness, or an abrupt change of subject. Only a few patients express anger or hostility when asked questions about lifestyle. As noted earlier, the clinician's reflection and validation of the patient's feelings will often overcome this resistance. It is, however, the patient's right to terminate discussion of difficult topics. The clinician should respect those preferences and move on to other subjects.

Communication barriers can include deafness, language and literacy barriers, cognitive limitations, and cultural differences. Information about risk factors can be obtained from deaf patients by relying on lip reading, written questionnaires, handwritten notes, or sign language. Clinicians who cannot speak the patient's language may require the aid of a translator to ask questions. If patients have partial command of the clinician's language, it is easy to mistakenly assume that the patient understands questions or instructions. A patient may nod in response to a yes/no question without truly understanding what was asked. For example, a Vietnamese-speaking patient who says "no" when asked whether she has ever had "hepatitis B" might answer "yes" if the disease was named in her language. Patients with cognitive limitations, due either to inadequate education or limited intelligence, may have difficulty in understanding complex words or sentences. The clinician should be careful to avoid sophisticated terminology (e.g., *saturated fats, hypertension, and monogamous relationships*) and should verify that the patient truly understands the questions. Even the most highly educated patients can get confused when presented with complex medical jargon.

Even if they have complete command of the clinician's language, patients with different *cultural background* may assign different meanings and weights to given risk factors or they may be offended by certain questions. It is therefore important for the clinician to be culturally competent: familiar with and sensitive to the attitudes and health belief model of the patient's culture. For example, the very concept of prevention may not be meaningful if patients believe that diseases develop from sinful behavior, rather than medical risk factors, or that suffering from disease leads to spiritual growth. Patients from certain ethnic or minority communities may be confused by the clinician's choice of words. For example, they may view a *"negative* test result" as unfavorable news. They may deny a history of "diabetes" or "hypertension" but admit to having "sugar" or "high blood."

Screening Questionnaires

Many practices ask patients to complete a medical history form at their first visit. If they ask questions about relevant risk factors, these forms can provide the clinician with useful risk assessment information and save time during the interview by identifying which topics require further investigation. They can also stimulate the patient's thinking, prompting the patient to bring up certain issues with the clinician that would otherwise be forgotten. The role of such questionnaires as a systematic tool to help practices deliver preventive care is discussed further in Chapter 21.

One limitation of such forms is that patients may not answer the questions honestly or may leave the questions unanswered. More comprehensive screening forms will take longer for patients to complete, increasing the likelihood of a patient not completing the questionnaire. The forms may not be understandable, especially if the patient speaks a different language or has difficulty reading. Finally, patients may become frustrated with the redundancy of completing multiple questionnaires over time, yet reserving such forms solely for new encounters may miss changes in a patient's modifiable risks. Therefore, clinicians must be careful to supplement and update risk factor information obtained from medical history forms.

As noted earlier, screening questionnaires, standardized instruments that have been validated as screening tools for specific conditions, have been developed for the detection of depression, alcohol abuse, cognitive impairment, and other health problems. These instruments have been designed out of concern that routine questions by clinicians have poor sensitivity and specificity in detecting these conditions. Unfortunately, most screening questionnaires also have limited sensitivity and specificity. That is, a patient with an abnormal score may not have the condition (false positive) and a patient with a normal score may have the condition (false negative). For example, the MMSE has a reported sensitivity and specificity of 87% and 82%, respectively (8,9). This means that, in a person with a 5% probability of having dementia, an abnormal score on the questionnaire has a positive predictive value of 20%: four people without dementia will score falsely positive on the questionnaire for every true case detected. An expert panel judging the accuracy of 19 screening questionnaires for childhood developmental delay gave its highest rating to instruments with a sensitivity and specificity approaching 80% and 90%, respectively (10). This means that the best performance of such instruments (assuming a sensitivity and specificity of 80% and 90%, respectively, and a 5% pretest probability of a developmental disorder) would be to falsely label 2 children as developmentally delayed for every true case detected; if the pretest probability is 1%, 12 children would be mislabeled for every true case detected.

In addition to their poor predictive value, completion of questionnaires is often too time consuming to be done during the clinical interview. Common solutions are to ask patients who are at risk for the problem to complete the questionnaires before meeting with the clinician, either in the waiting room or before the appointment. If the need for using the questionnaire first becomes apparent during the clinical interview, the patient can be asked to complete the form while the clinician moves on to another patient. The clinician can then return to the patient's room to discuss the results. Another solution is to send the patient home with the questionnaire with instructions to mail it to the clinician when completed or to provide the patient with the means to complete the survey electronically.

With technological advances, innovative new tools are emerging that link screening questionnaires with individualized risk factor profiles, personal guidelines on recommended services, patient information resources, and self-management tools. A unique aspect of these tools is that their use not only results in the collection of historic information but also initiates the delivery of care and empowers patients to assume active roles. The content of the screening questionnaires can range from the identification of a single target condition, as described in the preceding text, to more global assessments of preventive care needs. Frequently, these tools are electronic, rather than paper based, allowing for automated risk assessment calculations and automated delivery of information to the patient and/or clinician; the delivery systems can include websites, portable laptops, personal digital assistants (PDAs), and computer kiosks, all of which can be accessed in the clinician's office, elsewhere in the community, or at the patient's home. Examples of these innovative tools include www.HowsYourHealth.org and www.MyPreventiveCare.net (see Fig. 2.1). Linking this technology with electronic health records maintained by the practice and personal health records maintained by the patient can further enhance the efficient collection of information and foster patient-clinician communication. The information

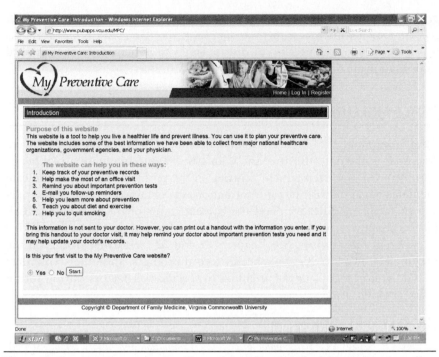

Figure 2.1 • "My Preventive Care" is a web-based personal health record used to collect the patient's prevention related history and to offer individualized recommendations.

and advice generated by these tools can be powerful motivators for patients attempting lifestyle change. The clinician and patient can together review the information these systems generate as part of their discussion of health maintenance.

CONCLUDING THE RISK ASSESSMENT INTERVIEW

As noted earlier, the clinician can continue to collect elements of the history during the physical examination. This may be particularly useful if the clinician finds any abnormalities on examination that prompt further questions. Regardless, the focused encounter period for discussions about risk factors should be concluded with the courtesies that are extended at the end of any clinical interview. Patients should be asked whether they have any additional concerns that they would like to discuss. They should be provided a transition to the next stage of the encounter by being told what to expect. If the interview is to be followed by a physical or laboratory examination, a helpful statement may be: *"I want to talk with you further about the health issues that we have discussed. But before we do that, I'd like to examine you and perform a few tests so that we will have a complete picture of your risk factors. I'll step out for a few minutes so that you can change into this gown. Is that ok?"*

Risk factors and preclinical disease states to anticipate in the physical examination are discussed in the next chapter.

OFFICE AND CLINIC ORGANIZATION

At a minimum, the clinician should document which risk factors were discussed in the notes for the visit. Clinicians should maintain a risk factor "problem list" for each patient. Entries on the problem list should indicate the dates when the risk factor information was obtained, previous attempts at risk factor modification, and the current status of the risk factor. Risk factors about which no information has been obtained should be flagged for attention at future visits. See Chapters 21 and 22 for further details on the use of alert stickers, electronic health record prompts, and other reminders in the medical record to call attention to specific risk factors during future office or clinic visits.

SUGGESTED READINGS

Bickley LS, Szilagi PG. *Bates' guide to physical examination and history taking*, 3rd ed. Philadelphia: JB Lippincott Co, 2002.

Coulehan JL, Block MR. *The medical interview: mastering skills for clinical practice*, 5th ed. Philadelphia: FA Davis Co, 2006.

Golden AS, Bartlett E, Barker LR. The doctor-patient relationship: communication and patient education. In: Barker LR, Burton JR, Zieve PD, eds. *Principles of ambulatory medicine*, 4th ed. Baltimore: Williams & Wilkins, 1995:30–41.

National Institute on Aging. *Working with your older patients: a clinician's handbook*. Bethesda: National Institute on Aging, Available at http://www.niapublications .org/pubs/clinicians2004/index.asp. 2004.

Stewart M, Brown JB, Weston WW, et al. *Patient-centered medicine: transforming the clinical method*. Thousand Oaks: Sage Publications Inc, 1995.

References

1. Mokdad AH, Marks JS, Stroup DF, et al. Actual causes of death in the United States, 2000. *JAMA* 2004;291:1238–1245.
2. Woodwell DA, Cherry DK. National ambulatory medical care survey: 2002 summary. *Adv Data* 2004;346:1–44.
3. Glasgow RE, Orleans CT, Wagner EH. Does the chronic care model serve also as a template for improving prevention? *Milbank Q* 2001;79:579–612, iv–v.
4. Boekeloo BO, Marx ES, Kral AH, et al. Frequency and thoroughness of STD/HIV risk assessment by physicians in a high-risk metropolitan area. *Am J Public Health* 1991;81:1645–1648.
5. Centers for Disease Control and Prevention. Trends in sexual risk behaviors among high school students–United States, 1991–2001. MMWR Morb Mortal Wkly Rep 2002:51:856–9.

6. U.S. Preventive Services Task Force. *Guide to clinical preventive services*. Available at http://www.ahrq.gov/clinic/pocketgd.htm. 2006.

7. Centers for Disease Control and Prevention. *Childhood lead poisoning prevention programs*. Available at: http://www.cdc.gov/nceh/lead/grants/contacts/CLPPP%20Map .htm. Accessed January, 2006.

8. Anthony JC, LeResche L, Niaz U, et al. Limits of the 'Mini-Mental State' as a screening test for dementia and delirium among hospital patients. *Psychol Med* 1982;12:397–408.

9. Palmer K, Backman L, Winblad B, et al. Detection of Alzheimer's disease and dementia in the preclinical phase: population based cohort study. *Br Med J* 2003; 326:245.

10. American Academy of Pediatrics Committee on Children with Disabilities. Developmental surveillance and screening in infants and young children. *Pediatrics* 2001; 108:192–196.

CHAPTER 3

The Physical Examination: Where to Look for Preclinical Disease

Alex H. Krist, Janelle Guirguis-Blake, Steven H. Woolf, and Robert S. Lawrence

The physical examination is an important part of the delivery of preventive care. There are limitations to its direct value, as discussed in the subsequent text. It can be very beneficial, however, if performed in a skillful manner, integrated with other essential elements of the encounter, and used to support counseling and motivate patients to improve health behaviors. In the context of this chapter, the physical examination refers to the direct inspection, auscultation, percussion, and palpation of the patient's body. Other elements of an encounter—for example, obtaining the history (see Chapter 2), performing laboratory tests (see Chapter 4), counseling the patient (see Section II)—may occur during the physical examination but are discussed separately in other chapters.

This chapter focuses on physical examination procedures to screen for asymptomatic disease or risk factors rather than on the physical diagnosis of patients with symptomatic disease. Patients who present with complaints or abnormal physical findings require careful, focused examination techniques to make the correct diagnosis. Physical examination procedures that qualify as preventive interventions (as opposed to a diagnostic workup) are those that detect abnormalities in the absence of symptoms.

When seeing a clinician for preventive care, most patients expect to have and most clinicians expect to perform a physical examination. It is an opportunity to detect abnormalities that the patient may not recognize, that the clinician may not have suspected based on historical information, or that may not be revealed by laboratory screening tests. Examination can potentially detect concerning signs of unhealthy behaviors (e.g., wheezing in a smoker suggesting early airway disease). Findings from an examination may also be necessary to properly interpret abnormal laboratory values; obtaining this information before the laboratory results may help to prevent unnecessary patient or clinician anxiety. For example, a slightly elevated prostate-specific antigen (PSA) test may be less concerning if the patient has a uniformly enlarged prostate consistent with benign prostatic hypertrophy.

TABLE 3.1 The Comprehensive Physical Examination

Skin

Head, scalp, face, nares

Pupils, sclera, conjunctiva, retina, extraocular muscles

Buccal mucosa, teeth, gums, tongue, pharynx

Ear, tympanic membranes

Neck, cervical lymph nodes, jugular veins, carotid arteries

Thoracic and lumbar spine

Posterior lung fields

Breasts, axillae

Precordial impulse, heart sounds

Shoulders, upper arms, elbows, forearms, hands, fingernails

Abdominal viscera

Genitalia, rectum, inguinal canal, femoral pulses

Hips, thighs, knees, lower legs, ankles, feet, toenails

Peripheral pulses

Mental status and central nervous system

Cranial and peripheral nervous system

While virtually any component of the physical examination (Table 3.1) can detect early-stage disease in the absence of symptoms, there is little scientific evidence that healthy persons experience better outcomes because of head-to-toe physical examinations. Conducting studies to evaluate definitively the effectiveness of physical examination procedures is difficult because of the required size, logistics, expenses, and possibly, ethical considerations associated with such studies. Even for physical examination elements for which there is evidence of health benefits, the likelihood that an individual patient will have an abnormality during a specific examination is low (e.g., there is a low probability that a woman aged 50–55 years will have a palpable breast mass on physical examination).

The time required for a thorough physical examination is an important opportunity cost. Busy clinicians often have only a few minutes to spend with each patient. Leveraging that time for counseling or other preventive interventions has a much greater likelihood of improving the patient's health than spending that same time doing a head-to-toe examination. Many clinicians react to these time constraints by making the physical examination more focused and cursory (1). Little may be gained by performing examination procedures in a cursory manner (e.g., examining only a small portion of the patient's skin, briefly palpating for breast masses), which is often ineffective and therefore makes poor use of limited time.

An appropriate way to focus the routine physical examination, however, is to emphasize examination procedures that have demonstrated potential benefit as screening procedures in asymptomatic patients. Ensuring that these selected procedures are performed well helps to maximize the value of the prevention focused physical examination. The history can help to guide the clinician in selecting additional examination procedures that may be indicated for a given patient based on individual risks. Because patients have come to expect clinicians to perform a comprehensive physical examination, the clinician may wish to explain the value of the focused physical examination and to highlight specific preventable conditions that merit attention.

Findings from the physical examination should be reviewed with the patient and used to inform and individually tailor counseling messages for patients. For example, the detection of wheezing in a smoker may prompt the clinician to say during their smoking cessation counseling, *"You know Mr. Smith, I can hear wheezing in your lungs. This is a sign that your smoking is damaging your lungs. It may be an early indication of something like emphysema."*

This chapter focuses on the physical examination procedures for which there is at least some scientific evidence that routine screening may be beneficial. These include sphygmomanometry; routine measurement of height, weight, and head circumference; testing for abnormal hearing and visual acuity; oral cavity examination; clinical breast examination (CBE); digital rectal examination (DRE); and skin examination. See Chapter 17 for discussion of specific examination procedures for children (e.g., newborn examination for the pupillary light reflex). The reader should consult the suggested readings at the end of this chapter for information about other preventive examination procedures not discussed here (e.g., auscultation of the heart or carotid arteries, palpation for abdominal aortic aneurysms or thyroid nodules, testicular examination, or congenital hip dislocation). Other references should be consulted regarding examination procedures to screen for occupational illnesses and injuries.

The discussion of each examination procedure that follows includes a brief introduction describing the target condition and the rationale for the screening test, guidelines on how often screening should be performed and on which patients, a summary of official guidelines issued by major organizations and agencies, and suggestions on patient preparation and technique. (The sources of the recommendations in the "Official Guidelines" sections are listed under "Suggested Readings" later in this chapter.) The discussion of each examination procedure also includes sections on the potential adverse effects of screening, the accuracy of the examination procedure, and suggestions on how to organize the office or clinic and maintain medical records for optimal screening. Data cited in the "Accuracy and Reliability as Screening Test" sections of this chapter and Chapter 4 are drawn from a large body of evidence. The hundreds of studies on which these estimates are based are not cited explicitly in these chapters due to space limitations. The reader interested in the source of the data is referred to other texts (1) that discuss the individual studies in more detail.

Because routine physical examination procedures usually detect no abnormalities, their most important value may lie in providing a setting for counseling patients about primary and secondary prevention of the target condition. Each section of this chapter therefore includes a "Standard Counseling" discussion of the reminders that clinicians should give all patients, even if no abnormality is detected, about how to prevent the target condition and when to return for additional screening. This section also refers readers to other relevant chapters in Section II of the book, which discuss in more detail how to counsel patients about specific health behaviors. This chapter does not discuss how to manage abnormal findings. For those instances the reader should refer to Chapter 18 for an overview of follow-up testing and treatment options.

SPHYGMOMANOMETRY

Introduction

Over the last three decades, substantial improvements have been made in the awareness and control of hypertension, a major risk factor for the development of cardiovascular disease. Unfortunately, approximately 50 million Americans are hypertensive, only 35% of whom have well-controlled blood pressure (2). Studies have consistently shown that the early detection and treatment of hypertension can reduce all-cause mortality as well as the incidence of cardiac and cerebrovascular events (2). Screening for hypertension is performed by periodic sphygmomanometry. In the typical office or clinic, this measurement is obtained when routine vital signs are taken before the clinician's examination.

Screening Guidelines. **All adults should undergo periodic screening for hypertension. The evidence is weaker for blood pressure screening of children and adolescents.**

Official Guidelines. The U.S. Preventive Services Task Force (USPSTF) recommends periodic measurement of blood pressure in adults. The USPSTF states that there is insufficient evidence to recommend routine screening under the ages of 18 years and 21 years, respectively. The American Academy of Family Physicians (AAFP) recommends periodic blood pressure measurement after age 18 years. On the basis of expert opinion and the potential to detect treatable causes of secondary hypertension (up to 28% of children with elevated blood pressure have secondary hypertension),

the American Academy of Pediatrics (AAP), the National Heart, Lung, and Blood Institute, and the American Heart Association recommend annual screening of children
aged 3 years and older. The Joint National Committee on Detection, Evaluation, and
Treatment of High Blood Pressure recommends that screening be repeated in adults
every 2 years if the previous reading was in a normotensive range (less than 120/80)
and every year if the reading was in a prehypertensive range (120–139/80–89).
Patients with stage 1 or 2 hypertension need more frequent monitoring.

Patient Preparation

Accurate blood pressure measurement is a *sine qua non* of diagnosing
hypertension. The patient should be seated for 5 minutes before blood
pressure is measured. Relaxation should be encouraged. The arm should
be at the level of the heart, comfortably supported on a firm surface, and
slightly flexed. Clothing with constricting arm sleeves should be removed.
The patient should not have exercised, smoked, or ingested caffeine for
30 minutes before measurement.

The examiner should select the proper cuff size to accommodate the
size of the patient's arm (Table 3.2). A normal-sized adult cuff will produce
falsely elevated pressures on an obese arm and falsely low pressures on a thin
arm or on that of a child. Therefore, choose a cuff with a bladder width
that is 20% wider than the diameter of the arm or 40% of the circumference
of the arm. The length of the bladder should be approximately 80% of the
circumference so that it does not completely encircle the limb. In children,
the bladder width should not exceed two-thirds the length of the upper arm
and the bladder length should not encircle more than three-fourths of the
circumference of the arm.

TABLE 3.2   Proper Bladder Dimensions for Blood Pressure
Measurement

Patient	Bladder Width (cm)	Bladder Length (cm)	Arm Circumference Range at Midpoint (cm)
Newborn	3	6	<6
Infant	5	15	6–15
Child	8	21	16–21
Small adult	10	24	22–26
Adult	13	30	27–34
Large adult	16	38	35–44

Adapted from American Heart Association. *Human blood pressure determination by
sphygmomanometry.* Dallas: American Heart Association, 1994.

Technique

The cuff should be placed snugly around the upper arm, with the lower edge approximately 1 in. above the antecubital fossa, the bladder over the brachial artery, and the tubing over the medial aspect of the arm. For a manual measurement, both the palpable systolic pressure and the audible Korotkoff sounds should be determined. Electronic devices automate this process and do not require audible or manual assessment. At least two measurements should be made and the average of the two should be recorded as the patient's blood pressure. If an abnormality is detected, the blood pressure can be compared in both arms in supine, sitting, and standing positions; in children, blood pressure can be measured in the lower extremities to rule out aortic coarctation. Differences of up to 10 mm Hg between arms are within the normal range.

For adults, blood pressure is considered *elevated* if it exceeds 120/80. The threshold for *prehypertension* is 120–129/80–89 and for *hypertension* is 140/90. For children and adolescents, hypertension is defined as being at the 95th percentile or greater for age, height, and gender (values listed in Table 3.3 for the 50th and 75th percentiles of height). Isolated blood pressure elevations can be due to anxiety and other factors (e.g., "white coat" hypertension), and the diagnosis of hypertension should therefore not be made until the patient has had two consecutive visits in which elevated blood pressure has been documented.

TABLE 3.3   Criteria for Elevated Blood Pressure

Age	Girls' Systolic/ Diastolic Blood Pressure		Boys' Systolic/ Diastolic Blood Pressure	
	50th Percentile for Height	75th Percentile for Height	50th Percentile for Height	50th Percentile for Height
1 yr	104/58	105/59	102/57	104/58
3 yr	107/66	108/67	109/65	111/66
6 yr	111/73	112/73	114/74	115/75
9 yr	117/77	118/78	117/79	115/75
12 yr	123/80	124/81	123/81	125/82
15 yr	128/83	129/84	129/83	133/84
17 yr	129/84	130/85	136/87	138/88

Adapted from National High Blood Pressure Education Program Working Group on High Blood Pressure in Children and Adolescents. The fourth report on the diagnosis, evaluation, and treatment of high blood pressure in children and adolescents. *Pediatrics* 2004;114:555–576.

TABLE 3.4 Recommended Follow-up Interval Based on Initial Blood Pressure Level

Initial Blood Pressure	Follow-up Recommended
Normal (<120/80)	Recheck in 2 yr
Prehypertension (120–129/80–89)	Recheck in 1 yr
Stage 1 hypertension (140–159/90–99)	Confirm within 2 mo
Stage 2 hypertension (160–179/100–109)	Evaluate or refer to source of usual care within 1 mo. For those with pressures >180/110, evaluate and treat immediately

Adapted from Joint National Committee on Detection, Evaluation, and Treatment of High Blood Pressure. The seventh report of the Joint National Committee on Detection, Evaluation, and Treatment of High Blood Pressure (JNC VII). *JAMA* 2003;289:2560–2572.

Standard Counseling

Patients should be reminded that regular physical activity (see Chapter 6), adoption of the DASH diet—Dietary Approaches to Stop Hypertension—(see Chapter 7), weight management (see Chapter 8), and alcohol moderation (see Chapter 10) will help control blood pressure and that their blood pressure should be measured again in the appropriate interval (see Table 3.4). Patients with an isolated blood pressure elevation should be informed that the elevation is not considered "high blood pressure" until repeat measurements are obtained, but the importance of returning for repeat measurements should be emphasized.

Potential Adverse Effects

There are no direct adverse effects from measuring blood pressure, but the results can be inaccurate, producing psychological, behavioral, and even financial consequences if the results affect insurance or employment eligibility or require repeat office visits to rule out hypertension. Although patients may experience anxiety over the possibility of having high blood pressure, studies have inconsistently demonstrated higher rates of work absenteeism among persons who receive the label of "hypertension" (1). Antihypertensive medications may produce side effects. Inaccurate sphygmomanometry can also produce false-negative results, allowing hypertensive persons to escape detection.

Accuracy and Reliability as Screening Test

Office sphygmomanometry is less accurate than invasive techniques (e.g., intra-arterial monitoring) for measuring blood pressure, but its exact sensitivity and specificity are uncertain. The type of instrument, the technique of the examiner, and the physiologic state of the patient affect the accuracy and reliability of the test. Given that patients' blood pressure varies throughout the day, a single office-based measurement may not reflect a patient's average blood pressure over time. Some evidence suggests that continual ambulatory blood pressure monitoring, which provides an average blood pressure measured over 24 hours, more accurately predicts clinical cardiovascular outcomes. However, whether this information more effectively guides treatment decisions remains uncertain.

Office and Clinic Organization for Routine Screening

Intake procedures for obtaining vital signs should provide sufficient time to allow the patient to relax for several minutes before the blood pressure is measured. The office or clinic should be equipped with a variety of cuff sizes for adults and children. Sphygmomanometers become inaccurate over time and should be recalibrated periodically. Reminder systems (see Chapters 21 and 22) should be in place to ensure that patients return for routine screening, obtain consecutive repeat measurements for elevated values, and obtain appropriate counseling and treatment if hypertension is diagnosed.

Medical Record Documentation

The blood pressure recorded in the medical record should be the average of two blood pressure readings obtained during the office visit. If the blood pressure is measured in both arms and the readings are significantly different, the arm and recorded values should be documented. Until elevated blood pressure has been confirmed on two consecutive visits, the finding should be described in the medical record as "elevated blood pressure" and not as "hypertension" or even "high blood pressure." The follow-up plan for elevated blood pressure readings should be documented.

HEIGHT, WEIGHT, AND HEAD CIRCUMFERENCE

Introduction

More than 65% of adult Americans and 15% of adolescents are obese or overweight, representing a 30% increase from the previous decade (3). Being overweight or obese (see Chapter 8) and having an increased waist circumference are well-established risk factors for diabetes, hypertension, coronary artery disease, other chronic diseases, and premature mortality (4). Screening has been advocated as a means of detecting patients who are overweight and obese and of initiating exercise and nutritional interventions to prevent complications, which are discussed in Chapters 6–8. The principal screening tests are height, weight (used to calculate the body mass index [BMI]), and other anthropomorphic measurements. In infants and children, frequent height, weight, and head circumference measurements are used to screen for abnormal growth velocity (including both delayed growth and obesity) and to institute nutritional and social service interventions (see Chapter 17). Some screening tests for obesity (e.g., skinfold thickness and other measures of body fat, waist and limb circumference) are not reviewed here.

Screening Guidelines. **The height and weight of adults should be measured periodically and used to calculate the BMI, but there is no scientific evidence regarding the proper interval. The height, weight, and BMI (and head circumference of infants and small children) should be measured at every childhood visit (unless recent measurements have been obtained within the last few weeks) and should be plotted on an appropriate growth chart (see Chapter 17).**

Official Guidelines. The USPSTF and the AAFP recommend that clinicians screen all adult patients for obesity and offer intensive counseling and behavioral interventions to promote sustained weight loss for obese adults. The American Heart Association recommends that adults obtain body weight and waist circumference measurements periodically. The AAP recommends that infants undergo height, weight, and head circumference measurement at well child visits between the ages 0–24 months and annually from ages 2–6 years; it also recommends annual BMI measurements for all children and adolescents.

Patient Preparation
Patients should remove heavy clothing and shoes.

Technique
Height and weight are generally measured with a standing platform scale and a height attachment. Electronic scales are common and do not require calibration, but platform scales should be calibrated to zero before the patient is weighed. When height is measured, patients should stand erect with their back against the scale or measuring wall and with their feet together. They should look straight ahead, with the outer canthus of the eye on the same horizontal plane as the external auditory canal.

Infants and small children should be weighed on an infant platform scale. The height of infants and small children is measured by placing the child in a recumbent position on a measuring board, holding the feet against a fixed foot piece, and moving the headpiece to touch the vertex. Head circumference should be measured by wrapping a measuring tape around the child's head at the level of the occipital protuberance and the supraorbital prominence. See Chapter 17 for more details on the examination of infants and children.

The height and weight determine the BMI (Table 3.5), which in turn classifies patients as overweight (BMI = 25–29.9 kg/m^2) or obese (BMI greater than or equal to 30 kg/m^2) (see Chapter 8). There are three classes of obesity: class I (BMI = 30–34.9 kg/m^2), class II (BMI = 35–39.9 kg/m^2), and class III (BMI = 40 kg/m^2 and above). The BMI is calculated by dividing the patient's height in kilograms by the height in meters squared (kg/m^2). Many electronic health records, calculators on personal digital assistants, and website tools (www.nhlbisupport.com/bmi/) can make this calculation automatically.

For infants and young children, the height, weight, and head circumference are used to detect abnormal size and growth velocity by plotting the data on age and gender-specific growth curves that reflect population norms. Since 2000, the growth charts from the Centers for Disease Control and Prevention have included a BMI-for-age growth chart to help better identify obese children and those at risk for obesity. These growth charts are discussed in further detail in Chapter 17.

Obtaining regular body weights is not always easy to do with older or frail patients. If weight loss is suspected, repeat weighing should be done. For the BMI, the patient's height before age 50 years should be used as the reference height. Clinically significant weight loss is considered to be weight loss exceeding 2% of baseline in 1 month, 5% in 3 months, or 10% in 6 months. The importance of the relationship of lean body mass and excess body fat should be taken into account. Less technical measurements such as BMI and waist circumference correlate well to total body fat but are not good indicators of visceral fat stores.

Standard Counseling

Patients should be counseled about the healthful benefits of regular physical activity (see Chapter 6), dietary modifications (see Chapter 7), and weight management through lifestyle modifications (see Chapter 8).

Potential Adverse Effects

There are no direct adverse effects from measuring height and weight, but the results can produce psychological, behavioral, and even financial consequences if they affect insurance and employment eligibility and can incur inconvenience and costs to have the abnormality evaluated. Significant social stigma exists for patients with obesity, although it is unclear whether defining and medicalizing obesity by clinical measurement increases this stigma. Some aggressive treatments for obesity, such as medications, very-low calorie diets, and bariatric surgery are associated with significant potential side effects and complications (e.g., 1–2% postoperative mortality for weight reduction surgery). False-positive results in measurements of infants and small children can create unnecessary parental anxiety about the possibility of a growth disorder.

TABLE 3.5 Table of Body Mass Indices

	Normal						Overweight					Obese										Extreme obesity														
BMI kg/m²	19	20	21	22	23	24	25	26	27	28	29	30	31	32	33	34	35	36	37	38	39	40	41	42	43	44	45	46	47	48	49	50	51	52	53	54
Height (inches)															Body weight (pounds)																					
58	91	96	100	105	110	115	119	124	129	134	138	143	148	153	158	162	167	172	177	181	186	191	196	201	205	210	215	220	224	229	234	239	244	248	253	258
59	94	99	104	109	114	119	124	128	133	138	143	148	153	158	163	168	173	178	183	188	193	198	203	208	212	217	222	227	232	237	242	247	252	257	262	267
60	97	102	107	112	118	123	128	133	138	143	148	153	158	163	168	174	179	184	189	194	199	204	209	215	220	225	230	235	240	245	250	255	261	266	271	276
61	100	106	111	116	122	127	132	137	143	148	153	158	164	169	174	180	185	190	195	201	206	211	217	222	227	232	238	243	248	254	259	264	269	275	280	285
62	104	109	115	120	126	131	136	142	147	153	158	164	169	175	180	186	191	196	202	207	213	218	224	229	235	240	246	251	256	262	267	273	278	284	289	295
63	107	113	118	124	130	135	141	146	152	158	163	169	175	180	186	191	197	203	208	214	220	225	231	237	242	248	254	259	265	270	278	282	287	293	299	304
64	110	116	122	128	134	140	145	151	157	163	169	174	180	186	192	197	204	209	215	221	227	232	238	244	250	256	262	267	273	279	285	291	296	302	308	314
65	114	120	126	132	138	144	150	156	162	168	174	180	186	192	198	204	210	216	222	228	234	240	246	252	258	264	270	276	282	288	294	300	306	312	318	324
66	118	124	130	136	142	148	155	161	167	173	179	186	192	198	204	210	216	223	229	235	241	247	253	260	266	272	278	284	291	297	303	309	315	322	328	334
67	121	127	134	140	146	153	159	166	172	178	185	191	198	204	211	217	223	230	236	242	249	255	261	268	274	280	287	293	299	306	312	319	325	331	338	344
68	125	131	138	144	151	158	164	171	177	184	190	197	203	210	216	223	230	236	243	249	256	262	269	276	282	289	295	302	308	315	322	328	335	341	348	354
69	128	135	142	149	155	162	169	176	182	189	196	203	209	216	223	230	236	243	250	257	263	270	277	284	291	297	304	311	318	324	331	338	345	351	358	365
70	132	139	146	153	160	167	174	181	188	195	202	209	216	222	229	236	243	250	257	264	271	278	285	292	299	306	313	320	327	334	341	348	355	362	369	376
71	136	143	150	157	165	172	179	186	193	200	208	215	222	229	236	243	250	257	265	272	279	286	293	301	308	315	322	329	338	343	351	358	365	372	379	386
72	140	147	154	162	169	177	184	191	199	206	213	221	228	235	242	250	258	265	272	279	287	294	302	309	316	324	331	338	346	353	361	368	375	383	390	397
73	144	151	159	166	174	182	189	197	204	212	219	227	235	242	250	257	265	272	280	288	295	302	310	318	325	333	340	348	355	363	371	378	386	393	401	408
74	148	155	163	171	179	186	194	202	210	218	225	233	241	249	256	264	272	280	287	295	303	311	319	326	334	342	350	358	365	373	381	389	396	404	412	420
75	152	160	168	176	184	192	200	208	216	224	232	240	248	256	264	272	279	287	295	303	311	319	327	335	343	351	359	367	375	383	391	399	407	415	423	431
76	156	164	172	180	189	197	205	213	221	230	238	246	254	263	271	279	287	295	304	312	320	328	336	344	353	361	369	377	385	394	402	410	418	426	435	443

Source: Adapted from Clinical Guidelines on the Identification, Evaluation, and Treatment of Overweight and Obesity in Adults: The Evidence Report. NIH Publication No.98-4083. Bethesda, MD: National Heart, Lung, and Blood Institute in cooperation with The National Institute of Diabetes and Digestive and Kidney Diseases; 1998.

Accuracy and Reliability as Screening Test

Height, weight, and BMI are easy to measure and highly reliable. The body fat percentage calculated from BMI correlates with directly measured body fat with an estimation error of only 4%. Additionally, the BMI has been linked with a wide range of health outcomes. The BMI does not account for body fat distribution or the relative weight of muscle versus fat, which are also independent predictors of health outcomes.

Office and Clinic Organization for Routine Screening

Offices and clinics should be equipped to measure height and weight for adults and to calculate BMIs easily with conveniently posted BMI conversion tables or automated BMI calculators (see page 59). Likewise, offices with pediatric patients should be equipped with infant platform scales, measuring boards, measuring tape, and a complete supply of pediatric growth charts for boys and girls of all ages. The office should have reminder systems (see Chapters 21 and 22) in place to ensure that parents of children with abnormal growth velocity keep appointments for follow-up visits and that the children receive appropriate evaluation and treatment.

Medical Record Documentation

Height, weight, BMI, and other anthropometric data should be recorded in an area of the medical record that allows easy comparison with previous measurements and early detection of important trends. The appropriate age- and gender-specific growth chart should be prominently displayed in the medical record of pediatric patients and should be filled out at each visit. The follow-up plan for abnormal height and weight should be documented in the medical record.

HEARING TESTING

Introduction

Approximately 28 million Americans have chronic hearing impairment, more than 1 million of whom are younger than 18 years (5). Approximately 5 million Americans cannot hear and understand normal speech, and approximately 10 million persons have noise-induced hearing loss. Screening for hearing impairment is performed because it has the potential to improve communication skills and functional status and because it may improve language development when detected in infants and young children. Screening tests to assess hearing can include simple physical examination techniques, which are discussed in this section, and laboratory tests (e.g., audiometry, auditory-evoked responses, otoacoustic emissions testing).

Screening Guidelines. **Clinicians should inquire periodically about difficulties with hearing in children and in the elderly. There is little evidence to support routine screening of adolescents and adults. Physical examination findings may further corroborate positive responses to inquiries about hearing difficulties.**

Official Guidelines. The AAFP recommends periodic inquiry about hearing difficulties in the elderly, but does not make recommendations supporting objective measurements for any age-group. The AAP recommends periodic historical inquiry about hearing during infancy and childhood and objective hearing testing by a "standard testing method" at ages 4, 5, 6, 8, 10, 12, and 18 years. Newborn hearing screening is discussed further in Chapter 17. In 1996 and 2001, the USPSTF found insufficient evidence to recommend for or against routine hearing screening of infants, children, and adults, but the recommendations are currently under reevaluation. Hearing screening is required by law in some states.

Patient Preparation

Hearing should be examined in a quiet area with minimal background noise.

Technique

Simple physical examination tests of hearing include the whispered voice and watch-tick tests. In the whispered voice test, the examiner softly whispers words from a distance of 1–2 ft while the patient blocks the opposite ear by placing a finger on the tragus; the patient should be able to repeat at least half the words correctly. In the watch-tick test, the examiner checks high-frequency hearing by moving a ticking watch toward the patient's ear and noting the distance at which the sound is first heard.

The hearing of young children is tested qualitatively by observing their response to whispered voice or sounds and the progress of their developing speech skills (e.g., delayed vocalization). For example, the examiner can stand or crouch behind the child and whisper softly to determine whether the child turns to the sound or responds to a question (e.g., "Do you like ice cream?"). See Chapter 17 regarding otoacoustic emissions and audiometry screening of newborns and young children.

Standard Counseling

Parents should be encouraged to contact the clinician if they or teachers note that the child has poor hearing, speech, or language skills. All patients, especially adolescents and young adults, should be reminded that occupational or recreational exposure to loud noise increases the risk of hearing loss. Older adults should be counseled that while loss of hearing is common with increasing age, it should not be accepted as "normal," can compromise their quality of life, and is often treatable with hearing aids.

Potential Adverse Effects

There are no known adverse effects from hearing testing, but inaccurate results may produce unnecessary anxiety, especially among the parents of young children; may affect insurance and employment eligibility; and may incur cost and inconvenience for appointments and testing to rule out a disorder. Inaccurate testing may produce false-negative results, allowing hearing impairment to escape detection.

Accuracy and Reliability as Screening Test

There are few data available regarding the sensitivity and specificity of physical examination techniques for hearing.

Office and Clinic Organization for Routine Screening

Examination rooms in which hearing screening is performed should be located away from loud working areas or noisy machines. The office or clinic should have referral and reminder systems in place to ensure that patients with abnormal screening tests receive appropriate diagnostic studies (e.g., audiometry, tympanometry) either on site or through a referred specialist, and that patients found to have hearing disorders receive proper treatment. Patient education literature about hearing aids and the need to treat presbycusis can be helpful to older adults.

Medical Record Documentation

The results of hearing tests should be recorded for each ear. The data can include the proportion of correctly heard words (whisper test) or the distance to hear watch sounds (watch-tick test). The follow-up plan for abnormal hearing should be documented.

VISUAL ACUITY TESTING

Introduction

Approximately 1–4% of American children have amblyopia, and an estimated 5–7% of preschool children have refractive errors (6). Screening for abnormal visual acuity is performed because the detection of amblyopia and amblyogenic risk factors can improve visual acuity through treatments such as surgery for cataracts or strabismus, use of glasses or refractive surgery treatments, and visual training to treat amblyopia (e.g., patching). Although 6% of adults have visual impairment, there is little evidence that early detection of visual impairment reduces morbidity for school-aged children, adolescents, and young adults. Detection of impairment in older adults, however, may prevent injuries and improve functional status. Testing for abnormal visual acuity can range from simple acuity testing by primary care clinicians to sophisticated refraction measurements by eye specialists. Chapter 17 provides further details on testing of visual acuity and screening tests for amblyopia and strabismus in young children.

Screening Guidelines.   Screening for amblyopia, strabismus, and defects in visual acuity is recommended for children younger than 5 years. Periodic screening for impaired visual acuity is appropriate in older adults, but there is no scientific evidence regarding the optimal interval. Asymptomatic adolescents and young adults do not require routine visual acuity screening.

Official Guidelines.   The USPSTF recommends visual acuity screening for children younger than 5 years, but reports insufficient evidence to determine the optimal screening tests and screening interval. The USPSTF is currently updating its recommendations on vision screening of older adults. The AAFP recommends screening for amblyopia, strabismus, and visual defects in children younger than 5 years and screening for visual difficulties in older adults. On the basis of expert opinion, the American Academy of Ophthalmology and the AAP recommend the following examinations at every well child visit between birth and age 3 years: an ocular history, vision assessment, external inspection of the eyes and lids, ocular motility assessment, pupil examination, and red reflex examination. Between age 3 and 5 years, these organizations recommend the above tests mentioned earlier along with age-appropriate visual acuity measurement (using HOTV or tumbling E tests) and ophthalmoscopy. They recommend annual screening of school children for visual acuity and ocular alignment. Vision screening of preschool and school children is also required by law in some states and in a number of federal programs. For adults, the American Academy of Ophthalmology recommends occasional examinations from puberty to age 40 years, and an examination at age 40 years, every 2–4 years until age 65 years, and every 1–2 years thereafter.

Patient Preparation

Individuals with a known refractive error and prescribed corrective lenses should wear their glasses or contact lenses for the examination.

Technique

To test visual acuity, the patient should sit or stand 20 ft from a standard Snellen eye chart. With one eye covered, the patient should read the letters aloud; moving from top to bottom, and then the test should be repeated with the other eye covered. The last full row of letters that the patient can read correctly indicates the acuity level. If the upper row of large letters cannot be seen at 20 ft, the patient should step forward until they become visible; the distance should be recorded in the upper figure (at a distance of 5 ft, the notation would be "5/200"). An acuity of 20/30 or better is generally considered normal for adults. If a standard Snellen wall chart is unavailable, acuity can be tested with pocket eye charts (Rosenbaum or Jaeger charts) held at a distance of 14 in. or, more approximately, by comparing the patient's ability to read printed material with that of the examiner. Illiterate and non–English speaking patients can be tested with the Snellen "E" chart (see Fig. 3.1) by asking whether the letter faces up, down, to the left, or to the right.

Chapter 17 discusses the evaluation of visual acuity in children, screening techniques for amblyopia and strabismus, and other examination procedures (e.g., detection of red reflexes).

Standard Counseling

Parents should be encouraged to contact the clinician if they or teachers note that the child has difficulty seeing or has poor school performance. Older adults should be reminded that although worsening vision is common with increasing age, it should not be accepted as "normal," can limit functional independence, increases the risk of falls and other unintentional injuries, and is often treatable with corrective lenses. Individuals with impaired vision may need to receive counseling about safe driving practices, ranging from modifying driving habits (e.g., reducing nighttime driving for older individuals with visual contrast impairment) to being advised to refrain from any future driving. Older adults at high risk for eye conditions, such as cataracts or glaucoma, or with early disease states (e.g., ocular hypertension) may also benefit from routine examinations by an eye specialist.

Potential Adverse Effects

There are no known adverse effects from visual acuity testing, but inaccurate results can produce unnecessary anxiety, especially among the parents of young children; may affect insurance and employment eligibility; and may incur costs and inconvenience for visits to eye care specialists to rule out a disorder. There is a potential for overly aggressive treatment of early disease or predisease, such as ocular hypertension, which may result in medication-related or surgical complications, with limited benefit. Conversely, inaccurate screening may produce false-negative results, allowing visual disorders to escape detection.

Accuracy and Reliability as Screening Test

Few studies have examined the sensitivity and specificity of visual acuity testing. In children, Snellen letters are estimated to have a sensitivity of 25–79% and a specificity of approximately 85%.

Office and Clinic Organization for Routine Screening

Offices and clinics should be equipped with a Snellen wall chart, a Snellen "E" chart, and eye covers. Visual acuity testing should not be performed in high-traffic areas, where the test is likely to be interrupted by the movement of staff or patients. A floor marker should identify the proper standing

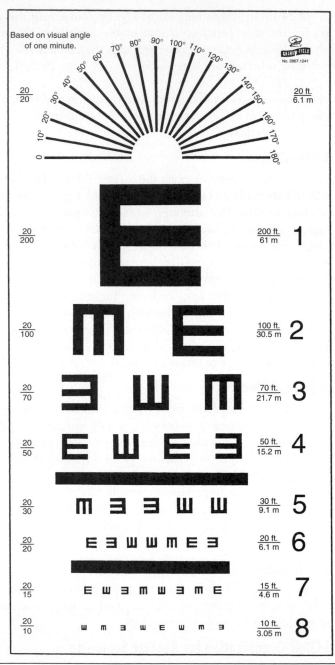

Figure 3.1 • Snellen "E" chart. The patient can be asked in which direction the "legs of the table" point. (Reprinted with permission from Seidel HM, Ball JW, Dains JE, et al. *Mosby's guide to physical examination*, Vol. 38, 2nd ed. St. Louis: Mosby-Year Book, 1991:389.)

position. Nurses and physician assistants can perform visual acuity testing before the clinician's examination. All staff performing the test should be trained in proper technique for performing the test and for recording the results. The office or clinic should have referral and reminder systems (see Chapters 21 and 22) in place to ensure that patients with abnormal visual acuity receive appropriate referrals to eye specialists and to verify that follow-up appointments are kept.

Medical Record Documentation

Visual acuity should be recorded for each eye. When the Snellen eye chart is used to determine the lowest row of letters that the patient can read correctly, indicate the number of letters from the next row that were read correctly (e.g., "20/25 + 2" means that the patient was able to read two letters from the 20/20 row). If strabismus is detected, indicate whether the eye is nasally deviated (esotropia) or temporally deviated (exotropia). The follow-up plan for abnormal visual acuity should be documented.

ORAL CAVITY EXAMINATION

Introduction

Approximately 30,990 new cases of oral cancer occur annually in the United States (7). An estimated 7,430 Americans died in 2006 from cancers of the oral cavity and pharynx. Screening the oral cavity for cancer is advocated because of the potential to improve outcomes through the detection of early-stage disease and because there is little harm or cost associated with the examination. There is little direct evidence, however, that screening for oral cancer results in improved outcomes. Conversely, targeted counseling for modifiable risk factors, such as smoking cessation or alcohol moderation, may be more effective uses of a clinician's limited time.

Screening Guidelines. **Oral cavity screening of asymptomatic persons may be indicated in patients who use tobacco, drink excessive amounts of alcohol, or have found suspicious lesions on self-examination. There is little scientific evidence, however, regarding the effectiveness of or optimal interval for oral cavity screening.**

Official Guidelines. The USPSTF and the AAFP conclude that there is insufficient evidence to recommend for or against routine screening for oral cancer for either high-risk or average-risk adults. The American Cancer Society (ACS) recommends including an oral cavity examination in the general periodic health examination, which it recommends at periodicities based on age-group.

Technique

The oral cavity cancer examination begins with the lips, a potential site of both oral cavity and skin cancer. Dental appliances such as dentures should be removed. Using a tongue blade and a light source, the examiner should systematically inspect the buccal mucosa, gums, dorsum of the tongue, and hard palate. A nodule or growth on the palate, especially if it is not in the midline, should be evaluated further. The teeth should be inspected for plaque and carious lesions and the gums should be inspected for signs of inflammation, bleeding, or recession. The posterior pharynx should be inspected by depressing the tongue with a tongue blade and noting abnormalities in the tonsillar architecture. The hypopharynx can be viewed with a Number 5 mirror (or pharyngoscope).

Ask the patient to touch the tongue tip to the hard palate and inspect the floor of the mouth and the ventral surface of the tongue. Using a gloved hand, wrap the tongue with gauze, pull it to each side to inspect the lateral borders, and palpate the tongue for masses or nodules. White or red material should be scraped to distinguish between food particles and leukoplakia, a precursor to oral neoplasms. An ulcer, nodule, or thickened white patch on the lateral or ventral surface of the tongue may represent a malignancy. Leukoplakia should be suspected if an immovable white lesion resembling white paint is detected on the buccal mucosa, lower lip, tongue, or floor of the mouth.

Standard Counseling

Patients who use tobacco should be advised to stop smoking or chewing tobacco (see Chapter 9), and those who drink excessive amounts of alcohol should receive appropriate counseling (see Chapter 10). All patients should be counseled regarding preventive dental care.

Potential Adverse Effects

The only direct adverse effects of the noninvasive oral cavity examination are the minor discomfort associated with the gag reflex and manipulation of the tongue. The detection of suspicious lesions can produce anxiety until a tissue diagnosis is obtained, however, and follow-up appointments with specialists may incur costs and inconvenience.

Accuracy and Reliability as Screening Test

Few studies have examined the sensitivity and specificity of the oral cavity examination, and the results have been variable, depending on the population, the skills of the examiner, and the study design: a sensitivity of 56–94%, specificity of 73–99%, and positive predictive value of 15–91% have been reported in studies on screening for oral cancer. More comprehensive examinations are likely more sensitive than the brief visual inspection of the oral cavity that is commonly performed by busy clinicians, but they also represent a greater opportunity cost because of the time required to perform the examination. In eight reports of population-based screening interventions, the average yield for suspicious and cancerous lesions was 6 and 0.5%, respectively (8).

Office and Clinic Organization for Routine Screening

The examination room should be equipped with a good light source, tongue blades, and cotton gauze. Referral and reminder systems (see Chapters 21 and 22) should be in place to ensure that patients with abnormal findings receive appropriate referrals to otolaryngologists, dentists, and other appropriate specialists; that the appointments are kept; and that patients with documented disease receive appropriate counseling and treatment.

Medical Record Documentation

The examiner should document that an oral cavity examination was performed and should describe the location, size, and appearance of abnormal lesions. The follow-up plan for suspicious findings should be documented.

CLINICAL BREAST EXAMINATION

Introduction

More than 214,600 new cases of breast cancer are diagnosed each year in the United States (7). It is the second leading cause of cancer death in women, accounting for an estimated 40,970 deaths in 2006 (7). Large clinical trials have demonstrated that mortality from breast cancer can be reduced by 15–20% in women aged 40–69 years who receive routine screening consisting of an annual CBE (breast examination by a physician) and mammography every 1–2 years (1). The balance of benefits to potential harms improves with increasing age and with increasing risk for developing breast cancer (based on family history, personal history, and other risk factors). Although few studies have evaluated the effectiveness of CBE alone compared to no screening, the CBE is a component of most trials that evaluated mammography. Mammography is discussed in Chapter 4 and breast self-examination in Chapter 14.

Screening Guidelines. **CBE as an adjunct to mammography may be offered to all women aged 40 years or older for breast cancer screening.**

Official Guidelines. The USPSTF recommends screening mammography with or without the CBE every 1–2 years for women older than 40 years, but adds that there is insufficient evidence to recommend the CBE alone or to recommend the teaching of breast self-examination. The AAFP supports the Task Force's recommendation, adding the caveat that clinicians should inform patients about the risks and benefits of screening before testing. On the basis of expert opinion, the ACS, the American College of Obstetricians and Gynecologists (ACOG), and the American College of Radiology recommend CBE as part of the periodic health examination beginning at "periodic" intervals between age 20 and 40 years and annually thereafter. The ACOG recommends CBE in all women annually as part of their physical examination.

Patient Preparation

The examination room should have adequate lighting. The patient should disrobe to the waist, remove her brassiere, and dress in a gown. A female chaperone may be advisable, especially if the examiner is a man.

Technique

The clinician should be sensitive to the anxiety of patients undergoing this examination, who often have been sensitized to the risks of breast cancer through lay media or the illnesses of family or friends. The clinician should inspect the breasts for size, symmetry, contour, skin color, and obvious lesions. Dimpling or retractions of the skin, edema resulting in *peau d'orange* texture (appearance of thick skin with large pores and accentuated markings), visible venous networks in one breast, or an abnormal nipple (e.g., bleeding, discharge, ulceration, inversion, retraction) may suggest carcinoma (see Fig. 3.2). Breast inspection is best performed in different positions: first with the patient seated and arms at the side, then with the arms over the head, with the hands pressed against the hips (or palms pushed against each other) to contract the pectoralis muscles, and, finally, with the patient leaning forward to place traction on the suspensory ligaments (see Fig. 3.3).

The breasts (including the nipples and subareolar tissue), axillae, and supraclavicular areas should be palpated in a systematic manner, feeling for lumps, nodules, or lymphadenopathy, with the patient in upright and supine positions. Vertical, concentric, rotatory, and other methods have been recommended for breast palpation (see Fig. 3.4). The most important requirement is that each portion of the breast be fully examined in a systematic manner. Always palpate the tail of the breast, because 40% of malignancies occur in the upper-outer quadrant. The tail is made accessible to palpation by having the patient raise her arms over her head. The entire axilla and supraclavicular areas should be palpated for lymphadenopathy, including the lateral portion along the undersurface of the arm, the anterior wall along the pectoralis muscles, and the posterior portion along the scapular border. Supraclavicular nodes are best palpated by having the patient turn her head toward the side being examined while raising the shoulder and bending the head forward to relax the sternocleidomastoid muscle.

If a breast mass is palpated, the examiner should note its location, size, shape, consistency, tenderness, mobility, and borders. In premenopausal

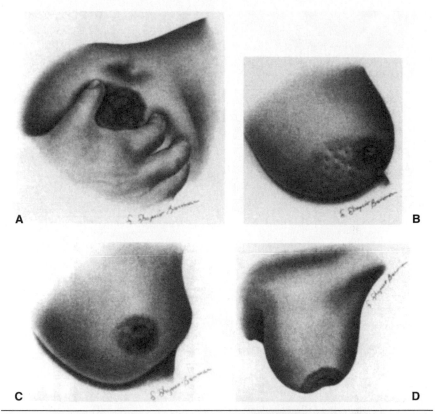

Figure 3.2 • Physical findings on inspection of the breasts. **A:** Skin dimpling. **B:** Edema (*peau d'orange*). **C:** Abnormal contour. **D:** Nipple retraction and deviation. (Reprinted with permission from Bates B. *A guide to physical examination*, 5th ed. Philadelphia: JB Lippincott Co, 1991:336.)

women, it is also important to note the stage of the patient's menstrual cycle. Breast carcinoma is more likely to be firm, nontender, and to produce dimpling or edema of the skin. Breast enlargement, nodularity, and tenderness that occur in monthly cyclical patterns and in different locations of the breast are often related to fibrocystic disease. These patterns are not consistent, however, and malignancy generally cannot be ruled out without careful documentation, repeat examinations, imaging studies, cyst aspiration, and/or tissue biopsy (see Chapter 18). Although small, 3–5 mm mobile axillary lymph nodes are common in adults, the examiner should note the location, size, consistency, and degree of fixation of any palpable nodes.

Standard Counseling

Women aged 40 years and older should be advised about obtaining a screening mammogram every 1–2 years (see page 115). The CBE may be repeated

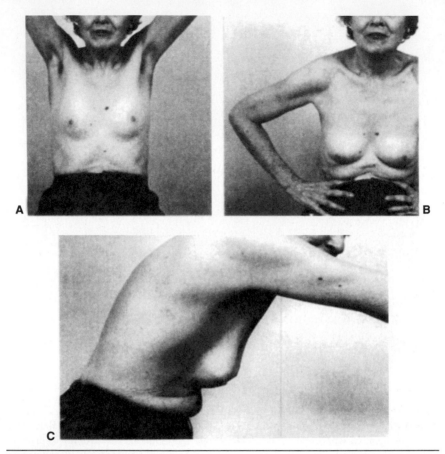

Figure 3.3 • Patient positions for breast inspection. **A:** Arms extended overhead. **B:** Hands pressed against hips. **C:** Leaning forward to place traction on the suspensory ligaments. (Reprinted with permission from Willms JL, Schneiderman H, Algranati PS. *Physical diagnosis: bedside evaluation of diagnosis and function.* Baltimore: Williams & Wilkins, 1994:226.)

annually, but the clinician should ensure that the patient understands its limitations, risks, and potential benefits. Women should be advised to notify the clinician if suspicious masses or lesions are noted on self-examination. If women are performing breast self-examinations they should be counseled on the appropriate technique. See Chapter 14 for further information about breast self-examination.

Potential Adverse Effects

The direct adverse effects of the CBE are embarrassment and discomfort during palpation. The detection of suspicious masses can produce significant anxiety until a tissue diagnosis is obtained and can lead to invasive and

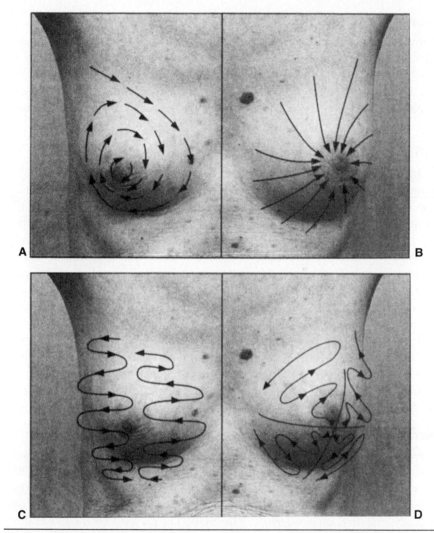

Figure 3.4 • Four alternative methods for systematic palpation of breast. **A:** Spiral, beginning with the tail. **B:** Spokes, periphery to center. **C:** Back-and-forth method. **D:** Quadratic, that is, palpation of each quadrant from areola to periphery. (Reprinted with permission from Willms JL, Schneiderman H, Algranati PS. *Physical diagnosis: bedside evaluation of diagnosis and function.* Baltimore: Williams & Wilkins, 1994:230.)

uncomfortable procedures such as needle aspiration and biopsy. Up to 80% of abnormal CBEs represent false positives. The costs and inconvenience associated with repeat office visits and appointments with specialists can be significant. Inaccurate or incomplete examinations can produce false-negative results, allowing premalignant and malignant lesions to escape detection.

Accuracy and Reliability as Screening Test

Comparing CBE alone to mammography and interval cancer development, CBE (without mammography) has a sensitivity of 40–69%, a specificity of 86–99%, and a positive predictive value of 4–50%. The accuracy and reliability of CBE are affected by the skills of the examiner and the age of the patient: as patients age, fatty tissue replaces fibrocystic tissue and the CBE becomes more accurate.

Office and Clinic Organization for Routine Screening

Examination rooms used for CBE should offer complete privacy, comfortable temperature, and good lighting. The CBE provides an important opportunity for recommending mammography (see Chapter 4) and, if advocated by the clinician, for teaching breast self-examination (see Chapter 14). The office or clinic should therefore have systems in place (see Chapter 21) to easily provide referrals for screening mammograms at the time of the breast examination and, if breast self-examination is recommended, to provide instructions and printed materials on proper technique. The office or clinic should have reliable referral and reminder systems in place to ensure that women return for their next breast examination within 1–2 years; that patients with abnormal findings on breast examination return for follow-up evaluations and, when indicated, receive referrals to surgeons or radiologists; that appointments with outside specialists are kept; and that women found to have breast disease receive appropriate counseling and treatment (see Chapters 21 and 22).

Medical Record Documentation

The examiner should document that a complete breast examination was performed. If a breast lesion is found on examination, the clinician should document the location by noting the quadrant, its diagonal relationship to the nipple ("3 o'clock, 3 cm from the nipple"), its size in centimeters, and the consistency, mobility, and tenderness of the mass. The presence or absence of skin, nipple, and lymph node findings should also be documented. A diagram of the breast, indicating the specific location of the mass, may be helpful for future reference and for describing the findings to other examiners. The follow-up plan for abnormal findings should be documented in the medical record.

PELVIC EXAMINATION

Introduction

The pelvic examination is part of the screening procedure for cervical cancer. It provides a means to visualize the cervix, which is necessary both to collect the Pap smear and to inspect for cervical lesions. The pelvic examination also allows for visualization of labial or vaginal lesions, such as squamous carci-nomas, and palpation of masses that could be suggestive of uterine or ovarian pathology. In 2006, an estimated 9,710 cases of cervical cancer, 41,200 cases of uterine cancer, 20,180 cases of ovarian cancer, and 6,160 cases of vulvar and vaginal cancer were diagnosed (7). Aside from its role in cervical cancer screening, there is little evidence that the pelvic examination is beneficial in detecting other pathology. Vaginal cancers are uncommon and often present symptomatically at an early stage. The pelvic examination is an insensitive means to detect early-stage ovarian or uterine pathology. Chapter 4 reviews the Pap smear, whereas this chapter focuses on the pelvic examination itself.

Screening Guideline. **The pelvic examination is recommended in conjunction with the Pap smear to screen for cervical cancer. Such screening should occur in sexually active women with a cervix, beginning 3 years after the onset of sexual activity or at age 21 years (whichever comes first) and should continue until age 65 years. There is little evidence to support doing a pelvic examination without a Pap smear as a means to screen for cervical, ovarian, uterine, or vaginal cancers.**

Official Guidelines. The AAFP and the USPSTF make similar recommendations as part of their cervical cancer screening guidelines; they do not recommend pelvic examination as a means to screen for ovarian cancer. The ACOG and the ACS recommend a periodic pelvic examination for women older than 19 or 20 years, respectively, or 3 years after the onset of sexual activity.

Patient Preparation

Patient preparation for the pelvic examination involves disrobing from the waist down and donning a gown or drape, lying supine on the examining table, and placing the legs in stirrups. A chaperone is recommended for this physical examination, especially if the examiner is a man.

Technique

A speculum of appropriate size and shape for the patient's vagina should be lubricated and warmed with warm water; jelly lubricants may interfere with cytologic studies for standard Pap smears. With two fingers placed at the introitus, the examiner should gently press down on the perineum and, with the other hand, slowly and gently introduce the closed speculum over the fingers (see Fig. 3.5). The discomfort of pressing on the urethra can be minimized by holding the blades of the speculum obliquely and advancing them along the posterior vaginal wall. Once the speculum enters the vagina, the fingers of the other hand should be removed from the introitus and the blades rotated to a horizontal position. When the speculum is fully advanced, the blades of the speculum should be opened, and the speculum should be maneuvered until the cervix comes into view.

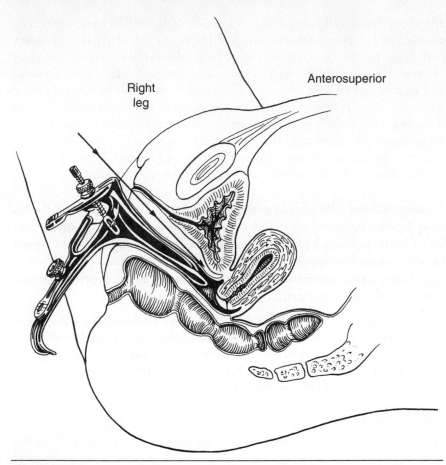

Figure 3.5 • Introduction of the speculum through the introitus. (Reprinted with permission from Willms JL, Schneiderman H, Algranati DS, eds. *Physical diagnosis: bedside evaluation of diagnosis and function*. Baltimore: Williams & Wilkins, 1994:574–575.)

The examiner should inspect the cervix and external os for ulcerations, nodules, masses, bleeding, leukoplakia, or discharge. The squamocolumnar junction (or transformation zone), the region from which 90–95% of cervical cancers arise, should be visualized. The squamocolumnar junction is located on the ectocervix or in the endocervical canal. It often migrates inward with age, so that visualization in older women can be difficult. Any discharge obscuring the view of the cervix should be wiped away. See Chapter 4 for details on performing the Pap test at this stage of the examination.

After removing the speculum the examiner can perform a bimanual examination. Lubricant should be placed on the index and middle finger of the examiner's dominant hand and the fingers should be inserted into the vagina until the tips touch the cervix. The examiner should place the nondominant hand on the patient's suprapubic region. The examiner should then palpate the cervix, uterus, and both adnexa between the two hands, feeling for consistency, mobility, tenderness, and masses.

Standard Counseling

The patient should be advised to return for repeat screening at the recommended interval and should be encouraged to reduce risks of unplanned pregnancy (see Chapter 11) and sexually transmitted infections (see Chapter 12), should these apply to the patient.

Potential Adverse Effects

The pelvic examination and Pap smear can be both embarrassing and uncomfortable. Falsely positive results can generate unnecessary anxiety and follow-up testing, including colposcopy, endocervical curettage, and other procedures. Women incur costs and inconvenience for follow-up cervical examinations. Falsely negative results may allow women with preventable cancers to escape detection.

Accuracy and Reliability as Screening Test

Chapter 4 discusses the accuracy and reliability of the Pap smear, in conjunction with the pelvic examination, in screening for cervical cancer. There is little evidence about the accuracy and reliability of the pelvic examination by itself. In general, however, the isolated pelvic examination is a poor means to identify cervical, ovarian, uterine, or vaginal cancers.

Office and Clinic Organization for Routine Screening

The routine performance of a pelvic examination for cervical cancer screening requires examination rooms with comfortable examination tables equipped with stirrups, good lighting, specula of varying sizes and shapes (including both Graves and Pedersen specula), gloves, lubricant, and gowns or other coverings. Reminder systems (see Chapters 21 and 22) should be in place to ensure that patients return for repeat screening at the recommended interval and that women with abnormal results receive appropriate follow-up and treatment.

Medical Record Documentation

The date and results of the pelvic examination should be placed in the medical record, preferably on a health maintenance flow sheet. The clinician should describe the appearance of the cervix and whether menstruation was noted. For future reference, it may be helpful to note in the medical record whether the uterus is retroverted and if a special speculum was required to visualize the cervix.

DIGITAL RECTAL EXAMINATION

Introduction

Prostate and colorectal cancers together account for more than 83,000 deaths and more than 387,700 new cases of malignancy in the United States each year (7). Colorectal cancer is the second leading cause of cancer death among Americans, and prostate cancer is the second leading cause of cancer deaths among American men. DRE is among the oldest of the screening tests that have been recommended to detect these malignancies, but other tests discussed in Chapter 4 (e.g., PSA for prostate cancer and fecal occult blood testing and endoscopy for colorectal cancer) are far more sensitive. For example, only 3% of colorectal cancers are palpable on DRE. To date, no studies have demonstrated that performing a DRE leads to decreased mortality from prostate cancer or colorectal cancer or improved quality of life. Many clinicians are accustomed to performing the DRE for screening based on their training and their belief that it has benefits and few adverse effects. Additionally, based on past experience, many patients expect a DRE as part of a comprehensive physical examination. The following explanation of how to perform the screening DRE does not necessarily imply an endorsement of the practice by the authors or editors.

Screening Guidelines. **It is reasonable for clinicians to defer a DRE, particularly after discussing its risks and benefits with the patient. Clinicians who do advocate routine DRE as a screening test recommend that the procedure be performed annually after age 50 years — or after age 40 years for individuals at higher risk of developing prostate cancer.**

Official Guidelines. The AAFP and the USPSTF have concluded that there is insufficient evidence to recommend for or against the DRE to screen for prostate cancer. The ACS and American Urological Association recommend that a DRE be offered annually to screen for prostate cancer for men older than 50 years and who have minimum life expectancy of at least 10 years or for men older than 40 years at high risk for prostate cancer (African American men and men with a family history of prostate cancer). Most organizations, whether they recommend DRE or take neutral positions, recommend that clinicians engage patients in a shared decision-making process before performing any prostate cancer screening examination or test. Further details about shared decision making are provided on pages 91–92. No organizations endorse DRE as a means to screen for colorectal cancer.

Patient Preparation

The examination can be performed in the Sim's (lying on left side with hips and knees flexed) or standing position. Explain to the patient why a DRE is indicated and acknowledge that it may be uncomfortable. The patient should be told that a cold-feeling lubricant will be used, that there may be a feeling of urgency for a bowel movement or to urinate, but that neither will occur. A chaperone may be advisable.

Technique

The gloved and lubricated examining finger is inserted through the anus and advanced along the anterior wall of the rectum to the prostate. The examiner should palpate the prostate gland and seminal vesicles across the anterior wall of the rectum. The finger may feel more of the prostate if the examiner's body is turned slightly away from the patient. The examiner should feel the median furrow and middle lobe of the prostate and then sweep the finger across the lateral lobes, noting whether the surface is smooth or nodular, as well as the consistency, shape, size, and mobility of the gland. The normal prostate gland is smooth, rubbery (consistency of a pencil eraser), and nontender, with well-defined borders. The normal size is approximately 3–4 cm in diameter (ordinarily twice the width of the examining finger), with less than 1 cm protrusion into the rectum; size generally increases with age. Prostatic carcinoma can present as one or more posterior nodules, which are often stony hard and painless. With more advanced disease, the entire gland may be stony hard and the median furrow may be obliterated. The patient should be given tissues to remove the lubricant from the perianal area and should be invited to assume a more comfortable position.

As explained in Chapter 4, testing for occult blood after a DRE (as opposed to home testing) does not constitute adequate fecal occult blood testing for colorectal cancer screening and therefore should not be routinely employed. Doing so can increase the likelihood of false-positive results, originating from the trauma of examination, and has a much higher false-negative rate than utilizing three samples collected after normal bowel movements (see page 111). The sensitivity of home occult blood testing on three samples is 23% whereas that of a single post-DRE test is less than 5%.

Standard Counseling

Patients who receive a DRE should be advised that the examination can be repeated annually to rescreen for prostate cancer and that shared decision making should occur before future prostate examinations. Patients should be advised that the in-office DRE does not qualify as a screening test for colorectal cancer and should be encouraged to obtain the screening tests that are recommended in Chapter 4.

Potential Adverse Effects

The direct adverse effects of the DRE are embarrassment and discomfort (e.g., the sensation of having to defecate or urinate, mucosal irritation, anal sphincter spasm, pain from hemorrhoidal disease or anal fissures). If a suspicious prostate mass is detected, the patient may experience considerable anxiety until further testing is completed and may incur costs and inconvenience for follow-up office visits and procedures. Some follow-up tests, such as prostate needle biopsy, have more substantial adverse effects. Such testing may reveal nonaggressive (latent) prostate cancers that pose no risk to health but result in complications from treatments (see Chapters 4 and 19).

Accuracy and Reliability as Screening Test

The sensitivity of the DRE in detecting prostate cancer is limited because the examining finger can only palpate the posterior and lateral aspects of the gland and because stage A tumors—the stage for which screening is intended—are, by definition, nonpalpable. The reported sensitivity of the DRE in detecting prostate cancer in asymptomatic men is approximately 55–68%, but in some studies, it is as low as 18–22%. Moreover, interexaminer reliability—the consistency of findings between examiners—is poor. DRE does enhance the accuracy of the PSA test when performed together—increasing the yield of screening by 26%—but doing so also increases the rate of false-positive findings. Only 6–33% of men with suspicious findings on DRE have histologic evidence of prostate cancer on needle biopsy (1). As already noted, only 3% of colorectal cancers are detectable by DRE.

Office and Clinic Organization for Routine Screening

Examination rooms used for routine screening should offer complete privacy and should be equipped with dressing gowns, gloves, and lubricant. The office or clinic should have reliable referral and reminder systems (see Chapters 21 and 22) in place to ensure that the DRE is repeated at the interval recommended by the clinician, that patients with abnormal rectal examinations receive appropriate follow-up diagnostic studies and consultations with specialists, that appointments are kept, and that patients found to have documented disease receive appropriate counseling and treatment. Home stool testing kits and appropriate referral information for endoscopy should be available to help patients obtain colorectal cancer screening.

Medical Record Documentation

The examiner should document that a DRE was performed. Prostatic enlargement can be graded on the basis of diameter in finger breadths (e.g., 1+ = three fingerbreadths, 2+ = four fingerbreadths, 3+ = five fingerbreadths, 4+ occupies most of the anterior outlet with encroachment of the rectal wall) or of depth of protrusion into the rectum: grade I (1–2 cm), grade II (2–3 cm), grade III (3–4 cm), and grade IV (more than 4 cm). The follow-up plan for abnormal findings should be documented.

SKIN EXAMINATION

Introduction

Skin cancer, including malignant melanoma and squamous and basal cell carcinoma, is the most commonly diagnosed cancer in the United States, with more than 800,000 new cases diagnosed annually. Approximately 62,190 of these cases are malignant melanomas, which claimed an estimated 7,910 lives in 2006 (7). The outcome of malignant melanoma and other skin cancers can be improved significantly if detected early—for example, the mean thickness of melanomas is a predictor of survival—and comprehensive skin cancer screening examinations have therefore been recommended by some organizations. Direct evidence that such examinations reduce the morbidity or mortality of skin cancer is limited, however.

Screening Guidelines. **Although clinicians should remain alert for malignant skin changes in all patients, comprehensive screening examinations of the skin are recommended primarily for persons with a personal history of skin cancer, clinical evidence of precursor lesions (e.g., dysplastic nevi, actinic keratoses, certain congenital nevi), and those with increased occupational or recreational exposure to sunlight. There is no scientific evidence regarding the optimal interval for skin screening.**

Official Guidelines. The USPSTF and the AAFP found insufficient evidence to recommend for or against routine skin cancer screening by total-body skin examination. The ACS recommends including a skin examination in the general periodic health examination.

Patient Preparation

Patients undergoing a comprehensive skin examination should be asked to remove street clothing. The patient should wear a gown during the examination, and skin surfaces should be covered after they are examined.

Technique

For patients undergoing a comprehensive skin examination, the entire skin surface should be examined in a systematic manner to ensure that all areas are inspected. Particular attention should be paid to sun-exposed areas (scalp, face, neck, shoulders, extensor surfaces of arms and hands) and to areas that are easily overlooked during routine self-examination (axillae, buttocks, perineum, backs of thighs, inner upper thighs, intertriginous surfaces). The skin cancer screening examination should search for evidence of basal cell carcinoma, squamous cell carcinoma, and malignant melanoma.

Basal cell carcinoma can be nodular, pigmented, cystic, sclerosing, or superficial, and it usually occurs on the head (especially the face), neck, and back. It may have a translucent, smooth, "pearly" appearance with a central

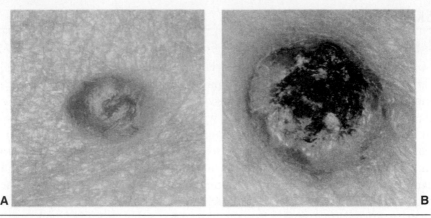

Figure 3.6 • **A**: Basal cell carcinoma. This lesion does not metastasize but it can extend below the skin to the bone. **B**: Squamous cell carcinoma. This lesion can increase in size, developing into large masses, and it can metastasize. (Reprinted with permission from the American Academy of Dermatology.) (See Color Plate.)

depression (see Fig. 3.6A) but can also be pigmented or hyperkeratotic. *Squamous cell carcinoma* often presents as a soft, mobile, elevated mass with a surface scale or a crusting nodule or plaque (Fig. 3.6B), but it can also have other appearances (e.g., the red–brown lesion of squamous cell carcinoma *in situ*, Bowen's disease). It usually occurs on sun-exposed areas such as the scalp, dorsal aspect of the hands, lower lip, and ear. *Malignant melanomas* include superficial spreading, nodular, lentigo, and acral-lentiginous forms. A pigmented lesion is more likely to be malignant if it is asymmetric, rapidly changes in size, or has irregular borders, variegated colors, or a diameter greater than 6 mm (see Fig. 3.7A–D). If suspicious lesions are discovered, the examiner should note the number, location, distribution, and physical characteristics of the lesion, including its size, shape, color, texture, and borders.

Patients with unusual bruises, lacerations, abrasions, or other signs of trauma with an unexplained etiology should be evaluated for a potential history of abuse.

Standard Counseling

Patients (and the parents of pediatric patients) should be reminded about the importance of limiting exposure to ultraviolet light (e.g., limiting time outdoors when ultraviolet light exposure is greatest, wearing hats and clothing covering arms and legs when outdoors, and applying SP 40/50 sunblock). Patients should be counseled to advise the clinician if a skin lesion changes in size, appearance, becomes tender, or starts bleeding; see Chapter 14 for further details about skin self-examination.

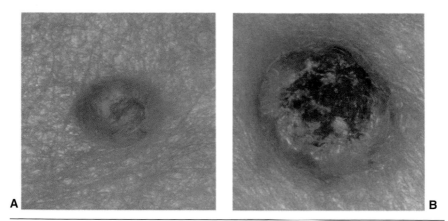

Figure 3.6 • **A**: Basal cell carcinoma. This lesion does not metastasize but it can extend below the skin to the bone. **B**: Squamous cell carcinoma. This lesion can increase in size, developing into large masses, and it can metastasize. (Reprinted with permission from the American Academy of Dermatology.)

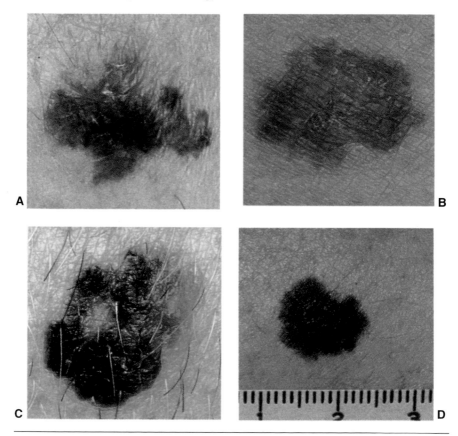

Figure 3.7 • The ABCDs of melanoma: **A**: Asymmetry—one half unlike the other half. **B**: Border—irregular, scalloped, or poorly circumscribed border. **C**: Color—varied from one area to another: shades of tan and brown; black; sometimes white, red, or blue. **D**: Diameter—larger than 6 mm, the diameter of a pencil eraser. (Reprinted with permission from the American Academy of Dermatology.)

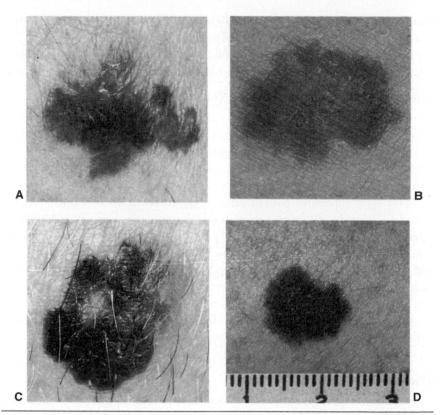

Figure 3.7 • The ABCDs of melanoma: **A:** Asymmetry—one half unlike the other half. **B:** Border—irregular, scalloped, or poorly circumscribed border. **C:** Color—varied from one area to another: shades of tan and brown; black; sometimes white, red, or blue. **D:** Diameter—larger than 6 mm, the diameter of a pencil eraser. (Reprinted with permission from the American Academy of Dermatology.) (See Color Plate.)

Potential Adverse Effects

The only adverse effect of the comprehensive skin examination is the embarrassment associated with being disrobed. Screening can result in unnecessary treatments such as skin biopsies, which can be uncomfortable, may leave a scar, and may require a return office visit for suture removal. The patient may experience anxiety while awaiting the pathology report. Incomplete or inaccurate skin examinations may overlook important lesions and allow cancers to escape detection.

Accuracy and Reliability as Screening Test

Factors affecting the accuracy and reliability of the skin examination include the proportion of the body examined (only 20% of malignant melanomas occur on exposed skin surfaces), the frequency of the examination, the skills of the examiner, and the type of cancer being sought. The positive predictive value of a suspicious lesion detected on screening skin examination is 21–58% for any skin cancer and 6–19% for melanoma. Primary care clinicians may be less accurate than dermatologists in diagnosing preselected abnormal skin lesions.

Office and Clinic Organization for Routine Screening

Examination rooms used for routine skin cancer screening should offer complete privacy, dressing gowns, comfortable temperature, good lighting (preferably daylight or fluorescent lighting), and a magnifying lens or hand-held light source to inspect lesions closely. Because the skin examination provides an important opportunity to counsel patients about avoiding ultraviolet light exposure, patient education literature on this topic can be made available. In offices or clinics in which suspicious lesions are biopsied, equipment for performing biopsies and submitting pathology specimens should be easily accessible. Referral and reminder systems (see Chapters 21 and 22) should be in place to ensure that patients return for repeat skin examinations at the interval recommended by the clinician, that patients with suspicious lesions obtain skin biopsies on site or receive referrals to a physician who performs them, that the results of skin biopsies are obtained from the pathologist and documented in the medical record, and that patients found to have skin disease receive appropriate counseling and treatment.

Medical Record Documentation

The examiner should document that a skin examination was performed and should describe which skin surfaces were inspected. The location, size, color, distribution pattern, and other physical characteristics of suspicious lesions should be described. Standard terms for skin lesions should be used (e.g., macule, patch, papule, nodule, tumor, plaque). A body diagram may be useful in mapping the exact location of lesions. Newer technologies allow clinicians to photograph lesions and incorporate them into the patient's medical record for more accurate longitudinal tracking. If a skin biopsy was performed, the clinician should describe the details of the procedure, including the size of the biopsy specimen (e.g., 3-mm punch), the section of the lesion that was taken (e.g., border, total excision), and the depth of the lesion that was excised (e.g., shave biopsy, full thickness). The follow-up plan for suspicious lesions should be documented.

CONCLUDING REMARKS

The prevention visit goes by many colloquialisms such as the "physical," "wellness examination," "health maintenance examination," or "checkup." These terms echo clinicians' and patients' frequent expectation that the key element of the visit will be a physical examination. While some elements of the examination are important, a thorough head-to-toe examination in asymptomatic individuals has low yield. The time it requires might be more effectively spent counseling patients about modifiable risk factors or arranging indicated screening tests and immunizations (9). Conversely, performing validated examination elements in a hurried, cursory manner may leave important findings undetected. A beneficial prevention examination requires an appropriately systematized, deliberate, focused, and individually risk-based approach. Adopting such an approach is an essential skill set for clinicians who deliver preventive care.

RESOURCES—PATIENT EDUCATION MATERIALS

Sphygmomanometry

National Heart, Lung, Blood Institute
The DASH Eating Plan
http://www.nhlbi.nih.gov/health/public/heart/hbp/dash/

American Academy of Family Physicians
High Blood Pressure: Things You Can Do to Help Lower Yours
http://familydoctor.org/092.xml

Height, Weight, and Head Circumference

American Academy of Family Physicians
Working with Your Doctor to Overcome Overweight and Obesity
http://familydoctor.org/788.xml

National Heart, Lung, and Blood Institute
Aim for a Healthy Weight: Information for Patients and the Public
http://www.nhlbi.nih.gov/health/public/heart/obesity/lose_wt/patmats.htm

Hearing Testing

American-Speech-Language-Hearing Association
Speech and Language Development
http://www.asha.org/public/speech/development/

National Institute on Aging
AgePage: Hearing Loss
http://www.niapublications.org/agepages/hearing.asp

Visual Acuity Testing

American Academy of Family Physicians
Strabismus
http://www.aafp.org/afp/980901ap/980901a.html

American Academy of Pediatrics
Children's Eye Health and Safety
http://www.aap.org/healthtopics/visionhearing.cfm

American Optometric Association
Eye Health
http://www.aoa.org/

National Institute on Aging
AgePage: Aging and Your Eyes.
http://www.niapublications.org/agepages/eyes.asp

Oral Cavity Examination

Oral Cancer Foundation
Oral Cancer Facts
http://www.oralcancerfoundation.org/facts/

American Cancer Society
Learn About Oral Cavity and Oropharyngeal Cancer
http://www.cancer.org/docroot/lrn/lrn_0.asp

Clinical Breast Examination

American Academy of Family Physicians
Breast Cancer: Steps To Finding Breast Lumps Early
http://familydoctor.org/018.xml

American Cancer Society
Learn About Breast Cancer
http://www.cancer.org/docroot/lrn/lrn_0.asp

National Cancer Institute
What You Need to Know About Breast Cancer
http://www.cancer.gov/cancertopics/wyntk/breast

Digital Rectal Examination

American Cancer Society
Learn About Prostate Cancer
http://www.cancer.org/docroot/lrn/lrn_0.asp

Centers for Disease Control and Prevention
Prostate Cancer Screening: A Decision Guide
http://www.cdc.gov/cancer/prostate/publications/decisionguide/

National Cancer Institute
Prostate Cancer Screening
http://www.nci.nih.gov/cancertopics/pdq/screening/prostate/patient/
    allpages

Virginia Commonwealth University
Should You Get a PSA Test? A Patient-Doctor Decision
http://www.acorn.fap.vcu.edu/psa/

Skin Examination

American Academy of Family Physicians
Skin Cancer: Saving Your Skin From Sun Damage
http://familydoctor.org/159.xml

American Cancer Society
Learn About Skin Cancer—Melanoma
http://www.cancer.org/docroot/lrn/lrn_0.asp

American Cancer Society
Learn About Skin Cancer—Nonmelanoma
http://www.cancer.org/docroot/lrn/lrn_0.asp

SUGGESTED READINGS

American Academy of Family Physicians. *Age charts for clinical preventive services and recommended immunization schedules for children and adults*. American Academy of Family Physicians, Available at: http://www.aafp.org/x28209.xml. Last updated March 2007.

American Academy of Pediatrics Committee on Practice and Ambulatory Medicine Section on Ophthalmology, American Association of Certified Orthoptists, American Association of Pediatric Ophthalmology and Strabismus, American Academy of Ophthalmology. Eye examination in infants, children, and young adults by pediatricians: policy statement. Vision screening guidelines. *Pediatrics* 2003;111(4):902–907.

American Cancer Society. *Finding cancer early: ACS guidelines*. Available at: http://www.cancer.org/docroot/PED/content/PED_2_3X_ACS_Cancer_Detection_Guidelines_36.asp?sitearea=PED. Accessed July, 2007.

American College of Obstetricians and Gynecologists. *Primary and preventive care: periodic assessments*. AGOG Committee Opinion No. 246. Washington, DC: American College of Obstetricians and Gynecologists, 2000.

American College of Obstetricians and Gynecologists. Primary and preventive care: periodic assessments. ACOG Committee Opinion No. 292.. *Obstet Gynecol* 2003;102:1117–1124.

American College of Physicians. *Current ACP guidelines*. Available at: http://www.acponline.org/clinical/guidelines/. Accessed January, 2006.

Bickley LS, Szilagi PG. *Bates' guide to physical examination and history taking*, 3rd ed. Philadelphia: JB Lippincott Co, 2002.

Canadian Task Force on the Periodic Health Examination. *CTFPHC systematic reviews and recommendations*. Available at: http://www.ctfphc.org/. Accessed January, 2006.

Committee on Practice and Ambulatory Medicine. *Recommendations for preventive pediatric health care (RE9535). American Academy of Pediatrics*. Available at: http://www.medicalhomeinfo.org/publications/screening.html#general. Last reviewed January 2006.

DeGowin RL, Brown DD. *DeGowin and Dewogin's bedside diagnostic examination*, 7th ed. New Baskerville: The McGraw-Hill Companies, 2000.

Joint National Committee on Detection, Evaluation, and Treatment of High Blood Pressure. *The seventh report of the Joint National Committee on Detection, Evaluation, and Treatment of High Blood Pressure (JNC VII)*. Available at http://www.nhlbi.nih.gov/guidelines/hypertension/jnc7full.htm. Accessed January, 2006.

National Institutes of Health Consensus Development Conference. Diagnosis and treatment of early melanoma. *JAMA* 1992;10:1–26.

Seidel HM, Ball JW, Dains JE, et al. *Mosby's guide to physical examination*, 5th ed. St. Louis: Mosby–Year Book, 2002.

Swartz MH. *Textbook of physical diagnosis: history and examination*, 5th ed. Philadelphia: WB Saunders, 2005.

U.S. Preventive Services Task Force. *Agency for healthcare research and quality*. Available at: http://www.ahrq.gov/clinic/uspstfix.htm. Accessed January, 2006.

References

1. U.S. Preventive Services Task Force. *Agency for healthcare research and quality.* Available at: http://www.ahrq.gov/clinic/uspstfix.htm. Accessed January, 2006.
2. Joint National Committee on Detection, Evaluation, and Treatment of High Blood Pressure. The seventh report of the Joint National Committee on Detection, Evaluation, and Treatment of High Blood Pressure. The JNCVII report. *JAMA* 2003;289: 2560–2572.
3. Flegal KM, Carroll MD, Ogden CL, et al. Prevalence and trends in obesity among US adults, 1999–2000. *JAMA* 2002;288(14):1723–1727.
4. U.S. Department of Health and Human Services. *Healthy people 2010: understanding and improving health*, 2nd ed. Washington, DC: U.S. Government Printing Office, Available at: http://www.healthypeople.gov/, 2000.
5. Caba AJ, Lee DJ, Gomez-Marin O, et al. Prevalence of concurrent hearing and visual impairment in US adults: The National Health Interview Survey, 1997–2002. *Am J Public Health* 2005;95:1940–1942.
6. Kemper A, Harris R, Lieu T, et al. Screening for Visual Impairment in Children 0 to 5 Years. Systematic Evidence Review No. 27 (Prepared by the Research Triangle Institute-University of North Carolina Evidence-based Practice Center under Contract No. 290-97-0011). Rockville, MD: Agency for Healthcare Research and Quality. May 2004. (Available on the AHRQ Web site at: www.ahrq .gov/clinic/serfiles.htm).
7. Jemal A, Siegel R, Ward E, et al. Cancer statistics, 2006. *CA Cancer J Clin* 2006; 56(2):106–130.
8. Canadian Task Force on the Periodic Health Examination. *CTFPHC systematic reviews and recommendations.* Available at: http://www.ctfphc.org/. Accessed January, 2006.
9. Stange KC, Zyzanski SJ, Jaen CR, et al. Illuminating the 'black box.' A description of 4454 patient visits to 138 family physicians. *J Fam Pract* 1998;46(5):377–389.

CHAPTER 4

Laboratory Screening Tests

Janelle Guirguis-Blake, Alex H. Krist, and Steven H. Woolf

Laboratory screening tests include blood work, tests performed at the bedside (e.g., Pap smear), imaging studies, and other laboratory procedures (e.g., audiometry) performed on asymptomatic[a] persons for the early detection of risk factors and preclinical disease. These tests are best used as an adjunct to the focused history and physical examination, rather than in lieu of them. Over time, largely due to time constraints and a cultural emphasis on the value of technology, testing became the central focus of the prevention visit, supplanting the role of the history and physical examination. Even now, many clinicians and patients equate the periodic health examination with a battery of screening tests: for example, obtaining an electrocardiogram, chest radiograph, urinalysis, and a comprehensive panel of blood tests. Many patients inappropriately judge the quality of their clinician by the number of tests that they order.

Several factors have contributed to the prominent role of laboratory screening in the periodic health examination. First, most patients and many clinicians believe that any noninvasive screening test can only be of benefit to a patient (1). Issues about test accuracy (e.g., false positives or false negatives) and the downstream harms and costs of diagnostic workups are rarely considered when ordering what appears to be a "simple laboratory test" (see Chapter 19). For selected laboratory screening tests such as mammography and Pap smears, there is good evidence that periodic screening reduces morbidity and mortality. In many other cases, there is limited evidence about the benefits of the screening tests, but the voices of advocacy organizations and shared anecdotal experiences have led clinicians and patients to assume that screening is better than waiting for a disease to present clinically. Laboratory tests appeal to clinicians for other reasons. Although they are often no more accurate than a careful history and physical examination, test results may be perceived as more reliable because they are generated by

---

[a]"Asymptomatic persons" refers to patients who lack signs or symptoms of the target condition, although they may be symptomatic for other reasons. Therefore, a woman with ulcerative colitis may be asymptomatic with respect to hyperlipidemia. "Asymptomatic" also excludes persons with a prior history of the target condition, such as a healthy woman with a prior history of breast cancer.

sophisticated technologies or because the results are quantitative. Numbers *seem* more accurate than subjective impressions, even if the numbers are inaccurate. Practical factors also promote overuse of screening tests. These include concerns about patient expectations, malpractice liability if tests are not ordered, local and state regulations for screening, and potential financial gain. Laboratory tests are convenient: it is often easier to simply order a battery of tests than to perform a methodical history and physical examination.

The potential harm of ordering laboratory screening tests extends beyond the financial and time costs to the patient and health care system. As discussed in detail in Chapter 19, laboratory screening tests can harm patients through direct physical complications, by generating inaccurate test results, and by setting off a cascade of follow-up tests and procedures that carry additional risks. These risks are influenced by the sensitivity, specificity, and positive predictive value (PPV) of the screening test.[b]

The PPV, the probability of true disease if a screening test is positive, depends on the prevalence, or pretest probability, of the disease. The PPV decreases, and the probability of producing falsely positive results increases, when patients at low risk of disease are tested, a common occurrence with screening. For example, if the pretest probability of disease is 1%, a test with a sensitivity and specificity of 90% has a PPV of 8.3%;[c] 11 patients will receive falsely positive results (and may require workups) for every true case of disease detected. If the probability is only 0.1%, the PPV falls to 0.9%; 111 patients will receive falsely positive results for every true case.

For many blood tests, the "normal range" is defined on the basis of population statistics. These tests are usually flagged as "abnormal" on laboratory printouts if they fall outside the 95% confidence interval (i.e., if less than 5% of the normal population would have the result), not because the result is necessarily pathologic. Because "normal" is defined statistically, if the same test is repeated on 100 healthy persons, an abnormal result will occur an average of five times. For statistical reasons, the probability of such results increases when multiple tests are performed at once, as in blood chemistry panels that combine more than 20 tests at once. For example, when 20 independent variables are tested at once on a chemistry panel, there is a 64% probability of an "abnormal" result, even when no abnormality exists. When such tests are ordered routinely on healthy persons receiving periodic health examinations, the probability of false-positive results is high and the clinician faces an ethical obligation to consider the potential adverse effects.

---

[b] *Sensitivity* is the proportion of persons with disease who correctly test positive. *Specificity* is the proportion of persons without disease who correctly test negative.

[c] The disease would affect 1,000 persons in a population of 100,000 (prevalence = 1%), meaning that 900 (1,000 × 90%) persons with disease would correctly test positive, and 9,900 (1 − [99,000 × 90%]) persons without disease would incorrectly test positive. Thus, only 8.3% (900/9,900 + 900) of positive test results would reflect true disease.

Given these concerns, what laboratory screening tests should clinicians perform routinely in the periodic health examination? With advances in medical technology, clinicians now have at their disposal hundreds of blood tests, imaging technologies, and other modalities that can detect diseases in asymptomatic persons. Since the late 1970s, authorities such as the Canadian Task Force on Preventive Health Care—CTF (formally known as the *Canadian Task Force on the Periodic Health Examination, see page xxxi*) the U.S. Preventive Services Task Force (USPSTF), and the American Academy of Family Physicians (AAFP) have used formal criteria and scientific evidence to weigh the benefits of such tests against their potential harms. In general, screening tests are not recommended unless there is (a) scientific evidence that the test can detect early-stage disease accurately (generating relatively few false-positive results) and (b) that early detection improves the clinical outcome. If the false-positive rate is unacceptably high for universal screening (i.e., because of low disease prevalence, test specificity, or PPV), *selective screening* may be recommended for specific high-risk groups rather than for all patients. Although restrictive recommendations for targeted screening are often viewed as a cost-control policy, their most important benefit often lies in protecting healthy patients from the psychological and physical morbidity associated with inaccurate test results and unnecessary workups. See Chapter 19 for more on the reasons to eschew certain preventive services see Appendix A for a general list of preventive services recommended by the USPSTF, and see Chapter 20 for guidance on which services a practice should adopt in its standard health maintenance schedule.

SHARED DECISION MAKING

Shared decision making, also commonly referred to as *informed decision making*, or *evidence-informed patient choice*, is a patient-centered process in which both the patient and clinician exchange information with each other, jointly contribute to the decision-making process, and come to a conclusion about a plan of action (2). Specifically, the USPSTF defines the goals of shared decision making as helping the patient to do the following:

1. Understand the seriousness of the illness or preclinical disease to be prevented.
2. Understand the preventive service, including the harms, benefits, alternative options, and uncertainties.
3. Weigh his or her values regarding potential benefits and harms associated with the service.
4. Engage in the decision at the desired level.

It takes more time for a clinician to engage in shared decision making than to check boxes on a laboratory requisition form, accompanied by the parting words "you should get these tests." It is important, however, for clinicians to use a consistent, evidence-based approach to offering and discussing preventive screening tests. From a health perspective, evidence that shared decision making improves health outcomes is indirect and mixed; however, the ethical, practical, and educational reasons to engage in shared decision making are compelling. The informed decision-making approach promotes patient autonomy, fosters trust in the patient–clinician relationship, and may increase adherence to care plans. As Chapter 19 discusses in more detail, the scientific evidence for some preventive services is incomplete and the balance of benefits and harms is uncertain or "too close to call." In such situations, including patient values and preferences clarifies the balance of harms and benefits for the individual patient. Even for those preventive screenings grounded in good quality evidence of benefit in population level studies, the benefit to individual patients must incorporate their values about quality of life issues and their willingness and ability to comply with follow-up diagnostic and treatment interventions. With patients' often unrealistic expectations about the ability of medicine to prevent all disease, shared decision making acknowledges the inherent limitations of technology and fosters a more realistic understanding about the harms and benefits of preventive care.

There are several barriers to shared decision making including: patients' limited ability to understand complex medical topics, clinicians' uncertainty about the evidence for the benefit of a preventive service, limited time during clinical encounters, and lack of reimbursement for such discussions (3). Concise decision aids (focused patient education materials) about specific choices in preventive care can help the patient to consider complex medical issues outside of the clinic visit setting and to return to the clinician in follow-up to ask informed questions and make decisions. Resources listed at the end of this chapter include decision aids on specific screening tests, as well as a useful web site (the Cochrane Inventory of Patient Decision Aids) where many other decision aids can be located and evaluated.

Using evidence-based clinic protocols (see Chapter 20), which can be programmed into electronic medical record systems (see Chapter 22), nurses can follow a routine procedure to identify those tests for which a patient may benefit from shared decision making and give such patients appropriate decision aids for review while awaiting the clinician (see also Chapter 21 for the role of nurses and other staff in making these resources available systematically).

CONTENTS OF THIS CHAPTER

This chapter reviews the laboratory screening tests that are commonly recommended for asymptomatic persons (see Appendix A). Research has demonstrated that screening with these tests improves health outcomes (e.g., morbidity, mortality) or has other compelling scientific support. The chapter discusses tests that should be offered to all patients and tests that should be performed on a routine basis only in select subgroups of patients with risk factors, due to low PPV in the general population or other concerns. These recommendations generally conform to the guidelines of evidence-based groups such as the USPSTF. The scientific evidence of the effectiveness of these tests and the arguments for why screening should be limited to selected populations or omitted completely are beyond the scope of this chapter. The reader should consult the references for more information about the scientific evidence for or against screening tests (4). The information in this chapter about screening tests of unproven effectiveness is provided as a guide for those clinicians who choose to use them, but such tests are not necessarily advocated by the editors. The editors specifically discourage the routine use of the screening tests discussed in Chapter 19.

The discussion of each screening test includes a brief introduction describing the target condition and the rationale for the test, a summary of official guidelines issued by major organizations and agencies, and detailed instructions on patient preparation and technique. (The sources of the recommendations in the "Official Guidelines" sections of this chapter are listed under "Suggested Readings" later in this chapter.) Although routine screening rarely detects clinically significant abnormalities, it does provide a setting for counseling patients about primary and secondary prevention of the target condition. Each section of this chapter therefore includes a "Standard Counseling" discussion of the reminders that clinicians should give all patients, even if no abnormality is detected, about how to prevent the target condition, and when to return for screening. This section also refers readers to relevant chapters in Section II of this book, which discuss in more detail how to counsel patients about specific health behaviors. Readers should consult Chapter 18 for guidance on proper follow-up of patients with abnormal results from the screening tests discussed in this chapter.

The discussion of each screening test also addresses the potential adverse effects of screening and the accuracy of the test, and suggestions on how to document screening in the medical record. Data cited in the "Potential Adverse Effects" and "Accuracy and Reliability as Screening Test" sections are drawn from a large body of evidence. The hundreds of studies on which these estimates are based are not cited explicitly in these chapters due to space limitations. The reader interested in the source of these data is referred to other texts that discuss the individual studies in more detail, such as the USPSTF *Guide to Clinical Preventive Services* (4).

To help address patients' questions or their anxiety about the risk of disease, clinicians may wish to provide educational materials such as those listed in the "Resources" section of this chapter, which can explain the meaning of a normal examination and encourage health behaviors for the primary prevention of the conditions for which the patients are being screened. Patient education materials for patients in whom screening tests are *abnormal* are listed in Chapter 18 and elsewhere in this book. The screening recommendations made in this chapter apply only to asymptomatic persons and therefore assume that the patient lacks clinical evidence of the target condition. Thus, for example, recommendations to limit chlamydia screening to persons with risk factors assume that the patient lacks signs or symptoms of infection. This chapter does not address laboratory tests performed in prenatal screening, occupational screening, preemployment screening, or screening for admission to schools.

This chapter encourages clinicians to establish reminder systems in the office or clinic to ensure that patients receive recommended screening tests on time and return for repeat screening at the appropriate interval. See Chapter 21 for detailed recommendations on how to design office systems and routines for this purpose, and see Chapter 22 for specific suggestions about automated reminder systems.

SCREENING BLOOD TESTS

Blood Glucose
INTRODUCTION

Within the chemistry panel, the glucose measurement is the only test for which there is even indirect evidence that screening improves health. Evidence indicates that that early detection and treatment of diabetes when patients also have hyperlipidemia or hypertension may lead to improved health outcomes. In the general population, there is insufficient evidence that screening for diabetes is beneficial in averting either microvascular complications (e.g., nephropathy, retinopathy, neuropathy) or cardiovascular disease. See Chapter 19 for more details.

Screening Recommendations **Screening for diabetes in patients with hypertension or hyperlipidemia should be routinely offered as a part of an integrated approach to reduce cardiovascular risk. Screening those with risk factors for diabetes (e.g., obesity, family history of diabetes, certain racial/ethnic minorities) may be considered. There is limited evidence about the optimal frequency for screening.**

Official Guidelines The USPSTF recommends routine screening in patients with hyperlipidemia and hypertension and concludes that there is insufficient evidence to recommend routine screening in the general population. The American Diabetes Association (ADA) notes that data from prospective studies are insufficient to determine the benefits of routine diabetes screening in the general population and recommends that the decision to test for diabetes should be based on clinical judgment and patient preference. On the basis of expert consensus and epidemiologic evidence that 50% of individuals diagnosed with diabetes have end-organ damage, the ADA recommends that clinicians consider screening for diabetes every 3 years with the fasting plasma glucose (FPG) test beginning at age 45 years and at a younger age for individuals with such risk factors as family history, overweight, and hypertension. The American College of Obstetricians and Gynecologists (ACOG) endorses the ADA recommendations. The American Heart Association recommends measuring FPG in persons aged 20 years and older according to the patient's risk for diabetes, as part of overall risk assessment for cardiovascular disease.

STANDARD COUNSELING

Regardless of whether the clinician and patient decide to screen for diabetes, all patients should be advised to exercise, eat a healthy diet, and maintain a normal weight (body mass index [BMI] of 20–25 kg/m^2) (see Chapters 6–8). More aggressive interventions to establish and maintain these behaviors should be considered for patients at increased risk for developing diabetes, especially those who are overweight or obese, have a family history of diabetes, or have a racial or ethnic background associated with an increased risk (e.g., Native Americans). Intensive dietary and physical activity programs should also be considered for patients who have impaired fasting glucose or impaired glucose tolerance, because good quality evidence from large trials has demonstrated that these programs can reduce the incidence of diabetes in these patients.

DEFINITION OF ABNORMAL RESULT

Three tests have been used to screen for diabetes: FPG, 2-hour postload plasma glucose (2-hour PG), and hemoglobin A1c (HbA1c). As defined by the ADA, an abnormal FPG test suggests diabetes with a value greater than or equal to 126 mg/dL and impaired fasting glucose with a value of 110–125 mg/dL (5). Guidelines advocate FPG for screening because it is easier to perform, more convenient for patients, and less expensive than other screening tests. The FPG is more reproducible than the 2-hour PG test, has less variation, and has similar predictive value for the development of microvascular complications. Compared with the FPG test, the 2-hour PG test may lead to more individuals being diagnosed with diabetes. HbA1c is less sensitive in detecting lower levels of hyperglycemia.

The random capillary blood glucose (CBG) test has been shown to have reasonable sensitivity in detecting persons who have either an FPG level greater than or equal to 126 mg/dL or a 2-hour PG level greater than or equal to 200 mg/dL, provided the results are interpreted according to age and the length of time since the last meal. The random blood glucose test can be used for screening but FPG is preferable.

The ADA recommends confirmation of a diagnosis of diabetes with a repeated FPG test on a separate day, especially for patients with borderline FPG results and patients with normal FPG levels for whom suspicion of diabetes is high.

POTENTIAL ADVERSE EFFECTS

A diagnosis of diabetes could potentially cause "labeling" in asymptomatic individuals (e.g., anxiety, a negative change in self-perception, stigma) and could lead to social consequences (e.g., loss of insurability). Screening can produce false-positive results and subsequent psychological distress, especially in those with "borderline" abnormal results. Medications for diabetes and glucose intolerance can produce side effects (e.g., hypoglycemia, weight gain, gastrointestinal symptoms). For those identified as having impaired glucose tolerance, 30–50% of whom will become euglycemic and not develop diabetes, the side effects of medication could easily outweigh its benefits.

ACCURACY AND RELIABILITY AS SCREENING TESTS

The sensitivity and specificity of the FPG, 2-hour PG, and HbA1c screening for detecting patients with retinopathy are approximately 75–80% at the following thresholds: FPG greater than or equal to 126 mg/dL, 2-hour PG greater than or equal to 200 mg/dL, or HbA1c greater than or equal to 6.4%.

Total Cholesterol and Lipid Profiles
INTRODUCTION

Coronary heart disease is the leading cause of morbidity and mortality in the United States, responsible for approximately 500,000 deaths each year. The risk for coronary heart disease increases with increasing levels of total cholesterol (TC) and low-density lipoprotein cholesterol (LDL-C), and declining levels of high-density lipoprotein cholesterol (HDL-C), in a continuous and graded manner with no clear threshold of risk. See Chapter 1 for web-based tools to calculate a patient's 10-year risk of experiencing a coronary heart disease event, which influences the appropriateness of advising patients to consider aspirin prophylaxis (see Chapter 15).

Screening Guidelines **All high-risk men and women age 20 years and older and average risk men age 35 years and older should be offered periodic TC and HDL-C measurements. Screening may be considered for average-risk women age 45 years and older, although**

there is insufficient evidence that primary prevention in this group improves health outcomes. Those at heightened risk of coronary heart disease include individuals with a personal history of coronary disease, peripheral atherosclerotic disease, or diabetes; those with a family history of premature coronary events; or those with hypertension, tobacco use, or obesity. The optimal interval and stopping age for screening are not certain. The benefits of screening adolescents and children younger than 20 years are also uncertain.

Official Guidelines The USPSTF recommends TC and HDL-C measurement in men aged 35 years and older and high-risk men and women age 20 and older. The National Cholesterol Education Program's Adult Treatment Panel III (ATP III), sponsored by the National Institutes of Health, recommends a fasting lipoprotein profile (TC, LDL cholesterol, HDL-C, and triglyceride) in all adults older than 20 years once every 5 years (6). This recommendation is endorsed by the American Heart Association and the ACOG. The AAFP suggests periodic cholesterol measurement in men aged 35–65 years and in women aged 45–65 years (see Chapter 17 for pediatric guidelines).

STANDARD COUNSELING

All patients, regardless of their lipid levels, should be advised regarding the health benefits of a diet low in saturated fat and high in fruits and vegetables, regular physical activity, avoiding tobacco use, and maintaining a normal weight (see Chapters 6–9).

DEFINITION OF ABNORMAL RESULTS

TC and HDL-C can be measured on nonfasting or fasting samples. For nonfasting measurements, a TC greater than or equal to 200 mg/dL or HDL-C less than 40 mg/dL requires a follow-up lipoprotein profile to determine appropriate management. Optimal LDL, HDL-C and TC as defined by ATP III are listed in Table 4.1.

Abnormal results should be confirmed by a repeated sample on a separate occasion, and the average of both results should be used for risk assessment.

POTENTIAL ADVERSE EFFECTS

Screening for and identifying lipid disorders in adults do not appear to have important psychological sequelae or to produce important changes in indices of mental health although labeling remains a potential harm. Screening low-risk individuals could lead to the costs and inconvenience of treatment with resultant small benefits. Statin therapy is associated with known adverse effects including rhabdomyolysis, increased liver transaminase levels, neuropathy, and other rarer events.

ACCURACY AND RELIABILITY AS SCREENING TESTS

The National Cholesterol Education Program has laboratory requirements for LDL-C testing to ensure precision (coefficient of variance less than 4%) and

TABLE 4.1   Adult Treatment Panel III (ATP III) Classification of Low-density Lipoprotein (LDL), Total, and High-density Lipoprotein (HDL) Cholesterol (mg/dL)

LDL Cholesterol

<100 Optimal

100–129 Near optimal/above optimal

130–159 Borderline high

160–189 High

>190 Very high

Total Cholesterol

<200 Desirable

200–239 Borderline high

>240 High

HDL Cholesterol

<40 Low

>60 High

accuracy (bias less than 4%). Those laboratories meeting these requirements report highly accurate cholesterol values. At least two measurements are necessary to ensure that true values are within 10% of the mean of the measurements. Although most laboratories calculate LDL values, many offer direct LDL measurement, which is highly accurate and can be ordered on nonfasting samples.

Human Immunodeficiency Virus
INTRODUCTION

As of 2004, there were a reported 495,000 persons living in the United States with human immunodeficiency virus (HIV-1) infection or acquired immunodeficiency syndrome (AIDS). One fourth of these individuals were unaware of their HIV status. Those at increased risk for HIV infection include men who have had sex with men after 1975; men and women having unprotected sex with multiple partners; past or present injection drug users; men and women who exchange sex for money or drugs or have sex partners who do; individuals whose past or present sex partners were HIV-infected, bisexual, or injection drug users; persons being treated for sexually transmitted infections (STIs); and persons with a history of blood transfusion between 1978 and 1985. Individuals receiving care in certain high- risk settings are also at increased risk (e.g., STI clinics, correctional facilities, homeless shelters). Since the late 1990s, treatment with highly active antiretroviral therapy (HAART) regimens has markedly reduced the morbidity and mortality associated with HIV. In pregnant women, early identification of maternal HIV seropositivity through universal screening and early antiretroviral treatment with multidrug regimens have been shown to significantly reduce maternal–infant transmission of HIV.

Screening Guidelines **All individuals at high risk for HIV (see risk categories in preceding text) and those who receive medical care in high-risk settings should be offered HIV screening. Universal screening should be routinely offered to all pregnant women in the first trimester and rapid screening for those women who present in labor with unknown HIV status.**

Official Guidelines The USPSTF recommends HIV screening in all adolescents and adults at increased risk for HIV infection and in all pregnant women, and they make no recommendation for or against routinely screening for HIV in adolescents and adults who are not at increased risk for HIV infection. The AAFP, American College of Physicians, and ACOG recommend counseling and HIV testing of high-risk individuals. The Centers for Disease Control and Prevention (CDC) recommends universal HIV screening in patients in all health care settings after patient notification (opt-out screening) and that persons at high risk for HIV infection should be screened for HIV at least annually. The CDC recommends that separate written consent for HIV testing should not be required; general consent for medical care should be considered sufficient to encompass consent for HIV testing. The American Academy of Pediatrics (AAP) considers all sexually active adolescents to be a high-risk group and recommends they be counseled and offered HIV testing.

STANDARD COUNSELING

HIV testing should be accompanied by pretest and posttest counseling. Ideally, the clinician should disclose all HIV results in person, regardless of whether the test is positive or negative.

All sexually active individuals should be counseled regarding the importance of prevention of STIs; such preventive measures include counseling regarding abstinence, consistent condom and spermicide use, and maintenance of mutually monogamous relationships (see Chapter 12). All sexually active adolescents and adults should be made aware of the contribution of alcohol in risky sexual practices. Prevention of HIV transmission in individuals who use injection drugs includes referral to drug rehabilitation programs, use of clean needles and paraphernalia, and education regarding the dangers of impaired judgment leading to risky sexual activity while intoxicated.

DEFINITION OF ABNORMAL RESULTS

The standard test for diagnosing HIV infection includes the repeatedly reactive enzyme immunoassay followed by confirmatory Western blot or immunofluorescent assay. A positive result on both the enzyme assay and confirmatory test identifies those individuals with HIV.

POTENTIAL ADVERSE EFFECTS

Since false-positive test results are rare, harms associated with HIV screening are minimal. Potential harms of positive test results include increased anxiety, labeling, and effects on close relationships. Documented HIV infection can also influence insurance coverage and employment opportunities.

Accuracy of Screening Tests

Standard testing for HIV infection with the repeatedly reactive enzyme immunoassay followed by confirmatory Western blot or immunofluorescent assay, has a sensitivity and specificity greater than 99%. False-positive test results are rare, even in low-risk settings. Compared with standard HIV testing, the reported sensitivities of rapid tests on blood specimens range from 96–100%, with specificities greater than 99.9%. Reported sensitivities and specificities of oral fluid HIV tests are also high (greater than 99%).

Syphilis
INTRODUCTION

In 2004, the reported nationwide incidence rate of primary and secondary syphilis infection was 2.7 per 100,000 persons. Syphilis, an infectious disease caused by the bacterium *Treponema pallidum*, causes a variety of symptoms depending on the stage of infection (primary, secondary, tertiary) and no symptoms during latent stages. Congenital syphilis results in fetal or perinatal death, as well as serious complications in surviving newborns. Populations at increased risk for syphilis infection include men who have sex with men and engage in high-risk sexual behavior, commercial sex workers, persons who exchange sex for drugs, and those in adult correctional facilities. There is no evidence to support screening for syphilis among individuals currently or previously infected with another sexually transmitted organism.

Screening Guidelines   **All high-risk adolescents and adults (see preceding discussion of high-risk groups) and all pregnant women should be offered syphilis screening.**

Official Guidelines The USPSTF strongly recommends screening persons at increased risk for syphilis infection and all pregnant women and recommends against routine screening of asymptomatic persons who are not at increased risk for syphilis infection. The AAFP clinical policy statement concurs with the USPSTF recommendations. The AAP and ACOG recommend prenatal screening for syphilis. The CDC recommends screening in all pregnant women at the first prenatal visit, and repeat screening early in the third trimester and at delivery for all high-risk women (e.g., those who live in areas of excess syphilis morbidity, are previously untested, or have positive serology in the first trimester). The CDC also recommends screening in all sexually active men who have sex with other men and in those individuals with HIV infection.

STANDARD COUNSELING

All sexually active individuals should be counseled regarding the importance of prevention of STIs; such preventive measures include counseling regarding abstinence, consistent condom and spermicide use, and maintenance of mutually monogamous relationships (see Chapter 12).

DEFINITION OF ABNORMAL RESULTS

Nontreponemal tests commonly used for initial screening are the Venereal Disease Research Laboratory (VDRL) or Rapid Plasma Reagin (RPR) tests, followed by a confirmatory fluorescent treponemal antibody absorption assay (FTA-ABS) or *Treponema pallidum* particle agglutination (TP-PA) test. Positive results on the confirmatory FTA-ABS or TP-PA identify those individuals with *T. pallidum* infection. See Chapter 12 for proper follow-up and treatment of patients with abnormal results from screening.

ADVERSE EFFECTS

Potential harms of screening may include opportunity costs to the clinician and patient (time, resources, and inconvenience). False-positive results may lead to stress, labeling, concerns about fidelity, and further testing. Harms of treatment include drug-related side effects including penicillin allergy and the Jarisch-Herxheimer reaction (febrile reaction with headache, myalgia, and other symptoms), which may occur within the first 24 hours of any therapy for syphilis.

ACCURACY OF SCREENING TESTS

The sensitivity of the RPR and VDRL tests is estimated to be 78–86% for detecting primary syphilis infection and 95–100% for later stages. Specificity ranges from 85–99% and may be reduced in individuals who have certain preexisting conditions (e.g., collagen vascular disease, pregnancy, injection drug use, advanced malignancy, tuberculosis, malaria, viral and rickettsial diseases). The confirmatory FTA-ABS test has a specificity of 96%. The PPV and number needed to screen (NNS, see page 499 in Chapter 19) are highly dependent upon the population prevalence of syphilis. For example, in a low-risk population, the NNS to detect a single case of syphilis is 24,000 whereas in a high-risk population of incarcerated women, the NNS would be only 10.

Prostate Cancer Screening with Prostate-Specific Antigen

INTRODUCTION

Prostate cancer is the second leading cause of cancer deaths in men. Incidence increases with age, and more than 75% of cases occur in men older than 65 years. Other risk factors include being African American and having a family history of a first-degree relative with prostate cancer. While prostate cancer is a major cause of cancer death in males, many more men are diagnosed with the disease than die from it. Men in the United States have a 15% lifetime risk of being diagnosed with prostate cancer, but only a 3% lifetime risk of dying from the disease. Prostate-specific antigen (PSA) and digital rectal examination (DRE) are the two predominant screening modalities for prostate cancer. Although it is certain that screening can detect prostate cancer in early stages, research has not proved whether screening reduces the death rate from prostate cancer. Given the known harms of the diagnostic workup that follows an abnormal PSA and the harms of treatment, the balance of the benefits and harms is uncertain.

Screening Guidelines **Clinicians should not order the PSA test without first engaging the patient in a shared decision-making process (see "Shared Decision Making" on pages 91–92). The population most likely to benefit from screening is average-risk men between the ages of 50 and 70 years with at least a 10-year life expectancy and high-risk men (African Americans or men with a first-degree relative with prostate cancer) between the ages of 45 and 70 years.**

Official Guidelines The USPSTF concluded in 2002 that the evidence was insufficient to recommend for or against routine screening for prostate cancer using PSA or DRE but acknowledged that some clinicians and patients may elect screening for other reasons. The AAFP concurs with this recommendation. The American Cancer Society (ACS) and American Urologic Association advise clinicians to discuss the potential harms and benefits with patients and to offer the test to all men aged 50 years and older who have at least a 10-year life expectancy, and to younger men (approximately age 45 years) at higher risk (African American men and men with a first-degree relative with prostate cancer).

STANDARD COUNSELING

Before ordering PSA testing, shared decision making should include the following: (a) discussion of the potential benefits and possible harms of PSA screening including the false- negative and false-positive results, the downstream adverse effects of the diagnostic workup (pain, bleeding, infection following biopsy) and treatments (erectile dysfunction, urinary incontinence, bowel dysfunction following radical prostatectomy), (b) consideration of patient preferences with respect to the adverse effects of treatments, and (c) agreement as to whether or not to screen. Such counseling and the agreed upon decision should be documented in the medical record.

DEFINITION OF ABNORMAL RESULTS

A PSA value greater than or equal to 4.0 ng/mL is generally considered abnormal. PSA density (the PSA concentration divided by gland volume), percent free PSA (the proportion of PSA that is unbound), PSA velocity (the rate of increase in PSA per unit of time), and age-specific and race-specific normal references have been proposed to improve the sensitivity or specificity of total serum PSA measurement. It is uncertain whether these other measurements improve the detection of clinically significant disease and whether they reduce unnecessary biopsies from false-positive results.

POTENTIAL ADVERSE EFFECTS

An abnormal screening test for prostate cancer often produces some anxiety. Less than 10% of men experience interference with daily activities as a result of prostate biopsy, a common feature of the diagnostic workup of an abnormal PSA. Fewer than 1% of patients undergoing biopsy have serious complications, including infections. Screening may lead to surgery, radiotherapy, or other treatments that carry a significant risk for complications, such as erectile, urinary, and bowel dysfunction. For indolent cancers, these adverse treatment effects occur without the benefit of a reduction in the risk of progressive prostate cancer.

ACCURACY AND RELIABILITY

A PSA greater than or equal to 4.0 ng/mL has an estimated sensitivity of 63–83% and a specificity of approximately 90% in the first screening. Specificity decreases with increasing age and the presence of benign prostatic hyperplasia. The combination of DRE and PSA increases the sensitivity of screening, but it also increases the rate of false-positive results.

OTHER LABORATORY SCREENING TESTS

Pap Smears
INTRODUCTION

The Pap smear is performed routinely to detect cervical dysplasia, carcinoma *in situ*, and invasive carcinoma. In the United States, it is estimated that approximately 10,000 new cases of cervical cancer were diagnosed in 2006, and 3,700 patients died from this disease. Women who have never been screened account for most invasive cervical cancers and cervical cancer-related mortality. Infection with human papillomavirus (HPV), a sexually transmitted organism, is a major risk factor for cervical cancer. HPV types 16 and 18 are known to be oncogenic. Other risk factors for cervical cancer include early onset of intercourse, a large number of sexual partners, and cigarette smoking.

Screening Guidelines **All sexually active adolescent and adult women with an intact cervix should be routinely offered Pap smear screening (regardless of HPV vaccination status). Those at low risk for cervical cancer can undergo screening every 2–3 years following three normal annual Pap smears. Women at high risk for HPV and cervical dysplasia (e.g., documented HPV infection, history of abnormal Pap smears, early onset of intercourse, large number of sexual partners, and cigarette smoking) should undergo annual screening. Women who have had adequate screening with normal smears can discontinue Pap smear at age 65 years. Pap screening is unnecessary after a hysterectomy for a nonmalignant indication. There is no role for HPV testing as a screening test (it may be appropriate as part of *a diagnostic workup* for an abnormal Pap smear—see page 477). See Chapter 16 regarding HPV vaccination for the primary prevention of cervical cancer.**

Official Guidelines The USPSTF strongly recommends screening for cervical cancer in women who have been sexually active and have a cervix; recommends against routinely screening women older than 65 years for cervical cancer if they have had adequate recent screening with normal Pap smears and are not otherwise at high risk for cervical cancer; and recommends against routine Pap smear screening in women who have had a total hysterectomy for benign disease. The USPSTF concludes that the evidence is insufficient to recommend for or against the routine use of new technologies (e.g., liquid-based methods or thin layer cytology [ThinPrep, AutoCyte PREP]) to screen for cervical cancer or routine HPV testing as a primary screening test for cervical cancer. The ACS and ACOG both recommend initiating screening 3 years after a woman becomes sexually active or at age 21 years; screening should entail annual Pap tests (or biannual if using a liquid-based prep) until age 30 years and can then be repeated every 2–3 years thereafter. The AAFP, ACOG, American College of Preventive Medicine, American Medical Association, and AAP recommend beginning screening at the onset of sexual activity or at age 18 years. They recommend that initial screening be conducted annually, or less frequently after three or more normal annual smears, based on patient risk factors and the discretion of the patient and clinician. The ACS and AAFP recommend discontinuing screening, or offering the option for patients to discontinue screening, after age 65 or 70 years provided there is documented evidence of adequate past screening.

PATIENT PREPARATION

The Pap smear is usually obtained during the pelvic examination (see Chapter 3 for further discussion of the pelvic examination).

TECHNIQUE

The selection and insertion of the speculum are discussed in Chapter 3. The examiner should inspect the cervix and external os for ulcerations, nodules, masses, bleeding, leukoplakia, or discharge. The clinician should visualize the squamocolumnar junction or transformation zone, located on the ectocervix or in the endocervical canal, where 90–95% of cervical cancers arise. Current evidence is equivocal as to whether the detection of cervical cancer is increased by sampling endocervical cells, but many laboratories consider smears inadequate if these cells are absent. The squamocolumnar junction often migrates inward with age, so that visualization in older women can be difficult. Any discharge obscuring the view of the cervix should be wiped away.

To maximize the likelihood of obtaining endocervical cells from the squamocolumnar junction, a complete Pap test requires the collection of specimens from the endocervical canal and the ectocervix. The two common collection techniques available at this time include (a) the wooden Ayre or extended tip spatula and endocervical brush (see Fig. 4.1), and (b) the cervical broom (e.g., Cervex-Brush or Papette [see Fig. 4.2]). The adequacy of sampling is improved by using the cervical broom. In the first technique, the endocervical sample is obtained by inserting the endocervical brush into the canal and rotating it 180 degrees between the fingers. The ectocervical specimen is typically obtained with a wooden Ayre spatula or extended type spatula. (A plastic spatula is used with liquid-based technologies.) The longer end of the spatula is placed in the os, and the spatula is rotated in a circular manner so that a full scraping of the squamocolumnar junction is obtained. The second technique, in which the cervical broom is inserted and rotated five complete turns, allows simultaneous sampling of endocervical and ectocervical cells.

Conventional Pap smear techniques involve spreading specimens (obtained by either spatula/brush or broom) onto one or more glass microscope slides and immediately applying either 95% ether-alcohol or a spray fixative. When using liquid-based technologies, the samples are then placed into a vial containing an alcohol-based preservative.

After plating the Pap smear and completing the examination, the patient should be told that the speculum will be removed; the speculum should be returned to the oblique angle before being gently withdrawn. Details about the patient's history (age, last menstrual period, type of contraception, previous cervical diagnoses or treatment) and relevant physical findings should be noted for the cytopathologist on the laboratory requisition form.

STANDARD COUNSELING

The patient should be advised to return for repeat screening at the recommended interval and should be encouraged to reduce risks of acquiring STIs (see Chapter 12).

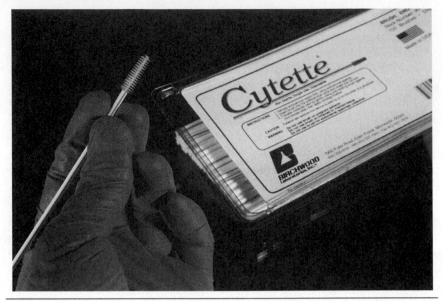

Figure 4.1 • Endocervical brush. Cytette, Birchwood Laboratories, Inc., Eden Prairie, MN, USA.

DEFINITION OF ABNORMAL RESULTS

The Pap smear may suggest the presence of cancer or its precursors if the laboratory reports squamous intraepithelial lesions, atypia including atypical squamous cells of unknown significance (ASCUS), dysplasia, cervical intraepithelial neoplasia (CIN), squamous cell carcinoma, or adenocarcinoma. The presence of HPV is also abnormal, and many laboratories automatically perform HPV testing (commonly referred to as *reflex HPV testing*) when liquid-based Pap smears are abnormal. Cervical samples that are identified by the laboratory as inadequate (e.g., due to absence of endocervical cells) may necessitate repeat testing, but there is little evidence regarding how many attempts should be made to obtain adequate specimens or whether the effort will result in improved cancer detection.

POTENTIAL ADVERSE EFFECTS

The pelvic examination and Pap smear can be both embarrassing and uncomfortable. False-positive results can generate unnecessary anxiety and follow-up testing, including colposcopy with biopsy, endocervical curettage, and other procedures that carry associated risks (e.g., bleeding, infection, uterine perforation, cervical stenosis or cervical incompetence). Women incur costs and inconvenience from follow-up cervical examinations. False-negative results may allow preventable cervical cancers to escape detection.

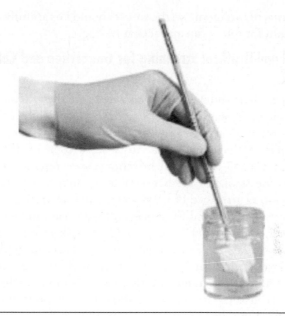

Figure 4.2 • Cervical broom. Papette, Wallach Surgical Devices, Inc., Orange, CT, USA.

ACCURACY AND RELIABILITY AS SCREENING TEST

Older studies reported that the Pap smear had a sensitivity of 47% (confidence interval = 30–87%) and a specificity of 95% (confidence interval = 86–100%) in detecting low-grade squamous intraepithelial lesions and CIN 2–3; this wide range in reported accuracy reflects limitations in study quality and heterogeneity in reference standards and disease prevalence rates. Recent trials comparing the Pap smear and liquid-based cytology suggest that sensitivity is similar, while the specificity of liquid based cytology is lower for detecting CIN 2 or greater. Some studies performed outside the United States suggest that liquid based cytology may yield superior specimens but these conclusions may not be generalizable to the U.S.

MEDICAL RECORD DOCUMENTATION

The date and results of the Pap smear should be documented in the medical record, preferably on a health maintenance flow sheet. The clinician should describe the appearance of the cervix and whether menstruation was noted. For future reference, it may be helpful to note in the medical record whether the uterus is retroverted and if a special speculum was required to visualize the cervix. When the Pap smear results are available, the presence of cellular atypia, dysplasia, or carcinoma on the smear should be carefully documented, along with plans for follow-up and repeat testing.

Endocervical and Urethral Screening for Gonorrhea and Chlamydia
INTRODUCTION

Chlamydia trachomatis and *Neisseria gonorrhoeae* are the two most commonly reported notifiable diseases in the United States. While chlamydia and gonorrhea are often considered similar STIs, chlamydia is far more common and underreported than gonorrhea. In 2002, a total of 351,852 cases of gonorrhea and 834,555 chlamydial infections were reported in the United States. Age is the strongest predictor of both chlamydial and gonorrheal infection: adolescent girls aged 15–19 years and men aged 20–24 years have the highest rates of chlamydia and women aged 15–24 years and men aged 20–24 years have the highest risk of gonorrhea. Other risk factors include having multiple or new sexual partners, inconsistent use of barrier contraceptives, and a history of previous or concurrent STI. In women, chlamydial and gonorrheal infection cause urethritis, cervicitis, and pelvic inflammatory disease. In men, infection results in acute urethritis, epididymitis, or prostatitis, and rarely chronic complications including chronic prostatitis and reactive arthritis. Treatment is highly effective.

Screening Recommendations **All sexually active women age 24 and younger, women at high risk (see preceding text for risk factors), and pregnant women should be offered screening for chlamydia and gonorrhea. Screening of nonpregnant women should be offered annually. Screening of pregnant women should be offered in the first trimester, followed by repeat screening in the third trimester for those at high risk. In areas with low prevalence of gonorrhea, clinicians may choose to screen only for chlamydia. Routine screening of men is not recommended.**

Official Guidelines
Chlamydia. The USPSTF and AAFP recommend that clinicians routinely screen for chlamydia infection in all sexually active women younger than 25 years (including pregnant women) and all other asymptomatic women at increased risk. They make no recommendation for or against screening asymptomatic low-risk women (pregnant or non-pregnant) and conclude that there is insufficient evidence to recommend for or against routine screening in men. ACOG recommends routine screening for chlamydial infection for all sexually active adolescents and other asymptomatic women at high risk for infection and all pregnant women. The CDC recommends annual chlamydia screening for sexually active women younger than 20 years and for older women who meet specific risk criteria.

Gonorrhea. The USPSTF recommends that clinicians screen all sexually active women including pregnant women who are at increased risk for gonorrheal infection; recommends against routine screening for gonorrhea infection in men and women who are at low risk for infection; and concludes that there is insufficient evidence to recommend screening in high-risk men and low-risk pregnant women. The AAFP and ACOG recommend screening sexually active women, including adolescents, at high risk for gonorrhea. The AAFP, ACOG, and AAP recommend screening pregnant women at risk for gonorrhea. The CDC recommends that clinicians screen all sexually active men who have sex with men for genital gonorrhea at least annually. Screening for rectal and pharyngeal gonorrhea is also recommended if there is a risk of exposure.

Complete treatment guidelines for chlamydia and gonorrheal infection are available from the CDC (7). See Chapter 12 for more details.

PATIENT PREPARATION

In women, the chlamydia and gonorrhea specimen is usually obtained during the pelvic examination. However, urine specimens can also be collected if a pelvic examination is not performed. For cervical collection, the patient must disrobe from the waist down, don a gown or drape, lie supine on the examining table, and place the legs in stirrups. Men must lower their trousers and briefs and should sit or lie supine to prevent falls from vasovagal reactions. The patient should be cautioned that the procedure may be uncomfortable. A chaperone may be advisable, especially if the patient is of the opposite sex of the examiner.

TECHNIQUE

Screening can be accomplished using culture, nucleic acid amplification tests, and nucleic acid hybridization tests (nucleic acid probes). Culture isolates can be collected from endocervical swabs in women and urethral swabs in men. Chlamydia and gonorrhea screening are often performed with a single specimen collection. In many circumstances based on local epidemiology, clinicians may choose to screen for only one of these infections.

In women, the technique for cervical specimens (whether sent for culture, nucleic acid amplification tests, or nucleic hybridization tests) is similar: the specimen is obtained by inserting and rotating the swab or cytology brush in the endocervical canal; depending on the type of laboratory test, the duration that the swab should remain in the endocervical canal may vary. Instructions are available from swab manufacturers. Newer DNA amplification tests can be used with urine samples and cervical swabs. If urine is used, a midstream sample is sent to the laboratory for analysis; cervical swabs can be collected as described earlier.

In men, the urethral specimen is obtained by advancing the culture swab approximately 2–3 cm into the urethra. Just as in women, urine samples can be used for screening.

STANDARD COUNSELING

All sexually active patients should be counseled to maintain safe sexual practices and should receive instructions on the correct use of condoms and spermicides (see Chapter 12). Women at increased risk should receive information about the early signs and symptoms of pelvic inflammatory disease. Adolescents should be advised that abstinence from sexual intercourse is the most effective preventive strategy.

POTENTIAL ADVERSE EFFECTS

Specimen collection can be uncomfortable, in both men and women. This is especially so when specimens are obtained from the urethra of men, who can experience vasovagal reactions. False-positive results can cause unnecessary anxiety, concerns about infidelity, and unnecessary treatment. False-negative results can result in treatment delays and inadvertent transmission to other sexual contacts.

ACCURACY AND RELIABILITY AS SCREENING TEST

Chlamydia screening tests that utilize amplified DNA assays (such as polymerase chain reaction and ligase chain reaction) have demonstrated sensitivity ranging from 81–100% and specificity ranging from 96–100% when compared to endocervical culture. For gonorrhea, sensitivity for nucleic acid amplification tests ranges from 67–100%, with specificity ranging from 94–100%. Nucleic acid amplification tests may be used with urine specimens in addition to endocervical and urethral swabs, and single specimens can be used to test for chlamydia as well as gonorrhea.

MEDICAL RECORD DOCUMENTATION

The date and results of the tests should be documented in the medical record. If results are positive, partner treatment and public health department notification (see Chapter 12) should be arranged and documented in the medical record.

Colorectal Cancer Screening
INTRODUCTION

Colorectal cancer (CRC) is the fourth most common cancer in the United States and is the second leading cause of cancer deaths, claiming 55,000 lives in 2006. Incidence is low until 45 years of age after which the incidence increases with each year of life. A 50-year-old person has a 5% chance of being diagnosed with CRC and a 2.5% chance of dying from this disease. Risk factors for CRC include age (older than 50 years), first-degree relative with a history of CRC, a family history of hereditary nonpolyposis CRC or familial adenomatous polyposis, and a personal history of ulcerative colitis. However, most cases occur in persons of average risk with age older than

50 years as the sole risk factor. Studies demonstrate that screening reduces the incidence of and mortality from CRC. Screening facilitates the removal of premalignant adenomatous polyps and the detection of early-stage disease, which is more amenable to treatment. While most polyps will not progress to CRC, the benefits of removing larger adenomatous polyps outweigh the risks of doing so.

***Screening Guidelines* All adults age 50 years and older should be offered screening for CRC. Acceptable screening tests include any of the following five options: (a) home fecal occult blood test (FOBT) every year, (b) flexible sigmoidoscopy every 5 years, (c) the combination of home FOBT every year and flexible sigmoidoscopy every 5 years, (d) colonoscopy every 10 years, or (e) double-contrast barium enema every 5 years. Barium enema is rarely used for screening, however. Colonoscopy should be offered earlier and more frequently for high risk individuals (e.g., those with a first-degree family history of CRC or hereditary polyposis syndromes). See page 114 regarding newer screening technologies.**

Official Guidelines   The USPSTF recommends screening for CRC in men and women age 50 years and older, or earlier for those with risk factors. Screening methods include FOBT, sigmoidoscopy, colonoscopy, and double contrast barium enemas. The ACS recommends screening average risk adults beginning at age 50 years with either yearly FOBT, flexible sigmoidoscopy every 5 years, FOBT plus flexible sigmoidoscopy every 5 years, a double contrast barium enema every 5 years, or a colonoscopy every 10 years. For individuals with a first-degree relative with CRC, the ACS recommends beginning screening colonoscopy at age 40 years or 10 years before the family member's diagnosis, and repeating the colonoscopy every 5–10 years. For individuals at very high risk, colonoscopy should begin at an earlier age and should be repeated every 1–2 years. For example, individuals with familial adenomatous polyposis should have genetic testing and colonoscopy every 1–2 years beginning at puberty. The American Gastroenterological Association and a consortium of other gastroenterological associations, the AAFP, and the American College of Surgeons make similar recommendations.

Fecal Occult Blood Test
TECHNIQUE

The FOBT can be performed in the examination room along with the DRE (see Chapter 3), but in-office FOBT is discouraged for screening because it is less accurate than home testing by the patient (8). With home testing, patients are generally given three cards impregnated with guaiac and are asked to collect two specimens from three separate consecutive stool samples. The patient is given instructions to avoid eating red meat (beef, lamb, including processed meats and liver), fish, uncooked fruits, and vegetables (especially melons, radishes, turnips, and horseradish), foods or supplements containing large amounts of vitamin C, nonsteroidal antiinflammatory agents, corticosteroids, and other medications that can cause gastritis during the week before the specimens are obtained. Evidence regarding the need for these restrictions is limited. Menstruating women and patients with active bleeding from rectal disorders (e.g., hemorrhoids) should postpone specimen collection until 3 days after the bleeding has ended. The patient should then mail or deliver the cards to the clinician's office in the provided preaddressed envelope.

When the slides are received, a drop of developer fluid is applied to the specimens, with blue discoloration representing an abnormal result. Rehydration of the dried specimens increases sensitivity at the expense of specificity, thereby increasing the likelihood of false-positive results. See page 114 regarding newer stool testing technologies.

POTENTIAL ADVERSE EFFECTS

The FOBT can be distasteful and embarrassing. Some patients report that they find the FOBT unpleasant or difficult to perform. Potential harms arise when false-positive screens lead to unnecessary invasive testing or false negatives lead to false reassurance. Colonoscopy examinations precipitated by FOBT screening incur risks such as bleeding or bowel perforations. Those risks increase with therapeutic procedures, such as a polypectomy or biopsy.

ACCURACY AND RELIABILITY AS SCREENING TEST

The sensitivity of FOBT varies with the frequency of testing and the method. Sensitivity and specificity for unhydrated specimens have been estimated at 40% and 96–98%, respectively. Hydration of the specimen increases sensitivity (60%) but reduces specificity (90%), resulting in more false-positive results. In the key studies evaluating FOBT, the PPV for detecting cancer and large polyps was 2–18% and 8–40%, respectively.

Sigmoidoscopy and Colonoscopy
INTRODUCTION

Endoscopy (sigmoidoscopy or colonoscopy) is a principal screening test for detecting adenomatous polyps and CRC. Both sigmoidoscopy and colonoscopy have the potential to be diagnostic and, by removing precancerous polyps, therapeutic. Flexible sigmoidoscopes measuring 60–65 cm in length can inspect the distal third of the colon, the region in which colorectal malignancies are most likely to occur. Nonetheless, more proximal lesions (which have been diagnosed more frequently in recent years) are not detectable by sigmoidoscopy, and flat malignancies within reach of the sigmoidoscope may not be visualized. Case–control studies have suggested, however, that regular sigmoidoscopy screening reduces the risk of CRC mortality within reach of the scope by 60%. Colonoscopy has the potential to inspect the entire colon—to the cecum. Although there is no direct evidence that screening colonoscopy is effective in reducing CRC mortality, the efficacy of colonoscopy is supported by its integral role in trials of FOBT as well as extrapolation of evidence from sigmoidoscopy studies. It has been hypothesized that colonoscopy screening reduces CRC mortality by 60%.

PATIENT PREPARATION

Commonly, the role of the primary care clinician is in facilitating, rather than performing, endoscopy. Whereas endoscopy is usually performed by gastroenterologists or general surgeons, the role of the primary care clinician is to identify patients who are due for screening, help patients decide whether they prefer endoscopy over FOBT, refer patients to accredited endoscopy facilities, verify that the patient obtains the study, and ensure proper interpretation and follow-up of results. The patient should provide informed consent to the procedure after being advised of the potential benefits and risks. Preparation begins on the evening before the procedure, in which the bowel is evacuated. A variety of regimens are used, typically involving some combination of magnesium citrate, polyethylene glycol, enemas, and fasting. For sigmoidoscopy, anxiolytics or sedatives may be prescribed on the day of the procedure to reduce anxiety. Colonoscopy is typically performed under conscious sedation. Endocarditis prophylaxis with antibiotics may be prescribed for those with high-risk cardiac lesions (e.g., prosthetic heart valves, congenital cardiac malformations, etc.) but is unnecessary for patients with moderate-risk lesions such as mitral valve prolapse with regurgitation.

TECHNIQUE

The techniques for performing flexible fiberoptic sigmoidoscopy and colonoscopy and for obtaining biopsies, which are learned through supervised training and practical experience, are beyond the scope of this chapter.

DEFINITION OF ABNORMAL RESULTS

Large or adenomatous polyps, masses, diverticula, and areas of inflammation or bleeding are considered abnormal.

POTENTIAL ADVERSE EFFECTS

A serious complication of endoscopy is bowel perforation, which occurs in approximately 0.01% of sigmoidoscopies and in up to 0.1–0.2% of colonoscopies. Bleeding from biopsy sites or mucosal injuries, moderate pain, and flatus are common. Transmission of infectious diseases is also possible but uncommon. Endoscopy may be inappropriate or may need reconsideration in patients with severe anal strictures or fissures, inadequate bowel preparation, recent pelvic or bowel surgery, active inflammatory bowel disease, toxic megacolon, acute diverticulitis, or immune deficiency, but many of these conditions are unlikely in asymptomatic patients undergoing screening. False-positive results are uncommon with endoscopy, but detected polyps, even if adenomatous, may not be destined to progress to cancer. Patients can incur costs, inconvenience, discomfort, and complications from the removal of these growths and for subsequent surveillance. False-negative results can occur if polyps or cancers are obscured from view or are located beyond the reach of the scope.

ACCURACY AND RELIABILITY AS SCREENING TEST

Sigmoidoscopy only visualizes the lower half of the colon but has been estimated to identify 50–92% of all patients with significant findings in the colon and rectum, depending on whether sigmoidoscopy alone or sigmoidoscopy combined with annual FOBT is compared to colonoscopy. This is because abnormal findings ("sentinel lesions") on sigmoidoscopy or abnormal FOBTs trigger examination of the entire colon with colonoscopy. Sensitivity and detection rates vary depending on the depth of insertion. The 60 and 65 cm flexible sigmoidoscopes can reach the splenic flexure in 80% of examinations and can thereby detect 40–65% of CRCs. The specificity of endoscopic screening approaches 100% for detection of significant polyps and cancers.

MEDICAL RECORD DOCUMENTATION

The date and results of the endoscopic examination should be placed in the medical record, preferably on a health maintenance flow sheet. The appearance and location of polyps, diverticula, areas of inflammation, or other abnormalities should be carefully described. If equipment is available, a videotape recording or photograph of abnormal findings should be included. The medical record should also indicate the type and length of the endoscope, the type and adequacy of the bowel preparation and medications, depth of insertion, difficulties in advancement or visualization, reason for stopping, and discomfort or complications experienced by the patient. The record should specify whether biopsies were obtained, the specific pathology results, and the plans for follow-up and repeat testing.

ADDITIONAL COLORECTAL CANCER SCREENING METHODS

Stool DNA and immunochemical testing and "virtual" colonoscopy (computed tomography) are emerging technologies for screening that may be more acceptable to patients. New stool tests do not require dietary restrictions, and virtual colonoscopy is non-invasive. However, there is currently limited information on accuracy, effectiveness in reducing CRC mortality, and harms of these services when performed in the general population.

STANDARD COUNSELING

Clinicians should educate patients about the options for CRC screening and their associated risks and benefits to help patients choose which test they prefer. Patients undergoing endoscopy should be advised of potential symptoms that may be experienced following the procedure (e.g., flatus, cramps). Following FOBT, endoscopy, or other forms of CRC screening, the patient should be reminded to return for repeat screening at the recommended interval, to undergo colonoscopy if their home FOBT is positive, and to contact the clinician if changes in bowel habits, stool color, or rectal bleeding occur. Patients can also be advised that reducing dietary fat and/or increasing dietary fiber intake may reduce the risk of developing CRC.

Mammography
INTRODUCTION

Breast cancer is the second leading cause of cancer deaths in women in the United States, claiming more than 40,000 lives in 2006. Major risk factors include age, early age of menarche, previous breast biopsies showing atypical hyperplasia, late age at first pregnancy or no pregnancy, and family history of breast cancer in first-degree relatives (mother, sister, and daughter) (9). Trials evaluating the efficacy of mammography have some limitations, but have reported reductions in mortality of up to 32% (10).

Screening Guidelines **All women aged 50 years and older should be offered annual or biennial mammography. Clinicians should discuss the risks and benefits of mammography screening for women between 40–50 years of age. The exact age to stop mammography screening is uncertain, but screening offers limited value in those patients with an average life expectancy of less than 10 years. Women should be referred for genetic counseling if they report a family history suspicious for the BRCA mutation (e.g., Ashkenazi Jewish women with one first-degree relative or two second-degree relatives with breast or ovarian cancer; non–Ashkenazi Jewish women with two first-degree relatives with breast cancer, one of whom received the diagnosis at 50 years or younger; a combination of three or more first- or second-degree relatives with breast cancer regardless of age at diagnosis; a combination of both breast and ovarian cancer among first- and second-degree relatives; a first-degree relative with bilateral breast cancer; a combination of two or more first- or second-degree relatives with ovarian cancer regardless of age at diagnosis; a first- or second-degree relative with both breast and ovarian cancer at any age; and a history of breast cancer in a male relative).**

Official Guidelines The USPSTF recommends screening mammography, with or without clinical breast examination (CBE), every 1–2 years for women aged 40 years and older. Most organizations recommend screening mammography, but they may differ in the recommended starting age and the interval. The USPSTF recommends genetic counseling for women whose family history suggests an increased risk of *BRCA1* or *BRCA2* mutations. The AAFP recommends screening average risk women at age 50 years and counseling women aged 40–49 years about the potential benefits and harms of earlier screening. For women age 40–49 years, the American College of Physicians recommends that clinicians should periodically perform individualized risk assessment for breast cancer and should base screening mammography decisions on the benefits and harms of screening, the woman's preferences, and her individual risk profile. The ACOG and the ACS recommend screening with mammography and CBE beginning at age 40 years. The ACS recommends magnetic resonance imaging in addition to mammography screening for women with at least a 20–25% greater risk of breast cancer (e.g., those with a personal or first-degree family history of a *BRCA1* or *BRCA2* mutation).

TECHNIQUE

Radiographic methods for performing mammography are the domain of the radiologist and are not discussed here. As with endoscopy screening, the role of the primary care clinician in providing mammographic screening is to identify women who are due for screening, refer patients to accredited mammographic facilities, verify that the patient obtains the study, and ensure proper interpretation and follow-up of results. In placing the requisition, the referring clinician should remember that a screening mammogram typically includes only oblique and craniocaudal views. Magnification views, spot compression films, and other special imaging techniques may be needed to evaluate abnormal screening studies and for women with palpable masses, a previous history of breast cancer, or breast augmentation. Digital mammography techniques (filmless mammography), which provide computerized acquisition and storage of mammographic images, are available at some mammography centers. While this technology is more expensive, it allows for easier storage, transferability, and comparison of films over time. Ultrasonography and magnetic resonance imaging of the breasts are indicated in certain circumstances; for example, magnetic resonance imaging of the breasts has been recommended for women at very high risk of breast cancer.

STANDARD COUNSELING

Patients should be reminded to wear two-piece clothing and to not apply topical agents (e.g., deodorants) to the breasts on the day of the study. See Chapters 3 and 14 regarding CBE and breast self-examination, respectively. The patient should be advised to contact the clinician if she detects a breast lump, tenderness, or another abnormality, even if her mammogram is normal. The importance of regular breast cancer screening (which includes mammography plus CBE) should be emphasized, and the patient should receive specific instructions about when to return for the next mammogram.

DEFINITION OF ABNORMAL RESULTS

Radiographic features associated with malignancy include irregular margins, spiculations, and clustered microcalcifications. Indirect radiographic signs can include localized distortion of breast architecture, developing neodensities, asymmetric breast tissue, and single dilated ducts.

POTENTIAL ADVERSE EFFECTS

Patients can experience discomfort from breast compression during imaging, and it is therefore preferable that they not obtain the study during menstruation. Risks from radiation exposure are minimal, totaling only a fraction of the radiation exposure used in other x-ray procedures such as lumbar spine radiography. As discussed further in Chapter 19, the potential harms of breast cancer screening include the generation of false-positive results and the overdiagnosis and overtreatment of lesions of uncertain clinical significance (e.g., ductal carcinoma *in situ*). Screening may also precipitate further diagnostic testing (mammography with spot views, invasive biopsies with either needle or open surgical procedures), anxiety, and additional medical expense. False-negative results may allow women with breast cancer to escape detection.

ACCURACY AND RELIABILITY AS SCREENING TEST

The sensitivity of mammography ranges from 77–95% for cancers diagnosed over the following year, and specificity ranges from 94–97%. Recent studies report false-positive rates of 3–6%. Owing to increased breast tissue density, sensitivity is lower in women younger than 50 years and in women who are taking hormone replacement. Specificity increases with shorter screening intervals and access to prior mammograms for purposes of comparison.

Tuberculin Skin Testing
INTRODUCTION

An estimated 9.6–14.9 million persons residing in the United States have latent tuberculosis (TB) infection. Those individuals at high risk for TB include persons infected with HIV, close contacts of persons known or suspected of having TB, persons with medical conditions that increase the risk of infection (e.g., immunosuppressed patients, those with leukemia, lymphoma, diabetes, chronic renal failure), immigrants from countries with a high prevalence of TB, medically underserved low-income populations (including high-risk racial or ethnic groups), patients suffering from alcohol abuse, injection drug users, residents of long-term institutions (e.g., nursing homes, prisons), and persons who work in health care facilities. Tuberculin skin testing is most commonly performed using the Mantoux test, in which a known quantity of purified protein derivative (PPD) is injected intradermally.

Screening Guidelines **Adolescents and adults at high risk for TB (see preceding text for those at high risk and Table 18.11 on page 489) or who live in high prevalence areas for**

TB should be routinely screened with the Mantoux intradermal test or the QuantiFERON-TB Gold Test.

Official Guidelines The USPSTF, AAFP, AAP, and CDC recommend tuberculin skin testing of persons with risk factors for acquiring TB. The CDC recommends that either the tuberculin skin test or QuantiFERON-TB Gold Test may be used for screening.

TECHNIQUE

In the Mantoux test, a tuberculin syringe is used to inject 0.1 mL of five tuberculin units (TUs) of PPD intradermally on the volar surface of the forearm. The injection should produce a skin weal measuring 6–10 mm. If the patient is anergic, control sites of mumps, *Candida,* or tetanus should be placed on the opposite arm. A circle should be placed around the injection site(s). The patient should return to the office or clinic in 48–72 hours, at which time the site is inspected for induration. (Erythema alone is an insignificant finding.) If induration is palpated, pen marks placed at the margins of induration can be helpful in measuring the diameter.

Infected persons can have false-negative tuberculin skin tests because of anergy, but anergy is disproved if the control sites are indurated. Infected persons may also have negative tuberculin skin tests if immunity has waned over time. In what is known as the *booster effect*, such persons may subsequently have a positive skin test if a PPD is placed a second time. In health care and other institutional settings (e.g., nursing homes), "two-step testing," in which persons with negative tuberculin skin tests are retested in 1–2 weeks, is commonly advised to distinguish persons with booster reactions related to old infections from persons who are new converters.

The QuantiFERON-TB Gold Test, which requires a serum blood sample, is an enzyme-linked immunosorbent assay test that detects the release of interferon-γ in fresh heparinized whole blood from sensitized persons.

DEFINITION OF ABNORMAL RESULTS

According to the CDC and the Prevention Advisory Committee for Elimination of Tuberculosis, an induration greater than 5, 10, or 15 mm is abnormal, depending on the risk category of the patient (see Table 18.11 on page 489). Induration should not be attributed to prior Bacille de Calmette-Guérin (BCG) vaccination. The QuantiFERON-TB test results are reported as positive, negative, or indeterminate.

POTENTIAL ADVERSE EFFECTS

There is a small amount of discomfort and local erythema associated with PPD injection. Rarely, patients experience hypersensitivity reactions, ulcerated or vesicular eruptions, lymphadenopathy, or fever. Patients with false-positive results may receive unnecessary antibiotic therapy, with potentially serious adverse effects (e.g., hepatotoxicity), and restrictions on job and insurance eligibility. They may also undergo unnecessary diagnostic procedures (e.g., chest radiography). False-negative results may cause patients with TB to escape detection.

ACCURACY AND RELIABILITY AS SCREENING TEST

For persons who have not contacted an active case, the reported probability of infection is approximately 5% for 5–9 mm induration, 25% for 10–13 mm induration, 50–80% for 14–21 mm induration, and 100% for more than 21 mm induration. The validity of these estimates depends heavily on the geographic area, the local prevalence of atypical mycobacteria, and the type of population being tested. False-positive results can be caused by improper measurement of induration (e.g., measuring erythema), cross-reactivity with atypical mycobacteria, hypersensitivity to PPD constituents, and Arthus reactions. False-negative results occur in 5–10% of patients due to testing in the early stages of infection, anergy, or improper technique. The QuantiFeron test has a similar sensitivity and higher specificity compared with the tuberculin skin test; it is unaffected by prior BCG vaccination and is less likely than the tuberculin skin test to be influenced by previous infection with nontuberculous mycobacteria.

MEDICAL RECORD DOCUMENTATION

The patient's risk factors for TB should be described. The date, type of tuberculin test (Mantoux, QuantiFeron), location of testing, and, if positive, the diameter of induration should be noted in the medical record. It is often helpful to use a diagram to mark the location of the tuberculin and control injections. Plans for follow-up treatment of new converters should be described.

Abdominal Ultrasonography for Abdominal Aortic Aneurysm
INTRODUCTION

Approximately 9,000 people die each year from large abdominal aortic aneurysms (AAAs). Most victims are older than 65 years. Major risk factors include age greater than or equal to 65 years, smoking history, and male sex. Family history also increases the risk but to a lesser extent. The diameter of the AAA is the main risk factor for rupture. Abdominal ultrasonography offers a noninvasive and accurate means to identify AAAs. Population-based studies have shown that screening programs reduce mortality from AAAs in older men; whether screening impacts all cause mortality is uncertain. Screening studies have not shown a benefit for women.

Screening Guidelines **Males between age 65 and 75 years with a current or past history of smoking should be offered one-time abdominal ultrasonography to screen for AAA.**

Official Guidelines The USPSTF recommends screening for AAA in men aged 65 to 75 years who have ever smoked; makes no recommendation for or against screening men in this age-group who never smoked; and recommends against routine screening in women. The Society for Vascular Surgery recommends screening all men aged 60 to 85 years; women aged 60 to 85 years with risk factors for coronary artery disease; and men and women aged 50 years and older with a family history of AAA.

TECHNIQUE

Imaging techniques for abdominal ultrasonography are the domain of the radiologist and are not discussed here. Adequate quality assurance and certification are important to ensure test accuracy. The role of the primary care clinician in providing AAA screening is to identify women who are due for screening, refer patients to accredited ultrasonography facilities, verify that the patient obtains the study, and ensure proper interpretation and follow-up of results.

DEFINITION OF ABNORMAL RESULTS

By definition, an AAA is present when the infrarenal aortic diameter exceeds 3 cm. An AAA larger than 5 cm is considered at increased risk for rupture.

ACCURACY OF SCREENING TESTS

Abdominal ultrasonography is 95% sensitive and 100% specific for AAA when appropriately performed.

ADVERSE EFFECTS

Screening itself can cause short-term anxiety. Those patients found to have an intermediate-sized AAA and who undergo longitudinal surveillance may experience more prolonged stress. Surgical AAA repair carries an average mortality risk of up to 5%. Furthermore, perioperative and postoperative cardiac and pulmonary complications are common in association with AAA repair.

OFFICE AND CLINIC ORGANIZATION FOR ROUTINE SCREENING

Practices participating in routine screening should be properly stocked with appropriate collection instruments, culture and transport media, and storage facilities. Clinicians and staff involved with the collection, plating, and handling of specimens should be trained in proper technique, and offices that send specimens to outside laboratories should maintain transport conditions that protect the quality of the specimen.

Cervical cancer screening requires specula of varying sizes and shapes (including both Graves and Pedersen specula), specimen collection equipment (e.g., spatulas, cytobrushes, and cotton swabs); slides, fixatives, or liquid-based cytology collection vials; gloves, lubricant, and gowns or other coverings.

Home FOBT screening requires a supply of preaddressed stool card packets that can be given to patients. In addition to three stool cards and a collection instrument (e.g., wooden spatula), the packet should include clearly written instructions on dietary restrictions and on how to collect the specimens. The envelopes used to mail the specimens must be approved by the U.S. Postal Service. Practices that perform or refer patients for endoscopy screening require bowel preparation kits (or standard prescriptions for the regimen). Offices and clinics that perform tuberculin testing should maintain a fresh supply of PPD and at least two controls (e.g., mumps, *Candida*, tetanus), tuberculin syringes, and a ruler that measures millimeters. A body diagram that can be inserted in the medical record may be helpful in marking the location of the injections.

Examination rooms should be outfitted with comfortable examination tables and good lighting. The practice should also provide a quiet discussion area where clinicians and patients can review the benefits and risks of tests before screening is conducted.

Reminder and referral systems should be in place to identify patients overdue for screening and to ensure that the clinician receives test results, that patients return for repeat screening at recommended intervals, and that patients with positive results receive appropriate follow-up and treatment. For practices that offer home FOBT screening, reminder systems should ensure that FOBT packets are mailed and returned to the office. For patients screened for infectious diseases, reminder systems should also ensure that infected patients receive appropriate antibiotic therapy; that potential contacts of infected patients are notified, tested, and treated according to guidelines; and that the public health department is notified of reportable cases. For patients screened for TB, reminder systems should ensure that patients return in 48–72 hours to have the site(s) read.

Ideally, a list of recommended preventive services should be programmed into electronic medical record systems, as discussed in Chapter 22. Appropriate data fields should automatically be populated with the dates and results of previous screening tests. As discussed further in Chapter 21, reminder letters or e-mail notices can alert patients when the next preventive service is due. Electronic medical records can automate such correspondence and can also facilitate tracking of test orders, results, and follow-up testing. Likewise, the electronic medical record can also facilitate public health department notification of reportable diseases.

The office or clinic should maintain a complete list of accredited screening facilities in the community (e.g., mammography centers), including high-quality facilities that will accept low-income or uninsured patients or that provide low-cost screening. The office should have access to the performance record and certification status of the laboratories to which specimens are sent.

CONCLUSIONS

In the face of competing demands and limited time, clinicians should focus on screening tests for which net benefit has been demonstrated in the scientific literature. As noted at the outset of this chapter, screening tests are not always beneficial. A "simple blood test" can incur harms by setting off a cascade of events. Shared decision making before ordering these tests helps to engage patients in their own care, clarify realistic expectations about the harms and benefits of completing and deferring tests, and facilitate adherence with testing and follow-up. Once the clinician is convinced that the patient is fully informed about these services, the patient's choice to forego screening should be respected. At future visits, the decision to undergo screening can be revisited.

The latter point emphasizes the importance of continuity in the provision of quality preventive care. Primary care clinicians who maintain a long-term relationship with patients can provide longitudinal monitoring of the performance of screening and the follow-up of results. The broad scope of testing outlined in this chapter is too extensive to compress into a single office visit. Unlike clinicians who see patients for single consultations or time-limited relationships, or who specialize in specific disorders, primary care clinicians can organize and monitor the delivery of a range of services over time to ensure a comprehensive approach to health maintenance.

RESOURCES — PATIENT EDUCATION MATERIALS

Decision aids clearinghouse

University of Ottawa
Cochrane Inventory of Patient Decision Aids
http://decisionaid.ohri.ca/cochinvent.php

Diabetes

National Institutes of Health/National Diabetes Education Program
Am I at risk for type 2 diabetes and other prevention materials in Spanish
    and English
http://www.ndep.nih.gov/diabetes/prev/prevention.htm

Cholesterol and cardiovascular health

National Institutes of Health
Live Healthier, Live Longer an interactive web program
http://www.nhlbi.nih.gov/chd/index.htm

National Institutes of Health/NHLBI
Protect Your Heart—Lower Your Blood Cholesterol
http://www.nhlbi.nih.gov/health/public/heart/other/sp_chol.htm

HIV

Centers for Disease Control and Prevention
HIV and AIDS- Are you at risk? and other patient brochures in English and Spanish about HIV
http://www.cdc.gov/hiv/pubs/brochure.htm

Syphilis

Centers for Disease Control and Prevention
Syphilis—CDC Fact Sheet
http://www.cdc.gov/std/syphilis/STDFact-Syphilis.htm

Prostate cancer screening

American Cancer Society
Can prostate cancer be found early?
http://www.cancer.org/docroot/CRI/content/CRI_2_4_3X_Can_prostate_cancer_be_found_early_36.asp?rnav=cri

Centers for Disease Control and Prevention
Prostate cancer screening- A decision guide
http://www.cdc.gov/cancer/prostate/decisionguide/index.htm

American Academy of Family Physicians
Prostate Cancer: What You Need to Know
http://familydoctor.org/361.xml

Cervical cancer

American Cancer Society
Overview: Cervical Cancer
http://www.cancer.org/docroot/CRI/CRI_2_1x.asp?dt=8

National Institutes of Health/National Cancer Institute
Pap Tests and Cervical Health: A Healthy Habit for You
http://www.cancer.gov/cancertopics/pap-tests-cervical-health

Gonorrhea

Centers for Disease Control and Prevention
Gonorrhea—CDC Fact Sheet in English and Spanish
http://www.cdc.gov/std/Gonorrhea/STDFact-gonorrhea.htm

Chlamydia

Centers for Disease Control and Prevention
Chlamydia—CDC Fact Sheet in English and Spanish
http://www.cdc.gov/std/chlamydia/STDFact-Chlamydia.htm

Colorectal cancer

American Cancer Society
Colorectal Cancer Consumer Brochure
http://www.cancer.org/colonmd/pdfs/consumer_brochure.pdf

NIH/NCI
Colorectal Cancer (PDQ): Screening
http://www.cancer.gov/cancertopics/pdq/screening/colorectal/patient

Centers for Disease Control and Prevention
Colorectal (Colon) Cancer: Screening
http://www.cdc.gov/cancer/colorectal/basic_info/screening/

Mammography

American Academy of Family Physicians
Breast Cancer: Steps To Finding Breast Lumps Early
http://familydoctor.org/018.xml

American Cancer Society
Learn About Breast Cancer
http://www.cancer.org/docroot/lrn/lrn_0.asp

National Institutes of Health/National Cancer Institute
What You Need to Know About Breast Cancer
http://www.cancer.gov/cancertopics/wyntk/breast

Tuberculosis screening

Centers for Disease Control and Prevention
Questions and Answers About TB 2005
http://www.cdc.gov/nchstp/tb/faqs/qa_introduction.htm

American Academy of Family Physicians
Tuberculosis: The Meaning of a Positive Test
http://familydoctor.org/120.xml

SUGGESTED READINGS

American Academy of Family Physicians. *Summary of Policy Recommendations for Clinical Preventive Services*. Available at http://www.aafp.org/online/en/home/clinical/exam .html. Accessed July 27, 2007.

American Cancer Society. *Finding cancer early: ACS guidelines*. Available at: http://www .cancer.org/docroot/PED/ped_2_1_introduction.asp?sitearea=PED. Accessed January, 2006.

American College of Obstetricians and Gynecologists. *Primary and preventive care: periodic assessments*. ACOG Committee Opinion No. 246. Washington, DC: American College of Obstetricians and Gynecologists, 2000.

American College of Obstetricians and Gynecologists. Primary and preventive care: periodic assessments. ACOG Committee Opinion No. 292. *Obstet Gynecol* 2003;102: 1117–1124.

American College of Physicians. *Current ACP guidelines*. Available at: http://www .acponline.org/sci-policy/guidelines/recent.htm. Accessed January, 2006.

American Thoracic Society. Diagnostic standards and classification of tuberculosis in adults and children. American Thoracic Society Tuberculosis Guidelines. *Am J Respir Crit Care Med* 2000;161:1376–1395.

Centers for Disease Control and Prevention. Sexually transmitted diseases treatment guidelines–2002. *MMWR* 2002;51(RR06):1–80.

Expert Panel on Detection, Evaluation, and Treatment of High Blood Cholesterol in Adults. Executive summary of the third report of the National Cholesterol Education Program Expert Panel on Detection, Evaluation, and Treatment of High Blood Cholesterol in Adults (ATP III). *JAMA*. 2001;285:2486–2497.

Gordis L. *Epidemiology*, 2nd ed. New York: WB Saunders, 2000.

Harris RP, Helfand M, Woolf SH, et al. Current methods of the U.S. Preventive Services Task Force: a review of the process. *Am J Prev Med* 2001;20(Suppl 3):21–35.

Nelson HD, Huffman LH, Fu R, et al. Genetic risk assessment and BRCA mutation testing for breast and ovarian cancer susceptibility. *Ann Intern Med* 2005;143:362–379.

Qasseem A, Snow V, Sherif K, et al. Screening mammography for women 40 to 49 years of age: a clinical practice guideline from the American College of Physicians *Ann Intern Med* 2007;146:511–5.

Taylor Z, Nolan CM, Blumberg HM. American Thoracic Society; Centers for Disease Control and Prevention; Infectious Diseases Society of America. Controlling tuberculosis in the United States: recommendations from the American Thoracic Society, CDC, and the Infectious Diseases Society of America. *MMWR* 2005;54(RR12): 1–81.

U.S. Preventive Services Task Force. *The guide to clinical preventive services 2006: recommendations of the U.S. Preventive Services Task Force. Agency for Healthcare Research and Quality. AHRQ pub no. 06–0588.* Also available at: http//:www .preventiveservices.ahrq.gov. Accessed March, 2007.

Welch HG. Informed choice in cancer screening. *JAMA* 2001;285(21):2776–2778.

Woolf SH, Chan EC, Harris R, et al. Promoting informed choice: transforming health care to dispense knowledge for decision making. *Ann Intern Med* 2005;143(4): 293–300.

References

1. Schwartz LM, Woloshin S, Fowler FJ Jr, et al. Enthusiasm for cancer screening in the United States. *JAMA* 2004;291:71–78.
2. Sheridan SL, Harris RP, Woolf SH. Shared Decision Making Workgroup. Shared decision making about screening and chemoprevention: a suggested approach from the U.S. Preventive Services Task Force. Third U.S. Preventive Services Task Force. *Am J Prev Med* 2004;26(1):56–66.
3. Woolf SH, Krist A. The liability of giving patients a choice: shared decision making and prostate cancer. *Am Fam Physician* 2005;71:1871–1872.
4. US Preventive Services Task Force. *Guide to clinical preventive services 2005*. Accessed February 1, at www.preventiveservices.ahrq.gov. 2006.
5. American Diabetic Association. Diagnosis and classification of diabetes mellitus. *Diabetes Care* 2006;29(Suppl 1):S43–S48.
6. Expert Panel on Detection, Evaluation, and Treatment of High Blood Cholesterol in Adults. Executive summary of the third report of the National Cholesterol Education Program Expert Panel on Detection, Evaluation, and Treatment of High Blood Cholesterol in Adults (ATP III). *JAMA* 2001;285:2486–2497.
7. Centers for Disease Control and Prevention. Sexually transmitted diseases treatment guidelines 2002. *MMWR* 2002;51(RR06):1–80.
8. Collins JF, Lieberman DA, Durbin TE, et al. Accuracy of screening for fecal occult blood on a single stool sample obtained by digital rectal examination: a comparison with recommended sampling practice. *Ann Intern Med* 2005;142:81–85.
9. Humphrey LL, Helfand M, Chan BKS, et al. Breast cancer screening: summary of the evidence. *Ann Intern Med* 2002;137:344–346.
10. Olsen O, Gotzsche PC. Cochrane review on screening for breast cancer with mammography. *Lancet* 2001;358:1340–1342.

II

What to Do with the Information– Designing A Health Maintenance Plan Targeted to Personal Health Behaviors and Risk Factors

CHAPTER 5

Introduction to the Principles of Health Behavior Change

Russell E. Glasgow and Michael G. Goldstein

Much has changed since the first edition of this book was published in 1996. Now there is far more evidence about the effectiveness of health behavior change interventions and the factors that enhance their effectiveness (1,2). Currently many more clinicians accept the premise that patient-centered health behavior change counseling is both important and efficacious.

The "5 A's" (1,2) (see pages 134–138) and motivational interviewing (MI) have been "packaged" and adapted to primary care, and training and resources to help clinicians counsel patients have become more widely accessible (3). Computer-assisted tools for health behavior change are becoming more sophisticated and patient centered (4,5). These technologies have the potential to inform patients and make their interactions with clinicians more efficient and productive.

We have also seen the general acceptance of the Chronic Care Model (6,7) as an alternative to the traditional acute illness care model. Self-management support—the use of patient-centered assessment, collaborative goal setting, problem solving, and coordinated follow-up—is central to the Chronic Care Model (8). These elements have enhanced the credibility of and clinician interest in patient-centered health behavior change.

Although these advances are encouraging, health behavior counseling by clinicians remains less than ideal (9,10). Some primary care clinicians mistakenly assume that they are doing a good job when the reality is otherwise. Others acknowledge the deficit but question the feasibility of implementing such strategies in the current primary care environment. In general, clinicians are faced with expectations to do more and more (e.g., implement guidelines for numerous conditions) in less and less time, and often without adequate reimbursement for "doing the right thing" in terms of health behavior counseling (11,12).

Despite these challenges, there are a number of reasons to pursue health behavior assessment and counseling in primary care. Patients still view *their* physician as being the most credible source on health matters (13), and patients who are successful in changing their behaviors often cite advice

129

from their physician as an important motivating factor. Each year, 83% of the U.S. population makes at least one visit to a physician's office or emergency department (14). Older patients and those having one or more chronic illnesses generally make even more visits. Therefore, the primary care practice provides an important setting to reach patients and to encourage health promotion and other preventive services (11,15).

The purposes of this chapter are to provide a context and overview for the chapters that follow on specific health behaviors. The chapter summarizes general principles of patient–clinician communication and explains the 5 A's framework for promoting health behavior change strategies. The discussion explores some of the complexities and emerging issues in health behavior counseling, including patient "resistance," addressing multiple behaviors, and contextual factors that influence health behavior counseling.

PRINCIPLES OF EFFECTIVE CLINICIAN–PATIENT COMMUNICATION

The landmark 2001 report by the Institute of Medicine, "*Crossing the Quality Chasm*," called for redesign of the U.S. health care system. The report stated that health care must be patient centered as well as safe, effective, timely, efficient, and equitable (6).

Effective clinician–patient communication is an essential ingredient of patient-centered care (6,16). The key components of a patient-centered approach include developing a common, shared understanding of the problem or illness; addressing the patient's feelings, beliefs, expectations, and concerns; knowing the "whole person" as well as the patient's family and social context; and collaboratively choosing among options for treatment, behavior change, and follow-up (16).

Leopold et al. (17) use the term *sustained partnership* to emphasize qualitative and structural aspects of the patient-centered clinician–patient relationship that distinguish it from "continuity" or simply seeing the same clinician over time.

Substantial research supports the relationships between patient-centered clinician–patient communication and a wide range of desirable clinical outcomes, including diagnostic accuracy, effective management of symptoms, patient satisfaction, and patient adherence to treatment and health behavior change recommendations (1,18,19). Core relationship-building skills, including open-ended inquiry, responding to patients' feelings, and expressing both empathy and respect are particularly important when addressing the issues of adherence to treatment plans and health behavior change (19–21). Moreover, patient satisfaction and adherence to preventive care recommendations appear to be more strongly linked to patients' perception that their clinician knows them as a person, and to their trust in the clinician, than to other defining elements of primary care (i.e., accessibility, continuity, comprehensiveness, integration, and clinical interaction) (22).

Patient-centered approaches that promote patient activation and self-management skills are key to achieving productive interactions and desirable health outcomes among patients with chronic illnesses (8,19). Lorig et al. have identified five core skills that patients should master to effectively self-manage: problem-solving; decision-making; finding and accessing community resources; forming a patient–clinician partnership; and taking action (23). Lessons learned from the Chronic Illness Care Breakthrough Series and other efforts to integrate self-management support into health care settings suggest that the following elements are critical to success: (a) assessment of patient beliefs, behavior, and knowledge; (b) collaborative goal setting; (c) identification of personal barriers and supports; (d) problem solving to overcome barriers; and (e) developing a personal action plan that is based on the previous four steps (24).

In a review of evidence-based self-management interventions in diabetes care, Roter and Kinmonth identified several overarching principles for promoting productive clinician–patient communication (19). Table 5.1 presents an adapted version of these principles. They are based on findings from research in clinician–patient communication, health behavior counseling, and self-management support. They may be used to address health behavior change issues across a variety of medical conditions and patient populations. The patient centered, collaborative nature of these principles is evident in the emphasis placed on understanding and empathizing with the patients' experience, negotiating goals, and helping patients to identify and overcome barriers to adherence and behavior change.

TABLE 5.1 Principles of Effective Communication

- Explore and hear the patient's perspective
- Provide emotional support and express empathy
- Share information that is useful and relevant
- Negotiate a plan
- Anticipate problems and barriers and identify potential solutions
- Offer ongoing follow-up and monitoring of the plan

Modified from Roter D, Kinmonth AL. What is the evidence that increasing participation of individuals in self-management improves the processes and outcomes of care? In: Williams R, Kinmonth A, Wareham N, et al. eds. *The evidence base for diabetes care*. John Wiley and Sons, 2002.

MODELS OF HEALTH BEHAVIOR CHANGE AND BRIEF HEALTH BEHAVIOR COUNSELING

Several models of health behavior change have informed the development of effective health behavior counseling. *Social Cognitive Theory* (also known as *Social Learning Theory*) posits that behavior change and maintenance are a function of an individual's: (a) outcome expectations (i.e., beliefs about outcomes that result from engaging in a behavior), and (b) efficacy expectations (self-efficacy) (i.e., beliefs and confidence in one's capacity to carry out specific behaviors in specific situations) (25,26). Therefore, interventions that increase a person's feelings of self-efficacy (e.g., skills training with an opportunity to practice in real-world settings) will improve behavioral outcomes. *Reciprocal determinism*, another principle of Social Cognitive Theory, holds that there is interdependence among personal factors, behavior, and the environment such that a change in any one of these elements has an influence on the others. Therefore, success resulting from a behavior (e.g., relaxation techniques for smoking withdrawal symptoms associated with cessation) may increase self-efficacy, which will in turn improve one's subsequent ability to remain abstinent from smoking. The environment exerts an effect on behavior in a variety of ways, including modeling, a powerful determinant of behavior change. Therefore, repeated exposure to positive role models, such as clinicians who engage in healthy behaviors or peers, with effective coping repertoires promotes adoption of healthy behaviors.

The *Self-determination Theory* of human motivation distinguishes between motivations that are *autonomous* versus those that are *controlled* by external conditions or persons other than oneself (27). Autonomous, or internal, motivation is associated with improved adherence and improvements in diabetes care (28,29). Moreover, clinicians who foster patient autonomy and offer advice and treatment options "without pressure or demand" in a noncontrolling, nonauthoritarian way promote enhanced adherence to treatment recommendations and healthy behaviors (28,29). See, for example, the discussion of shared decision making in Chapter 4 (see pages 91–92).

The *Transtheoretical Model* (TTM) of change (30) is based on empirical evidence that individuals progress through a series of stages when making lifestyle changes: precontemplation (unaware of a problem or no plan to change in the foreseeable future); contemplation (ambivalent about changing with no commitment to change); preparation (intends to take action within the next month); action (has made a commitment to change and is actively attempting to make behavior change); and maintenance (has successfully made a change but still needs to monitor behavior to prevent slips and relapse). A large proportion of individuals engaging in high-risk behaviors, as many as 80% in some cases (e.g., smoking), are in precontemplation or contemplation stages (31). A key principle of the TTM is that individuals at different stages of change utilize different behavioral and experiential change strategies and respond best to interventions that are tailored to their stage of change (31). Therefore, although "action" level interventions are appropriate for individuals in the action stage, they are not effective, and may backfire, if delivered to individuals at earlier stages of change. For example, as discussed in Chapter 9, many tobacco cessation quit lines discourage referrals of patients who have not reached the preparation stage.

By recognizing that many patients are in early stages of change and not ready to take action, clinicians may revise their initial expectations and goals, and redefine success as moving patients along the continuum of stages of change (e.g., thinking about change in the precontemplation stage), rather than as reaching a desirable final outcome (e.g., successfully abstaining from smoking). Such an orientation may help clinicians to reduce their own level of frustration in facilitating patient behavior change, which is an important barrier to delivering effective counseling and self-management support. More appropriate strategies for counseling patients in the precontemplation and contemplation stages include providing personalized information and feedback about the impact of the behavior on function, and helping patients to reflect upon both the pros and cons of a given change (32).

MI (21) is an approach to patient counseling that is compatible with the models noted earlier. Miller and Rollnick define MI "as a directive, client-centered counseling style for eliciting behavior change by helping clients to explore and resolve ambivalence" (21). Initially developed as an intervention for problematic alcohol and substance use, it has now been applied to a large range of health behavior change targets (21). The four general principles that underlie MI are (a) *express empathy*, (b) *develop discrepancy*, (c) *roll with resistance, and* (d) *support self-efficacy.*

Empathy is a key component of effective clinician–patient communication and perhaps the most important element of MI (21). Specific skills and strategies associated with expressing empathy include asking open-ended questions (particularly about the patient's beliefs, values, expectations, and feelings), reflective listening (an active process of seeking to understand and clarify the meaning of the patient's discourse), normalization of patients' feelings, affirmation of attempts to cope and manage, and support of the patient's autonomy and right to choose or reject change (21,33). Exploration of ambivalence is especially important as a tool for understanding the barriers and obstacles to change (21). The clinician's expression of empathy is facilitated by being genuinely curious about the patient and being willing to set aside one's agenda. *Developing discrepancy* is accomplished by raising patients' awareness of the consequences of their present behavior and highlighting the discrepancy between their present behavior and their own priorities, values, and goals (21,33). Patients are encouraged to identify their own reasons for making change. Clinician exhortations or arguments for change tend to build resistance. On the other hand, when "change talk" is elicited or spontaneously expressed by the patient, the clinician can then more easily provide affirmation and support to help build and deepen commitment (33,34). *Rolling with resistance* involves backing off when the patient expresses it, by acknowledging that change is difficult while also inviting the patient to consider new information or perspectives. The clinician *supports self-efficacy* by helping the patient to build on past successes, take achievable small steps toward change, and problem solve to overcome barriers (21).

Brief versions of MI have been developed for use by clinicians in primary care and other health care settings (3,33,35). These versions emphasize the MI strategies described earlier and the assessment of two specific dimensions of motivation: (a) *conviction or importance* regarding the need for change, and (b) *confidence or self-efficacy* about taking action. Assessment is followed by the tailoring of counseling to address the patient's level of conviction and confidence, agreeing on a realistic and achievable goal, and assisting the patient to develop a behavior change plan.

As a general rule, if both conviction and confidence are low, it is most efficient to first focus on enhancing conviction. For patients with low conviction levels, effective counseling strategies include providing information and feedback (after asking patients' permission), exploring ambivalence, and providing a menu of options for treatment and follow-up. Patients not ready to commit to action may agree to simply think about the possibilities for change or to seek assistance when they are ready to take action. For patients with low confidence, strategies include reviewing past experience, especially successes; teaching problem-solving and coping skills; and encouraging small steps that are likely to lead to initial success. For all patients, a follow-up plan is essential, as evidence suggests that follow-up is an important ingredient of successful health behavior change counseling interventions (2,36,37). See Table 5.2 for a summary of these strategies.

THE 5 A'S OF HEALTH BEHAVIOR COUNSELING—A UNIFYING FRAMEWORK

In 2002, The Counseling and Behavioral Interventions Work Group of the U.S. Preventive Services Task Force recommended adoption of the "5 A's" construct as a unifying conceptual framework for evaluating and describing health behavior counseling interventions in clinical settings (1). The 5 A's framework (**A**ssess, **A**dvise, **A**gree, **A**ssist, **A**rrange follow-up) was first developed for smoking-cessation counseling (38) (see Chapter 9). Since that time it has been utilized to address other health behaviors (1,20,39) and the

TABLE 5.2   Principles of Patient-Centered Counseling[a]

Assess (Before Telling)

- Strive to understand the patient's perspective (experience, feelings, ideas, function, expectations, and goals)
- Assess conviction and confidence

Build Rapport

- Engage in reflective listening
- Express empathy
- Provide affirmation and support

Tailor Counseling: Agree on Goals and Assist Based on Conviction and Confidence

For low conviction:
- Share information and feedback (with permission) (Advise)
- Explore ambivalence
- Provide a menu of options, agree on a realistic goal, and support choice and autonomy
- Arrange follow-up

For low confidence:
- Review successful past experience
- Agree on an achievable specific goal
- Teach problem-solving and coping skills
- Encourage small steps
- Arrange follow-up

[a] Adapted from Goldstein MG. Promoting self-management in primary care settings: limitations and opportunities: a commentary. In: Williams R, Herman W, Kinmonth AL, eds. *The evidence base for diabetes care*. West Sussex, England: John Wiley and Sons, 2002:701–710.

self-management component of chronic illness care (24,40). See Table 5.3 for a summary of the 5 A's construct, adapted from the U.S. Preventive Services Task Force Counseling and Behavioral Interventions Work Group report (1). Note that the 5 A's framework is closely linked to the Principles of Effective Communication (Table 5.1) and Principles of Patient-Centered Counseling (Table 5.2). An important difference is the absence of a specific relationship-building component among the 5 A's. As described earlier,

TABLE 5.3 The 5 A's for Behavioral Counseling and Health Behavior Change

Assess	Ask about and assess behavioral health risks and factors that affect choice of behavior change goals and methods • Assessing behavioral risk factors identifies patients in need of intervention and provides a basis for tailoring brief interventions for maximum benefit • Assess beliefs, behaviors, knowledge, motivation, and past experience (some recommend performing this step as part of "Agree")
Advise	Give clear, specific, well-timed, and personalized behavior change advice, including information about personal health harms and benefits • Clinician advice establishes behavioral issues as an important part of health care • Advise in a noncoercive, nonjudgmental manner that respects readiness for change and patient autonomy • Advice is most powerful when linked to the patient's own health concerns, past experiences, family/social situations, and level of health literacy
Agree	Collaboratively select appropriate goals and methods based on the patient's interest in and willingness to change the behavior • Collaborate to find common ground and to define behavior change goals and methods • Shared decision making (see Chapter 4) is especially recommended for interventions that involve significant risk–benefit tradeoffs • Shared decision making about behavior change results in a greater sense of personal control, choices based in realistic expectations and patient values, improved patient adherence, and time saved in the examination room
Assist	Using self-help resources and/or counseling, help the patient to achieve goals by acquiring skills, confidence, and social and environmental supports for behavior change • Health care staff provide motivational interventions, address barriers to change, and/or secure support needed for successful change • Effective interventions teach self-management and problem-solving or coping skills that enable patients to take the next immediate steps toward targeted behavior change

TABLE 5.3 *(Continued)*

	• An action plan is developed that lists goals, barriers and strategies, and specifies follow-up plans
Arrange	Schedule follow-up (in person or by telephone) to provide ongoing assistance and support and to adjust the plan as needed, including referral to more specialized intervention • Consider behavioral risk factors as chronic problems that change over time • Routine follow-up assessment and support through some kind of contact is usually necessary to promote and maintain behavior change

Adapted from Goldstein MG, Whitlock EP, DePue J. Multiple health risk behavior interventions in primary care: summary of research evidence. *Am J Prev Med* 2004;27(2 Suppl):61–79.

relationship skills (e.g., open-ended inquiry, reflective listening, and empathy) are essential elements of effective counseling interventions. However, the easily remembered and simple 5 A's framework has obvious advantages as a tool for learning and dissemination. Evidence supporting each of the elements of the 5 A's is reviewed elsewhere (1,2).

The *"Assess"* (or *"Ask"*) *component* refers to the determination of whether the patient engages in the behavior. This step is necessary to identify patients in need of behavioral interventions. Assessment can be addressed in a number of ways to avoid overburdening the primary care clinician, including use of previsit health risk appraisal instruments, questionnaires, or interactive computer-based systems (see Chapters 2 and 21). The importance of this initial step of documenting the status of patients' health behaviors has been emphasized by referring to such documentation as "the new vital sign" (41). Chapters 9 and 10 discuss the use of the "vital sign" approach to systematically identify patients who use tobacco and alcohol, respectively.

The *"Advise"* *component* refers to a brief, clear message by the clinician that emphasizes the importance of changing the behavior. Advice is most effective when it is personalized and relates to a patient's symptoms, values, and expressed concerns (20,21,40).

The *"Agree"* *component* is the essential step of collaboratively identifying behavioral and self-management goals and setting specific targets. Discussing the patient's knowledge, beliefs, attitudes, feelings, and preferences can help lay the foundation for an appropriate plan.

The *"Assist"* *component* includes working with patients to develop a specific behavioral action plan to address the patient's goals. The process includes helping patients to identify barriers; use problem-solving strategies

TABLE 5.4 Action Planning Tool

Action Plan

1. Goals: something you want to do:
   _____

2. Describe
   How: _____ Where: _____
   What: _____ Frequency: _____
   When: _____
3. Barriers: _____
4. Plans to overcome barriers: _____
5. Conviction___ and confidence___ratings (0–10)
6. Follow-up: _____

to overcome barriers; identify specific strategies, tools, and resources; and learn behavior-change skills. Through this process the clinician strives to enhance patient confidence to successfully change and maintain health behaviors. Problem solving associated with this step is at the heart of effective behavior change. A primary care clinician might hand off this step to a nurse or specially trained educator, especially when more intensive intervention is needed or desired. As discussed in Chapter 9, actions such as prescribing medications to aid with smoking cessation and making plans to have a quit line call patients are also examples of the Assist category. Table 5.4 presents a tool to assist with action planning.

The *"Arrange" component* includes making specific plans for follow-up contacts with the health care team (or with clinicians who have special expertise in addressing health risk behaviors and self-management). Follow-up might be provided through means other than office visits and other face-to-face encounters. Options include mailed reminders, e-mails, and telephone follow-up, including the use of interactive distance technologies (5,8,42,43).

Clinicians with strong long-term relationships with patients, such as those providing primary care, can leverage these relationships during multiple contacts over time. With multiple contacts, the clinician can build on previous progress while also taking advantage of teachable moments when the clinician can reference new symptoms or patient concerns that might be linked to problematic health behaviors or risk factors (44).

CAVEATS AND CAUTIONS

Our experience in training clinicians in the 5 A's is that clinicians who perceive themselves as being patient centered and collaborative are often humbled by

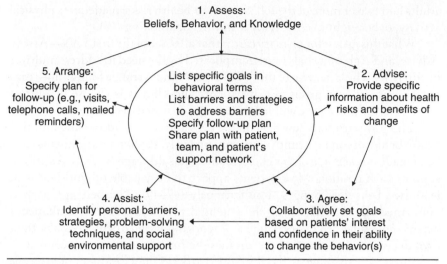

Figure 5.1 • Interactive process of 5 A's counseling.

reviewing video or audio tapes of their interactions with patients. Silence may well be golden in certain contexts; Chapter 2 discusses the utility of silence in drawing out sentiments that patients might otherwise not express. Unfortunately, in health care settings clinicians typically rush in to provide directive recommendations or attempt to solve problems *for* patients, rather than work with them to develop personalized action plans. Becoming truly patient centered and collaborative may require an investment in training and follow-up coaching (21).

A second caveat is that clinical experience, system supports, and research evidence (9,45) all support the notion that the fourth and fifth A's (problem-solving assistance and arranging follow-up and community support) are both critically important for long-term success. However, they are also challenging for busy clinicians and are implemented far less frequently than are the first three A's. Although each of the A's is important, *it is the level of integration, synthesis, and iterative refinement of all five that is the hallmark of successful counseling.* As shown in Figure 5.1, each step should contribute to development or updating of an action plan and should relate to and inform the other counseling steps.

MULTIPLE HEALTH BEHAVIOR CHANGES

Another of the complexities in primary care–based health behavior counseling is that many patients have more than one health behavior to address. Data from the 2001 National Health Interview Survey suggested that 58% of U.S.

adults had two or more of the following four health risks: inadequate physical activity, overweight/obesity, risky drinking, or smoking (46).

What this means for primary care is that all three of the first 5 A's—Assess, Advise, and Agree on goals—are complicated by the need to address multiple health risks. The latter two of the 5 A's—Assist and Arrange follow-up—may not be pursued at a given visit if patients and clinicians choose to address other behaviors, but they will be ultimately addressed over time.

There are currently few data on the pros and cons of addressing multiple health behaviors one at a time versus concurrently. Passionate arguments have been made on each side of this choice; some data, although far from definitive, support each position. Most patients appear to be capable of working on at least two behavior changes simultaneously (47–49). The best approach is "informed choice," discussing the potential pros and cons of simultaneous versus sequential behavior change and working with patients to make their own decision. The following reexamines the first three A's in this context.

Assess. A body of work has developed around the assessment of multiple risks, most commonly in the form of health risk appraisals. Most experience with health risk appraisals, however, comes from worksite and community settings, rather than primary care. Chapter 1 discusses the role of risk assessment tools that calculate the probability of a disease on the basis of multiple risk factors. Questionnaires and other tools for systematically collecting risk factor information before office visits are discussed further in Chapter 2.

Chapter 2 offers a short list of screening questions about health behaviors, but the Prescription for Health project (www.prescriptionforhealth.org) developed a somewhat longer list of questions that explores more carefully the patient's habits with regard to smoking, physical activity, diet, and alcohol use (see Fig. 5.2). The questions were designed to be simultaneously brief—a practical necessity to administer and score in primary care—yet reliable, valid, sensitive to change, and broadly applicable (50). Priority was also given to measures that addressed public health goals and could directly inform intervention. Many primary care offices may wish to enhance this list to address other dimensions of these behaviors or to screen for other problems, such as depression or medication adherence.

Advise and Agree. When patients present with multiple health risks, there is little evidence concerning the optimal approach to advising and collaborating with patients in prioritizing and selecting goals. The clinician should present patients with feedback in terms that they can understand, including which health behaviors place them at the highest risk (usually, this is smoking). The patient should decide which behavior(s) they are ready and willing to prioritize. Such an approach both addresses clinicians' responsibility to share risk information with patients (and where possible, to relate this to personal and family history) and is consistent with the principles of MI and the 5 A's. The discussion of exercise counseling in Chapter 6 provides a list

Physical Activity (IPAQ; short version)

Scoring: see **www.ipaq.ki.se**

We are interested in finding out about the kinds of physical activities that people do as part of their everyday lives. The questions will ask you about the time you spent being physically active in the **last 7 days**. Please answer each question even if you do not consider yourself to be an active person. Please think about the activities you do at work, as part of your house and yard work, to get from place to place, and in your spare time for recreation, exercise or sport.

Think about all the **vigorous** activities that you did in the **last 7 days. Vigorous** physical activities refer to activities that take hard physical effort and make you breathe much harder than normal. Think *only* about those physical activities that you did for at least 10 minutes at a time.

1. During the **last 7 days,** on how many days did you do **vigorous** physical activities like heavy lifting, digging, aerobics, or fast bicycling?

    _____ **days per week**

    ☐ No vigorous physical activities ➡ ***Skip to question 3***

2. How much time did you usually spend doing **vigorous** physical activities on one of those days?

    _____ **hours per day**
    _____ **minutes per day**

    ☐ Don't know/Not sure

Think about all the **moderate** activities that you did in the **last 7 days. Moderate** activities refer to activities that take moderate physical effort and make you breathe somewhat harder than normal. Think only about those physical activities that you did for at least 10 minutes at a time.

3. During the **last 7 days**, on how many days did you do **moderate** physical activities like carrying light loads, bicycling at a regular pace, or doubles tennis?

    _____ **days per week**

    ☐ No moderate physical activities ➡ ***Skip to question 5***

4. How much time did you usually spend doing **moderate** physical activities on one of those days?

    _____ **hours per day**
    _____ **minutes per day**

    ☐ Don't know/Not sure

Think about the time you spent **walking** in the **last 7 days**. This includes at work and at home, walking to travel from place to place, and any other walking that you might do solely for recreation, sport, exercise, or leisure.

5. During the **last 7 days**, on how many days did you **walk** for at least 10 minutes at a time?

    _____ **days per week**

    ☐ No walking ➡ ***Skip to question 7***

6. How much time did you usually spend **walking** on one of those days?

    _____ **hours per day**
    _____ **minutes per day**

    ☐ Don't know/Not sure

The last question is about the time you spent **sitting** on weekdays during the **last 7 days**. Include time spent at work, at home, while doing course work and during leisure time. This may include time spent sitting at a desk, visiting friends, reading, or sitting or lying down to watch television.

Figure 5.2 • Adult measures of behavior change.

7. During the **last 7 days**, how much time did you spend **sitting** on a **week day**?

_____ hours per day
_____ minutes per day

☐ Don't know/Not sure

Risky drinking (BRFSS 2003) Scoring–Number of drinks: Binge drinking = 5 or more drinks for men; 4 or more for women.

A drink of alcohol is defined as 1 can or bottle of beer, 1 glass of wine, 1 can or bottle of wine cooler, 1 cocktail, or 1 shot of liquor.

- During the past 30 days, how many days per week or per month did you have at least one drink of any alcoholic beverage? [if none, STOP]

- On the days when you drank, about how many drinks did you drink on average?

- Considering all types of alcoholic beverages, how many times during the past 30 days did you have 5 or more drinks on an occasion? (for women the threshold for binge drinking is 4 drinks).

Cigarette Smoking Scoring —— any current smoking, especially daily smoking as trigger for intervention

- Have you smoked at least 100 cigarettes in your entire life? [if no, STOP]

- Have you smoked at least part of a cigarette in the last 7 days? [if no, STOP]

- During a typical 7-day period how many cigarettes did you smoke?

Eating Patterns– (Starting the Conversation-Diet)

- How many times a week do you eat fast food meals or snacks?
  __ 1 time __ 2 times __ 3 or more times __ None ___Don't know/not sure

- How many servings of fruit or vegetables do you eat each day?
  __ 1 serving __ 2 servings __3 or more servings __ None __ Don't know/not sure

- How many regular sodas or glasses of sweet tea do you drink each day? (one glass is an 8 oz serving)
  __< 1glass __ 1 glass __ 2 glasses __ 3 glasses ___4 or more __ None __Don't know/not sure

- How many times a week do you eat beans (like pinto or black beans), chicken or fish?
  __1 time __ 2 times __ 3 or more times __ None ___Don't know/not sure

- How many times a week do you eat regular snack chips or crackers (not the low-fat variety)?
  __1 time __ 2 times __ 3 or more times __ None ___Don't know/not sure

- How many times a week do you eat desserts and other sweets?
  __ 1 time __ 2 times __ 3 or more times __ None ___Don't know/not sure?

- How much margarine, butter or meat fat do you use to season vegetables or put on potatoes, bread, or corn?
  __ Very little __ Some __ A lot

Figure 5.2 • (*Continued*)

of considerations (page 164–165) that clinicians should review to decide how strongly they wish to prioritize health behavior counseling in their practice.

OFFICE AND CLINIC ORGANIZATION

Abundant and ever-increasing evidence indicates that the 5 A's strategy, and the behavior change theories and principles that underlie them (1,2,42),

TABLE 5.5 Office Practice Planning Matrix for Implementing 5 A's

Component	Who	What	When	Where	Resources Needed	Notes
Assess						
Advise						
Agree						
Assist						
Arrange						

are most effective when implemented consistently. Unfortunately, there is also evidence and much clinical experience to suggest that it is challenging in busy primary care settings to routinely deliver care based upon these strategies—especially in an integrated, coordinated manner.

It is beyond the scope of this chapter to discuss practice redesign or office systems changes in detail (see Chapters 21 and 22), but three recommendations are offered here. The first is that the 5 A's need to be customized to individual practice settings. A simple tool, such as that shown in Table 5.5, can help a practice tailor its delivery of the 5 A's to its staffing pattern, resources, patient flow, culture, and priorities. Customizing the approach of a practice to health behavior counseling is consistent with the larger strategy advocated in Chapter 20, which details the need for practices to individually define the preventive services they wish to systematically offer patients.

The second, related recommendation is to distribute and share responsibility for 5 A's implementation among different members of the office staff. As discussed in Chapter 21, those practices that are successful in consistently delivering high-quality preventive care, behavioral counseling included, distribute the workload across staff members and take advantage of the special talents of different personnel (40,51). The physician is usually in a unique position of credibility to deliver Advice, but the other four A's can often be either automated or delivered by nonphysician staff, often with greater success.

The third recommendation is that practices develop strong partnerships with community resources in their area. This is consistent with both the 5 A's and with the Chronic Care Model emphasis on community resources to support self-management. Practices need to reach out beyond their walls to partner with community resources in order to provide counseling at the intensity that many patients require. Efforts under way to create systems that make it easy for clinicians to refer patients to tobacco quit lines, weight loss programs (e.g., Weight Watchers), and so on, are reflective of this trend (52).

The chapters that follow identify specific community resources with which clinicians can partner to help patients with various health behaviors.

CONCLUSIONS AND FUTURE DIRECTIONS

The communication and behavior change principles reviewed in this chapter have been successfully applied in almost every health care setting and across a wide variety of health conditions, health behaviors, and patient subgroups. However, it is challenging to find ways to consistently implement the 5 A's—especially the fourth and fifth ones—in a patient-centered manner in the current primary care world. To sustain implementation of behavioral counseling over the long term, it may be necessary to either redesign practice infrastructure (see Chapter 21) and/or for there to be significant health care policy changes beyond the capacity of the individual practice (e.g., "pay-for-performance" [see Chapter 23] that includes health behavior counseling). The prevalence of multiple unhealthy behaviors in the U.S. population presents a complex challenge. Exciting and innovative approaches to meeting this challenge bode well for the future (2).

SUGGESTED READINGS

Glasgow RE, Ory MG, Klesges LM, et al. Practical and relevant measures of health behavior for primary care settings. *Ann Fam Med* 2005;3:73–81.

Goldstein MG. Promoting self-management in primary care settings: limitations and opportunities: a commentary. In: Williams R, Herman W, Kinmonth AL, et al. eds. *The evidence base for diabetes care*. West Sussex, England: John Wiley and Sons, 2002:701–710.

Goldstein MG, Curry SJ, eds. Addressing multiple behavioral risk factors in primary care. *Am J Prev Med* 2004;27(2 Suppl).

Haas LJ. *Handbook of primary care psychology*. New York: Oxford University Press, 2005.

Rollnick S, Mason P, Butler C. *Health behavior change: a guide for practitioners*. New York: Churchill Livingstone, 1999.

Whitlock EP, Orleans CT, Pender N, et al. Evaluating primary care behavioral counseling interventions: an evidence-based approach. *Am J Prev Med* 2002;22:267–284.

References

1. Whitlock EP, Orleans CT, Pender N, et al. Evaluating primary care behavioral counseling interventions: an evidence-based approach. *Am J Prev Med* 2002;22:267–284.

2. Goldstein MG, Whitlock EP, DePue J. Multiple health risk behavior interventions in primary care: summary of research evidence. *Am J Prev Med* 2004;27(2 Suppl):61–79.

3. Rollnick S, Butler CD, McCambridge J, et al. Consultations about changing behavior. *Br Med J* 2005;331(7522):961–963.

4. Brug J, Oenema A, Campbell M. Past, present and future of computer-tailored nutrition education. *Am J Clin Nutr* 2003;77(4):1028S–1034S.
5. Glasgow RE, Bull SS, Piette JD, et al. Interactive behavior change technology: a partial solution to the competing demands of primary care. *Am J Prev Med* 2004;27(25): 80–87.
6. Institute of Medicine, Committee on Quality of Health Care in America. *Crossing the quality chasm: a new health system for the 21st century*. Washington, DC: National Academy Press, 2001.
7. Wagner EH, Austin BT, Davis C, et al. Improving chronic illness care: translating evidence into action. *Health Aff* 2001;20:64–78.
8. Bodenheimer TS, Lorig K, Holman H, et al. Patient self-management of chronic disease in primary care. *JAMA* 2002;288(19):2469–2475.
9. Glasgow RE, Eakin EG, Fisher EB, et al. Physician advice and support for physical activity: results from a national survey. *Am J Prev Med* 2001;21(3):189–196.
10. McGlynn EA, Asch SM, Adams J, et al. The quality of health care delivered to adults in the United States. *N Engl J Med* 2003;348(26):2635–2645.
11. Stange KC, Woolf SH, Gjeltema K. One minute for prevention: the power of leveraging to fulfill the promise of health behavior counseling. *Am J Prev Med* 2002;22:320–323.
12. Yarnell KS, Pollack KI, Ostbye T, et al. Primary care: is there enough time for prevention? *Am J Public Health* 2003;93(4):635–641.
13. Davis D, Schoenbaum SC, Collins KS, et al. *Room for improvement: patients report on the quality of their health care*. Report No.: Publication Number 534. New York: The Commonwealth Fund, 2002.
14. National Center for Health Statistics. *Health, United States, 2003*. Report No.: DHHS Publication No. 2003–1232. Hyattsville: National Center for Health Statistics, 2003.
15. Woolf SH, Chan EC, Harris R, et al. Promoting informed choice: transforming health care to dispense knowledge for decision making. *Ann Intern Med* 2005;143(4): 293–300.
16. Stewart M, Brown J, Weston W, et al. *Patient-centered medicine: transforming the clinical method*. Thousand Oaks: Sage Publications Inc, 1995.
17. Leopold N, Cooper J, Clancy C. Sustained partnership in primary care. *J Fam Pract* 1996;42(2):129–137.
18. Ockene JK, Zapka JG. Provider education to promote implementation of clinical practice guidelines. *Chest* 2000;118(2 Suppl):33S–39S.
19. Roter D, Kinmonth AL. What is the evidence that increasing participation of individuals in self-management improves the processes and outcomes of care? In: Williams R, Kinmonth A, Wareham N, et al. eds. *The evidence base for diabetes care*. John Wiley and Sons, 2002.
20. Goldstein MG, DePue J. Models for provider-patient interaction: applications to health behavior change. In: Shumaker S, Schron EB, McBee WL, eds. *The handbook of health behavior change*. New York: Springer-Verlage New York, 1998: 85–113.
21. Miller WR, Rollnick S. *Motivational interviewing: preparing people for change*. New York: The Guilford Press, 2002.
22. Safran D, Taira D, Rogers W, et al. Linking primary care performance to outcomes of care. *J Fam Pract* 1998;47:213–220.
23. Lorig KR, Holman HR. Self-management education: history, definition, outcomes, and mechanisms. *Ann Behav Med* 2003;26:1–7.

24. Glasgow RE, Funnell MM, Bonomi AE, et al. Self-management aspects of the improving chronic illness care breakthrough series: implementation with diabetes and heart failure teams. *Ann Behav Med* 2002;24(2):80–87.

25. Bandura A. *Social foundations of thought and action: a social cognitive theory.* Englewood Cliffs: Prentice Hall, 1986.

26. Bandura A. Health promotion by social cognitive means. *Health Educ Behav* 2004;31(2):143–164.

27. Williams GC, Deci EL. The importance of supporting autonomy in medical education. *Ann Intern Med* 1998;129(4):303–308.

28. Williams GC, Freedman ZR, Deci EL. Supporting autonomy to motivate patients with diabetes for glucose control. *Diabetes Care* 1998;21(10):1644–1651.

29. Williams GC, Rodin GC, Ryan RM, et al. Autonomous regulation and long-term medication adherence in adult outpatients. *Health Psychol* 1998;17(3):269–276.

30. Prochaska JO, DiClemente CC. Toward a comprehensive model of change. In: Miller W, Heather N, eds. *Treating addictive behavior.* New York: Plenum Publishing, 1986.

31. Prochaska JO, Velicer WF, Rossi JS, et al. Stages of change and decisional balance for 12 problem behaviors. *Health Psychol* 1994;13(1):39–46.

32. Prochaska JO, Goldstein MG. Process of smoking cessation. Implications for clinicians. *Clin Chest Med* 1991;12(4):727–735.

33. Rollnick S, Mason P, Butler C. *Health behavior change: a guide for practitioners.* New York: Churchill Livingstone, 1999.

34. Miller WR, Rollnick S. *Motivational interviewing: professional training videotape series.* Directed by Theresa B Moyers, ed. 1998. Video Recording.

35. Goldstein MG. Promoting self-management in primary care settings: limitations and opportunities: a commentary. In: Williams R, Herman W, Kinmonth AL, eds. *The evidence base for diabetes care.* West Sussex, England: John Wiley and Sons, 2002:701–710.

36. Fiore MC, Bailey WC, Cohen SJ, et al. *Treating tobacco use and dependence: clinical practice guideline.* Rockville: U.S. Department of Health and Human Services, Public Health Service, 2000.

37. Norris SL, Nichols PJ, Caspersen CJ, et al. The effectiveness of disease and case management for people with diabetes. A systematic review. *Am J Prev Med* 2002;22 (4 Suppl):15–38.

38. Glynn TM, Manley MW. *How to help your patients stop smoking: a manual for physicians.* Report No.: NIH Publication #89–3064. Bethesda: Smoking, Tobacco and Cancer Program, Division of Cancer Prevention and Control, National Cancer Institute, 1989.

39. Ockene J, Adams A, Hurley T, et al. Brief physician- and nurse practitioner-delivered counseling for high-risk drinkers: does it work? *Arch Intern Med* 1999;159: 2198–2205.

40. Glasgow RE, Davis CL, Funnell MM, et al. Implementing practical interventions to support chronic illness self-management. *Jt Comm J Qual Saf* 2003;29(11):563–574.

41. Fiore MC. The new vital sign. Assessing and documenting smoking status (commentary). *JAMA* 1991;266:3183–3184.

42. Glasgow RE, Goldstein MG, Ockene J, et al. Translating what we have learned into practice: principles and hypotheses for addressing multiple behaviors in primary care. *Am J Prev Med* 2004;27(25):88–101.

43. Glasgow RE. Translating research to practice: lessons learned, areas for improvement, and future directions. *Diabetes Care* 2003;26(8):2451–2456.
44. Cooper GS, Goodwin MA, Stange KC. The delivery of preventive services for patient symptoms. *Am J Prev Med* 2001;21(3):177–181.
45. Glasgow RE, Wagner E, Schaefer J, et al. Development and validation of the patient assessment of chronic illness care (PACIC). *Med Care* 2005;43(5):436–444.
46. Fine LJ, Philogene GS, Grambling R, et al. Prevalence of multiple behavioral risk factors in the United States: results from the 2001 National Health Interview Survey. *Am J Prev Med* 2003;27(2S):18–24.
47. Vandelanotte C, De Bourdeaudhuij I, Sallis JF, et al. Efficacy of sequential or simultaneous interactive computer-tailored interventions for increasing physical activity and decreasing fat intake. *Ann Behav Med* 2005;29(2):138–146.
48. Glasgow RE, Strycker LA, King D, et al. Robustness of a computer-assisted diabetes self-management intervention across patient characteristics, healthcare settings, and intervention staff. *Am J Manag Care* 2006;12:137–145.
49. Toobert DJ, Strycker LA, Glasgow RE, et al. Effects of Mediterranean lifestyle trial on multiple risk behaviors and psychosocial outcomes among women at risk for heart disease. *Ann Behav Med* 2005;29(2):128–137.
50. Glasgow RE, Ory MG, Klesges LM, et al. Practical and relevant measures of health behavior for primary care settings. *Ann Fam Med* 2005;3:73–81.
51. Ockene IS, Hebert JR, Ockene JK, et al. Effect of physician-delivered nutrition counseling training and an office-support program on saturated fat intake, weight, and serum lipid measurements in a hyperlipidemic population: Worcester Area Trial for Counseling Hyperlipidemia (WATCH). *Arch Intern Med* 1999;159(7):725–731.
52. Woolf SH, Krist AH, Rothemich SF. *Joining Hands: Partnerships Between Physicians and the Community in the Delivery of Preventive Care.* Washington, D.C.: Center for American Progress, 2006, http://www.americanprogress.org/issues/2006/10/health_reports.html/pdf/health_woolf.pdf.

CHAPTER 6

Regular Exercise

Steven Jonas

INTRODUCTION

First Thoughts

Regular exercise provides many health benefits to those who engage in the activity (1–3). In addition to its direct benefits, regular exercise is an essential part of healthy weight management and any effective program to lose weight. The broad public health implications of exercise therefore include its pivotal importance in dealing with the obesity epidemic (see Chapter 8 for more details).

The following definitions apply to the commonly used term *exercise*.

Physical activity is "any body movement produced by skeletal muscles that results in a substantive increase over the resting energy expenditure."

Leisure-time physical activity is "an activity undertaken in the individual's discretionary time that leads to any substantial increase in the total daily energy expenditure."

Exercise is a form of leisure-time physical activity that is usually performed on a repeated basis over an extended period of time (exercise training) with a specific external objective such as the improvement of fitness, physical performance, or health" (1).

It is important to note that "regularity," exercising on a repeated basis over an extended period of time, is included in the standard definition for exercise. *Sessions, workouts* and *going to the gym* are terms that are used interchangeably with regular exercise throughout this chapter.

Counseling

The most recent U.S. Preventive Services Task Force (USPSTF) recommendation on counseling for regular exercise, issued in 2002 (4), concluded that "there is insufficient evidence to determine whether counseling patients in primary care settings to promote physical activity leads to sustained increases in physical activity in adult patients." More recent controlled studies suggested that counseling for regular exercise in clinical practice may be effective in helping patients to become regular exercisers (5–7). Whether there is high-quality evidence to support exercise counseling in the primary care setting, patients may request advice on how to become more physically active. The goal of this chapter is to guide clinicians on how to provide exercise counseling to their otherwise healthy patients: the sedentary person who wants to exercise; the sedentary person who needs to exercise for risk factor modification; and the exerciser who is looking for advice because of injury, burnout, or a need for consultation and reinforcement. This chapter presents a practical guide, based on 20 years of experience in the field and an extensive lay literature, on how to effectively offer physical activity counseling. The approach presented in subsequent text therefore reflects an experience-based consensus on fostering leisure-time, health-promoting, regular exercise, for its own sake.

This chapter does not specifically address the role of regular exercise in either the treatment or management of diseases or pathologic conditions (such as hypertension), or rehabilitation, although many of the basic principles for helping any patient to become a regular exerciser would hold true.

BASIC CONCEPTS IN EXERCISE

Epidemiology of Exercise

Epidemiologic data show that regular exercise promotes general health, while its lack, known variously as *physical inactivity* or *sedentary lifestyle*, increases the risk of a variety of diseases and negative health conditions. At the beginning of the chapter on Physical Activity and Fitness in *Healthy People 2010* (2) it is stated that:

> "Research has demonstrated that virtually all individuals will benefit from regular physical activity . . . . Moderate physical activity can reduce substantially the risk of developing or dying from heart disease, diabetes, colon cancer, and high blood pressure. Physical activity may also protect against lower back pain and some [other] forms of cancer (for example, breast cancer). On average, physically active people outlive those who are inactive. Regular physical activity also helps to maintain the functional independence of older adults and enhances the quality of life for people of all ages."

The 2004 "Best Practices Statement" of the American College of Sports Medicine (ACSM) (8) states:

> "Physical activity offers one of the greatest opportunities for people to extend years of active independent life and reduce functional limitations . . . . A substantial body of scientific evidence indicates that regular

physical activity can bring dramatic health benefits to people of all ages and abilities, with these benefits extending over the life span . . . . and improve the quality of life . . . "

The position taken in both of these reports was shaped by four important developments that have taken place over the past half century (9). First, the biomedical community identified and clearly described those aspects of physical fitness that are related to health. Second, the scientific knowledge base underlying the original hypothesis that regular physical activity benefits health became firmly established. Third, the epidemiology of physical activity and inactivity has been studied and described in increasing detail over the years. Fourth, it has been recognized that both moderate and intense physical activity benefit health.

A major challenge is how to use all of our knowledge and understanding to actually help patients become regular exercisers at a level that is both comfortable and useful to them. Sound clinical advice, provided in an appropriate way by clinicians, can help patients unleash their own motivational process to become regular exercisers.

There are no known clinical trials of different approaches to the "nuts and bolts" of regular leisure-time exercise. Controlled research comparing the effectiveness of one particular leisure-time exercise program versus another in fostering an ongoing pattern of regular exercise would be difficult to design and very expensive to conduct. On the other hand, there is research on various exercise programs used as therapeutic interventions for the treatment of specific diseases and disorders. Therapeutic exercise regimens (and there are many very useful ones) are beyond the scope of this chapter.

Exercise: Aerobic and Nonaerobic

There are two types of regular exercise based on level of intensity: "aerobic" and "nonaerobic." Exercise is considered aerobic when it is intense enough to lead to a significant increase in muscle oxygen uptake. Nonaerobic exercise is any physical activity above the normal resting state involving one or more major muscle groups that is sustained but not so intense as to cause a significant increase in muscle oxygen uptake.

(Anaerobic exercise is intense physical activity, necessarily of very short duration [usually measured in seconds], fueled by energy sources within the contracting muscles, without the use of inhaled oxygen, most often incurred in competitive sports. It is not a factor in regular exercise.)

The heart rate is a simple measure to distinguish aerobic exercise from nonaerobic exercise. The exercise is considered to be aerobic when the pulse reaches or exceeds a level of 60% of the theoretical maximum normal, age-adjusted heart rate (220 − the person's age); 0.6 (220 − age). It is important to note that this commonly used formula roughly approximates the true degree of increased oxygen uptake by the muscles (10) and is more accurate for measuring the intensity of exercise in beginners than in conditioned athletes. Most regular exercisers do not routinely measure their heart rate during their workouts, relying instead on subjective measures, such as deep breathing and sweating, to know when they are *in the zone*. Patients who are subject to extreme tachycardia should take their pulse while exercising. To assure that exercise intensity remains at a safe level, the pulse rate should remain below 85% of the person's theoretical maximum age-adjusted heart rate (220 − age).

Although the evidence to date shows that exercise must be aerobic for it to be beneficial in reducing long-term risk for coronary artery disease, exercise at *any* level above the sedentary state is helpful for weight loss and for producing the mental benefits associated with regular physical activity. An even modest level of regular exercise frequency (1 or 2 hours per week at nonaerobic intensity) probably reduces mortality. Moderate-intensity physical activity other than regular leisure-time exercise, the so-called lifestyle approach, may also be beneficial for improving health and reducing mortality.

Objectives for Regular Exercise

Given the known benefits of regular exercise and the harmful consequences of a sedentary lifestyle, the objectives for the activity can be set out in a straightforward manner. Regardless of the accumulated data about the long-term health benefits of regular exercise, most regular exercisers engage in the activity because of the immediate benefits of feeling good and feeling better about themselves. When counseling patients about regular exercise, it is very important to bear this in mind. Most regular exercisers do not engage in the activity in order to reduce their risk for future disease. Risk reduction does not motivate most nonexercisers to start exercising either, unless a negative health event such as a heart attack shocks them into appropriate action, or they are exercising to promote weight loss. When patients ask about the benefits of regular exercise, the clinician should stress the short-term gains: feeling good, improved personal appearance, and increased self-esteem. The clinician should point out though that most but not all sedentary people who become regular exercisers experience these gains. Long-term benefits will also motivate some patients and should be noted.

Risks of Regular Exercise in the Otherwise Healthy Patient

Regular exercise has its risks as well as its benefits. Virtually all of the risks are preventable or modifiable. The most common risk of exercise is injury. There are three types of injuries: intrinsic, extrinsic, and overuse. Intrinsic injury is that caused by the nature of the activity or sport, for example, shin splints in running. Extrinsic injury is that caused by an external factor, for example, a cyclist hit by an automobile. Overuse injury results from exercising too far, too fast, too frequently. The latter is the most common cause of injury in most of the activities and sports used for regular exercise, such as running, fast walking, cycling, and swimming.

Intrinsic injury can be prevented by the use of proper equipment and correct technique. The risk of extrinsic injury can be significantly diminished by taking certain, mainly common sense, safety precautions, such as always wearing a helmet and never wearing a radio headset while riding a bicycle. Overuse injury can be prevented by choosing a sport along with a workout schedule that are suitable to the exerciser, and by maintaining moderation in distance, intensity, and speed. The risk of a variety of pathologic problems is increased when a previously sedentary person engages suddenly in intense exercise or when a regular exerciser suddenly increases exercise intensity. Therefore moderation and gradual change, if changes are to be made, are as always, good counsel.

GETTING UNDERWAY

"Recommendation" versus "Prescription"

Many clinicians use the term *exercise prescription* when discussing regular exercise with their patients. The term hails from the disease and medical models and appeals to many clinicians, especially those new to using the intervention. "Prescription," however, usually means telling a patient to do something for a limited period of time. Regular exercise is by its very nature voluntary. No one can be forced to do it.

Regular exercise requires more than just the temporary extra expenditure of time required to establish most other positive lifestyle changes such as engaging in healthy eating, achieving weight loss, and stopping cigarette smoking. For example, all people spend time food shopping, cooking, and eating. After learning about what changes to make, healthy eating requires only that the time be spent differently. After undergoing smoking cessation counseling and quitting tobacco use, no extra time need be spent again, unless relapse occurs. In contrast, regular exercise requires a permanent commitment of time that would be otherwise spent doing something else. Of course, the maintenance of any successful behavior change requires constant attention for the rest of one's life, to a greater or lesser extent. However, in order to be most effective in counseling their patients to become regular exercisers, clinicians need to recognize the ongoing time commitment that regular exercise requires.

Therefore, because of its special nature, exercise cannot be prescribed like a drug. Rather, the clinician is *recommending* the effort to become a regular exerciser. The clinician's goal should be to develop a respectful and supportive partnership with their patients, using advice and counseling to assist them in the decision-making process. The primary need is for the clinician to spend time with patients communicating about regular exercise, recognizing obstacles to success, and equipping patients with the tools to overcome them.

Risk Assessment

The clinician should assess every patient before recommending a regular exercise program. Some will need a full medical examination (see subsequent text). Many otherwise healthy patients will not. According to the USPSTF, neither a resting electrocardiogram nor an exercise stress test provides information helpful in reducing the risk of an adverse outcome from regular exercise among asymptomatic persons. Although the USPSTF does not endorse them, these tests may be clinically indicated for men older than 40 years with two or more risk factors for coronary artery disease other than sedentary lifestyle. Coronary artery disease risk factors include elevated serum cholesterol, history of cigarette smoking, hypertension, diabetes, or a family history of early-onset coronary artery disease

Furthermore, the clinician should conduct a thorough clinical evaluation of patients for whom regular exercise presents a *definite* risk, before advising these patients to start exercising. These high-risk patients may have a history of one or more of the following diseases or conditions:

- Previous myocardial infarction
- Exertional chest pain or pressure, or severe shortness of breath
- Pulmonary disease, especially chronic obstructive pulmonary disease
- Bone, joint or other musculoskeletal diseases or other limitations

These conditions are not necessarily contraindications to regular exercise, but each patient's risk must be assessed on an individual basis.

Patients for whom regular exercise presents *a possible* risk may have a history of one or more of the following diseases or conditions:

- Hypertension
- Cigarette smoking
- Elevated serum cholesterol
- Prescription medication used on a regular basis
- Abuse of drugs or alcohol
- Any other chronic illness, such as diabetes
- Family history of heart disease
- Overweight in excess of 20 lb
- Current sedentary lifestyle

Regular exercise is very useful in the management of a number of these diseases and conditions (3). For example, regular physical activity has been shown to reduce the rate of progression of diabetes by more than 50% (11). In fact, regular exercise may be a pivotal force in changing the natural history of a number of disease processes and possibly even obviate the need for therapeutic interventions. As mentioned earlier, the presence of these diseases may well become a motivational factor in convincing a nonexerciser to get started. Regular exercise in high-risk patients is beyond the scope of this chapter. However, it is important to stress that in initiating exercise such patients must follow a slow, gradual, and careful regimen with close medical supervision.

COUNSELING

Getting Started
GOAL SETTING

In most cases, the first subject to discuss with patients is goal setting: why is the patient thinking about regular exercise? It may be because the clinician suggested it, but virtually no one becomes and remains a regular exerciser simply because they are told to do so. To succeed, the patient must mobilize internal motivation. What goals does the patient want to achieve, and why? Specifically, does the patient want to become fit, lose weight, look better and feel better, reduce future risk of various diseases and conditions, or join a friend or family member in a race? In both starting and staying with a regular exercise program, it is very helpful if patients have a good grasp of just why they are doing it in the first place. The same list can be used in the process of motivational interviewing with patients who are not yet prepared to make health-promoting lifestyle changes. Chapter 5 provides additional information about motivational interviewing and also discusses the "stages of change" delineated in Prochaska's Transtheoretical Model: *precontemplation, contemplation, preparation, action*, and *maintenance* (see pages 132–133). For patients currently in the precontemplation or contemplation stages of change, addressing the questions mentioned earlier may be helpful to patients in advancing to the next stage.

REALISM

The clinician should counsel patients to set realistic goals and define success for themselves. A good formulation of this concept is to "explore your limits and recognize your limitations." Consider the example of endurance versus speed. After some reasonable period of training, say 3–4 months, most people can improve endurance, but they may not be able to improve their speed. Speed is the product of speed-specific training plus natural ability. Many people will be able to train fairly easily for endurance, because for most people endurance is not simply the product of natural ability. On the other hand, because natural ability is such an important element in speed, many exercisers will not be able to improve their speed no matter how hard they try. Clinicians should stress this point to their patients in order to avoid frustration, injury, and quitting. On the other hand, if patients are encouraged to explore their limits gradually and carefully, they may discover abilities they never knew they had.

INNER MOTIVATION

As noted in Chapter 5, the literature regarding positive lifestyle and behavior change clearly shows that the only kind of motivation that works in the long run comes from within. The patient says, "*I want to do this for me, because I want to look better, feel better, and feel better about myself, not for anyone else.*" In contrast, a patient who is externally motivated says, "*I'm doing this to make my [spouse, boy/girl friend, children/parents, employer/coworkers] feel better, but I don't anticipate getting much out of it for me.*" External motivation almost invariably leads to guilt, anxiety, anger, frustration, and, quitting, and possibly even injury.

TAKING CONTROL

"Taking control" is an important concept to stress with patients. In this formulation, patients decide to engage in physical activity on a regular basis, perhaps in a physical activity that they have never done before or even contemplated doing. Many people find that "taking control" of the process for themselves, thinking "yes I can, because yes, *I* can do this" is an important motivator, both in starting a regular exercise program and sticking with it.

GRADUAL CHANGE

"Gradual change leads to permanent changes" is another basic element leading to success in becoming a regular exerciser, losing weight (see Chapter 8), and making other lifestyle changes. It is recommended that the previously sedentary person should start with ordinary walking, at a normal pace, for 10 minutes or so, three times a week (see Table 6.1). After a couple of weeks, the patient can increase the length of each session. After several more weeks, the patient can increase the frequency of sessions and the speed with which the exercise is performed. The hardier soul may move through this program more quickly, but all should be counseled against going out for an hour, at full tilt at the beginning. "Too much, too soon" may lead to muscle pain, injury, and an increased likelihood of quitting. Once again, a *gradual* increase in time spent, distance covered, and speed are the proven formula for adherence.

GETTING STARTED: "IT IS THE REGULAR, NOT THE EXERCISE"

Further, the clinician should recognize that, for most people, the first challenge of becoming a regular exerciser is the "regular," and not the "exercise." Indeed for most people who are regular exercisers, the hard part remains the regular, not the exercise. Most people are aware that exercise is *good for them* and that they will feel better and increase their self-esteem

TABLE 6.1 The Pace Walking Plan (Phase I: Introductory Program)

Week	Day							Total	Comments
	M	T	W	Th	F	S	S		
1	Off	10	Off	10	Off	Off	10	30	Ordinary walking
2	Off	10	Off	10	Off	Off	10	30	Ordinary walking
3	Off	20	Off	20	Off	Off	20	60	Ordinary walking
4	Off	20	Off	20	Off	Off	20	60	Ordinary walking
5	Off	20	Off	20	Off	Off	20	60	Fast walking
6	Off	20	Off	20	Off	Off	20	60	Fast walking
7	Off	20	Off	20	Off	Off	30	70	Fast walking
8	Off	20	Off	20	Off	Off	30	70	Fast walking
9	Off	20	Off	20	Off	Off	20	60	Pace walking
10	Off	20	Off	20	Off	Off	30	70	Pace walking
11	Off	20	Off	30	Off	Off	30	80	Pace walking
12	Off	20	Off	30	Off	Off	30	80	Pace walking
13	Off	30	Off	30	Off	Off	30	90	Pace walking

Times in minutes.

if they begin exercising. Despite these positive reinforcements, most people have busy schedules and other demands that make it difficult for them to make room in their lives for exercise on a regular basis.

The correct first step for many patients who are motivated to start exercising is to discover that they can indeed find and make the time in their lives for exercise on a regular basis. They should define success for themselves by setting reasonable goals, recognizing that change will not occur overnight, and placing themselves in control of the process. For most people, the focus of the first 2–4 weeks of an exercise program (Table 6.1) should include making the time to exercise and walking instead of learning a new sport or athletic activity.

Patients who live in poor neighborhoods or who have limited resources face special challenges in becoming physically active. They often lack a conducive and convenient place in their built environment or safe surroundings to engage in regular exercise of the type discussed here. Researchers and urban planners are beginning to deal with this important issue.

Duration and Frequency

The original regular exercise recommendation of the ACSM dates back to the early 1980s and stated that in order for exercise to have a health benefit, it should be performed continuously for a minimum of 20–60 minutes at least three times per week. As of 2005, the ACSM recommendation was to exercise for 30–60 minutes (including warm-up and cooldown) three to five times per week (12). This recommendation assumes that the exercise will be done at least at the lower end of the aerobic level of intensity. Some guidelines encourage even greater duration for daily exercise (e.g., 60 or more minutes). However, they are problematic in terms of patient adherence and the heightened risk of overuse injuries. In the tables for regular exercise schedules presented in this chapter (Tables 6.1–6.4), the recommended duration and periodicity are also based on the assumption that the exercise will be done at the aerobic level of intensity.

As previously noted, since the early 1990s it has been recognized that physical activity, even at a moderate level of intensity, can also be beneficial to health. The Centers for Disease Control and Prevention (CDC) and the ACSM (13) recommended that, for persons not engaging in regular aerobic exercise at the ACSM standard, an accumulated 30 minutes daily of moderate-intensity physical activity (below the aerobic level) should be performed on as many days of the week as possible. The so-called lifestyle

TABLE 6.2   The Pace Walking Plan (Phase II: Developmental Program)

Week	Day							Total
	M	**T**	**W**	**Th**	**F**	**S**	**S**	**Total**
1	Off	Off	Off	Off	Off	Off	Off	Off
2	Off	20	Off	20	Off	Off	20	60
3	Off	20	Off	20	Off	20	20	80
4	Off	20	Off	20	Off	20	30	90
5	Off	20	Off	30	Off	20	30	100
6	Off	20	Off	30	Off	20	40	110
7	Off	30	Off	30	Off	30	30	120
8	Off	30	Off	30	Off	30	40	130
9	Off	30	Off	40	Off	30	40	140
10	Off	30	Off	40	Off	30	50	150
11	Off	40	Off	30	Off	30	60	160
12	Off	40	Off	30	Off	40	60	170
13	Off	30	Off	40	Off	50	60	180

Times in minutes.

TABLE 6.3 The Pace Walking Plan (Phase III A: Maintenance—2 Hours per Week)

| Week | Day | | | | | | | Total |
	M	T	W	Th	F	S	S	
1	Off	Off	Off	Off	Off	Off	Off	Off
2	Off	30	Off	30	Off	40	Off	100
3	30	Off	40	Off	20	Off	40	130
4	Off	40	Off	30	Off	40	Off	110
5	30	Off	40	Off	20	Off	40	130
6	Off	40	Off	30	Off	60	Off	130
7	20	Off	30	Off	30	Off	40	120
8	Off	40	Off	30	Off	50	Off	120
9	20	Off	40	Off	20	Off	60	140
10	Off	30	Off	30	Off	40	Off	100
11	20	Off	30	Off	20	Off	40	110
12	Off	40	Off	30	Off	60	Off	130
13	20	Off	30	Off	30	Off	40	120

Times in minutes.

approach to exercising regularly includes such activities as ordinary walking, gardening, and housecleaning for a minimum of 10 minutes per session (14). The "lifestyle" approach can help some people get started exercising regularly. Counting and recording short sessions and trying to figure what does and does not "count" as exercise can become confusing and time consuming. Therefore, it is likely that most people who commit to exercising regularly will prefer the leisure-time, scheduled approach. Nevertheless, for some the lifestyle approach can be a very good way to get started.

Any amount of regular exercise at any level of intensity is better than no exercise at all. Whatever the recommendations suggest, the amount of time that an individual devotes to regular exercise must fit comfortably into that individual's overall lifestyle, whether it is 2 hours a week or 12. Otherwise, success is doubtful.

Choosing the Activity or Sport

Once the patient deals successfully with the problem of making exercise a *regular activity*, the patient will need to focus on choosing a specific sport or activity. Please see the list of suggested readings at the end of this chapter for details on a variety of sports options. The first point the clinician should

TABLE 6.4 The Pace Walking Plan (Phase III B: Maintenance Plus—3 Hours per Week)

Week	M	T	W	Th	F	S	S	Total
				Day				
1	Off	Off	Off	Off	Off	Off	Off	Off
2	Off	30	Off	40	Off	30	50	150
3	Off	30	Off	50	Off	40	60	180
4	Off	40	Off	40	Off	50	80	210
5	Off	30	Off	50	Off	40	60	180
6	Off	50	Off	30	Off	50	70	200
7	Off	40	Off	30	Off	30	60	160
8	Off	30	Off	50	Off	40	60	180
9	Off	30	Off	40	Off	30	50	150
10	Off	30	Off	50	Off	40	50	170
11	Off	40	Off	30	Off	50	70	190
12	Off	40	Off	40	Off	50	80	210
13	Off	30	Off	50	Off	40	60	180

Times in minutes.

stress is that regular aerobic exercise is not limited to running and aerobic dance. There is a wide range of activities or sports that can be used for regular exercise, whether aerobic or nonaerobic.

There are the "tried and true" sports, such as running, fast walking, bicycling, and aerobic dance. These are sports to which most people have ready access at home, where they may even exercise to the accompaniment of a video or television show. Less widely available are activities that often require an athletic facility, such as running and walking on a treadmill or indoor track, swimming, and group aerobic dance classes. Exercise machines such as treadmills, stair climbers, ellipticals, and stationary bicycles can be purchased for home use. For cycling, there are also "indoor trainer" devices on which road bicycles can be mounted for riding in place. Certain individual and team skill sports are often played at aerobic intensity and are useful for regular exercise. These sports include singles tennis, squash, racquetball, handball, and full-court basketball. They require an athletic facility with courts and at least one partner. Weight training, with free weights or a machine, can be done at home or in the gym and can also be performed aerobically. As contrasted with weight training for strength and bulk, aerobic routines stress lighter resistance, more repetitions and sets (groups of repetitions) of each program component, and less time between sets to keep the heart rate in the training range. Some health clubs feature "circuit training," utilizing a set of machines and stations offering different muscle resistance levels. Aerobic exercises are performed by participants in a series, following a timed schedule established by a prerecorded set of instructions broadcast in the circuit training room over the loudspeaker.

The choice of sports and activities for regular exercise is therefore very broad. No one sport is "better" than any other sport for regular exercise. The "best" sport or other physical activity is the one that gets the exerciser into a long-term regular schedule while hopefully achieving some level of enjoyment. The heart and muscles do not "know" what sport the exerciser is performing. If the activity increases heart rate and muscle oxygen uptake to a given level, the benefit will be the same, regardless of the sport. For example, pace walking—fast walking with a strong arm swing (see Fig 6.1)—is equivalent to running if each is done to the same level of aerobic intensity. Pace walking with a strong arm swing at a rate of 11–12 minutes per mile is usually as demanding on the cardiovascular system as running 8–9 minutes per mile.

After learning the "regular" part by engaging in ordinary walking, it is then time for the patient to choose a sport or other physical activity that he or she will enjoy. In fact, the likelihood of remaining a regular exerciser will be increased if the patient chooses two different sports or activities (e.g., going to the health club once or twice a week for low-impact aerobic dance, and pace walking once or twice a week). Once the exerciser is in a routine, the activities can be varied over the course of the year in order to further decrease the chance of boredom.

Making Exercise "Fun"

When contemplating regular exercise, many patients will say, "*Well, I know I should exercise, but I know it just isn't going to be fun*." In fact, some people find to their surprise that exercise is enjoyable, in and of itself. For those exercisers whose enjoyment from exercise lie in between, there are some techniques for making exercise more fun. Over the long run, the following techniques may also help all exercisers maintain the fun level:

- Let it be fun: positive anticipation is very important.
- Set appropriate goals, and avoid doing too much, too soon, as discussed previously.
- For the distance sports, train by minutes, not miles (see later in this chapter).
- Recognize that, in those distance sports in which concentration on technique is not required, exercise time is uniquely private and great

for thinking. (For safety considerations, road bicycling should not be viewed this way.)

- Listen to music, the news, or radio talk shows through a headset. (Appropriate safety measures must be taken, however. Outdoor use of in-the-ear headphones can block out the sounds of traffic, animals, and other individuals approaching. Rather, sponge phones mounted on the temple in front of the auditory canal should be used. Outdoor cyclists should never use headsets.)
- Set nonexercise-related goals like getting an errand or two completed in the course of a workout.
- Periodically, reward oneself with a new piece of clothing or a long-denied snack treat.
- Enjoy the rhythm, being outdoors, and the seasonal variation that is part of many of the sports done for aerobic exercise.
- Many regular exercisers find that a very useful way to stay on a program and enjoy it is to engage occasionally in racing, not for speed but for participation and feelings of personal achievement in terms of distance covered or time spent.
- Be sure to take a week or two off when needed, at least one to two times per year.

Generic Training Program

Tables 6.1–6.4 present a generic training program from the beginning phase through regular maintenance, at all levels up to the training level required for racing on a regular basis. Note that the workouts are measured in minutes instead of miles. Time rather than distance is a better way to define the workout because, in the end, what counts is the duration and not the speed: the mental and physical stressor of speed is not a factor for distance sports.

Psychologically, it is much easier to pace walk regularly for 40 minutes at a stretch than it is to cover 3 or 4 measured miles. If the person is feeling good and the weather is nice, he or she will go faster and cover more ground. A bit of stiffness on a given day will lead to a slower workout and therefore less distance covered. The benefit of focusing on time is that the workouts can be used for any sport or activity the patient decides to undertake. The minutes formula allows the person to easily mix and match sports or activities in a single program. The periodicity and duration of the sessions comprising the program recommended in these tables are based on the assumption that the person will be engaging in a *regular exercise* program, at a level of intensity eventually reaching the aerobic range. The objective is to help patients become regular exercisers at a comfort level that works for them.

The Introductory Program (Table 6.1) starts with ordinary walking and concludes with pace walking (see page 163 for a brief description of the technique). This program leads up to engaging in 1.5 hours of exercise per week. The Developmental Program (Table 6.2) provides for up to 3 hours of exercise per week. There are two Maintenance Programs: the program in Table 6.3 provides an average of 2 hours per week over a 13-week period, whereas that in Table 6.4 provides an average of 3 hours per week. The latter is the equivalent of 15–20 miles of running per week, which is all that is required to gain the maximum health benefits from regular exercise. Musculoskeletal fitness increases with exercise intensity, time, and distance, up to approximately 75 miles of running per week.

As noted, the current (2006) ACSM recommendation encourages working out 3–5 days per week. The total weekly allotted time for each pace walking program in the tables is distributed over 3–4 days per week. Obviously, the suggested times can be redistributed over 4–5 days per week, with shorter sessions for each workout. Some stretching after a brief warm-up is recommended. There are books devoted entirely to stretching (see "Resources" at the end of this chapter). Some sport-specific books also contain a section on stretching. Note that, once a 4-day-per-week level is reached, in either Phase II or Phase III B, more than half of the total workout time is scheduled for the weekends, making the program more convenient for most people. Phase III A is an every-other-day program, requiring an average of only 2 hours per week. These programs provide the framework in which virtually any motivated patient can become a regular exerciser—slowly, gradually, and without the need to make an overwhelming time commitment.

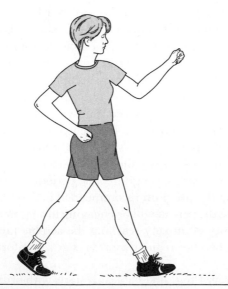

Figure 6.1 • Correct pace walking gait and arm swing.

Technique

The clinician need not be a technical expert in the sports or activities suitable for regular exercise. There are many good books written for the layman on the subject (see "Resources" for some examples). If exercise counseling becomes a regular part of the practice, the clinician may benefit from periodic visits to local bookshops and/or the popular web-based booksellers for an update on available books.

The technique for pace walking (Fig. 6.1), the recommended starting sport, is very simple. Sample instructions for the patient are provided in the sidebar (Box):

How to Pace Walk: Walk fast with a purposeful stride of medium length. With each step, land on your heel, then roll forward along the outside (lateral aspect) of your foot, and push off with your toes. Try to keep your feet pointed straight ahead, walking along an imaginary white line. This will help your balance and rhythm, and will allow you to increase your speed. Your back should be comfortably straight, but not rigidly so. Your shoulders should be dropped and relaxed, your head up. Swing your arms forward and back, strongly, with your elbows comfortably bent. (The elbow bend prevents the accumulation of fluid in the hands, which will happen if you swing your arms strongly while keeping them straight.) At the end of the back swing, you should feel a tug in your shoulder. On the fore swing, your hand should come up no further than mid-chest level. To stay in balance and maintain a smooth forward motion from the hips down, concentrate on the back swing, not the fore swing.

For most people, it is the strong arm swing that makes pace walking aerobic. If a person has been completely sedentary for some time, just walking quickly without the strong arm swing will most likely raise the heart rate into the aerobic range. When the exerciser has been working out more regularly though, walking fast alone will not be sufficient to raise the heart rate into the aerobic range. That is why if walking is to be used as the aerobic exercise on an ongoing basis (and many regular exercisers do so use it), a second major muscle group must be brought into play (i.e., swinging the arms strongly as in pace walking).

Equipment

As with technique, details on equipment can be found in various sport-specific books. Common to most regular exercise sports or activities is the need for properly fitting shoes in order to achieve success and avoid injury. Proper fit means that the shoe should conform to the shape of the exerciser's foot by touching the foot in as many places as possible, except over the toes. The shoe should be flexible under the ball of the foot, and it should have a firm vertical "heel counter" at the back end of the shoe to keep the heel down in the shoe. The design should be suited to the sport for which it will be used: that is, shoes for pace walking or running should facilitate forward motion, shoes for tennis or aerobic dance should facilitate lateral motion. Referral to a sports medicine orthopedist or podiatrist may be necessary for orthotics or special shoes in patients with a lower extremity disorder or a known foot deformity such as hallux valgus. In general, a person should be advised to buy equipment in a "pro shop" rather than in a department store. A pro shop is a store other than a sports "superstore" that is dedicated to sports equipment. In general, the more sport specific the focus of the store, the more likely the buyer will come away with suitable equipment. In a pro shop, the buyer is more likely to find salespeople who are knowledgeable about the sport for which they are selling equipment and more likely to actually engage in the sport themselves. Although "good buys" and high quality equipment can be found at sports "superstores," the quality of the advice received can be highly variable, if available at all. The cost of equipment for the regular exerciser can range from nothing (the person decides to pace walk or jog, and their wardrobe already includes an adequate pair of shoes and the necessary clothing), to hundreds or even several thousand dollars for a health club membership, high-performance athletic shoes, or a top-of-the-line bicycle. The best recommendation for beginners is to spend as little as possible, except on buying a good pair of shoes if they lack a pair, until they are convinced they are going to stay with the sport.

OFFICE AND CLINIC ORGANIZATION

These principles must be reduced to a counseling package that can be used successfully in clinical practice. First, of course, clinicians must decide whether exercise counseling is important for some or all of their patients. To do that, the clinician should follow the same goal-setting process that the potential exerciser undertakes as his or her first step. See the questions posed in the section on "Setting Reasonable Limits and Priorities in Risk Assessment" in Chapter 1 (pages 10–18). It will also be necessary for the clinician to answer the following questions:

- Is exercise promotion important in my practice? Why? For which patients?
- What are the goals, for the patients, the practice, and the clinician?
- Who should do the counseling: medical professionals or other staff members?
- How is exercise counseling going to be paid for?
- Is counseling groups of patients (group visits) a strategy worth trying?
- If so, when will they be offered and under what fee arrangements?
- How should the practice use community resources (e.g., classes offered by health systems and community centers, health clubs, sports clubs, gyms,

pools, tracks, bicycle routes, walking or running trails, courts, and pro shops), if at all?

- Are there other resources, such as Internet or telephone coaching services, which can be used in concert with the clinician?
- Is role modeling important?
- How should I learn the specifics of regular exercise counseling and incorporate them into my own knowledge base and skills?
- How much time am I willing to invest in developing an exercise promotion component in my practice?

It should be noted that asking and answering these questions for oneself, with certain variations to be sure, applies to the consideration of adding any health behavior counseling program/protocol to one's practice. In particular the list applies to weight management efforts for which a regular exercise component should surely be included. In many practices, group programs for promoting both regular exercise and healthy weight management will be at least in part integrated. Practices face opportunity costs in setting up a group class for every behavior, and therefore some parsimony is required. Although a practice would likely run separate group classes for smoking cessation or healthy sexual practices, an integrated program for exercise and weight management might come naturally because regular exercise is so central to effective weight management and because so many persons who first seek help with regular exercise are trying to lose weight. Indeed it would make sense for a practice to have an integrated approach to the triad of exercise, diet, and weight management, at least for "beginners." More advanced classes that focus on exercise might be considered for patients going on to higher levels of regular exercise for its own sake and perhaps competitive sports (e.g., racing).

Further, if it is decided to incorporate exercise promotion into one's routine clinical practice, it is worth spending time to learn about and evaluate the various community resources for promoting both regular exercise and weight management. This will save time and provides substantive assistance to patients. The clinician can consider setting up a formal referral relationship with respected community facilities and establishing convenient in-office systems (e.g., fax referral forms, automated referrals using an electronic health record) to facilitate the process (see Chapter 21 for more details on making use of these resources). By whatever method exercise counseling is accomplished the clinician should make it a regular part of the practice and be sure to document the exercise counseling in the patient's medical record. Finally, although not essential, clinicians who regularly exercise themselves can set examples for patients. Such clinicians can draw on their own experiences to counsel patients on the benefits and the drawbacks of being a regular exerciser.

RESOURCES—PATIENT EDUCATION MATERIALS

Organizations

American Academy of Family Physicians
http://www.aafp.org/
> *Exercise: a healthy habit to start and keep* at http://familydoctor.org/059.xml.
> Reviewed/Updated: 04/05; Created: 01/96.

American College of Sports Medicine
http://www.acsm.org/
> *ACSM guidelines for healthy aerobic activity* at http://www.acsm.org/pdf/
> Guidelines.pdf.

American Heart Association
http://www.americanheart.org/. July, 2007.
> *Exercise and fitness*. 2006 at http://www.americanheart.org/presenter.jhtml?identifier
> =1200013.

Centers for Disease Control and Prevention
http://www.cdc.gov/. Page last updated: May 22, 2007.
> *Physical activity for everyone* at http://www.cdc.gov/nccdphp/dnpa/physical/
> index.htm.

National Institute on Aging
http://www.nia.nih.gov/
> *Exercise for older adults* at http://nihseniorhealth.gov/exercise/toc.html. Last reviewed:
> 29 June 2005; First published: 19 March 2002.

Books

General

Jonas S. *Regular exercise: a handbook for clinical practice*. New York City: Springer-Verlag New York, 1996.

Thompson W, Jonas S, Bernadot D. American College of Sports Medicine. *ACSM fitness book*. Champaign: Human Kinetics Publishers, 2003.

Walking

Ikonian T. *Fitness walking*, 2nd ed. Champaign: Human Kinetics Publishers, 2005.

Jonas S. *Pace walking*. New York City: Crown, 1988.

Running

Brown RL, Henderson JK. *Fitness running*, 2nd ed. Champaign: Human Kinetics Publishers, 2003.

Fixx J. *The complete book of running*. New York: Random House, 1977. (An absolute evergreen).

Glover B, Shepherd J, Glover S-lF. *The Runner's handbook*, 2nd rev ed. New York: Penguin Publishing, 1996.

Hanc J. wrote both *The essential runner*. New York: Lyons and Burford, 1994; and *The essential marathoner*. New York: Lyons and Burford, 1996, both now available from Globe-Pequot Press.

Sheehan G. *Running and being: the total experience*, 2nd Wind II. New Jersey: Simon and Schuster, 1998. (This is a reissue of this classic work).

Bicycling

Barry DD, Barry M, Sovndal S. *Fitness cycling*. Champaign: Human Kinetics Publishers, 2006.

Swimming and Water Workouts

Katz J. *Swimming for total fitness, updated*. New York: Broadway Books, 2002.

Heart Rate Monitoring

Edwards S. *Heart rate monitor guidebook*. Sacramento: Heart Zones Publishing, 2005.

Weight Training

Baechle TR, Earle RW. *Fitness weight training*. Champaign: Human Kinetics Publishers, 2005.

Triathloning

Jonas S. *Triathloning for ordinary mortals, and doing the duathlon too*, 20th Anniv. 2nd ed. New York: WW Norton, 2006.

SUGGESTED READINGS

American College of Sports Medicine. *Guidelines for healthy aerobic exercise*. http://www.acsm.org/pdf/Guidelines.pdf. 2006.

Blair SN, Kohl HW, Paffenbarger RS, et al. Physical fitness and all-cause mortality. *JAMA* 1989;262:2395–2401.

Harris SS, Caspersen CJ, De Friese GH, et al. Physical activity counseling for healthy adults. *JAMA* 1989;261:3590–3598.

Paffenbarger RS, Hyde RT, Wing AL, et al. The association of changes in physical-activity level and other lifestyle characteristics with mortality among men. *N Engl J Med* 1993;328:538–545.

Pate RR, Pratt M, Blair SN, et al. Physical activity and public health: a recommendation from the Centers for Disease Control and Prevention and the American College of Sports Medicine. *J Am Med Assoc* 1995;273:402–407.

Sandvik L, Erikssen J, Thaulow E, et al. Physical fitness as a predictor of mortality among healthy, middle-aged Norwegian men. *N Engl J Med* 1993;328:533–537.

U.S. Department of Health and Human Services, Public Health Service. *Healthy people 2000: National Health Promotion and Disease Prevention Objectives*. DHHS Pub. No. (PHS) 91–50213. Washington, DC: Government Printing Office, 1991.

References

1. Bouchard C, Shephard RJ, Stephens T, eds. *Physical activity, fitness, and health: international proceedings and consensus statement*. Champaign: Human Kinetics Publishers, 1994:77–78.
2. U.S. Department of Health and Human Services, Healthy People 2010. *Physical activity and fitness*, chapter 22. Washington, DC: U.S. Department of Health and Human Services, 2000:22–21. Conference edition, in two volumes.
3. Blair SN, LaMonte MJ. How much and what type of physical activity is enough? *Arch Intern Med* 2005;165:2324–2325.

4. U.S. Preventive Services Task Force. *Behavioral Counseling in Primary Care to Promote Physical Activity: Recommendations and Rationale*, Rockville, MD. Agency for Healthcare Research and Quality, (see also http://www.ahrq.gov/clinic/3rduspstf/physactivity/physactrr.htm), July 2002.

5. Petrella RJ, Koval JJ, Cunningham DA, et al. Can primary care doctors prescribe exercise to improve fitness? *Am J Prev Med* 2003;24(45):316–322.

6. Elley CR, Kerse N, Arroll B, et al. Effectiveness of counseling in patients on physical activity in general practice: cluster randomized controlled trial. *Br Med J* 2003;326:793–799.

7. Pinto BM, Goldstein MG, Ashba J, et al. Randomized controlled trial of physical activity counseling for older primary care patients. *Am J Prev Med* 2005;29(4): 247–255.

8. Cress ME, Buchner DM, Prohaska T, et al. Physical activity programs and behavior counseling in older adult populations. *Med Sci Sports Exer* 2004;36: 1997–2003.

9. Paffenbarger RS. An introduction to the journal of physical activity and health. *J Phys Act Health J* 2004;1:1–3.

10. Wier LT, Jackson AS. Exercise intensity: misleading measurements. *Running FitNews* 1993;11(2):1.

11. Diabetes Prevention Program Research Group. Reduction in the incidence of type 2 diabetes with lifestyle intervention or metformin. *N Engl J Med* 2002;346: 393–403.

12. American College of Sports Medicine. Guidelines for healthy aerobic exercise. http://www.acsm.org/pdf/Guidelines.pdf. 2006.

13. Pate RR, Pratt M, Blair SN, et al. Physical activity and public health: a recommendation from the Centers for Disease Control and Prevention and the American College of Sports Medicine. *J Am Med Assoc* 1995;273:402–407.

14. Fogelholm M, Suni J, Rinne M, et al. Physical activity pie: a graphical representation integrating recommendations for fitness and health. *J Phys Act Health* 2005;2(4):391–396.

CHAPTER 7

Nutrition

Roger A. Shewmake

The goal of this chapter is to provide evidence-based information to help clinicians counsel patients regarding the latest nutritional approaches to disease prevention and health promotion. It also attempts to clarify the strong relationships between nutrition and the prevention of chronic disease and the important influence of nutrient deficiencies and excesses.

For a large majority of the population, the food choices made daily, over time, will either benefit or impair health. Food choices and habits are very complex and personal issues that reflect preferences developed through association with family and friends, as well as habits developed through one's ethnic heritage, culture, traditions, ethnicity, religion, and social interactions. Food is used for celebrations of all aspects of life and therefore can serve as "comfort foods," especially at emotionally stressful times. In the current rushed environment, the availability, convenience, and economy of food often sway personal choices. Individuals select foods for a variety of reasons but the diet ingested over time can make important contributions to health.

Nutrient effects are a common thread that runs through many of the chronic diseases that affect populations. Consuming a diet high in refined carbohydrates and fat, along with low-fiber intake, high caloric density, low nutrient density, and inadequate physical activity, are common risk factors for cardiovascular disease, diabetes, obesity, and hypertension among other diseases and negative health conditions. As discussed in Chapter 8, the prevalence of overweight and obesity is increasing in the United States, which in turn increases the risk of many chronic diseases (e.g., hypertension, diabetes, and some forms of cancer) and of premature death. See Chapter 8 for further details on the assessment and treatment of overweight and obesity.

According to the American Heart Association (AHA) (1):

1. *"There are dietary and other lifestyle practices that all individuals can safely follow throughout the lifespan as a foundation for achieving and maintaining cardiovascular and overall health."*
2. *"Healthy dietary practices are based on one's overall pattern of food intake over an extended period of time and not on the intake of a single meal."*

3. *"The guidelines form a framework within which specific dietary recommendations can be made for individuals based on their health status, dietary preferences, and cultural background."*

This chapter focuses on the components of a healthy diet. It includes a practical discussion of the influence of macronutrients, vitamins, and minerals upon health, with special emphasis on nutrition's effect upon lipoproteins, blood pressure, diabetes, and the lifecycle. Chapter 6 discusses the important role of physical activity, which must generally be combined with the nutrition interventions discussed here to promote wellness and reduce weight.

NUTRITIONAL ASSESSMENT

Dietary Assessment

Chapter 2 discusses screening and exploratory questions that clinicians can use in the periodic health examination to quickly assess a patient's dietary habits. The 24- to 72-hour dietary recall has also been a useful tool in evaluating normal habits, intakes, and evidence of possible deficiencies in the diet. An ongoing record or a checklist that is possibly completed at mealtime may be one of the better methods of completing a dietary recall. Limited memory, cognitive impairment, increased time to complete the recall, and other difficulties created by health problems may make it difficult to obtain representative information without multiple sampling.

Anthropometric Assessments

See Chapter 3 (pages 57–61) regarding the measurement of height and weight to calculate the body mass index (BMI).

Biochemical Assessment of Nutritional Status

Serum prealbumin has a half-life of 2 days and is more sensitive than albumin in evaluating nutritional changes. Improved nutritional intake can increase prealbumin levels by approximately 10 mg/L/day. A lower increase may indicate inadequate nutritional support, poor response, and a poor prognosis. Low levels of insulin-like growth factor 1, another very sensitive indicator of nutritional change, is associated with increased morbidity. Evidence does not support the use of either serum prealbumin or insulin-like growth factor 1 as a single marker of nutritional status.

Nutrition Screening of Older Adults

Nutritional screening of seniors has gained in popularity as an effort to identify individuals who are at risk and need further intervention. The Nutrition Screening Initiative, a project of the American Academy of Family Physicians, American Dietetic Association, and the National Council on Aging, provides a "Determine Your Nutrition Health" checklist. The National Screening Initiative is targeted for identification of elderly individuals who are at nutritional risk. Using the mnemonic D-E-T-E-R-M-I-N-E, it provides a list of warning signs for malnutrition that should be addressed (see Tables 7.1 and 7.2).

Subjective Global Assessment

The Subjective Global Assessment of Nutritional Status (see Table 7.3) does not employ objective biochemical and anthropometric measurements. It is a screening tool that requires clinical judgment to interpret information collected by interviews and observations. The instrument correlates well with other more objective measures and is cost effective (2).

THE IMPORTANCE OF NUTRITION COUNSELING

A clinician's advice on nutrition is of great importance in helping patients to modify dietary practices. This chapter provides detailed guidance, but the science of healthy living needs to be made practical for patients. Short and useful recommendations can be as simple as: (a) do not crash diet, (b) eat real foods, (c) watch your portion size, and (d) eat breakfast. Eating breakfast is a caloric plus in that it increases the metabolic rate and can provide nutrients needed for the day.

Adopting a healthy diet can be simple but is not always easy. Patients can easily become discouraged when they attempt to change too many eating habits at once. Clinicians can advocate small steps, perhaps through a "nutrition prescription" of adding one fruit or vegetable today or changing to 1% milk. Remind patients that healthy living is not defined by just one meal or 1 day but the accumulation of small changes; these changes become habits over time. Behavior modification can begin with modest steps, such as not bringing foods home that are too tempting or replacing them with better choices. "Choose/do not choose" lists are often excellent tools to change behavior. The short but essential admonition to watch portions and be active can sum up basic first steps to meeting healthy nutrition goals (see Table 7.4).

THE DIETARY GUIDELINES FOR AMERICANS

In 2005, the Food and Nutrition Board of the Institute of Medicine (IOM), along with Health Canada, released the sixth in a series of reports on dietary reference values for the intake of macronutrients and energy (U.S. Dietary Guidelines). This report established Dietary Reference Intakes (DRIs) for carbohydrates, fiber, fatty acids, cholesterol, protein, amino acids, energy, and physical activity, replacing older

TABLE 7.1 Checklist to Help Older Adults Assess Their Nutritional Health

The warning signs of poor nutritional health are often overlooked

	Yes
I have an illness or condition that made me change the kind and/or amount of food I eat	2
I eat fewer than two meals per day	3
I eat few fruits or vegetables, or milk products	2
I have three or more drinks of beer, liquor, or wine almost every day	2
I have tooth or mouth problems that make it hard for me to eat	2
I don't always have enough money to buy the food I need	4
I eat alone most of the time	1
I take three or more different prescribed or over-the-counter drugs a day	1
Without wanting to, I have lost or gained 10 lb in the last 6 months	2
I am not physically able to shop, cook and/or feed myself	2
Total	

Total your nutritional score. If it is:

0–2   **Good**! Recheck your nutritional score in 6 months

3–5   **You are at moderate nutritional risk.** See what can be done to improve your eating habits and lifestyle. Your area's office on aging, senior nutrition program, senior citizens center, or health department can help. Recheck your nutritional score in 3 months.

6 or more   **You are at high nutritional risk.** Bring this checklist the next time you see your doctor, dietician, or other qualified health or social service professional. Talk with them about any problems you may have. Ask for help to improve your nutritional health.

Remember that warning signs suggest risk, but do not represent diagnosis of any condition.

The "Determine Your Nutritional Health" checklist was developed by the Nutrition Screening Initiative, a project of the American Academy of Family Physicians, the American Dietetic Association and the National Council on the Aging, Inc. First published: June 1998. Revised: April 2005.

TABLE 7.2   D-E-T-E-R-M-I-N-E Checklist to Help Older Adults Identify Symptoms of Nutritional Problems

The Nutrition Checklist is Based on the Warning Signs Described Below. Use the Word D-E-T-E-R-M-I-N-E to Remind You of the Warning Signs

☐ *Disease* Any disease, illness, or chronic condition that causes you to change the way you eat, or makes it hard for you to eat, puts your nutritional health at risk. Four out of five adults have chronic diseases that are affected by diet. Confusion or memory loss that keeps getting worse is estimated to affect one out of five or more of older adults. This can make it hard to remember what, when, or if you have eaten. Feeling sad or depressed, which happens to about one in eight older adults, can cause big changes in appetite, digestion, energy level, weight and well-being.

☐ *Eating poorly* Eating too little and eating too much both lead to poor health. Eating the same foods day after day or not eating fruit, vegetables, and milk products daily will also cause poor nutritional health. One in five adults skip meals daily. Only 13% of adults eat the minimum amount of fruit and vegetables needed. One in four older adults drink too much alcohol. Many health problems become worse if you drink more than one or two alcoholic beverages per day.

☐ *Tooth loss/mouth pain* A healthy mouth, teeth, and gums are needed to eat. Missing, loose or rotten teeth, or dentures which do not fit well or cause mouth sores, make it hard to eat.

☐ *Economic hardship* As many as 40% of older Americans have incomes of less than $6000 per year. Having less—or choosing to spend less—than $25–30 per week for food makes it very hard to get the foods you need to stay healthy.

☐ *Reduced social contact* One-third of all older people live alone. Being with people daily has a positive effect on morale, well-being, and eating.

☐ *Multiple medicines* Many older Americans must take medicines for health problems. Almost half of older Americans take multiple medicines daily. Growing old may change the way we respond to drugs. The more medicines you take, the greater the chance of side effects, such as increased or decreased appetite, change in taste, constipation, weakness, drowsiness, diarrhea, nausea, and others. Vitamins or minerals, when taken in large doses, act like drugs and can cause harm. Alert your doctor to everything you take

(continued)

TABLE 7.2 *(Continued)*

☐ **Involuntary weight loss/gain** Losing or gaining a lot of weight when you are not trying to do so is an important warning sign that must not be ignored. Being overweight or underweight also increases your chance of poor health.

☐ **Needs assistance in self-care** Although most older people are able to eat, one out of every five has trouble walking, shopping, or buying and cooking food, especially as they get older.

☐ **Elderly, age above 80 years** Most older people lead full productive lives. But as age increases, the risk of frailty and health problems increases. Checking your nutritional health regularly makes good sense.

Adapted from materials developed by the Nutrition Screening Initiative, Washington, DC 2007.

recommended dietary allowances (RDAs) last updated in 1989. The DRIs are based on scientific relationships between nutrient intake, chronic disease, and health status. The new dietary guidelines, which provide evidence-based nutritional guidance for ages 2 years and older, have the goals of inspiring individuals to seek more information about healthy eating, communicating scientifically accurate but understandable information, and guiding federal policy and programs. Public confusion around nutrition is fostered by terms commonly used in commercials and food labels (e.g., whole grain, organic, fat-free, no trans-fats, all natural, rich in fiber, low glycemic index, lowers cholesterol). The guidelines make 41 key recommendations, 23 for the general public and 18 for special populations. Clinicians should refer to the Dietary Guidelines for Americans 2005 Toolkit for Health Professionals (http://www.health.gov/dietaryguidelines/dga2005/toolkit/), which compiles the latest evidence-based nutrition and physical activity recommendations.

Food Groups to Encourage

A key theme in the guidelines is the consumption of adequate nutrients within caloric needs. This should be accomplished by consuming a variety of nutrient-dense foods and beverages within and among the basic food groups while choosing foods that limit intake of saturated and trans-fat, cholesterol, added sugars, salt, and alcohol. Diets should emphasize a variety of fiber-rich fruits, vegetables, and whole grains, staying within one's energy needs. Five servings of fruits and vegetables per day is recommended. Patients should consume 3 oz equivalents of whole grains daily (at least half whole grains

TABLE 7.3 Subjective Global Assessment Summary

HISTORY

1. Weight change
   Overall loss in past 6 months: amount = _____ kg _____ %
   Change in past 2 weeks: _____ increase
   _____ no change
   _____ decrease
2. Dietary intake change (relative to normal)
   _____ no change
   _____ change
   Duration: _____ weeks
   Type: _____ suboptimal solid diet
   _____ full liquid diet
   _____ hypocaloric liquids
   _____ starvation
3. Gastrointestinal symptoms (persisting for >2 weeks)
   ___ none ___ nausea ___ vomiting___ diarrhea ___ anorexia
4. Functional capacity
   _____ no dysfunction (e.g., full capacity)
   _____ dysfunction
   Duration: _____ weeks
   Type: _____ working suboptimally
   _____ ambulatory
   _____ bedridden

PHYSICAL EXAMINATION

For each trait, specify a rating as follows:

0 = normal, 1+ = mild, 2+ = moderate, 3+ = severe
_____ loss of subcutaneous fat (triceps, chest)
_____ muscle wasting (quadriceps, deltoids)
_____ ankle edema
_____ sacral edema
_____ ascites

SUBJECTIVE GLOBAL ASSESSMENT RATING (select one)
_____ A = well nourished
_____ B = moderately (or suspected of being) malnourished
_____ C = severely malnourished

From Detsky AS, McLaughlin JR, Baker JP, et al. What is subjective global assessment? *J Parent Ent Nutr* 1987;11(1):8.

TABLE 7.4 Behavioral Steps for a Healthy Diet

Food Preparation

Preplan your meals
Learn to cook the calorie-reduced way
Include low-calorie foods at each meal
Shop when your control is highest and have a list

Mealtime

Preload your stomach with liquids and drink ample liquids during meals
Use smaller plates, bowls, glasses, and serving spoons
Do not keep serving dishes on the table
Stop eating for a minute during the meal
Leave a little food on your plate (doggy bag)

Snacking at Home

Keep tempting foods out of the house
Eat three healthy meals a day
Brush your teeth after every meal and use mouthwash
Preplan snacks into your eating plan
Try sugar-free gum, hard candy, diet soda, or fruit when craving sweets
Exercise every day
Ask family and friends not to offer you snacks
Talk to yourself

Emotional Snacking

Use relaxation exercises
Take a warm bubble bath
Listen to relaxing music
Get out of the house

and the rest should be enriched) and three cups per day of fat-free, low-fat, or equivalent milk products. Children aged 2–8 years should consume two cups of fat-free or low-fat milk or equivalent milk products per day. Other key recommendations include consuming two servings of fish per week (approximately 8 oz total) to help reduce risks from cardiovascular disease, reducing the intake of sugars especially through sweetened beverages, and consuming less than 2,300 mg of sodium with an increase in foods rich in potassium. See Figure 7.1 for an example of how to accomplish all of this within the limits of a 2,000-cal diet.

CARBOHYDRATES

Patients should consume 130 g/day of carbohydrates. Carbohydrates should provide 50–60% of total daily calories and should emphasize complex carbohydrates that include dietary fiber (see subsequent text). The intake of refined carbohydrates and sugars should be limited to reduce the risk of caries.

Glycemic index is a measure of how quickly carbohydrates enter the blood stream and then elevate blood sugar levels. In general, most refined foods in the United States have a high glycemic index, whereas nonstarchy vegetables, fruits, and legumes seem to have a lower glycemic index. Although some hypothesize that long-term consumption of high-glycemic index foods may increase the risk of obesity, diabetes, and heart disease, others argue that the index is studied primarily under artificial laboratory conditions and does not accurately portray the mixed meals that most individuals consume. The American Diabetes Association states that there is insufficient evidence to use glycemic index in the management of diabetes. Clinicians should at least be aware of the glycemic index of certain foods, and that it may cause spikes in blood sugar levels, especially among patients with diabetes (*www.glycemicindex.com*).

FIBER

Individuals older than 4 years should consume at least 25 g of fiber each day (see Table 7.5), yet 50% of women consume fewer than 13 g a day and 50% of men consume fewer than 17 g a day (3). Fiber includes two main types: soluble and insoluble. *Insoluble fiber*, an important aid in normal bowel function, is provided in high concentrations in whole wheat breads, wheat cereals, wheat bran, rye, rice, barley, cabbage, beets, carrots, Brussels sprouts, turnips, cauliflower, and apple skins. Sources of *soluble fiber* include oat bran, oatmeal, beans, peas, rice bran, barley, citrus fruits, apple pulp, psyllium, carrots, strawberries, peaches with skin, and apples with skin. Most fiber-rich foods contain a mixture of both soluble and insoluble fibers. The AHA recommends eating a variety of food fiber sources (1).

Fiber, especially insoluble fiber, helps promote bowel regularity. Individuals should start slowly and gradually increase their fiber intake over time, while also making sure to increase their intake of fluids. Foods high in fiber tend to be lower in total calories, saturated fat, and cholesterol. Fiber may also help to curb appetite and can be an important adjunct to weight management plans.

MyPyramid.gov
STEPS TO A HEALTHIER YOU

Sample Menus for a 2000 Calorie Food Pattern

Averaged over a week, this seven day menu provides all of the recommended amounts of nutrients and food from each food group. (Italicized foods are part of the dish or food that precedes it.)

Day 1

BREAKFAST

Breakfast burrito
1 flour tortilla (7" diameter)
1 scrambled egg (in 1 tsp soft margarine)
*1/3 cup black beans**
2 tbsp salsa
1 cup orange juice
1 cup fat-free milk

LUNCH

Roast beef sandwich
1 whole grain sandwich bun
3 ounces lean roast beef
2 slices tomato
1/4 cup shredded romaine lettuce
1/8 cup sautéed mushrooms (in 1 tsp oil)
1 1/2 ounce part-skim mozzarella cheese
1 tsp yellow mustard
3/4 cup baked potato wedges*
1 tbsp ketchup
1 unsweetened beverage

DINNER

Stuffed broiled salmon
5 ounce salmon filet
1 ounce bread stuffing mix
1 tbsp chopped onions
1 tbsp diced celery
2 tsp canola oil
1/2 cup saffron (white) rice
1 ounce slivered almonds
1/2 cup steamed broccoli
1 tsp soft margarine
1 cup fat-free milk

SNACKS

1 cup cantaloupe

Day 2

BREAKFAST

Hot cereal
1/2 cup cooked oatmeal
2 tbsp raisins
1 tsp soft margarine
1/2 cup fat-free milk
1 cup orange juice

LUNCH

Taco salad
2 ounces tortilla chips
2 ounces ground turkey, sautéed in 2 tsp sunflower oil
*1/2 cup black beans**
1/2 cup iceberg lettuce
2 slices tomato
1 ounce low-fat cheddar cheese
2 tbsp salsa
1/2 cup avocado
1 tsp lime juice
1 unsweetened beverage

DINNER

Spinach lasagna
1 cup lasagna noodles, cooked (2 oz dry)
2/3 cup cooked spinach
1/2 cup ricotta cheese
*1/2 cup tomato sauce tomato bits**
1 ounce part-skim mozzarella cheese
1 ounce whole wheat dinner roll
1 cup fat-free milk

SNACKS

1/2 ounce dry-roasted almonds*
1/4 cup pineapple
2 tbsp raisins

Day 3

BREAKFAST

Cold cereal
1 cup bran flakes
1 cup fat-free milk
1 small banana
1 slice whole wheat toast
1 tsp soft margarine
1 cup prune juice

LUNCH

Tuna fish sandwich
2 slices rye bread
3 ounces tuna (packed in water, drained)
1 tbsp mayonnaise
1/2 tsp diced celery
1/4 cup shredded romaine lettuce
2 slices tomato
1 medium pear
1 cup fat-free milk

DINNER

Roasted chicken breast
*3 ounces boneless skinless chickenbreast**
1 large baked sweet potato
1/2 cup peas and onions
1 tsp soft margarine
1 ounce whole wheat dinner roll
1 tsp soft margarine
1 cup leafy greens salad
3 tsp sunflower oil and vinegar dressing

SNACKS

1/4 cup dried apricots
1 cup low-fat fruited yogurt

Day 4

BREAKFAST

1 whole wheat English muffin
2 tsp soft margarine
1 tbsp jam or preserves
1 medium grapefruit
1 hard-cooked egg
1 unsweetened beverage

LUNCH

White bean-vegetable soup
1 1/4 cup chunky vegetable soup
*1/2 cup white beans**
2 ounce breadstick
8 baby carrots
1 cup fat-free milk

DINNER

Rigatoni with meat sauce
1 cup rigatoni pasta (2 ounces dry)
*1/2 cup tomato sauce tomato bits**
2 ounces extra lean cooked ground beef (sautéed in 2 tsp vegetable oil)
3 tbsp grated Parmesan cheese
Spinach salad
1 cup baby spinach leaves
1/2 cup tangerine slices
1/2 ounce chopped walnuts
3 tsp sunflower oil and vinegar dressing
1 cup fat-free milk

SNACKS

1 cup low-fat fruited yogurt

Figure 7.1 • Sample menus for a 2,000-cal food pattern. (Reproduced with permission from www.mypyramid.gov/downloads/sample _menu.pdf. Accessed 2005.)

Sample Menus for a 2000 Calorie Food Pattern

Averaged over a week, this seven day menu provides all of the recommended amounts of nutrients and food from each food group. (Italicized foods are part of the dish or food that precedes it.)

Day 5

BREAKFAST
Cold cereal
1 cup shredded wheat cereal
1 tbsp raisins
1 cup fat-free milk
1 small banana
1 slice whole wheat toast
1 tsp soft margarine
1 tsp jelly

LUNCH
Smoked turkey sandwich
2 ounces whole wheat pita bread
1/4 cup romaine lettuce
2 slices tomato
3 ounces sliced smoked turkey breast*
1 tbsp mayo-type salad dressing
1 tsp yellow mustard
1/2 cup apple slices
1 cup tomato juice*

DINNER
Grilled top loin steak
5 ounces grilled top loin steak
3/4 cup mashed potatoes
2 tsp soft margarine
1/2 cup steamed carrots
1 tbsp honey
2 ounces whole wheat dinner roll
1 tsp soft margarine
1 cup fat-free milk

SNACKS
1 cup low-fat fruited yogurt

Day 6

BREAKFAST
French toast
2 slices whole wheat French toast
2 tsp soft margarine
2 tbsp maple syrup
1/2 medium grapefruit
1 cup fat-free milk

LUNCH
Vegetarian chili on baked potato
1 cup kidney beans*
1/2 cup tomato sauce w/ tomato tidbits*
3 tbsp chopped onions
1 ounce low-fat cheddar cheese
1 tsp vegetable oil
1 medium baked potato
1/2 cup cantaloupe
3/4 cup lemonade

DINNER
Hawaiian pizza
2 slices cheese pizza
1 ounce Canadian bacon
1/4 cup pineapple
2 tbsp mushrooms
2 tbsp chopped onions
Green salad
1 cup leafy greens
3 tsp sunflower oil and vinegar dressing
1 cup fat-free milk

SNACKS
5 whole wheat crackers*
1/8 cup hummus
1/2 cup fruit cocktail (in water or juice)

Day 7

BREAKFAST
Pancakes
3 buckwheat pancakes
2 tsp soft margarine
3 tbsp maple syrup
1/2 cup strawberries
3/4 cup honeydew melon
1/2 cup fat-free milk

LUNCH
Manhattan clam chowder
3 ounces canned clams (drained)
3/4 cup mixed vegetables
1 cup canned tomatoes*
10 whole wheat crackers*
1 medium orange
1 cup fat-free milk

DINNER
Vegetable stir-fry
4 ounces tofu (firm)
1/4 cup green and red bell peppers
1/2 cup bok choy
2 tbsp vegetable oil
1 cup brown rice
1 cup lemon-flavored iced tea

SNACKS
1 ounce sunflower seeds*
1 large banana
1 cup low-fat fruited yogurt

* Starred items are foods that are labeled as no-salt-added, low-sodium, or low-salt versions of the foods. They can also be prepared from scratch with little or no added salt. All other foods are regular commercial products that contain variable levels of sodium. Average sodium level of the seven day menu assumes no-salt-added in cooking or at the table

Figure 7.1 • *(Continued)*

179

Sample Menus for a 2000 calorie food pattern

Averaged over a week, this seven day menu provides all of the recommended amounts of nutrients and food from each food group.

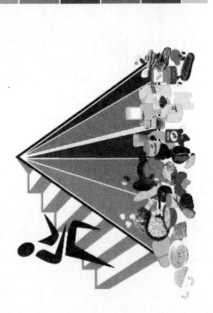

Food Group		Daily Average Over One Week
GRAINS	Total Grains (oz eq)	6.0
	Whole Grains (oz eq)	3.4
	Refined Grains (oz eq)	2.6
VEGETABLES*	Total Veg* (cups)	2.6
FRUITS	Fruits (cups)	2.1
MILK	Milk (cups)	3.1
MEAT & BEANS	Meat/ Beans (oz eq)	5.6
OILS	Oils (tsp/grams)	7.2 tsp/32.4 g

*Vegetable subgroups (weekly totals)

Dk-Green Veg (cups)	3.3
Orange Veg (cups)	2.3
Beans/ Peas (cups)	3.0
Starchy Veg (cups)	3.4
Other Veg (cups)	6.6

Nutrient	Daily Average Over One Week
Calories	1994
Protein, g	98
Protein, % kcal	20
Carbohydrate, g	264
Carbohydrate, % kcal	53
Total fat, g	67
Total fat, % kcal	30
Saturated fat, g	16
Saturated fat, % kcal	7.0
Monounsaturated fat, g	23
Polyunsaturated fat, g	23
Linoleic Acid, g	21
Alpha-linolenic Acid, g	1.1
Cholesterol, mg	207
Total dietary fiber, g	31
Potassium, mg	4715
Sodium, mg*	1948
Calcium, mg*	1389
Magnesium, mg	432
Copper, mg	1.9
Iron, mg	21
Phosphorus, mg	1830
Zinc, mg	14
Thiamin, mg	1.9
Riboflavin, mg	2.5
Niacin Equivalents, mg	24
Vitamin B6, mg	2.9
Vitamin B12, mcg	18.4
Vitamin C, mg	190
Vitamin E, mg (AT)	18.9
Vitamin A, mcg (RAE)	1430
Dietary Folate Equivalents, mcg	558

* Starred items are foods that are labelled as no-salt-added, low-sodium, or low-salt versions of the foods. They can also be prepared from scratch with little or no added salt. All other foods are regular commercial products which contain variable levels of sodium. Average sodium level of the 7 day menu assumes no-salt-added in cooking or at the table.

Figure 7.1 • *(Continued)*

TABLE 7.5 Recommended Fiber Intake

Children		
1–3 yr	Boys and girls	19 g/d
4–8 yr	Boys and girls	25 g/d
9–13 yr	Boys	31 g/d
	Girls	26 g/d
14–18 yr	Boys	38 g/d
	Girls	26 g/d
Adults		
19–50 yr	Men	38 g/d
	Women	25 g/d
>50 yr	Men	30 g/d
	Women	21 g/d

Institute of Medicine: Dietary Reference Intakes for Energy, Carbohydrate, Fiber, Fat, Fatty Acids, Cholesterol, Protein, and Amino Acids. Washington, DC: National Academy of Sciences, 2002.

FATS

Total fat intake should not exceed 20–30% of total calories, and saturated fats should contribute less than 10% of calories. Fats consumed should eschew trans-unsaturated fatty acids and emphasize polyunsaturated fatty acids and monounsaturated fatty acids such as those found in fish, nuts, and vegetable oils (canola, olive oil, and the fat in peanut butter). For meats, poultry, dried beans, milk or milk products, the varieties should be selected that are low-fat or fat-free, with a limited intake of fats and oils high in saturated or trans-fatty acids. As discussed in Chapter 8, reducing fat intake is a basic principle of weight control, but overrestriction of dietary fat to less than 20% of caloric intake may compromise the overall quality of the diet. Patients should consume less than 300 mg/day of cholesterol.

Heart-Healthy Dietary Practices

To help control blood pressure, the AHA recommends a diet that limits intake of sodium (see subsequent text) and alcohol (no more than two drinks per day for men and one drink per day for women) and maintenance of a daily pattern that emphasizes fruits, vegetables, and low-fat dairy products (see Table 7.6). Recommendations also emphasize the need for normal body weight and physical activity (see Chapters 6 and 8).

To achieve and maintain a desirable blood cholesterol and lipoprotein profile, patients should limit intake of saturated fatty acids, trans-unsaturated fatty acids, and cholesterol. Dietary factors that lower low-density lipoprotein (LDL) cholesterol and raise high-density lipoprotein (HDL) include intake of polyunsaturated fatty acids, monounsaturated fatty acids, soluble fiber, soy protein, and Omega-3 fatty acids (4–6). Nondietary measures to control serum lipids include the interrelated tasks of aerobic exercise and weight loss (see Chapters 6 and 8).

TRIGLYCERIDES

Factors that increase triglyceride levels include excess body weight, reduced physical activity; increased intake of sugar and refined carbohydrates, particularly in the setting of insulin resistance and glucose intolerance; and increased alcohol intake. High triglycerides are often associated with low HDL cholesterol, obesity, diabetes, and high blood pressure (see Table 7.7).

SODIUM AND POTASSIUM

Sodium intake should be limited to less than 2,300 mg (approximately one teaspoon of salt)/day. This can be accomplished by choosing and preparing foods with little salt and at the same time consuming potassium rich foods such as fruits and vegetables. Table 7.8 lists food rich in sodium.

The AHA recommends limiting sodium intake to approximately 1.5 g/day for those with or without hypertension. The reduction of salt intake is most effective in lowering blood pressure in older individuals and in those with hypertension, diabetes, or chronic kidney disease. The AHA recommends eating eight to ten servings of fruits and vegetables daily to increase potassium intake, which effectively reduces blood pressure in both normotensive and hypertensive individuals.

Specifically, the AHA recommends the use of the Dietary Approaches to Stop Hypertension (DASH) diet, which emphasizes fruits, vegetables and low-fat dairy products and no more than 1,500 mg of sodium per day (see Table 7.9). It includes whole-grain products, fish, poultry, nuts, and reduced intake of red meat, sweets, and sugar containing beverages. The DASH diet contains higher amounts of magnesium, potassium, calcium, protein, and fiber as compared to the average American diet. Owing to its relatively high content of potassium, phosphorus, and protein, the DASH diet is not recommended for those individuals with chronic kidney disease, that is, an estimated glomerular filtration rate lower than 60 mL/minute/1.73 m^2.

The National Heart, Lung, and Blood Institute Health Information Center has produced an informative booklet entitled *The DASH Eating Plan*. The guide provides examples of the DASH diet on a daily basis, information

TABLE 7.6 Nutrients and Food Sources Associated with Reduced Cardiovascular Disease Risk[a]

Nutrient	Foods
Omega-3 fatty acids	Fatty fish (salmon, sword, mackerel, sardine, trout, tuna), walnuts, flax seed oil, canola oil
Monounsaturated fats[b]	Canola, olive, avocado, peanut oil
Polyunsaturated fats[b]	Sunflower seed oil, corn oil, vegetable oil
Whole grains	Hundred percent whole-grain breads, cereals, grain products (check ingredient list for first ingredient mentioned)
Soluble fibers	Beans, oats, lentils, apple, pears, many vegetables
Insoluble fibers	Bran, whole grains, the outer layer of vegetables and fruits
Vitamin E	Whole grains, wheat germ, plant oils, asparagus, shrimp, nuts
Ascorbic acid (vitamin C)	Citrus fruits, kiwi, strawberries, tomatoes, broccoli, cauliflower, peppers, potatoes
Folate	Fruits (including citrus), green vegetables
Pyridoxine (vitamin B_6)	Whole grains, bananas, meats, nuts, peanuts, legumes
Cobalamin (vitamin B_{12})	Fish, poultry, meats, eggs, dairy foods
Carotenoids	Orange, yellow, red, green fruits and vegetables (except citrus)
Phytonutrients	Vegetables, fruits, soy and other legumes, whole grains, egg yolks
Potassium	Bananas, citrus fruits, vegetables, potatoes, dairy products
Magnesium	Fruits and vegetables, whole grains, fish and seafood, nuts, legumes
Calcium	Dairy products, fish with bones, almonds, green vegetables

[a]Data support the health effects of consuming these nutrients from foods, not supplements.
[b]Most data support the concept that benefits will be gained when these fatty acids are used to replace saturated fat.

TABLE 7.7 Nonpharmacologic (Lifestyle) Methods to Lower Triglyceride Levels

- Eat fewer high-fat foods
- Total amount of fat should be 30% or less of total calories
- Substitute unsaturated fat for saturated fat. Unsaturated fats come from plants and are liquid at room temperature
- Eat smaller amounts of low-fat dairy products, lean meats, fish, and poultry
- Limit cholesterol to 300 mg or less per day
- Eat fewer calories if overweight
- Exercise to use up excess calories and help achieve a healthy body weight
- Eat less sugar and fewer sugar-containing foods. Substitute with artificially sweetened beverages labeled sugar-free or other nonalcoholic drinks
- Follow your doctor's advice on alcohol (alcohol increases triglyceride levels for some individuals)

Adapted by author from materials developed by the Cleveland Clinic Foundation.

on lowering calories, finding sodium in the diet, reducing use of sodium in food preparation and when dining, and a week's worth of DASH eating plans to help guide patients through the process (www.nhlbi.nih.gov).

ALCOHOLIC BEVERAGES

For those who choose to drink alcoholic beverages, the U.S. Dietary Guidelines 2005 recommend to do so sensibly and in moderation, defined as the consumption of up to one drink per day for women and up to two drinks per day for men. A standard drink is considered to be 12 oz of beer,

TABLE 7.8 Sodium Content of Various Foods

Food	Portion	Sodium (mg)
Parmesan cheese	1 oz	528
Instant chocolate pudding	1/2 cup	470
Herring, smoked	3 oz	5,234
Ham	3 oz	1,114
Chicken noodle soup	1/2 cup	387
Tomato soup	1/2 cup	696
Beef Jerky	1 oz	627

TABLE 7.9 The Dietary Approaches to Stop Hypertension (DASH) Diet

The meal pattern shown below, from the "Dietary Approaches to Stop Hypertension" (DASH) study, is rich in low-fat dairy foods, fruits, and vegetables. The study was based on a 2000 calorie diet that contained the number of servings from each of the food groups shown in the chart below. For many people, following the DASH meal pattern can be an important and easy step in preventing or managing high blood pressure.

The DASH Eating Style

Food Group	Daily Servings	1 Serving Equals
Milk and Dairy Foods	3	8 oz milk 1 C yogurt 1.5 oz cheese
Fruits	4–5	1 medium fruit ¼ C dried fruit ½ C frozen or canned 6 oz fruit juice
Vegetables	4–5	1 C raw leafy ½ C cooked 6 oz vegetable juice
Grain Foods	7–8	1 slice bread ½ C dry or hot cereal ½ C cooked rice/pasta
Meat, Fish Poultry	2 or less	3 oz cooked meat poultry, or fish
Nuts, Seeds, Legumes	4-5 per week	1/3 C nuts 2 tbls seeds ½ C cooked legumes

10 Ways to DASH Up your Dining

1. **Re-think your drink!** Make milk your beverage of choice: put a pitcher on the dinner table

2. **Pizza!** Combine a pre-made pizza crust with pizza sauce, mozzarella and lots of veggie toppings

3. **Pudding Anyone?** Make creamy banana pudding treat by adding fresh banana chunks to instant pudding mix made with milk

4. **Make It With Milk!** Use milk in place of water when cooking, especially for boxed rice and pasta dishes and other mixes

5. **For That Snack Attack:** Serve cereal with milk and fresh fruit. Substitute flavored yogurt for milk to create yogurt sundaes

(continued)

185

TABLE 7.9 (Continued)

Sample DASH Menu

Breakfast
1 C cornflakes (1 tsp sugar)
8 oz low-fat milk
1 banana
1 slice whole wheat toast
1 tbls jelly
6 oz orange juice

Lunch
2 oz sliced turkey
1.5 oz part skim mozzarella
1 pita bread
1 tbls low-fat mayonnaise
Raw vegetable medley
  3–5 carrot sticks/2 radishes
  2 loose leaf lettuce leaves
½ C fruit cocktail in light syrup

Snack
¼ C dried apricots
¾ C mini pretzels
1/3 C mixed nuts

Dinner
3 oz grilled lean beef
1 C scallion rice
1 C steamed broccoli
Spinach salad with:
  ½ C raw spinach
  2 cherry tomatoes
  2 cucumber slices
  1 tbs light Italian
    dressing
8 oz low fat chocolate
    milk

6. **Make Souper Soup!** Add canned, fresh, or frozen veggies to the family's favorite soups (made with milk)

7. **Shake 'em Up!** Go creative in the kitchen with blender drinks. Start with a base of milk, add frozen fruit chunks and flavorings to make your own signature drink

8. **Create a Baked Potato Bar**–Serve baked potatoes with a variety of toppings like chili, salsa, shredded cheese, and broccoli

9. **Encourage Big Dippers!** People love to eat raw fruits and veggies–if they can dip them. Make a fruit dip by sprinkling cinnamon into vanilla yogurt.

10. **Get Fresh and Freezer Friendly!** Choose pre-cut veggies and salad mixes to freshen up your meals in minutes. Stock up on frozen fruits and veggies so that they're always handy.

Developed from source materials provided by the National Heart, Lung, and Blood Institute (www.nhlbi.gov). See http://www.nhlbi.nih.gov/hbp/prevent/h_eating/h_eating.htm (accessed August 2007) for more details.

1.5 oz of distilled spirit, or 5 oz of wine. Alcohol should not be consumed by some individuals, including pregnant women, and should be avoided by individuals engaging in activities that require attention, skill, or coordination (7). Further information is available at http://www.niaaa.nih.gov/FAQs/General-English/default.htm.

There is a dose–response relationship between alcohol and blood pressure, especially in people drinking more than two drinks daily. Meta-analysis has shown that consuming less alcohol reduces both systolic and diastolic blood pressure. Moderating alcohol intake may lower blood pressure by an average of 2–4 mm of mercury.

CALCIUM AND VITAMIN D

The National Osteoporosis Foundation estimated in 2004 that 10 million Americans had osteoporosis (80% are women) and 34 million more were estimated to have low bone mass. Risk factors that can be altered include inadequate intake of calcium and vitamin D, as well as inadequate weight-bearing exercise (see Chapter 6) and excessive consumption of alcohol (see Chapter 10). Weight-bearing exercises done on a regular basis, working against gravity, contribute to the development of a higher peak bone mass and may reduce the risk of falls because of increased strength in muscle, bone, and balance.

Table 7.10 lists current age-specific recommendations on calcium intake. More than 70% of adults and 60% of adolescents do not consume these amounts of calcium. Healthful sources of calcium include low-fat dairy products such as milk, yogurt, cheese, and ice cream. Milk and dairy products provide 72% of the calcium available in the U.S. food supply. A minimum of three servings of dairy products per day is recommended to consume sufficient calcium. The American Academy of Pediatrics (AAP) recommends milk, cheese, yogurt, and other calcium-rich foods in the diets of children to help build bone mass and prevent rickets. An 8 oz serving of milk provides approximately 35% of the 800 mg calcium recommended for children aged 4 through 8 years. Another contributing factor to lower calcium intake is the perception that dairy products and milk have a higher caloric content and are, therefore, foods that should be avoided in order to "lose weight."

Other sources of calcium are listed in Table 7.11. They include dark leafy green vegetables such as spinach, turnip greens, and broccoli; tofu made with calcium; almonds; and certain fish, such as sardines, mackerel, perch, and salmon with the bones. Food processors have fortified many foods with calcium, including orange juice, breakfast cereals, and breads. Patients who do not consume sufficient calcium in foods may consider taking calcium supplements (see Table 7.12). If calcium supplementation is needed, an additional calcium supplement should be taken in addition to

TABLE 7.10 Calcium Guidelines

Age (yr)	Calcium Goal (mg/d)
1–3	500
4–8	800
9–18	1,300
19–50	1,000
51+	1,200
Pregnant or Lactating	
≤18	1,300
19–50	1,000

Food and Nutrition Board, Institute of Medicine. Dietary Reference Intakes for Calcium, Magnesium, Vitamin D, and Fluoride. Washington, DC: National Academy of Sciences, 1997.

the low amount provided in most multivitamin and mineral supplement preparations.

Vitamin D is essential for calcium absorption and bone health. The RDA for vitamin D is 200–400 IUs daily; one should not exceed 2,000 IUs daily. One cup of milk provides 51 IUs of vitamin D. Other good sources include cod liver oil, egg yolks, and fatty fish.

TABLE 7.11 Calcium Content of Selected Foods

Source	Calcium Content (mg)	Percentage (%) of DRI
Yogurt (1%, 1C)	452	45.2
Sardines (8 md)	354	35.4
Milk (1%, 1C)	300	30.0
Swiss cheese (1 oz)	259	25.9
Broccoli (1 stalk)	103	10.3
Spinach (3.5 oz, raw)	93	9.3
Shrimp (fried, 3.5 oz)	72	7.2

DRI = dietary reference intake. Percentages are based on the 1,000 mg that are recommended for adults age 19–50 yr.

TABLE 7.12 Common Calcium Supplements

Product	Source and mg of Elemental Calcium/Tablet	Number of Tablets for 900–1,000 mg Dose of Calcium
Caltrate 600	Carbonate (600)	1.5
Os-Cal	Carbonate (500)	2
Posture (600 mg)	Phosphate (600)	1.5
Citracal	Citrate (200)	5
Citracal Liquitab	Citrate (500)	2
Tums 500 mg	Carbonate (500)	2
Tums E-X 300 mg	Carbonate (300)	3.5
Tums Ultra	Carbonate (400)	2.5
Fosfree	Carbonate, gluconate, lactate (175)	6

MAGNESIUM

Magnesium is a required cofactor for several essential metabolic reactions including those that involve adenosine triphosphate and guanosine triphosphate. Magnesium consumption may improve bone density and reduce fracture rates. Hypermagnesemia can also contribute to chronic constipation. Foods high in magnesium include beans, broccoli, mackerel, nuts and seeds, okra, oyster scallops, soy milk, spinach, tofu, whole grain and fortified breads, and cereals.

IRON

Iron plays an important role in hemoglobin synthesis and in supporting immune responses. The current RDA, 8 mg/day, is generally met in the diets of healthy populations. Inadequacies may occur in certain high-risk subgroups. Anemia, the most common hematologic disorder, is usually caused by inadequate iron intake. If patients do not consume sufficient iron from good food sources (see Table 7.13), the clinician can prescribe iron sulfate (325 mg three times daily).

For persons with poor digestive-tract iron absorption due to low gastric acidity, serum iron levels can drop if dietary sources are mainly "nonheme" iron (from vegetables and fruits). *Heme iron* derives from animal products (meat, fish, and poultry); its absorption does not require stomach acid and is therefore unaffected by higher gastric pH. Although heme iron is more readily absorbed, nonheme iron contributes the larger portion of available iron in the average diet.

TABLE 7.13 Foods High in Iron

Liver	3 oz	7.5 mg
Dried beans	1 cup	4.9 mg
Green peas	1 cup	3.2 mg
Dark molasses	1 tbsp	3.2 mg
Hamburger meat	3 oz	3 mg
Spinach	1 cup	1.7 mg
Prunes	5 large	1.7 mg
Collard greens	1 cup	1.5 mg
Chicken	2.8 oz (1 breast)	1.3 mg
Eggs	1 egg	1 mg
Wheat bread	1 slice	0.8 mg
Raisins	$\frac{1}{2}$ oz	0.5 mg

ZINC

Sources of zinc are listed in Table 7.14. Zinc intake declines with age and among those who avoid meats. Some evidence suggests that zinc improves immune function and, in the elderly, reduces pressure ulcers. After 50 years of age, the RDA for zinc is 8 mg for women and 11 mg for men, but most persons older than 70 years have inadequate intake (8). High-dose zinc supplementation can induce copper deficiency and suppress the immune system. Unless an individual is being monitored closely for copper status, doses of zinc supplements should be 40–50 mg/day.

NUTRITIONAL SUPPLEMENTS

A large proportion of persons in the United States use vitamins and other nutrient supplements. For example, in 1997, approximately 12% of the population used herbal medications. When patients report current medications to their clinician, they often do not mention the use of such supplements. A vitamin/mineral supplement that does not exceed 100% of the DRI for any components may be helpful if an individual is on a very low-calorie weight loss diet; elderly and not eating as much as needed; a strict vegetarian; or does not consume milk, cheese, or yogurt.

Overuse of multivitamin and mineral preparations is a policy concern. For example, excessive vitamin A intake can increase the risk of hip fractures, and high iron intake can aggravate hemochromatosis. Large amounts of folate can mask vitamin B_{12} deficiency. Supplementation of single nutrients can

TABLE 7.14 Zinc Content
of Selected Foods

Oysters	21–113 mg
3 oz ground beef—lean	4.6 mg
3 oz turkey—dark meat, baked	3.8 mg
Beef enchilada	2.3 mg
$\frac{1}{4}$ cup dry roasted peanuts	1.4 mg
1 cup 1% milk	1.0 mg
$\frac{1}{4}$ cup walnuts, English	0.8 mg
1 egg	0.6 mg
3 oz salmon, baked	0.4 mg

sometimes have adverse effects on the absorption and utilization of other nutrients. Treatment with beta-carotene, vitamin A, and vitamin E may increase mortality. 124-Dehydroepiandrosterone (DHEA) is being marketed as the "fountain of youth" but is generating concern regarding its metabolism to sex steroids in target tissues (brain, bone, adipose, and skin) (9).

Until 2007, vitamins, herbal medications, and other nutritional supplements are regulated under the Dietary Supplement Health and Education Act of 1994. This law exempted these products from the safety and efficacy requirements and regulation of marketing claims that prescription and over-the-counter drugs must fulfill. Between January 1993 and October 1998, a total of 2,621 adverse events, including 101 deaths, associated with dietary supplements were reported to the U.S. Food and Drug Administration (FDA).

The guidelines of the supplement act are often circumvented and the law provided no mechanism for postmarketing surveillance. Plants may be misidentified or replaced with cheaper or more readily available alternatives. The potency of herbal medication can vary from manufacturer to manufacturer and from lot to lot. Some herbals have been adulterated with heavy metals, pesticides, and even conventional drugs. Since herbal medications cannot be patented, manufacturers are discouraged from performing the costly type of research to assure efficacy and safety as is done for manufactured pharmaceuticals.

In 2007, the FDA established a final rule requiring "good manufacturing practices" for dietary supplements to ensure that supplements contain what is on the label and no contaminants or impurities. The rule requires manufacturers to evaluate the identity, strength, purity, and composition of the supplements.

Clinicians should advise patients to avoid taking "mega" doses of supplements and to use products that provide no more than 100% of the daily value of all the vitamins. They should check for the United States Pharmacopeia symbol on the product label, indicating that the product contains the advertised amount of the nutrient and will dissolve in 60 minutes. Patients should also be aware that many supplements now have added herbs, enzymes, or amino acids that may interfere with medications such as anticoagulants. Botanicals such as garlic, ginseng, inositol, nicotinate, and onions may have fibrinolytic properties. Botanicals with coagulant properties include agrimony, mistletoe, goldenseal, and yarrow (10). Botanicals containing salicylate or that have antiplatelet properties include aloe gel, black cohosh, onion, dandelion, feverfew, wintergreen, ginseng, licorice, and garlic. Botanicals containing coumarins with potential anticoagulant effects include anise seed, meadow sweet, dandelion, fenugreek, horseradish, licorice, celery, parsley, and red/sweet clover.

PREPREGNANCY AND PREGNANCY

Nutritional status before and during pregnancy can affect the health of the mother, the growth and development of the fetus, and the risk of birth defects and future health in the parturient. Risk factors that may be apparent before pregnancy include poor eating habits and an increased need for nutrients (a special concern with adolescent mothers), and a history of three or more pregnancies in the last 2 years (especially miscarriages) or of poor obstetrical outcomes. Overweight and obese mothers are at higher risk for gestational diabetes and its complications (e.g., macrosomia); see Chapter 8 for guidance on weight management. The clinician should be alert for the "food faddist": individuals who have made diet modifications for chronic disease, have a BMI less than 20 or greater than 25 kg/m^2, or have low hemoglobin/hematocrit concentrations. Nutritional issues of concern during pregnancy include poor intake of energy and important nutrients (especially magnesium, zinc, calcium, iron, vitamin A, vitamin D, iodine, and magnesium) and those on a poorly managed vegetarian diet. As noted in the preceding text, pregnant women should also avoid alcoholic beverages.

In 1990, the IOM published weight gain recommendations for pregnancy based on prepregnancy BMI (see Table 7.15). Folic acid supplementation is important before and during pregnancy to reduce the risk of neural tube and other birth defects. The dose is 400 mg/day of folic acid in addition to the folate provided through foods. Because many pregnancies are unplanned, it is recommended that women of reproductive age increase the folic acid content of their diet, "just in case." Preexisting chronic diseases such as diabetes increase the risk of birth defects, especially those involving the heart and

TABLE 7.15 Weight Gain Recommendations for Pregnancy Based on Prepregnancy Body Mass Index

Prepregnancy Body Mass Index (kg/m²)	Recommended Total Gain (kg)	Recommended Rate of Gain (kg/wk)
<19.8	12.5–18	0.5
19.8–26.0	11.5–16	0.4
>26.0–29.0	7–11.5	0.3
>29.0	≥7	—

Institute of Medicine. Nutrition during pregnancy part l: weight gain. Washington: National Academy Press, 1990.

central nervous system. Vegan vegetarians (see page 198) will most likely need a vitamin B_{12} supplement and perhaps zinc, calcium, and vitamin D. Women with phenylketonuria must resume a low-protein amino acid modified diet during pregnancy.

Breastfeeding

Breastfeeding is strongly endorsed by the world's health and scientific community. Benefits for children include fewer infectious illnesses (e.g., diarrhea, otitis media, and respiratory tract infections), higher scores on cognitive and intelligence tests, and lower incidence of sudden infant death syndrome, juvenile onset diabetes, asthma, and eczema. There is some evidence that breastfed infants are at lower risk of childhood obesity and dental disease. The breastfeeding mother benefits from a greater feeling of bonding with the child, a reduced risk of postpartum bleeding, more rapid uterine involution, an earlier return to prepregnancy weight, and earlier resumption of the menstrual cycle with decreased menstrual blood loss and anemia.

The U.S. Breastfeeding Committee recommends exclusive breastfeeding for at least the first few weeks of life. Breastfeeding for the first 6 months of life with gradual introduction of solid foods after 6 months is preferred. The AAP recommends delaying the introduction of solid food until 4–6 months of age and avoiding cow's milk until after 12 months of age (11).

A Cochrane Review found that breastfeeding initiation and duration could be effectively increased by changes in institutional policy in maternity care practices. The Baby Friendly Hospital Initiative, established by the World Health Organization, consists of a structured comprehensive set of policy changes to help promote breastfeeding. Institutions that have adopted

TABLE 7.16 Ten Steps to Successful Breastfeeding

1. Have a written breastfeeding policy that is routinely communicated to all healthcare staff
2. Train all health care staff in skills necessary to implement this policy
3. Inform all pregnant women about the benefits and management of breastfeeding
4. Help mothers initiate breastfeeding within a half hour of birth
5. Show mothers how to breastfeed and how to maintain lactation even if they should be separated from their infants
6. Give newborns no food or drink other than breast milk unless medically indicated
7. Practice rooming-in. Allow mothers and infants to remain together 24 hr a day
8. Encourage breastfeeding on demand
9. Give no artificial teats or pacifier (also called *dummies* or *soothers*) to breastfeeding infants
10. Foster the establishment of breastfeeding support groups and refer mothers to them on discharge from the hospital or clinic

this initiative typically experience higher breastfeeding rates. Table 7.16 lists institutional breastfeeding promotion policies.

INFANCY AND CHILDHOOD

Rapid growth and development of infants and children provide a higher turnover of nutrients and a unique set of nutrient needs for growth and development. Caloric needs during childhood are approximately 100 kcal/kg and gradually decrease to approximately 55 kcal/kg by the teen years.

Fat should account for 30–35% of the child's diet. Assuming a proper growth rate, high fat foods can be replaced with lower fat foods after 2 years of age. Calcium and phosphorus intake should be similar to assure optimum bone formation and density. Calcium sources that children often prefer include milk, yogurt, cheeses, and calcium fortified juices. Exposure to sunlight and intake of vitamin D food sources are encouraged.

Water, milk, and 100% fruit and vegetable juices are preferred fluids; parents should introduce vegetable juices before fruit juices to keep children from acquiring preferences for sweets. Parents should discourage overconsumption of juices to avoid displacing other foods that are more energy and nutrient dense. Artificially sweetened beverages should be avoided. Children can obtain appropriate dietary fiber by consuming fruits, vegetables, and whole grain breads and cereals (see Figure 7.2).

ADOLESCENCE

Accelerated growth during adolescence may result in nutritional deficiencies with resultant loss of height, osteoporosis, and delayed maturation. Inappropriate food choices, poorly selected vegetarian diets, food faddism, and dieting to lose weight can easily lead to health complications. Nutritional concerns also include inadequate intake of: (a) protein (recommendations for males are 45–60 g daily; for females 44–46 g daily) (b) calcium (Table 7.10), (c) iron, and (d) vitamins A, C, and D. As with other age-groups, adolescents should be encouraged to consume a wide variety of foods, including five servings of fruits and vegetables daily. Vegetarians should be encouraged to consume adequate sources of vitamin B_{12}, riboflavin, zinc, iron, calcium, protein, and energy.

Obsession with weight or dieting should be discouraged. Regular meal patterns that include breakfast and no skipping of meals should be encouraged. The teen years are a critical time for evaluation of eating habits and the tendency toward eating disorders.

OLDER ADULTS

The goals of good nutrition in the elderly are to maintain adequate weight and appetite and to avert complications from nutrition-related disorders (e.g., osteoporosis, fractures, anemias, obesity, diabetes, heart disease, and cancers). Older individuals are the largest demographic group at disproportionate risk for nutritional deficiencies, inadequate diet, and malnutrition. The Nutrition Screening Initiative reports that 24% of elderly individuals are at high risk of suboptimal nutrition whereas 38% are at moderate risk (12). Malnutrition affects 5–10% of independently living older individuals, 30–60% of those institutionalized, and 35–65% of hospitalized patients (13–15). Poor nutritional status may often go unrecognized until pronounced changes are evident. Unintended weight loss, in particular, may herald a terminal downward spiral if weight loss is not identified and addressed.

Nutritional deficiencies occur among older adults because of physical health problems, medications, poverty, ignorance, food anxieties, depression, grief, and dementia. Food information labels that are difficult to read or interpret can contribute to inappropriate food purchases. The elderly are also susceptible to the misleading claims of advertisers, and many unnecessarily use nutritional supplements and other over-the-counter therapies, which can be costly and may lead to adverse effects.

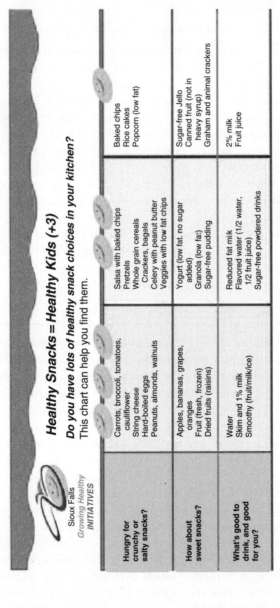

Sioux Falls
Growing Healthy
INITIATIVES

Healthy Snacks = Healthy Kids (+3)

Do you have lots of healthy snack choices in your kitchen?
This chart can help you find them.

Hungry for crunchy or salty snacks?	Carrots, broccoli, tomatoes, cauliflower String cheese Hard-boiled eggs Peanuts, almonds, walnuts	Salsa with baked chips Pretzels Whole grain cereals Crackers, bagels Celery with peanut butter Veggies with low fat chips	Baked chips Rice cakes Popcorn (low fat)
How about sweet snacks?	Apples, bananas, grapes, oranges Fruit (fresh, frozen) Dried fruits (raisins)	Yogurt (low fat, no sugar added) Granola (low fat) Sugar-free pudding	Sugar-free Jello Canned fruit (not in heavy syrup) Graham and animal crackers
What's good to drink, and good for you?	Water Skim and 1% milk Smoothy (fruit/milk/ice)	Reduced fat milk Flavored water (1/2 water, 1/2 fruit juice) Sugar-free powdered drinks	2% milk Fruit juice

3 Family Faces – Best Snack / **2 Family Faces** – Better Snack / **1 Family Face** – Good Snack
And remember: Healthy Snacks + Healthy Activity = Healthy Kids. So go out and walk, run, and play
For more healthy ideas go to **www.healthysiouxfalls.org**

Figure 7.2 • Parent guide for choosing healthy snacks for children. (Reproduced with permission from www.healthysiouxfalls.org. Accessed 2006.)

Seniors' diets also reflect their environment and social support system: who shops and cooks, finances, the number of meals per day, and where they are eaten. Social isolation, lack of family support, loss of a significant other or caregiver, and the decreased mobility that results from physical disabilities or from social isolation can lessen the availability of foods. The elderly at high risk are most often dependent on others for care, and this dependency may result in the potential for abuse. Home visits and direct conversations with caregivers often provide a different picture of the ability to care for the patient than that reported in the office visit. Physical activity, especially resistance training, is an important objective to maintain lean body mass and muscle tone and to help constipation.

Changes in the basal metabolic rate associated with aging reduce the need for calories by as much as 10% at ages 50–70 years and by 20–25% thereafter. Nonetheless, seniors who consume less than 1,500 cal/day are likely to develop poor nutritional status unless closely supervised. Because their caloric needs diminish but nutrient requirements do not, older adults are in greater need of high nutrient density in their diets. Nutrition is affected further by the complications of chronic illness. Dysphasia, slow eating, low protein intake, and anorexia (often accompanying depression) can also compromise nutrition. Of those 75 years and older, two-thirds are edentulous. The elderly often have decreased salivation and absorption accompanied with changes in taste and smell acuity.

Older patients are at high risk of adverse food–drug interactions. Seniors often take multiple medications (engaging in "polypharmacy") for multiple chronic medical conditions. It is estimated that more than 30% of all prescription drugs are taken by older adults. Use of over-the-counter drugs is also highest in older adults (16). Aging alters drug absorption, distribution, metabolism, and excretion. Aging affects gastric emptying and intestinal motility, lowers the ratio of lean body weight to body fat, diminishes binding of drugs by serum protein, and reduces renal and hepatic function.

Food interactions can further potentiate these drug effects. Drugs may also reduce appetite, taste, or smell. Polypharmacy, depression, and underlying medical illnesses may produce a situation very similar to "failure to thrive" in infants. When assessing nutritional status, clinicians should therefore be careful to obtain an accurate drug history. They should also ask about vitamin, mineral, and other dietary supplements, which are widely used by seniors as a form of "nutritional insurance" and perceived by them as safe. Clinicians should consider potential interactions between these supplements and prescribed medications.

The American Dietetic Association holds that liberalization of the diet prescription can enhance the quality of life and nutritional status of older residents in long-term care. An unacceptable or unpalatable diet can lead to lessened food and fluid intake. It may not be advantageous to initiate a medically or self-imposed restrictive nutrition prescription if it may suppress appetite and cause substantial, unintentional weight loss. Foods offered to the elderly may often need enhancements to achieve proper consistency and to accommodate their taste acuity.

Clinicians should monitor older patients for both laxative and alcohol abuse and for major changes in body weight, as well as the maintenance of adequate hydration. Fluid intake is essential for good health, especially for seniors who consume large amounts of protein, use laxatives or diuretics, or live in warm climates. Dehydration is one of the most common causes of fluid and electrolyte imbalances in the elderly (17). Many elderly have a reduced fluid intake which may arise from a decreased thirst sensation, limited access to water, or limited water conservation by kidneys. Conversely, excessive water consumption may result in dilutional hyponatremia (water intoxication) and increased nocturia (18). Generally, fluid intake of 30–35 mL/kg of actual body weight and a minimum of 1,500 mL/day or 1.0–1.5 mL/kcal of food intake is adequate. More fluid intake is necessary for stressful situations that might increase fluid loss such as severely hot weather or heavy exertion. In addition to water and other beverages (e.g., coffee, tea), fluids may derive from soups, vegetables, and fruits.

SELECTED SPECIAL APPROACHES TO HEALTHY EATING

The Mediterranean Diet

The "Mediterranean" type diet includes an increased amount of vegetables, legumes, fruits, and cereals (mostly unrefined); a low to moderate intake of dairy products; a moderate to high intake of fish; a meal pattern characteristically low in saturated fats and high in unsaturated fats (olive oil); relatively low meat intake; and moderate intake of ethanol, usually in the form of wine (19) (see Figure 7.3). Such dietary patterns—emphasizing plant foods and unsaturated fats—are associated with a lower risk of developing cardiovascular disease and longer life expectancy. The Mediterranean Diet also utilizes foods high in Omega-3 fatty acids, specifically eicosadienoic acid and docosahexaenoic acid, which confer cardioprotective effects. See Table 7.6 for food sources of Omega-3 fatty acids.

Vegetarianism

Vegetarian diets are plant-based diets that emphasize eating fruits, vegetables, legumes, seeds, and nuts. There are three major categories of vegetarianism, as follows:

- Vegan—a very strict vegetarian food pattern ("pure" vegetarianism)
- Lacto—a vegetarian food pattern that includes milk and milk products
- Lacto-ovo—a vegetarian food pattern that includes milk and eggs as well (20)

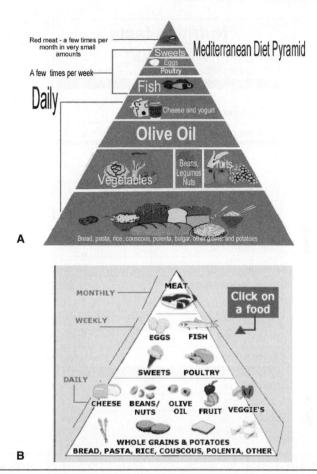

Figure 7.3 • Mediterranean diet pyramids. Adapted from Consumer Reports. NOV 94. Source: Oldways Preservation and Exchange Trust. *A nonprofit organization promoting healthy eating using traditional food from many cultures.* The Word Health Organization, and Harvard School of Public health. 1994. (Reproduced with permission from www.womensheart.org/content/nutrition/mediterranean.asp. Accessed 2007.)

Carefully planned and monitored vegetarian diets can be healthful. Such diets may reduce the risk of obesity, coronary heart disease, diabetes, hypertension, diverticular disease, and constipation. Potential complications of a vegetarian diet include iron-deficiency anemia, vitamin B_{12} deficiency, and vitamin D deficiency or rickets. Intake of Omega-3 fatty acids, essential amino acids, and calcium may be compromised. A carefully planned vegetarian diet should encourage a wide variety of foods and nutritionally adequate menus with sufficient calories. Such diets need careful monitoring when the patient is an infant, child, pregnant or lactating woman, or an older adult.

Nutrition facts

Serving size 1 cup (228 g)
Serving per container 2

Amount per serving	
Calories 250	Calories from fat 110

	% Daily Value*
Total fat 12 g	18%
Saturated fat 3 g	15%
Trans-fat 3 g	
Cholesterol 30 mg	10%
Sodium 470 mg	20%
Total carbohydrate 31 g	10%

Dietary fiber 0 g	0%
Sugars 5 g	
Protein 5 g	

Vitamin A	4%
Vitamin C	2%
Calcium	20%
Iron	4%

Figure 7.4 • Sample label for macaroni and cheese. (Reproduced with permission from http://www.cfsan.fda.gov/dms/foodlab.html. Accessed 2007.)

FOOD LABELS

A new general guide to calories has been provided by the U.S. Dietary Guidelines to aid consumers. Food labels indicate that 40 cal is considered low consumption, 100 cal is moderate, and 400 cal is high, all based on a 2,000-cal diet. The new food label recommendations offer consumers advice on which nutrients to increase and which to limit. The label is also helpful in indicating whether a product is a good source of nutrients (see Figure 7.4).

OFFICE AND CLINIC ORGANIZATION

The practice should display patient education materials and/or posters that may stimulate questions about healthy diets. These materials should be readily available to reinforce discussions and provide an opportunity for the patient to learn more at a later time. The reception area is an excellent place to educate patients.

Many practices give patients pedometers as a means of emphasizing the need for physical activity. Clinics that do not have the services of a registered dietitian or licensed nutritionist should develop a referral system so that patients can obtain the help they need to meet the dietary goals recommended by the clinician. Internet access to appropriate nutritional resources can also be provided in the reception area, or a listing of useful websites can be supplied to patients.

SUMMARY

A healthy diet coupled with appropriate food choices is an essential component of health promotion and disease prevention. Eating well and physical activity help slow the progression of chronic disease. Substantial amounts of health care resources could be saved by expanding health promotion and disease prevention programs that target dietary changes. The U.S. Surgeon General's report states "for two out of three adult Americans who do not smoke and do not drink excessively, one personal choice seems to influence long-term health prospects more than any other: what we eat" (21).

SUGGESTED READINGS

Academy of Breastfeeding Medicine. www.bfmed.org. See Academy of Breastfeeding Medicine Model Breastfeeding Policy: www.bfmed.org/protocol/mhpolicy ABM.pdf. Accessed 2007.

Adams KF, Schatzkin A, Harris TB, et al. Overweight, obesity, and mortality in a large prospective cohort of persons 50 to 71 years old. *N Engl J Med* 2006;355(8): 763–778.

Alfenas RC, Mattes RD. Influence of glycemic index/load on glycemic response, appetite, and food intake in healthy humans. *Diabetes Care* 2005;28:2123–2129.

Amato P, Morales AJ, Yen SS. Effects of chromium picolinate supplementation on insulin sensitivity, serum lipids, and body composition in healthy, nonobese, older men and women. *J Gerontol A Biol Sci Med Sci* 2000;55(5):M260–M263.

American Academy of Pediatrics. Policy statement: breastfeeding and the use of human milk. *Pediatrics.* 2005;115:496–506.

American Diabetes Association. Nutrition principles and recommendations in diabetes. *Diabetes Care* 2004;27(suppl 1):S36–S46.

American Dietetic Association. Position of the American Dietetic Association promoting and supporting breastfeeding. *J Am Diet Assoc* 2005;105:810–818.

Appel LJ, Brands MW, Daniels SR, et al. Dietary approaches to prevent and treat hypertension: a scientific statement from the American Heart Association. *Hypertension* 2006;47:296–308.

Appel LJ, Moore TJ, Obarzanek E, et al. DASH Collaborative Research Group. A clinical trial of the effects of dietary patterns on blood pressure. *N Engl J Med* 1997;336:1117–1124.

Ascherio A, Rimm EB, Hernan MA, et al. Relation of consumption of vitamin E, vitamin C, and carotenoids to risk for stroke among men in the United States. *Ann Intern Med* 1999;130:963–970.

Baby Friendly USA: www.babyfriendlyusa.org.

Beaudry M, Dufour R, Marcoux S. Relation between infant feeding and infection during the first six months of life. *J Pediatr (Rio J)* 1995;126:191–197.

Bjelakovid G, Dimitrinka N, Gluud L, et al. Mortality in randomized trials of antioxidant supplements for primary and secondary prevention. *JAMA* 2007;297:842–857.

Blumberg J. Nutritional needs of seniors. *J Am Coll Nutr* 1997;16:577.

Bogden JD, Bendick A, Kemp FW, et al. Daily micronutrient supplements enhance delayed-hypersensitivity skin test responses in older people. *Am J Clin Nutr* 1994; 60(3):437–447.

Bogden JD, Oleske JM, Munves EM, et al. Zinc and immunocompetence in the elderly : baseline data on Zinc nutriture and immunity in unsupplemented subjects. *Am J Clin Nutr* 1987;46(1):101–109.

Boukaiba N, Flament C, Acher S, et al. A physiological amount of Zinc supplementation: effects on nutritional, lipid, and thymic status in an elderly population. *Am J Clin Nutr* 1993;57(4):566–572.

Breastfeeding Coalition of the Inland Empire Model Hospital Policy Recommendations: www.breastfeeding.org/articles/modelpolicy.pdf.

Brownie S. Why are Elderly individuals at risk for nutritional deficiency. *Intl J Nursing Prac* 2006;12:110–118.

Bryant RJ, Cadogan J, Weaver CM. The new dietary reference intakes for calcium: implications for osteoporosis. [Review]. *J Am Coll Nutr* 1999;18(5 suppl):406S–412S.

Campbell W. Dietary protein requirements of older people: is the RDA adequate? *Nutr Today* 1996;31:192.

Centers for Disease Control and Prevention. *2003 National immunization survey*. Available at: http://www.cdc.gov/breastfeeding/NIS_data Accessed December 16, 2004.

Chobanian AV, Bakris GL, Black HR, et al. Seventh report of Joint National Committee on Prevention, Evaluation, and Treatment of High Blood Pressure. *JAMA* 2003;289(19):2560–2571.

Christen Y. Oxidative stress and Alzheimer disease. *Am J Clin Nutr* 2000;71(2):621S–629S.

Conlan D, Korula R, Tallentire D. Serum copper levels in elderly patients with femoral-neck fractures. *Age Aging* 1990;19(3):212–214.

Cumming RG, Klinieberg RJ. Breastfeeding and other reproductive factors and the risk of hip fractures in elderly women. *Int J Epidmiol* 1993;22:884–891.

Dawson-Hughes B, Dallal GE, Krall EA, et al. A controlled trial of the effect of calcium supplementation on bone density in postmenopausal women. *N Engl J Med* 1990;323(13):878–883.

DeLorgeril M, Renaud S, Mamelle N, et al. Mediterranean alpha-linoleic acid-rich diet in secondary prevention of coronary heart disease. *Lancet* 1999;343:1454–1459.

Dewey KG, Heinig MJ, Nommsen-Rivers LA. Differences in morbidity between breast-fed and formula-fed infants. *J Pediatr (Rio J)* 1995;126:696–702.

Ervin RB, Wright JD, Kennedy-Stephenson J. Use of dietary supplements in the United States, 1988–94. *Vital Health Stat 11* 1999;(244):i–ii, 1–14.

Escott-Stump S. *Nutrition and diagnosis related care*, 5th ed. Lippincott Williams & Wilkins, 2002.

Evans WJ, Cyr-Campbell D. Nutrition, exercise, and healthy aging. *J Am Diet Assoc* 1997;97:632.

Fisher JO, Birch LL, Smiciklas-Wright H, et al. Breastfeeding through the first year predicts maternal control in feeding and subsequent toddler energy intakes. *J Am Diet Assoc* 2000;100:641–646.

Food and Nutrition Board, Institute of Medicine. *Dietary Reference Intakes for Calcium, Magnesium, Vitamin D, and Fluoride*. Washington, DC: National Academy of Sciences, 1997.

Food and Nutrition Board, Institute of Medicine. *Dietary, functional and total fiber, dietary reference intakes for energy, carbohydrate, fiber, fat, fatty acids, cholesterol, protein, and amino acids*. Washington, DC: National Academy Press, 2002.

Gaziano JM, Manson JE, Branch LG, et al. A prospective study of consumption of carotenoids in fruits and vegetables and decreased cardiovascular mortality in the elderly. *Ann Epidemiol* 1995;5:255–260.

Geerling JH. Natural family planning. *Am Fam Physician* 1995;52:149–156.

Gillman MW, Cupples LA, Gagnon D, et al. Protective effect of fruits and vegetables on development of stroke in men. *JAMA* 1995;273:1113–1117.

Girodon F, Galan P, Monget AL, et al. Impact of trace elements and vitamin supplementation on immunity and infections in institutionalized elderly patients: a randomized controlled trial. *Arch Intern Med* 1999;159(7):748–754.

Glycemic Index. www.glycemicindex.com. Accessed 2007.

Goulding MR, Rogers ME, Smith SM. Public health and aging: trends in aging-United States and worldwide. *MMWR* 2003;52:101–106.

Guallar E, Aro A, Jimenez FJ, et al. Omega-3 fatty acids in adipose tissue and risk of myocardial infarction: the EURAMIC Study. *Arterioscler Thromb Vasc Biol* 1999;19:1111–1118.

Harris WS. N-3 Fatty acids and serum lipoproteins: human studies. *Am J Clin Nutr* 1997;65:1645S–1654S.

Harris TB, Visser M, Everhart J, et al. Waist circumference and sagittal diameter reflect total body fat better than visceral fat in older men and women. The Health, Aging and Body Composition Study. *Ann NY Acad Sci* 2000;904:462–473.

Heinig MJ, Nommsen-Rivers LA, Peerson JM, et al. Factors related to duration of postpartum amenorrhea among USA women with prolonged lactation. *J Biosoc Sci* 1994;26:517–527.

High KP. Nutritional strategies to boost immunity and prevent infection in elderly individuals. *Clin Infect Dis* 2001;33(11):1892–1900.

Infant Feeding Action Coalition (INFACT) Canada. http://www.infactcanada.ca. Accessed 2007.

Institute for Reproductive Health/IMPACT. *Breastfeeding: protecting a natural resource*. Washington, DC, 1990.

Jones G, Steketee R, Black R, et al. Bellagio Child Survival Study Group. Child survival II: how many child deaths can we prevent this year? *Lancet* 2003;362:65–71.

Joshipura KJ, Ascherio A, Manson JE, et al. Fruit and vegetable intake in relation to risk of ischemic stroke. *JAMA* 1999;282:1233–1239.

Kang JX, Leaf A. Effects of long-chain polyunsaturated fatty acids on the contraction of neonatal rat cardiac myocytes. *Proc Natl Acad Sci U S A* 1994;91:9886–9890.

Keller H, Brockest B, Haresign H. Building capacity for nutrition screening. *Nutr Today* 2006;41(4):164–170.

Key TJA, Thorogood M, Appleby PN, et al. Dietary habits and mortality in 11,000 vegetarians and health conscious people: results of a 17 year follow up. *Br Med J* 1996;313:775–779.

Klevay LM. Lack of a recommended dietary allowance for copper may be hazardous to your health. *J Am Coll Nutr* 1998;17(4):322–326.

Knekt P, Reunannen A, Javinen R, et al. Antioxidant vitamin intake and coronary mortality in the longitudinal population study. *Am J Epidemiol* 1994;139:1180–1189.

Kreft B, Fischer A, Kruger S, et al. The impaired immune response to diptheria vaccination in elderly chronic hemodialysis patients is related to zinc deficiency. *Biogerontology* 2000;1(1):61–66.

Law MR, Morris JK. By how much does fruit and vegetable consumption reduce the risk of ischaemic heart disease? *Eur J Clin Nutr* 1998;52:549–556.

Lowik MR, van Dokkum W, Kistemaker C, et al. Body composition, health status and urinary magnesium excretion among elderly people (Dutch Nutrition Surveillance System). *Magnes Res* 1993;6(3):223–232.

Luptor J, Trumbo P. Dietary fiber. *Modern nutrition*, 10 ed. Lippincott Williams & Wilkins, 2006:83.

Marshall TA, Stumbo PJ, Warren JJ, et al. Inadequate nutrient intakes are common and are associated with low diet variety in rural, community-dwelling elderly. *J Nutr* 2001;131(8):2192–2196.

Martin BJ. The magnesium load test: experience in elderly subjects. *Aging (Milano)* 1990;2(3):291–296.

McClain CJ, McClain M, Barve S, et al. Trace metals and the elderly. *Clin Geriatr Med* 2002;18:801–818.

McKay DL, Perrone G, Rasmussen H, et al. Multivitamin/mineral supplementation improves plasma B-vitamin status and homocysteine concentration in healthy older adults consuming a folate-fortified diet. *J Nutr* 2000;130(12):3090–3096.

McVea KLSP, Turner PD, Peppler DK. The role of breastfeeding in sudden infant death syndrome. *J Hum Lact* 2000;16:13–20.

Montgomery DL, Splett PL. The economic benefit of breast-feeding infants in the WIC program. *J Am Diet Assoc* 1997;97:379–385.

Mori TA, Beilin LJ, Burke V, et al. Interactions between dietary fat, fish, and fish oils and their effects on platelet function in men at risk of cardiovascular disease. *Arterioscler Thomb Vasc Biol* 1997;17:279–286.

National Alliance for Breastfeeding Advocacy. http://www.naba-breastfeeding.org/nabareal.htm. Accessed 2007.

National Osteoporosis Foundation. *Physician's guide to prevention and treatment of osteoporosis*. Washington, DC: National Osteoporosis Foundation, 2006. http://www.nof.org/physguide/index.asp. Accessed 2007.

Ness AR, Powles JW. Fruit and vegetables and cardiovascular disease: a review. *Int J Epidemiol* 1997;26:1–13.

Newcomb PA, Storer BE, Lonnecker MP, et al. Lactation and a reduced risk of pre-menopausal breast cancer. *N Engl J Med* 1994;330:81–87.

Palmer B. The influence of breastfeeding on the development of the oral cavity: a commentary. *J Hum Lact* 1998;14:93–98.

Port FK, Eknoyan G. The Dialysis Outcomes and Practice Patterns Study (DOPPS) and the Kidney Disease Outcomes Quality Initiative (K/DOQI): a cooperative initiative to improve outcomes for hemodialysis patients worldwide. *Am J Kidney Dis* 2004;44(5 Suppl 2):1–6.

Position paper; liberalization of the diet prescription improves quality of life for older adults in long-term care. *J Am Diet Assoc* 2005;105(12):1955–1965.

Prasad AS, Fitzgerald JT, Hess JW, et al. Zinc deficiency in elderly patients. *Nutrition* 1993;9:218–224.

Radford A. The ecological impact of breastfeeding. *Baby Milk Action Coalition, XIII IOCU World Congress*. Hong Kong, 1991.

Recommended dietary allowance, 10th ed. Washington, DC: National Academy Press, 1989.

Rimm EB, Ascherio A, Giovannucci E, et al. Vegetable, fruit, and cereal fiber intake and risk of coronary heart disease among men. *JAMA* 1996;275:447–451.

Robertsen SB. High-glycemic index foods, hunger, and obesity: is there a connection? *Nutr Rev* 2000;58:163–169.

Robinson MK, Trujillo EB, Mogensen KM, et al. Improving nutritional screening of hospitalizad patients: the role of prealbumin. *JPEN J Parenter Enteral Nutr* 2003;27(6):389–395.

Rosenblatt KA, Thomas DB. Lactation and the risk of epithelial ovarian cancer. The WHO Collaborative Study of Neoplasia and Steroid Contraceptives. *Int J Epidemiol* 1993;22:192–197.

Saari JT. Copper deficiency and cardiovascular disease: role of peroxidation, glycation, and nitration. *Can J Physiol Pharmacol* 2000;78(10):848–855.

Sakurai Y, Teruya K, Shimada N, et al. Association between duration of obesity and risk of non-insulin-dependent diabetes mellitus: the Sotetsu Study. *Am J Epidemiol* 1999;149:256.

Singhal A, Cole TJ, Fewtrell M, et al. Breastmilk feeding and lipoprotein profile in adolescents born preterm: follow-up of a prospective randomized study. *Lancet* 2004;363:1571–1577.

Smigh MM, Durkin M, Hinton VJ, et al. Influence of breastfeeding on cognitive outcomes at age 6–8 years: follow-up of very low birth weight infants. *Am J Epidemiol* 2003;158:1075–1082.

Sorensen JM. Herb-drug, food-drug, nutrient-drug, and drug-drug interactions: mechanisms involved and their medical implications. *J Altern Complement Med* 2002;8(3):293–308; and *JAMA* 1998;279:1200–1205.

Splett PL, Montgomery DL. *The economic benefits of breastfeeding an infant in the wic program: twelve month follow-up study*. Final Report submitted to USDA Food and Consumer Service, March 1998.

Squitti R, Pasqualetti P, Cassetta E, et al. Elevation of serum copper levels discriminates Alzheimer's disease from vascular dementia. *Nueurology* 2003;60(12): 2013–2014.

Strause L, Saltman P, Smith KT, et al. Spinal bone loss in postmenopausal women supplemented with calcium and trace minerals. *J Nutr* 1994;124(7):1060–1064.

Sullivan DH, Bopp MM, Roberson PK. Protein-energy, undernutrition and life-threatening complications among the hospitalized elderly. *J Gen Intern Med* 2002; 17(12):923–932.

Texas Ten-step Hospital Program: www.dshs.state.tx.us/wichd/lactate.

Thorogood M, Hillsdon M, Summerbell C. Lifestyle interventions for sustained weight loss. In: Clinical evidence. London: BMJ Publishing, 2003.

U.S. Census Bureau. *Statistical Abstract of the United States*. 122nd ed. www.census.gov/prod/2003pubs/02statab/opo.pdf. 2002.

U.S. Department of Health and Human Services. *CDC guide to breastfeeding interventions*. U.S. Department of Health and Human Services, http://www.CDC.gov/breastfeeding. To obtain the CDC Breastfeeding Guide go to www.cdc.gov/breastfeeding and go to bfguide@CDC.gov. Accessed 2007.

U.S. Department of Health and Human Services. *Healthy people 2000: national health promotion and disease prevention objectives*. Washington, DC: US Department of Health and Human Services, 1990, DHHS (PHS) publication No 91–50213.

United States Breastfeeding Committee. *Benefits of breastfeeding*. Raleigh, NC: United States Breastfeeding Committee, 2002. http://www.usbreastfeeding.org/Issue-Papers/Benefits.pdf. Accessed 2007.

Weimer J. *The economical cost of breastfeeding: A review and an analysis*. ERS Food Assistance and Nutrition Research Report No. 13. Washington, DC: Economic Research Services, US Department of Agriculture, 2001.

World Health Organization. *Community-based strategies for breastfeeding promotion and support in developing countries*. Geneva, Switzerland: World Health Organization, 2003.

Wright A, Holberg C, Martinez F. Breastfeeding and lower respiratory tract illness in the first year of life. *Br Med J* 1989;299:945–949.

Zawada ET Jr. Malnutrition in the elderly. Is it simply a matter of not eating enough? *J Postgrad Med* 1996;100:207–222.

References

1. Krauss RM. AHA dietary guidelines, revision 2000; a statement for healthcare professionals from the Nutrition Committee of the American Heart Association. *Circulation* 2000;102:2284–2299.

2. Detsky AS, McLaughlin JR, Baker JP, et al. What is subjective global assessment of nutritional status? *JPEN J Parenter Enteral Nutr* 1987;11:8–13.

3. Wakimoto P, Block G. Dietary intake, dietary patterns, and changes with age: an epidemiological perspective. *J Gerontol A Biol Sci Med Sci* 2001;56(2):65–80.

4. Slavin J. Why whole grains are protective: biological mechanisms. *Proc Nutr Soc* 2003;62:129–134.

5. Ludwig DS, Pereira MA, Kroenke CH, et al. Dietary fiber, weight gain, and cardiovascular disease risk factors in young adults. *JAMA* 1999;282:1539–1546.

6. Naidu KA. Vitamin C in human health and disease is still a mystery? An overview. *Nutr J* 2003;2:7.

7. U.S. Department of Health and Human Services. *Dietary guidelines for Americans*. Available at: www.healthierus.gov/dietaryguidelines. 2005.

8. Briefel RR, Bialostosky K, Kennedy-Stephenson J, et al. Zinc intake of the U.S. population: findings from the third National Health and Nutrition Examination Survey, 1988–1994. *J Nutr* 2000;130(5S Suppl):1367S–1373S.

9. Nair KS, Rizza RA, O'Brien P, et al. DHEA in elderly women and DHEA or testosterone in elderly men. *N Engl J Med* 2006;355:1647–1659.

10. *Physician's desk reference*, 61st ed. Montvale, NJ: Thompson PDR, 2007.

11. Kleinman RE, ed. Committee on Nutrition. *Pediatric nutrition handbook*, 4th ed. American Academy of Pediatrics, 1998:43–53.

12. Nutrition Screening Initiative. *Nutrition screening manual for professionals caring for older Americans*. Washington, DC: Nutrition Screening Initiative, 1991.

13. Chen CC, Schilling LS, Lyder CH. A concept analysis of malnutrition in the elderly. *J Adv Nurs* 2001;36:131–142.

14. Gilford A, Khun RK. Development of nutritional risk screening in the community. *Brit J Comm Health Nursing* 1996;1:335–336.

15. Vellas B, Lauque S, Andrieu S, et al. Nutrition assessment in the elderly [Review]. *Curr Opin Clin Nutr Metab Care* 2001;4:5–8.

16. DeBrew JK, Barba BE, Tesh AS. Assessing medication knowledge and practices of older adults. *Home Healthc Nurse* 1998;16:686–691.

17. Chernoff R. Thirst and fluid requirements. *Nutr Rev* 1994;52(8, Part II):S3.

18. Morley J. Water, water everywhere and not a drop to drink. *J Gerontol A Biol Sci Med Sci* 2000;55:M359–M360.

19. Trichopoulou A, Orfanos P, Norat T, et al. Modified Mediterranean diet and survival: EPIC-elderly prospective cohort study. *Br Med J* 2005;330(7498):991.

20. Escott-Stump S. *Nutrition and diagnosis–related care*, 5th ed. Lippincott Williams & Wilkins, 2002:56.

21. U.S. Department of Health and Human Services. *The surgeon general's report on nutrition and health*. Washington, DC: U.S. Dept of Health and Human Services 1988: 2998 DHHS(PHS) publication No. 88-50210.

CHAPTER 8

Weight Management

Steven Jonas and Kavitha Bhat Schelbert

The theory and practice presented in this chapter were originally developed for the book: Jonas S, and the Editors of Consumer Reports Books. *Take Control of Your Weight* (Yonkers, NY: Consumer Reports Book, 1993).

OBESITY, OVERWEIGHT, AND HEALTH

Overview

"Obesity has been steadily increasing in the United States for the past 3 decades. At present almost 65% of the population is overweight or obese, with the prevalence higher for minority populations. Obesity now is present in 31% of the population and overweight in 34%. Approximately 1% of the adult population is moving into the obese category (body mass index >30 kg/m²) every year. A similar increase is being seen among children and adolescents. This pattern is not confined to the United States, but is also occurring throughout the world, in both developed and less developed countries."

"Obesity is associated with several risk factors and diseases. These include insulin resistance, glucose intolerance, type 2 diabetes mellitus, hypertension, dyslipidemia, coronary heart disease, stroke, heart failure, and certain kinds of cancer, as well as earlier mortality. This has led to increasing costs. Obesity has been reported to be responsible for 5.5% to 7.8% of all health care costs, to lead to a loss of productivity by days lost from work, and to cause a great number of disabilities. These disabilities are expensive both financially and with respect to quality of life."

"The change in weight of the U.S. population has occurred without changes in the gene pool, suggesting that the root cause of the epidemic is change in lifestyle and environment rather than a biological genetic change in the population. This does not imply that genes are not important. Between 30% and 40% of the variance of weight is genetic. There is clearly a gene-environment interaction, with some

individuals being more sensitive than others to the "toxic" environment we now experience. The environmental determinants of weight gain in the population are diet and physical activity. Individuals are eating more and exercising less, and this imbalance between energy intake and energy expenditure leads to a situation in which adults between 20 and 40 years of age in this country gain about 1.8 to 2.0 pounds per year."

–Pi-Sunyer and Kris-Etherton, 2005 (1)

Obesity also increases the risk of developing a number of the possible complications of pregnancy, and is associated with gout and osteoarthritis (the latter through simple excess mechanical wear on the joints). As well, obesity can make simply moving about more difficult, and it can lead to negative self-image and depression. It can also confer the consequences of the unfortunate prejudice against overweight and obese people that, along with the obesity epidemic itself, is all too common in U.S. society. In addition to its role as a risk factor for specific diseases and negative health conditions, obesity is also considered to be a causal factor in overall mortality (2–5). Its continued growth as a risk factor puts obesity on track to replace smoking as the leading cause of death in the United States some time in the future. More than 100,000 excess deaths are thought to occur annually due to obesity (6).

Overweight and Obesity

The definitions of "overweight" and "obesity" in current use (2006) were established by the World Health Organization in 1997 (7). As noted in Chapter 3, an adult is "overweight" if the body mass index (BMI)[a] is 25–29.9 kg/m². *Mild or class I obesity* is defined as a BMI of 30–34.9 kg/m², *moderate or class II obesity* as a BMI of 35–39.9 kg/m², and *extreme, morbid, or class III obesity* as a BMI of 40 kg/m² or more (7).

These definitions have superseded their predecessors. "Overweight" formerly referred to any weight above that considered to be in the normal range by age, sex, and height. "Obesity" formerly referred to excess body fat, regardless of weight. The BMI is considered an indirect measure of body fatness. Research on the relationship of body composition and fat distribution suggests that visceral body fat percentage may be a better predictor of poor health than weight or percentage of body fat alone (8). The most common way to measure visceral fat in clinical practice is the waist circumference, but measurements of waist circumference vary with the examiner and are

---

[a]BMI is a measure of the relationship between weight and height that is associated with body fat proportion and health risk. BMI is equal to body weight in kilograms/height in meters squared. A simple BMI calculator may be found at: http://www.nhlbisupport.com/bmi/.

frequently inaccurate. According to current guidelines, a waist circumference of at least 35 in. (88 cm) in women and 40 in. (102 cm) in men is associated with increased cardiovascular risk (9).

Overweight and Obesity as Social Constructs

Regardless of the various medically defined categories, most people think of obesity as a matter of self-perception as well as of weight, height, and body fat ratios: that is, how one looks, feels, and thinks about one's body image. American society stresses thinness for women (10). Therefore, a 5-ft 7-in. tall woman weighing 125 lb, even if described by most observers as "attractive" may *think* of herself as "fat" if she carries some excess adipose tissue on, say, the lateral aspects of her thighs. In evaluating a patient for obesity, it is important to bear in mind not only what the tables say about the subject, but also what the patient has to say about it.

Given societal norms, certain patients will set their goals for weight loss not on the basis of health or other physical needs, but rather on the basis of perceived societal or other interpersonal demands. The clinician should recognize that patients who find it difficult if not impossible to lose weight for metabolic reasons may well experience serious conflict created by *societally* determined weight/fat desiderata (11).

There may well be a need to clarify whether the patients' goal concerns weight *per se* as a risk factor, or physical appearance (e.g., the fact that they do not resemble a fashion model despite being of normal weight), or body image (a mental construct that is often distorted even when the weight and appearance are excellent in the eyes of others). Knowing what the patient perceives as "the problem" is important for a variety of reasons. The first is to correct self-misperceptions, for example, the anorexic patient who thinks her 85-lb body is obese. The second is to clarify the reasons, health promoting or otherwise, why one might engage in a weight-loss program. For example, one can achieve physical health benefits through weight loss (risk reduction). One can also achieve psychological benefits both from simply accomplishing the often difficult task of losing weight and from improving one's looks and feeling better. The third is to ensure that the patient is setting a sensible weight loss target, an achievable BMI goal. Therefore, the clinician may be well advised to focus first not on weight loss *per se* but rather on self-acceptance, healthy eating for its own sake, and regular exercise for its own sake (see Chapters 6 and 7) (12).

Benefits and Risks of Weight/Fat Loss

In terms of physical health, the benefit of weight/fat loss is the reduction or elimination of risks associated with obesity. Modest weight loss, even of 5% of initial body weight, can significantly improve many comorbid conditions (13). As noted, the overweight person who manages to lose weight will often feel better physically and psychologically, will look better to self and others, will be more able to engage in regular physical activity, and will have dealt with the personal social negatives of being obese. But the attempt to lose excess weight and fat carries certain risks as well, primarily fear of failure and fear of success. Fear of failure often inhibits the initiation of weight loss, especially for persons who have experienced "yo-yo dieting" (see "Starvation Response and 'Yo-Yo' Dieting" on pages 212–213). Weight-loss therapists report that, for some patients, a major risk of success in weight loss concerns sexuality and relationships with the opposite sex. Many persons with adult-onset obesity report that their sex life has diminished or disappeared entirely over time. Weight loss may bring increased anxiety over the prospect of becoming sexually active once again. There are also medical risks from extreme weight loss measures, from related eating disorders such as anorexia and bulimia, and from becoming too thin, but these complications of weight loss are rare.

METABOLISM OF WEIGHT GAIN AND LOSS

Mechanisms for Saving Energy

When individuals consume food energy (calories) beyond their immediate needs, the body stores much of the excess as body fat. Body fat, other than that which plays a protective, cushioning function, serves mainly to store potential energy. A certain level of stored energy is healthy. But for many people, the storage capacity and the amount stored are both well above any potential need other than in the case of famine. That person is overweight or obese. Nevertheless, given the place that obesity occupies in our culture as well as its importance as a health risk, it can be helpful to share with patients the concept that excess body fat is nothing more than stored potential energy.

Metabolism versus Social Constructs

Although our culture often uses moralistic terms to refer to overeating/overweight (e.g., "I was *bad*; I ate too much," "I feel *guilty* for eating that hot fudge sundae"), obesity is obviously *not* caused by wickedness. Neither is overeating nor underexercising a sin. However, although the fact that overweight has nothing to do with immorality may seem obvious to the clinician, prevailing social attitudes toward overweight may make the distinction less obvious to patients. There is indeed a view in society that overeating, although not a sin or a sign of wickedness, is a sign of weakness or of lack of self-discipline, or is a reaction to unmet emotional needs. In this context, it is useful to review the metabolic origins of excess body fat. A formulation like "excess body fat is simply tomorrow's meal you ate 2 years ago" might prove to be helpful.

Dietary Fat is Calorie Rich

Patients should also be given two other relevant facts about fat metabolism. First, a gram of dietary fat contains approximately 9 cal of potential energy, whereas a gram of protein or carbohydrate contains only about 4. (This is one reason why low-fat eating is helpful for both weight loss and desired-weight maintenance.) Second, because of the energy requirements for internal carbohydrate and protein conversion to fat, excess calories presented to the body in the form of dietary fat are stored as body fat with much less extra energy expenditure than are excess carbohydrate or protein calories: approximately 3% of dietary fat calories are metabolized in the conversion to body fat; approximately 33% of carbohydrate or protein calories are metabolized to convert them to body fat (14).

Beginning with the so-called Scarsdale Diet that was popularized in the mid-1970s, certain weight-loss advocates have recommended some variation of a low-carbohydrate ("low carb") or ketogenic diet emphasizing high intake of protein and fat. The current prototype is the "Atkins Diet"; low "glycemic index" diets such as the South Beach and "Zone" Diets have also become popular. Such eating plans have been found to achieve greater weight loss over the first 6 months of dieting as compared with the traditional diet recommended in this chapter (and in Chapter 7), which limits fat and calorie intake and encourages moderate protein and proportionally higher carbohydrate intake.

Initially, low-carb diets tend to suppress the appetite better and can improve triglyceride and high-density lipoprotein (HDL) levels (15). However, they are ultimately no more effective than low-fat diets in achieving weight loss after 1 year of treatment (15–17). Unlike low fat diets, low glycemic index and ketogenic diets appear ineffective in reducing, and may even increase, low-density lipoprotein (LDL) cholesterol levels (18,19). These diets are quite difficult to sustain long term, and the dropout rates observed in these trials were quite high. Owing to these concerns and the lack of data regarding long-term safety, the authors choose not to advocate low-carb diets.

The Starvation Response and "Yo-Yo" Dieting

A critical metabolic factor in weight gain, especially relevant to our weight reduction, diet-conscious culture, is a phenomenon called the *starvation response*. Like the fat energy storage system, it is a mechanism to enhance the survival of the individual and species (20). If a person experiences a sudden decrease in caloric intake, the resting metabolic rate (RMR, the measure of energy required to maintain organ system function) will start to decrease, probably within 24–36 hours. During the course of species development, this process was originally designed to conserve energy. The RMR, which is normally approximately 75 cal/hour, can in the first instance drop to

60 cal/hour. A second exposure to sudden caloric deficit can lower RMR further to approximately 50 cal/hour. In some people, the RMR may drop to as low as 35–40 cal/hour.

The starvation response can be elicited by sudden calorie restriction dieting. Unfortunately, the metabolic system responds the same way to intentional caloric deficit as it does to externally induced deficits. The metabolic system cannot recognize that the immediate caloric deficit in this instance does *not* indicate that food might be in short supply for quite some time. Therefore, when the person finishes with a particular diet designed for short-term weight loss with no long-term healthy eating component and returns to his or her prediet eating pattern (as often happens), there is no available built-in "second signal" to stimulate an immediate return to normal RMR.

Usually, the sudden calorie restriction diets described in the lay literature contain little information about lifelong healthy eating and how to go about establishing that pattern. Many dieters using these methods lose some weight and then return to their normal eating pattern. If a person with a lowered RMR resumes normal eating without increasing energy expenditure, they will consume calories in excess of metabolic need. Most of the excess calories will be stored as body fat, and body weight will increase again. That outcome may well induce the person to try losing weight once more.

If the same sudden calorie-restriction dieting approach is followed, perhaps just formulated differently, the RMR may be further depressed. And again, even if some weight is lost on subsequent tries, unless the person has managed to change his or her regular eating pattern, the diet often produces immediate, sometimes significant, weight loss, followed by slow, but steady weight regain. This dieting-induced pattern is called *yo-yo dieting*. (After a number of such cycles, the RMR may be depressed to the point that the next episode of calorie restriction dieting has no effect on body weight at all, as well as having no further effect on an already greatly depressed RMR.)

There is one known mechanism by which a depressed RMR can be raised, however: engaging in regular exercise (21). Muscle requires more energy for maintenance of its basal functions than does fat. Regular exercise raises the RMR by gradually creating new muscle mass. For patients averse to regular exercise, this will be a "good news/bad news" message, but they should be encouraged to use this method to raise their RMR, if they feel that they can manage it (see Chapter 6 for more details about exercise).

Pathways to Overweight

It was formerly thought that body weight/fat proportion was simply the result of the interplay of caloric intake and caloric expenditure. According to this model, weight loss was simply a matter of taking in fewer calories than were required to satisfy a person's energy needs. It is now known that the process is not quite so simple as that described by the old "calories in/calories out" formula. The existence of the starvation response demonstrates that body weight/fat proportion is the product of the interplay among caloric intake, physical activity, *and* metabolic rate. Because this interplay exists, it is now apparent that there is more than a single pathway—overeating—to overweight/obesity. In addition to the relatively rare organic disease causes of overweight, such as hypothyroidism, the following four principal dietary/metabolic pathways to overweight have been hypothesized (22,23):

1. Adult-onset overeating: *high-calorie overweight*
2. Childhood-onset overeating, arising from familial eating patterns (which may result in a high or normal caloric intake in adult life): *familial overweight*
3. Dieting-induced, lowered RMR, with low caloric intake: *dieting-induced low calorie overweight* (DI-LCO)
4. Genetically-determined, lowered RMR, with low caloric intake: *genetic predisposition low calorie overweight* (similar in outcome to DI-LCO)

Although observational data support this theoretical construct, the epidemiology of the pathways to overweight, other than the genetically determined one, has not been studied with any rigor. Therefore, in the overweight/obese population, the distribution of the causes of overweight/obesity among the postulated four pathways is not known. Nevertheless, assuming that the pathways construct is correct, one of the first steps in helping patients find a successful long-term weight reduction plan is to determine which pathway led to overweight in the first place (see pages 216–218).

Achieving Success in Weight Loss

Weight loss success is measured not just by how much weight and body fat decrease, but by the extent to which one remains at or near the target weight/body fat level after the loss has occurred. Further, success is determined by whether that goal can be achieved without permanently "going on a diet." One of the keys to success is for the patient to understand that permanent weight loss is usually achieved not just by reducing caloric intake for a finite period of time, but also by changing one's *whole way of eating*, and, often, how energy is expended. As noted by Blair and Church (24):

> *"[T]he majority of studies show that regular physical activity has health benefits at any weight, and for those who want or need to lose weight, physical activity is a critical component of long-term weight management. Consequently, physical activity promotion should be a foundation of clinical therapy and public health policy, whether to promote health or weight control."*

To achieve *permanent* weight loss, a program must help the person to make *permanent* changes in eating habits and activity patterns. It must make normal, healthy eating part of the person's life *from the beginning of the program*, not something added on in a maintenance program after the weight is lost (see Chapter 7 for the principles and details of healthy eating). Carefully defining "success" in a manner that fits the patient can help him or her deal with both the fear of failure and the fear of success.

WEIGHT LOSS/MANAGEMENT PROGRAM DEVELOPMENT

U.S. Preventive Services Task Force Recommendations for Screening for Obesity in Adults

"The U.S. Preventive Services Task Force (USPSTF) recommends that clinicians screen all adult patients for obesity and offer **intensive counseling and behavioral interventions** *to promote sustained weight loss* **for obese adults** *[emphasis added]."* See Chapter 3 for further details.

"The USPSTF concludes that the evidence is insufficient to recommend for or against the use of **moderate- or low-intensity counseling** *together with behavioral interventions to promote sustained loss in obese adults [emphasis added]."*

"The USPSTF concludes that the evidence is insufficient to recommend for or against the use of counseling of any intensity and behavioral interventions to promote sustained weight loss in **overweight** *adults [emphasis added]"* (25).

Approaches to Healthy Weight Management

There are numerous approaches to weight management and weight loss (see "Resources—Patient Education" at the end of this chapter). The healthy ones all revolve in one way or another around healthy eating (as defined and described in Chapter 7) and regular exercise (as discussed in Chapter 6) (1). The program recommendations made in the balance of this chapter, based on experience and observation, constitute just one of a number of healthy protocols that can achieve the desired outcome.

Is Weight/Fat Loss Possible?

Before discussing with the patient the details of a program for weight loss, it is often necessary to deal with the question, is weight loss possible? In contrast with the situation faced, for example, when counseling patients about regular exercise, few patients need to be convinced of the benefits of weight loss or that they ought to try to lose weight if they are overweight. In fact, of the approximately 65% of the population who are either overweight or obese, at any one time an estimated 50% are trying to lose weight. For many, the big question is "can I succeed?"

It is well known that organized weight loss programs have long-term success rates of only 5–20%. Less well-recognized are the results of at least two early studies of self-directed weight loss regimens that showed a success rate of 60–75% (26,27). It stands to reason that self-directed regimens might work best, at least for those patients who are equipped to undertake them. Therefore, success is certainly possible. But patients have to get on the correct pathway for themselves (dealt with in the balance of this chapter) if the chance is to be a reasonable one. At the same time that the possibility of success is being considered, it should also be recognized that a variety of physiologic, metabolic, and psychological factors make it very difficult if not impossible for certain overweight persons to lose weight (28). It is important for these people to strive for self-acceptance (and for society to increase its tolerance of overweight people). Furthermore, for some patients for whom weight reduction to the "normal" range is not possible, partial weight reduction is a worthwhile goal (28). Such goals should be considered with the patient, including a determination of whether achieving them will provide self-acceptance. For some patients, striving to live a healthier lifestyle—healthful eating and exercise—without necessarily losing weight may be the appropriate goal (11).

The "Four Pathways Up/Three Pathways Down" Model

According to the Pathways hypothesis, depending upon which pathway a particular patient followed in gaining weight, he/she will have to accomplish one or more of the following in order to lose weight: reduce total caloric intake; lower the amount of dietary fat (both to reduce the ease with which the body can convert excess calories to body fat and to lower caloric intake); and engage in regular exercise (both to consume excess calories stored in body fat and to raise the RMR).

Three possible pathways to weight reduction can also be postulated (22):

1. For high-calorie overweight, reducing caloric intake is obligatory and regular exercise is desirable.
2. For normal calorie overweight, caloric intake reduction and regular exercise are both equally important.
3. For dieting-induced or genetically predisposed LCO, regular exercise is obligatory and low-fat eating is desirable (not only to lower caloric intake but also to maintain lean body mass as weight is lost and to establish a lifelong pattern of healthy eating).

Assessment

To choose the correct pathway to weight loss, it helps to know how the patient became overweight. The following questions will help make the correct determination, as well as provide the basis for making general eating habit recommendations. General questions on weight and eating history include: What is the patient's weight? Is the patient overweight or obese by BMI? By how much? For how long? Is the excess weight composed primarily of fat? Was the patient's weight ever in the normal range? What has the patient's adult weight range been? Is the patient really overweight, in the physical sense, or only by self-perception? Is body image adjustment possibly more appropriate than weight loss?

See Chapter 7 (pages 170–171) for information on how to assess eating habits. If the overweight/obese patient eats large amounts frequently and consumes foods that are high in fats and simple sugars, high calorie overweight is the probable etiology. If, on the other hand, the patient can truly say, "I don't eat, but I can't lose weight," either dieting-induced or genetically predisposed LCO is likely. In taking the history of overweight/obesity, the following questions may help distinguish between family-induced and genetically predisposed overweight (although such a distinction cannot always be determined): Is there a parental history of overweight? For all or part of their lives? Were the grandparents overweight? Are any siblings overweight? Was the patient overweight as a child? What were the childhood eating patterns? Were any other relatives morbidly obese? Is there an identifiable, perhaps cultural, attitude toward body size/shape, eating, and weight gain in the family? Was weight loss dieting common in the family during childhood?

In general, negative answers to these questions make either genetically predisposed or family-induced overweight unlikely. Positive answers generally indicate one of the two, but it can be difficult to distinguish between them, unless the patient clearly has DI-LCO. Genetic predisposition does not require the appearance of overweight in childhood. *If* the patient was overweight as a child, *and* the parents (and likely siblings as well) were overweight, *and* food and eating were a major center of family life, *and* the patient is currently eating a high or normal calorie diet, then the chances are good that the familial pathway is responsible for the obesity (unless adult-onset DI-LCO is superimposed on the familial overweight of childhood origin). *If* one or both parents were overweight (and possibly siblings as well), *and* food was not ample on the table during childhood, *and* weight loss dieting was common in the family, *and* the patient has had a great deal of difficulty losing weight as an adult, *and* has been eating a low-calorie diet for an extended period without seeing significant weight loss, then genetically predisposed LCO is the probable etiology.

To detect the presence of *dieting-induced* LCO, the following questions may be helpful. If the answer to more than half of them is yes, this is the likely pathway. Was the patient of normal weight until a particular point in adulthood, such as having her first child? Did the patient then become a chronic dieter? Was an attempt made to lose weight on one or more fad diets (such as a fruit only, grain only, or high protein/fat, "Atkins-type" diet)? Has the patient tried without success to lose weight on a very low-calorie diet (less than 1,000 cal/day), liquid or otherwise? Does the patient remain overweight despite regularly consuming less than 1,000 cal/day? On a crash diet, have 10 lb or more been lost in a short time, say 2–3 weeks, only to be regained within 2–3 months of completing the diet? Have major weight fluctuations been experienced more than twice? Is each diet thought of as a short-term but definitive solution?

Once the patient and clinician have agreed on the pathway that led to the patient's obesity and have together identified the correct pathway to weight reduction, program design can begin. (If regular exercise is to be part of the program, please refer to Chapter 6 for guidance in developing that component.)

Mental Approaches to Weight Loss

The difficulty inherent in successfully losing weight is well known. It is advisable for the clinician to address the fear of failure. It is useful to advise the patient that just as with many health-promoting behavior changes, it takes many people a number of tries before achieving success; achieving permanent weight-loss is one of the toughest lifestyle changes to make (although some significant number of those who try do make it); if permanent weight loss is not possible, it is possible to be overweight and relatively healthy at the same time by engaging in other health-promoting behaviors (11); and it is alright to fail—(a) it is difficult, and (b) one can always try again when one is again ready. It may be possible to deal with these fears early on in the assessment and goal-setting steps of the weight loss program. If the clinician senses that the fear is deep-seated and could be a significant barrier to success (and the health risks associated with obesity for that particular patient are substantial), a referral for psychotherapy might be in order.

Before undertaking any combination of healthy eating and exercise aimed at weight loss, the basic approach for engaging in behavior change is the same as for becoming a regular exerciser (see Chapter 6) or for engaging in most forms of behavior change (see Chapter 5). They are reviewed here only briefly.

The first step is *goal setting*, establishing what the patient wants to do and why. Patients should take some time to think carefully about this undertaking, considering the sacrifices necessary for reaching the desired goal and how prepared they are to make them, as well as what they want to achieve. Realism is essential. What is feasible, achievable, and desirable, given the identified pathway to overweight? Inner motivation is required for long-term positive results. External motivation, *"I'm doing this for my spouse (or boy/girl friend, children/parents, employer/coworkers)"* almost invariably leads to guilt, anxiety, anger, frustration, and quitting.

It is important to stress with patients the concept of *taking control* (10,22). *They* are deciding what they want to do with their bodies. Many people find that "taking control" is an important element both in starting a weight management program and in adhering to it. Rejecting both perfectionism and the "fat is sinful" concept is also very helpful. *Gradual change*, as in "gradual change leads to permanent changes," applies as much to achieving success in weight loss as it does to doing so in becoming physically active (see page 155) and any other behavior change endeavor.

Successful weight loss is not something that can be achieved in a hurry. Virtually all successful people achieve their goals gradually, at an average of 1–2 lb per week. Because weight normally varies up or down by 1–3 lb over the course of a week, for the first few weeks of any long-term program it will be impossible to tell if "anything is happening." In the absence of any immediate physical gratification (unless the patient happens to be one of those who retains excess amounts of water and loses it rapidly at the outset) one has to learn patience. Some persons find it helpful to deal with the loss of immediate physical gratification by replacing it with the immediate mental gratification that comes from taking control.

Admittedly, patience is a difficult skill to learn in our society, one that is so oriented towards instant gratification. Also, absolutism is not required for weight-loss dieting, and in fact it may be counterproductive. The *occasional* consumption of high-fat food, for example, can then become normal. Fat intake can be controlled because as eating habits change, tolerance for fatty foods often declines. Once gradual change is learned, however, the patient will come to see healthy eating and managing weight as a lifelong process. For many patients it is essential to recognize that for a variety of metabolic reasons, once they reach their goal, a lifetime program of healthy eating and exercise are likely to be essential if they are to maintain their new weight. Patience, an understanding of how they became overweight in the first place, an ongoing review of their goals, and a personal sense of commitment to their goals are important and central to making that lifelong change.

Approaches to Eating

The behavioral key to successful weight loss is learning a pattern of generally healthy eating that can be maintained for life. This principle cannot be repeated too often. One constant is that because fat is so calorie dense compared with carbohydrates and protein and because fat is so easily absorbed through the intestinal wall compared with carbohydrates and proteins, lowering the fat content of the diet is the long-term ingredient to success in weight-loss and lower-weight maintenance. As noted earlier, because of the higher caloric content of fat as compared with carbohydrates and protein, and because it requires significantly less energy for the body to convert excess dietary fat into body fat than it does to convert carbohydrates and protein into body fat, low-fat eating can most effectively achieve caloric restriction, if that is required. For the person with LCO, low-fat eating is particularly beneficial for several reasons: it will encourage the use of body fat to meet energy needs; as caloric needs increase secondary to the addition of muscle mass, low-fat eating will help prevent excess calorie consumption; and low-fat intake will reduce serum cholesterol and low-density lipoprotein levels.

Because most people select *types* of food to eat and generally do not physically count calories or fat grams on a regular, ongoing basis, the plan adopted for the long term should generally aim to achieve change *qualitatively* (by helping the patient to choose different *types* of foods), rather than *quantitatively* (by counting fat grams and/or calories). In addition to types of foods, the plan should address portion size (e.g., one meat serving is the size of a deck of cards, an oz of cheese is equal in size to 4 dice, and a serving of fruit or vegetables is the size of an average fist), the optimal frequency of eating, and daily/weekly eating patterns. This is not to say that at the beginning highly detailed calorie-restrictive diet plans formulated by dieticians/nutritionists cannot be useful to help patients get started. It is just that most people trying to lose weight will not adhere to such plans for any extended period of time. They need to learn how to make the necessary qualitative changes in their overall, long-term eating patterns, eating what they choose to eat.

Lowering Fat

Experience indicates that the best way to lower fat in the diet is by so-called food-substitution, implemented on a gradual basis. Patients learn to identify the high-fat foods in their regular diet, and choose for themselves which foods to gradually remove from their eating pattern. At the same time, the person chooses which low or lower fat foods to gradually substitute. In this approach, it is important for the patient to understand that healthy eating begins in the supermarket and continues in the food preparation process. Healthy food shopping and healthy cooking, the precursors to healthy eating, are essential to successful weight loss (see pages 222–224).

The goal of food substitution is to achieve *qualitative* change in eating. The recommended food substitution pattern is to take one small, dietary fat–lowering step at a time. The person does not have to stop eating chocolate, ice cream, red meat, cheese, and butter all at once, or eliminate them entirely.

As an example, let us say that the patient eats high-fat meats (e.g., sausage or luncheon meats) five times a week. He can first try reducing it to four times per week for the first 2 weeks of a new weight loss program. If that goes well, he can try reducing it to three times per week for the next 2 weeks. If the patient feels that ultimately he cannot do without high-fat meats less than two times a week that number should be set as the goal, achieved by substituting lower fat foods of the patient's own choice. The patient should repeat this process for all the identified major high-fat foods.

PLAN IMPLEMENTATION

Healthy Eating
LOW-FAT FOOD CHOICES SIMPLIFIED: SOME EXAMPLES

- The patient should substitute lower fat for higher fat milk, aiming towards 1% fat or skim milk. Low or nonfat yogurt is a very useful substitute for butter, margarine, or sour cream on baked potatoes and other foods normally eaten with a fatty softener, as a base for a vegetable spread, or with fresh fruit for a pleasing dessert.
- Fatty cuts of meat should be eaten sparingly (although as noted they do not have to be eliminated from the diet completely, and they should be reduced gradually, not all at once). It helps to choose lower fat cuts such as flank steak, pork tenderloin, or loin lamb chops, with visible fat trimmed off, and to limit portion size to approximately 3 oz. (Not all food descriptions have the same meaning. Approximately 60% of the calories in both "extra lean" and "lean" hamburger come from fat.) Sausages, hot dogs, and luncheon meats should be avoided (unless they are made from poultry *and* the label shows that they are low in fat. Not all poultry luncheon meats are low in fat.) Poultry cuts should be chosen carefully. White meat is much lower in fat content than dark meat; the skin should be removed. Ground turkey is usually high in fat.
- Prepared carbohydrates can be very tasty. Those that are high in fiber have the additional advantages of promoting satiety and reducing colorectal cancer risk. Patients can consider beans, rice, potatoes, legumes (such as garbanzos and lentils), pasta, whole grain cereals, bread and bread products (such as whole-grain bagels), green and orange vegetables, and fruit. High-fat toppings for these foods should be avoided. For patients who like the idea, adding spices is a noncaloric way to make such foods more interesting.
- The lower fat varieties of fish, such as cod, haddock, northern pike, flounder, grouper, halibut, red snapper, Dover sole, bass, bluefish, swordfish, and tuna are preferred. Fatty fish rich in Omega-3 fatty acids, such as mackerel, lake trout, herring, sardines, albacore tuna and salmon, reduce cardiovascular events, and can be consumed twice a week.
- Frozen "lite" meals (after checking the labels to make sure that they really are low in fat) can be recommended for easy dinner preparation.
- Frozen low or nonfat yogurt, ice milk, sherbet, fruit sorbets, and frozen fruit bars can be substituted for ice cream, but patients should be cautious about their sugar content.
- Food substitution in the gradual change mode is also useful to deal with the "fast-food" problem: pizza, hamburgers, cheeseburgers, French-fries, fried chicken, fried Tex-Mex, and similar foods, often washed down with high-calorie beverages.

- Encourage patients to choose their fats well. Have them shift from saturated fats and trans-fatty acids, which generally come from animal sources and prepared foods, to unsaturated fats from vegetables, nuts, and fish.

EATING OUT: ENJOYING RESTAURANT DINING AND REMAINING HEALTHY

- Size it down: Encourage patients to share the entrée with their dining partner, order the lunch portion, or ask for a take-home box when they first get the meal. If they are still hungry they should order a side salad, soup, or vegetable.
- Keep it light: Avoid menu items that are described as fried, battered, creamed, or smothered. Opt instead for grilled, baked, broiled, or steamed items. When ordering sautéed or stir-fried foods, ask that oil be used lightly. Get sauces and dressings on the side.

HEALTHY EATING PATTERNS

In addition to lowering fat in the diet, the patient can consider other aids to developing a healthy eating pattern. The old saw "eat three square meals a day" is especially valuable for weight loss. Many people think that skipping breakfast, and the calories and fat it might contain, is a good way to lose weight. There is evidence that both eating breakfast and eating at regular intervals are elements of successful weight loss that can be as important as the content of the meals.

Behavior modification is commonly recommended as a weight loss tool. By itself, however, it is not a method for weight loss but rather a means to an end. Although behavior modification techniques can be useful in helping the patient to implement a plan, developing the plan must come first. Useful behavioral techniques include keeping an eating log, controlling "mindless eating" (eating for reasons other than to satisfy hunger), not continuing to eat after feeling full, avoiding distractions and interruptions while eating, not eating too fast (taking smaller bites, chewing completely, putting the fork down between bites, etc.), and reducing portion size.

HEALTHY FOOD SHOPPING

There are three elements necessary for establishing a lifelong pattern of healthy eating: healthy eating itself but before it, healthy food shopping and healthy cooking. It can be said with some authority that healthy eating begins in the supermarket. Unless the patient is one of the relatively rare persons who can eat the same meals over and over again, he or she is not going to maintain a healthy eating pattern unless the menu is varied and appetizing. The patient's family members will also be unlikely to maintain healthy eating patterns, especially if they do not have a weight problem.

As for the shopping itself, most important is the simple but often ignored notion that an unhealthy food cannot be eaten if it is not in the refrigerator or pantry or on the kitchen counter or coffee table. When shopping, one has to be very aware of this fact. Among the other keys to health-conscious food shopping are these: not shopping when hungry; shopping with a list for the ingredients of planned low-fat dishes and for other low-fat foods; making sure that high-fat foods are not bought on impulse; learning the layout of one's supermarket, so that the high-fat food aisles can be avoided; and learning to read and use the U.S. Food and Drug Administration (FDA)-mandated food labels (see page 200).

HEALTHY COOKING

The second step in healthy eating, after the healthy shopping phase, is to make low-fat meals so satisfying that the customary high-fat foods are not missed. The preparation of low-fat foods can vary greatly. Chinese cuisine, for example, can take the same ingredients of chicken and vegetables and vary the seasonings, combinations, coatings, sauces, slicing, and mode of cooking to make vastly different dishes. Healthy foods can be prepared in so many different ways that in a month of dinners made from the same basic ingredients the same taste and texture need not be experienced twice. There are many low-fat cookbooks on the market (some of which are presented in the "Resources—Patient Education" section) and there are plenty of recipes, ranging from the simple to the complex, for healthy and tasty low-fat dishes. For example, a low-fat eating plan could include chicken (primarily white meat) three times a week; as long as a little time is taken in its preparation, the meals will never become boring. Chicken is indeed a staple of many low-fat diets. It is easy to prepare and cook.

As is well known, fish is very important to the low-fat eater too, but it should be prepared with a low-fat method such as broiling or grilling. Meat can be included if, as noted, low-fat varieties and cuts are chosen, all visible fat is trimmed off, and it is prepared in such a way as to remove as much of its intrinsic fat as possible. Vegetables form the centerpiece of any low-fat diet. Paying attention to cooking time (the less the better) and using imaginative recipes can overcome the reputation vegetables sometimes receive as being tasteless, soft, and overcooked. Salads are, of course, an important part of any low-fat diet, as long as fat is not added in the form of meat, cheese, mayonnaise, or oily or creamy dressings. Many tasty low-fat dessert ideas can also be found in low-fat cookbooks.

A variety of food preparation and cooking equipment can make low-fat cooking easier and can also help to produce the best flavor, texture, and appearance. Useful equipment includes a steamer for cooking vegetables; a greaseless frying pan or grill (e.g., George Forman grill); a greaseless/waterless cookware system; a microwave oven; an oriental wok; an automatic bread making machine; a food processor or blender (for making dressings, dips, toppings, and drinks from stock or nonfat yogurt); a bulb baster for removing fat from gravies and sauces; a gravy separator; and sharp knives and poultry shears (helpful for trimming visible fat from meat and removing poultry skin before cooking).

Several cooking ingredients can facilitate tasty low-fat cooking: herbs and spices used creatively; low-fat lubricants such as vegetable oil; a low-fat nonstick spray; wine; lemon juice; wine or herb vinegar; a low-fat broth; cooking soy sauce (low salt, if preferred); marinades for lower fat cuts of meat; and olive oil, used sparingly, for pan frying.

MEDICAL AND SURGICAL INTERVENTIONS

Aggressive lifestyle modification, including dietary intervention, exercise, and behavioral modification, will always remain the cornerstone of obesity and overweight management. However, like other chronic conditions, obesity can require multiple modalities for effective management, such as the addition of pharmacotherapy. In certain cases, bariatric surgery may be necessary to achieve success or prevent and treat comorbid conditions. It is unclear if pharmacotherapy treatment without lifestyle modification is effective in the treatment of obesity (29). Studies suggest that the addition of pharmacotherapy to aggressive lifestyle modification produces greater weight loss than either modality alone (30). According to guidelines issued in 1998 by the National Heart, Lung, and Blood Institute, candidates for pharmacotherapeutic treatment of obesity are those individuals whose BMI is greater than 30 kg/m^2 or whose waist circumference exceeds 35 in. (in men) or 40 in. (in women). Patients whose BMI is greater than 27 kg/m^2 and who also have an obesity-related comorbid condition are also candidates for pharmacotherapy (9).

Currently three medications—phentermine, orlistat, and sibutramine— have been approved by the FDA for the treatment of obesity: (see Table 8.1). Only the latter two are indicated for long-term use. Orlistat, a gastric and pancreatic lipase inhibitor, achieves significant weight loss over 2 years and reduces weight regain (29,31). It also improves LDL cholesterol, insulin, glycosylated hemoglobin, and fasting glucose levels, and glucose tolerance. However, its effectiveness in clinical practice is dampened by its significant adverse gastrointestinal effects, such as diarrhea (31). Sibutramine, a norepinephrine and serotonin reuptake inhibitor, also promotes weight loss and improves HDL cholesterol and triglyceride levels (31). This drug is contraindicated in patients already on selective serotonin reuptake inhibitors, may interact with other medications, and requires monitoring of blood pressure (31,32).

Many medications first introduced to treat other conditions have been shown to induce weight loss. Metformin, exenatide, and pramlinitide, used in the treatment of diabetes, may also be useful adjuncts in therapy

TABLE 8.1 Medications Currently Available for Use in the Treatment of Obesity

Drug	Mechanism of Action	Adverse Effects	Other Effects	Drug–Drug Interactions	Contraindications	Notes
			FDA Approved			
Phentermine 15–37.5 mg QD in single or divided doses	Amphetamine-like analog; release norepinephrine; thermogenesis, appetite suppressant	Increased blood pressure and heart rate, agitation, anxiety, insomnia	Potential for abuse	SSRIs, tricyclics, guanethidine,	Patients on sympathomimetics, MAO inhibitors, furazolidone; CAD, HTN	Not for long-term use (should be taken for <12 weeks)
Orlistat 120 mg TID with meals	Gastric and pancreatic lipase inhibitor; prevents 30% of dietary fat absorption	Gastrointestinal (oily stool, steatorrhea, increased fecal urgency; may worsen gallbladder disease or kidney stones	Improves fasting LDL and insulin, Hb A1c levels, and glucose tolerance additive weight loss effect with statins	Decreased absorption of fat-soluble vitamins	Malabsorption syndrome, cholestasis, pregnant/nursing women, drug hypersensitivity	Approved for use down to age 12 yr; currently FDA-approved for over-the-counter use at half the dosage

(continued)

TABLE 8.1 *(Continued)*

Drug	Mechanism of Action	Adverse Effects	Other Effects	Drug–Drug Interactions	Contraindications	Notes
Sibutramine 5–15 mg QD	Norepinephrine and serotonin reuptake inhibitor; enhances satiety (decreases food intake)	Increased blood pressure and heart rate; headache, dry mouth, anorexia, insomnia, constipation	Improves HDL, triglyceride, Hb A_{IC}, and fasting glucose levels	MAO inhibitors, sympathomimetics, SSRIs, lithium, antiepileptics, antimigraines; metabolism inhibited by CYP3A1 inhibitors	CAD, CHF, arrythmias, stroke, renal/hepatic impairment, poorly/uncontrolled HTN, anorexia nervosa,	Monitor blood pressure; intermittent treatment as effective as continuous
			Off-Label Medications			
Metformin 500–2,000 mg QD in single or divided doses	Insulin sensitizing agent; increased uptake of glucose by cells; decreased hepatic glucose output and free fatty acids	Nausea, diarrhea, bloating, flatulence	Improves fasting and 2-hr postprandial glucose levels; improves fertility	Sulfonylureas, insulin, furosemide, nifedipine, cimetidine, adrenergic blockers, alcohol, clomiphene	Renal or hepatic impairment, CHF, COPD, alcohol abuse; discontinue 48 hr before i.v. contrast administration or general anesthesia	Weight loss in patients with prediabetes, PCOS, HIV-related lipodystrophy

Exenatide	Incretin (glucagon-like peptide-1) mimetic agent; promotes gastric release	NCL	As a single agent, does not cause hypoglycemia	Monitor patients on insulin closely for hypoglycemia	NCL	NCL
Topiramate 25–100 mg QD in single or divided doses	GABAergic and antiglutamatergic antiepileptic agent	Paresthesias, liver function abnormalities, confusion, blood dyscrasias, dizziness, drowsiness, cognitive/memory impairment	Reduces binge episodes	NCL	NCL	Produces continued weight loss beyond 1 yr, unlike most other agents
Zonisamide 100–600 mg/d	Serotonergic and dopaminergic antiepileptic agent	Kidney stones, increased serum creatinine, somnolence, dizziness, headache, nausea, agitation; skin rash	NCL	NCL	Hypersensitivity to sulfonamides; renal/hepatic impairment	NCL

(continued)

TABLE 8.1 (Continued)

Drug	Mechanism of Action	Adverse Effects	Other Effects	Drug–Drug Interactions	Contraindications	Notes
Fluoxetine 60 mg QD	Selective serotonin reuptake inhibitors	Sexual dysfunction, somnolence, agitation, diarrhea, tremor	Approved for treatment of binge-eating disorder	NCL	NCL	Often used in combination with phentermine for short-term weight loss treatment
Bupropion Start 100 mg BID or 75 mg QD of extended release to 300–400 mg QD	Norepinephrine and dopamine uptake inhibitor	Dry mouth, agitation, anxiety, insomnia, nausea, vomiting, dizziness, constipation, sweating	NCL	MAO inhibitors, ritonavir	Renal/hepatic impairment; do not use with alcohol; may lower seizure threshold	Weight loss is dose related

Adapted from Ionaides-Demoss LL, Prioetto J, McNeil JJ. Pharmacotherapy for obesity. *Drugs* 2005;65(10):1391–1418 and Palamara KL, Mogul HR, Peterson SJ, et al. Obesity: new perspectives and pharmacotherapies. *Cardiol Rev* 2006;14:238–258.

CAD = coronary artery disease; CHF = congestive heart failure; COPD = chronic obstructive pulmonary disease; FDA = U.S. Food and Drug Administration; GABA = gamma aminobutyric acid; Hb A$_{1C}$ = hemoglobin A$_{1C}$; HDL = high- density lipoprotein; HIV = human immunodeficiency virus; HTN = hypertension; LDL = low-density lipoprotein; MAO = monoamine oxidase; NCL = none currently listed; PCOS = polycystic ovary syndrome; SSRI = selective serotonin reuptake inhibitor.

for obese patients with diabetes. Many medications that are currently experimental increase energy expenditure, decrease appetite, or increase satiety. Examples include selective B3 agonists, uncoupling protein homologs, and thyroid receptor agonists. Rimonabant, a selective CB1 endocannabinoid receptor antagonist, was expected to be approved at the time of writing, once certain safety considerations were satisfactorily addressed. Most currently available pharmaceutical agents prescribed without an accompanying program of behavior modification achieve no more than a 5–10% long-term weight loss reduction. Further, weight regain is likely if the medication is discontinued or when health-promoting behaviors are not maintained (29).

Bariatric procedures, of both the "restrictive" and the "malabsorptive" types, have become increasingly popular and available. Their safety profile has also improved, with 1–2% overall postoperative mortality, but the risk remains high enough to warrant scrutiny in selecting appropriate patients. The malabsorptive procedure with the greatest benefit and best safety profile in the United States is the open or laparoscopic Roux-en-Y gastric bypass (33). Indicated for those with class III obesity (BMI greater than or equal to 40 kg/m^2) or those with class II obesity (BMI greater than or equal to 35 kg/m^2) with comorbid conditions, bariatric surgery should be offered to patients in these categories who have been attempting medically supervised weight loss for at least 1–2 years without significant success (9). Bariatric surgery can improve or even resolve many comorbid conditions, including diabetes, hyperlipidemia, and hypertension (33). Patients considering this procedure should be reminded that strict adherence to intensive lifestyle changes will be required to prevent weight regain. Centers that include perioperative and postoperative psychological evaluation and long-term follow-up offer the greatest chance for long-term success.

COMMUNITY RESOURCES

One of the most important functions a primary care clinician can perform is to link patients with other weight-management resources outside of the clinic setting that may enhance patients' chances for success. Recommended programs should promote the diet and exercise principles outlined in this book (see this chapter and Chapters 6 and 7) and should teach the behavioral and cognitive skills that are essential if weight loss is to be achieved and then maintained.

Commercial weight loss programs and peer-led support groups, such as Weight Watchers and Take Off Pounds Sensibly (TOPS) Club, Inc., are widely available and can help patients achieve significant reductions in weight (34). Patients may also benefit from interactive online resources such as WebMD, biggestloserclub.com and eDiets. Programs that include online support and feedback for users to help them maintain motivation have been especially successful (35). Commercial portion-controlled meal plans, such as those offered by Seattle Sutton, Nutrisystem, Health Management Resources, and Jenny Craig, and liquid meal replacements, such as SlimFast or Optifast, have also been useful adjuncts in successful weight management (36–38).

The Centers for Disease Control and Prevention Task Force on Community Preventive Services (see page xxxvi) found sufficient evidence that worksite programs can produce significant weight loss (39). Multidisciplinary programs may also be offered through local health care facilities, health departments, fitness centers, and parks and recreation centers. These programs frequently offer professional guidance by dieticians, physical therapists, exercise physiologists, or other counselors and health educators, and may be found by contacting local dietitians and public health agencies.

CONCLUSION

Weight loss can be a complex, difficult, and frustrating process for both patient and clinician. Success can be achieved, however, especially if these principles are followed: both clinician and patient must understand overweight in general and the patient's type of overweight in particular; goal setting is essential and should be realistic; inner motivation is the only kind that works; patience is essential; doing it oneself while taking control is the guide; and gradual change is the route. Finally, clinicians should remind their patients that even modest weight loss of 5–10% is sufficient to improve physical health and prevent comorbid diseases from developing (13,40–42).

For matters related to office and clinic organization, please refer to pages 164–165 in Chapter 6. Of note here, having an "obesity-friendly" practice is important. Furniture should be wide enough for obese patients to sit comfortably and without embarrassment. Bariatric furniture is now available that will not only sustain extra weight and size, but can be decorative as well. Standard upright scales are not readily accessible to patients with large abdominal girth, whereas alternative scales are available that allow the patient to hold onto the scale as they are weighed. Scales should be located in a private room or area.

Finally, although not essential, clinicians engaging in weight loss counseling should consider their own weight. They will set an example for their patients by demonstrating healthy weight management by example. Clinicians who have dealt with weight loss can also talk from experience, knowing both the benefits and the difficulties of the process.

RESOURCES—PATIENT EDUCATION MATERIALS

American Academy of Family Physicians
www.aafp.org, see for example at http://familydoctor.org/

Working with Your Doctor to Overcome Overweight and Obesity—
familydoctor.org.
Information about obesity from the American Academy of Family Physicians.
http://familydoctor.org/788.xml 64 k.

Weight Control: The Power of Healthy Choices—familydoctor.org
Information about weight control from the American Academy of Family Physicians.
http://familydoctor.org/197.xml 26 k

American Heart Association:
http://www.americanheart.org

*American Heart Association Guidelines for Selecting a Weight Loss and Maintenance
Program*
http://www.americanheart.org/presenter.jhtml?identifier=2884

American Diabetes Association
http://www.diabetes.org/

Weight Loss Matters
http://www.diabetes.org/weightloss-and-exercise/weightloss.jsp

National Institute for Diabetes, Digestive, and Kidney Diseases
http://win.niddk.nih.gov/

Publications for Health Care Professionals
http://win.niddk.nih.gov/publications/index.htm#health

Cookbooks

The American Heart Association publishes an extensive list of weight-loss cookbooks. As
of 2006 that list included: *Love Your Heart, the American Heart Association No-Fad Diet,
The New American Heart Association Cookbook, Seventh Edition, the American Heart
Association Low-Fat, Low-Cholesterol Cookbook, Third Edition, the American Heart
Association Low-Calorie Cookbook, the American Heart Association One-Dish Meals
cookbook, and the American Heart Association Low-Fat and Luscious Desserts cookbook.*

Jonas S, Gordon SJ. 30 Secrets of the world's healthiest cuisines: global eating tips and
recipes from China, France, Japan, the Mediterranean, Africa, and Scandinavia. New
York City: John Wiley and Sons, 2000.

Interactive online diet programs:

http://www.webmd.com/
http://biggestloserclub.com/
http://www.ediets.com/
http://www.sonomadiet.com/
http://www.southbeachdiet.com/
http://www.weightwatchers.com/.

SUGGESTED READINGS

Bays H. Current and investigational antiobesity agents and obesity therapeutic treatment targets. *Obes Res* 2004;12:1197–1211.

Consumer Reports Web Watch. *Healthratings.org rates the 20 most-trafficked diet sites. Research conducted by: Consumer Reports WebWatch and the Health Improvement Institute (HII). Consumer Reports WebWatch, 101 Truman Ave., Yonkers, N.Y., USA 10703-1057.* Yonkers, http://www.consumerwebwatch.org/dynamic/health-report-diet-site-ratings.cfm. Accessed 10/10/06, September 28, 2006.

Garner DM, Wooley SC. Confronting the failure of behavioral and dietary treatments for obesity. *Clin Psychol Rev* 1991;11:729–780.

NAASO. *The Obesity Society.* http://www.naaso.org/education/. Accessed, 2007.

National Institutes of Health. Clinical guidelines on the identification, evaluation, and treatment of overweight and obesity in adults: the evidence report. *Obes Res* 1998;6 (Suppl 2):51S–209S.

Snow V, Barry P, Fitterman N, et al. Clinical Efficacy Assessment Subcommittee of the American College of Physicians. Pharmacologic and surgical management of obesity in primary care: a clinical practice guideline from the American College of Physicians. *Ann Intern Med* 2005;142:525–531.

References

1. Pi-Sunyer X, Kris-Etherton PM. Improving health outcomes: future directions in the field. *J Am Diet Assoc* 2005;105(5 Suppl 1):S14–S16.
2. Mokdad AH, Marks JS, Stroup DF, et al. Actual causes of death in the United States, 2000. *J Am Med Assoc* 2004;291(10):1238–1245.
3. Mokdad AH, Marks JS, Stroup DF, et al. Correction: actual causes of death in the United States, 2000. *J Am Med Assoc* 2005;293(3):293.
4. Flegal KM, Graubard BI, Williamson DF, et al. Excess death associated with underweight, overweight, and obesity. *J Am Med Assoc* 2005;293(15):1861–1874.
5. Couzin J. A heavyweight battle over CDC's obesity forecasts. *Science* 2005;308: 770–771.
6. Flegal KM, Graubard BI, Williamson DF, et al. Excess deaths associated with underweight, overweight, and obesity. *JAMA* 2005;293(15):1861–1867.
7. World Health Organization. *Preventing and managing the global epidemic of obesity. Report of the World Health Organization Consultation of Obesity.* Geneva: WHO,1997.
8. Gasteyger C, Tremblay A. Metabolic impact of body fat distribution *J Endocrinol Invest* 2002;25(10):876–883.
9. National Institutes of Health. Clinical guidelines on the identification, evaluation, and treatment of overweight and obesity in adults: the evidence report. *Obes Res* 1998;6(suppl 2):51S–209S.
10. Brownell KD. Dieting and the search for the perfect body: where physiology and culture collide. *Behav Ther* 1991;22:1–12.
11. Jonas S, Konner L. *Just the weigh you are: how to be fit and healthy whatever your size.* Shelburne: Chapters Publishing/Houghton-Mifflin, 1997.
12. Burgard D. Walking your inner dog. *Health at every size* 2004;18(4):61–63.
13. Pi-Sunyer FX. A review of the long-term studies evaluating the efficacy of weight loss in ameliorating disorders associated with obesity. *Clin Ther* 1996;18:1006–1035.

14. Flatt JP. The biochemistry of energy expenditure. In: Bjorntorp P, Brodoff BN, eds. *Obesity* New York: JB Lippincott Co, 1988.

15. Yancy WS Jr, Olsen MK, Guyton JR, et al. A low-carbohydrate, ketogenic diet versus a low-fat diet to treat obesity and hyperlipidemia: follow up of a randomized, controlled trial. *Ann Intern Med* 2004;140:769–777.

16. Stern L, Iqbal N, Seshadri P, et al. The effects of low carbohydrate versus conventional weight loss diets in severely obese adults: one-year follow up of a randomized trial. *Ann Intern Med* 2004;140:778–785.

17. Erlanson-Albertsson C, Mei J. The effect of low carbohydrate on energy metabolism. *Int J Obes (Lond)* 2005;29(Suppl 2):S26–S30.

18. McMillan-Price J, Petocz P, Atkinson F, et al. Comparison of 4 diets of varying glycemic load on weight loss and cardiovascular risk reduction in overweight and obese young adults: a randomized controlled trial. *Arch Int Med* 2006;166(14): 1466–1475.

19. Nordman AJ, Nordmann A, Briel M, et al. Effects of low-carbohydrate vs low-fat diets on weight loss and cardiovascular risk factors: a meta-analysis of randomized controlled trials. *Arch Intern Med* 2006;166(3):285–293.

20. Jonas S, Aronson V. *The "I don't eat (but I can't lose)" weight loss program*. New York: Rawson Associates, 1989.

21. Mole PA, Stern JS, Schultz CL, et al. Exercise reverses depressed metabolic rate produced by severe caloric restriction. *Med Sci Sports Exerc* 1989;21:29.

22. Jonas S. (and the Editors of Consumer Reports Books). *Take control of your weight*. Yonkers: Consumer Reports Books, 1993.

23. Jonas, S. The 'Dynamic Epidemiology" of obesity: knowledge to help improve our ability to manage the condition. *J Am Med Athletic Assoc* 2004;17(2):5–7, 17.

24. Blair SN, Church TS. The fitness, obesity and health equation: is physical activity the common denominator? *J Am Med Assoc* 2004;292(10):12323–11233.

25. U.S. Preventive Services Task Force. *Guide to clinical preventive services, 3rd edition: periodic updates, Vol. 1: methods and screening*. Rockville: Agency for Healthcare Research and Quality Screening for Obesity in Adults, 2003:413–414, www.ahrq.gov.

26. Kayman S, Bruvold W, Stern JS. Maintenance and relapse after weight loss in women: behavioral aspects. *Am J Clin Nutr* 1990;52:800–807.

27. Schachter S. Recidivism and self-cure of smoking and obesity. *Am Psychology* 1982; 37:436.

28. Brownell KD, Wadden TA. The heterogeneity of obesity: fitting treatments to individuals. *Behav Ther* 1991;22:153–177.

29. Li Z, Maglione M, Tu W, et al. Meta-analysis: pharmacologic treatment of obesity. *Ann Intern Med* 2005;142(7):532–546.

30. Wadden TA, Berkowitz RJ, Womble LG, et al. Randomized trial of lifestyle modification and pharmacotherapy for obesity. *N Engl J Med* 2005;353(20):2111–2120.

31. Palamara KL, Mogul HR, Peterson SJ, et al. Obesity: new perspectives and pharmacotherapies. *Cardiol Rev* 2006;14:238–258.

32. Ionnaides-Demoss LL, Prioetto J, McNeil JJ. Pharmacotherapy for obesity. *Drugs* 2005;65(10):1391–1418.

33. Brechner RJ, Farris C, Harrison S, et al. A graded, evidence-based summary for evidence for bariatric surgery. *Surg Obes Relat Dis* 2005;1:430–441.

34. Tsai AG, Wadden TA. Systematic review: an evaluation of major commercial weight loss programs in the United States. *Ann Intern Med* 2005;142(1):56–66.

35. Wantland DJ, Portillo CJ, Holzemer WL, et al. The effectiveness of Web-based vs. non-Web-based interventions: a meta-analysis of behavioral change outcomes. *J Med Internet Res* 2004;6(4):e40.

36. Wadden TA, Butryn ML, Byrne KJ. Efficacy of lifestyle modification for long-term weight control. *Obes Res* 2004;12(suppl):151S–162S.

37. Heymsfield SB, van Mierlo CAvan der Knaap HC, et al. Weight management using a meal replacement strategy: meta and pooling analysis from six studies. *Int J Obes Relat Metab Disord* 2003;27(5):537–549.

38. Huerta S, Li Z, Li HC, et al. Feasibility of a partial meal replacement plan for weight loss in low-income patients. *Int J Obes Relat Metab Disord* 2004;28(12):1575–1579.

39. Katz DL, O'Connell M, Yeh MC, et al. Public health strategies for preventing and controlling overweight and obesity in school and worksite settings: a report on recommendations of the Task Force on Community Preventive Services. *MMWR* 2005;54(RR-10):1–12.

40. Tuomilehto J, Lindstrom J, Eriksson JG, et al. Finnish Diabetes Prevention Study Group. Prevention of type 2 diabetes mellitus by changes in lifestyle among subjects with impaired glucose tolerance. *N Engl J Med* 2001;344:1343–1350.

41. Goldstein DJ. Beneficial health effects of modest weight loss. *Int J Obes Relat Metab Disord* 1992;16:397–415.

42. Knowler WC, Barrett-Connor E, Fowler SE, et al. Diabetes Prevention Program Research Group. Reduction in the incidence of type 2 diabetes with lifestyle intervention or metformin. *N Engl J Med* 2002;346:393–403.

CHAPTER 9

Tobacco Use

Stephen F. Rothemich

Tobacco use remains the leading cause of preventable death in the United States, a rank that it has held ever since deaths were first quantified by risk factors in the early 1990s (1,2). In the United States, cigarette smoking and exposure to tobacco smoke account for approximately one in five deaths (438,000 people) each year, as well as 5.5 million years of potential life lost (3). Although overweight (the product of a combination of poor diet and physical inactivity) runs a close second as a leading cause, tobacco use causes more than twice as many deaths as alcohol consumption, motor vehicle accidents, firearm use, unsafe sexual behavior, and illicit drug use combined. In addition to this staggering loss of life, as of 2001 tobacco use cost society more than $167 billion per year through smoking-attributable health care expenditures ($76 billion) and adult productivity losses ($92 billion). Helping smokers quit is ranked by the National Commission on Prevention Priorities as among the top three most effective and cost effective clinical preventive services that clinicians can offer patients (4).

Smoking harms nearly every organ of the body, has been causally linked to dozens of adverse health effects (see Table 9.1), and reduces overall health status (5). Cigarette smoking alone is responsible for more than 30% of U.S. cancer deaths (6). Smokeless tobacco use causes oral cancer and other oral lesions. Environmental tobacco smoke, a known human carcinogen, causes premature death and disease in children and in adults who do not smoke; scientific evidence indicates no risk-free level of exposure to secondhand smoke exists (7). Quitting smoking has both immediate and long-term benefits, reducing the risk of diseases caused by tobacco and improving health in general.

In 2004, 44.5 million Americans, or 20.9% of the adult population, smoked cigarettes; 23.4% of men smoked compared with 18.5% of women. Among whites, 22.2% smoked compared with 20.2% of blacks. The highest levels of smoking were among people aged 25–44 years (23.8%); American Indians and Alaskan Natives (33.4%); people who had earned a General Educational Development (GED) but not a standard high-school diploma (39.6%); and people living below the poverty threshold (29.1%) (8). Although

TABLE 9.1 Adverse Health Effects of Smoking Supported by Strong Evidence

Cancer

Bladder

Cervical

Esophageal

Kidney

Laryngeal

Leukemia

Lung

Oral

Pancreatic

Stomach

Respiratory Effects

Asthma (poor control)

Asthma-related symptoms

Chronic obstructive pulmonary disease

Impaired lung growth

Lung function decline

Pneumonia

Respiratory symptoms (coughing, phlegm, wheezing, dyspnea)

Cardiovascular Effects

Abdominal aortic aneurysm

Atherosclerosis

Cerebrovascular disease

Coronary heart disease

Reproductive Effects

Low birth weight

Placental abruption

Placenta previa

Preterm birth

Reduced fertility

Sudden infant death syndrome

TABLE 9.1 *(Continued)*

Other Effects

Cataract

Hip fractures

Increased absenteeism

Increased health services usage

Low bone density

Peptic ulcer disease (*Helicobacter pylori* positive)

Poor surgical outcomes

Poor wound healing

Adapted from U.S. Centers for Disease Control and Prevention. *The health consequences of smoking: a report of the surgeon general*. Atlanta: U.S. Department of Health and Human Services, Centers for Disease Control and Prevention, 2004:2–6.

the national smoking rate is slowly declining, it is still well above the national goals set in *Healthy People 2010:* less than 12% for adults and 16% for adolescents (9).

This chapter provides clinicians and their associates with the necessary information to institute effective smoking cessation techniques in their practices. Although this chapter emphasizes smoking cessation, these interventions may be used to help smokeless tobacco users quit as well. The interventions described are based on the U.S. Public Health Service (PHS) guidelines, with additional emphasis on the role of telephone "quit lines," now available in every state in the United States. Although one option for clinicians is to deliver intensive counseling as the primary focus of a series of clinic visits, an alternative is to offer simple advice to quit coupled with referral to a quit line, a 30-second option that many clinicians may find easier to incorporate into their daily practice.

BACKGROUND

Many clinicians recognize smoking as a major threat to a patient's health but do not feel confident in their ability to intervene effectively. Most clinicians have not experienced success in helping patients to stop smoking. Most have treated patients with significant tobacco-related diseases who have been unable to stop despite multiple attempts, even as they became sicker. Repeated failures to help patients stop smoking frequently cause clinicians to become discouraged and reinforce the belief that nothing can be done about smoking. Another barrier preventing clinicians from trying to help patients quit smoking includes a lack of formal training in tested cessation techniques. Perhaps most important, many office practices are not organized to support the delivery of smoking cessation interventions.

However, the evidence is clear: advice from clinicians helps smokers quit. Even providing brief, simple advice increases the likelihood that a smoker will successfully quit and remain abstinent 12 months later (10). The methods outlined here show how best to use the limited time available to impact smoking behavior among patients.

METHODS

Treating Tobacco Use and Dependence, which is available online in its entirety (11) and in a summary for clinicians (12), details the PHS clinical practice guidelines for promoting smoking cessation among patients.

Clinician Intervention

The clinician intervention recommended in the PHS guideline comprises five activities, each beginning with the letter "A" (often referred to as the *5 As,* as discussed in Chapter 5):

- *Ask* all patients about smoking
- *Advise* smokers to stop
- *Assess* if the smoker is willing to make a quit attempt
- *Assist* their efforts with self-help materials, a quit date, and possibly cessation medication
- *Arrange* follow-up

This intervention plan describes a general approach to patients who smoke and can be used in almost any outpatient encounter, whether the clinician and patient have 30 seconds or 30 minutes for the discussion (13).

Ask about smoking at every opportunity. For example, a nurse or other staff member should routinely ask patients *"Do you smoke?"* or *"Are you still smoking?"* at each visit, usually while measuring vital signs. Once it is known that a person smokes, an identifier should be placed prominently on the patient's chart to remind the clinician and staff to discuss smoking at each visit (see Fig. 9.1). (See Chapters 21 and 22 for further information about chart alert stickers, automated prompts, and other clinician reminder systems.) Patients who have never smoked or who formerly smoked should be congratulated on their decision.

Advise all smokers to stop. A clear statement of advice (e.g., *"As your physician, I must advise you to stop smoking now"*) is essential. Many patients do not recall receiving this advice from their clinician. Therefore, the statement must be

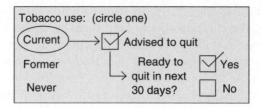

Figure 9.1 • A tobacco-use "vital sign" stamp, which can appear prominently on the patient's chart where vital signs are recorded to remind the clinician and staff to systematically assess smoking status at each visit. The traditional version, illustrated in the U.S. Public Health Service guideline (12), only contains the information in the left-most column of the version shown here (the first of the 5 *As*, "Ask"). This second generation stamp, courtesy of Stephen F. Rothemich, MD, MS, is designed for also obtaining and documenting the second and third *As* ("Advise" and "Assess").

short, clear, and memorable. Personalization of the message by referring to the patient's clinical condition or family history may add to the effectiveness of the advice. The type of motivation that will help smokers quit varies greatly from patient to patient. Although almost any clinical encounter provides an opportunity to discuss smoking, timing of the advice can be very important. The so-called teachable moment is that time when a patient's circumstances make him or her more receptive to advice. Teachable moments occur when patients are affected by diseases caused by smoking, but they may also occur following auscultation or pulmonary function testing, or when a friend or relative is ill.

Assess if *the smoker is willing to make a quit attempt.* Patients' level of interest in stopping smoking is usually evident in discussions with the clinician. If it is not, ask patients if they want to stop. See Chapter 5 for further information about the transtheoretical model and stages of readiness to change, which include precontemplation, contemplation, preparation, action, and maintenance (see pages 132–133).

Patients not ready to make a quit attempt (precontemplation or contemplation stages) may respond to a motivational intervention. The clinician can motivate patients to consider a quit attempt with the *5 Rs*:

- *Relevance*—encourage the patient to indicate why quitting is personally relevant
- *Risks*—ask the patient to identify potential negative consequences of tobacco use
- *Rewards*—ask the patient to identify potential benefits of stopping tobacco use
- *Roadblocks*—ask the patient to identify barriers or impediments to quitting
- *Repetition*—repeat motivational intervention at every clinic visit

Assist *the patient in stopping.* For those patients who express a sincere desire to stop smoking, the clinician should help them set a specific date for the next attempt. There is evidence that patients who set a "quit date" are more likely to make a serious attempt to stop than those who do not (14). This date should be in the near future (generally within 4 weeks), but not immediate, giving the patient the necessary time to prepare to stop. Patients should be encouraged to announce their "quit date" to family, friends, and coworkers. Once a patient has selected a specific date to stop, information must be provided so that he or she can prepare for that date. For patients who can read, this is easily accomplished by providing them with a self-help brochure. Effective brochures provide the patient with necessary information about smoking cessation (e.g., symptoms and time course of withdrawal, cessation tips, reasons to quit, answers to common questions). A list of print and online patient education materials is provided later in the "Resources-Patient Education Materials" section at the end of this chapter. Patients who cannot read need to acquire this information from other sources, such as audiotapes, video materials, or counseling by a clinician or health educator.

Arrange *follow-up visits.* When patients know that their progress will be reviewed, their chances of successfully stopping improve. This monitoring may include a letter or telephone call from the office staff just before the quit date, reinforcing the decision to stop. Most relapses occur in the first weeks after cessation. A person who comes to the office after being a nonsmoker for 1–2 weeks has a much improved chance of remaining abstinent than those without follow-up (15). For this reason, it is critical that patients be contacted during their first 2 weeks of abstinence to reinforce their decision to stop. Nurses or other clinicians as well as the physician may conduct this follow-up in the office or by telephone. It should consist of an assessment of the patient's progress, troubleshooting for any problems encountered or anticipated, and discussion of the effectiveness or side effects of cessation medications.

Although follow-up visits are critical during the first 2 weeks after cessation, clinic staff should remain in contact with the patient and schedule a formal follow-up visit in 1–2 months. For patients who cannot return for an appointment, contact by telephone or by mail may be helpful. Many patients can benefit from the social support and information offered through quit lines, Internet discussion sites, and local support group sessions offered by the American Cancer Society, the American Lung Association, or local churches or community organizations (see page 250). While only a small proportion of patients referred to such programs actually participate (16), these programs have the potential for large public health impact. However, for individual patients, clinicians should consider these referrals as augmenting, not replacing, a clinician's care.

Patients may also express interest in techniques such as hypnosis and acupuncture. These have not been proved to be effective through randomized, controlled trials but are probably not harmful. Informed patients who wish to try these techniques should not be discouraged from doing so.

Pharmacologic Agents

Clinicians should consider recommending over-the-counter nicotine replacement therapy or one of several prescription medications that can increase the success rate for quit attempts. Table 9.2 summarizes currently available pharmacologic adjuvants for smoking cessation. U.S. Food and Drug Administration (FDA)-approved pharmacotherapies recommended as first-line agents include bupropion, varenicline tartrate, nicotine gum, nicotine inhaler, nicotine nasal spray, nicotine patch, and nicotine lozenges. Secondary pharmacotherapy options, not FDA-approved for use in smoking cessation but of proven benefit, include nortriptyline and oral clonidine (17,18). A nicotine vaccine, which will prevent transfer of nicotine through the blood–brain barrier, is in early development.

Selection of an appropriate agent depends on patient contraindications, patient preference, cost/coverage issues, and clinician familiarity with the pharmacotherapy. Among over-the-counter options, patches offer simplicity, while lozenges or gum give patients more control over dosing schedules. All forms of nicotine replacement therapy can help patients stop smoking, almost doubling long-term success rates (19), with similar efficacy to prescription medication. The long-term use of nicotine replacement therapies does not pose a known health risk and may be helpful with smokers who report persistent withdrawal symptoms. However, use of any nicotine replacement therapy should be avoided for 1 month following myocardial infarction, serious arrhythmia, or unstable angina.

Clinical trial data suggest that bupropion and varenicline tartrate are effective aids to smoking cessation. Bupropion can be paired safely with nicotine replacement therapy, although blood pressure may need more careful monitoring. Even when used alone, bupropion use leads to quit rates about double those achieved with the nicotine patch. The effects of bupropion go beyond antidepressant activity, but its mechanism of action in smoking cessation remains unknown. Additionally, the FDA has approved the use of bupropion sustained release for long-term maintenance. The more recently approved varenicline tartrate appears to be even more effective than bupropion. Nortriptyline and clonidine have smoking cessation efficacy, and while these may produce a number of unpleasant side effects, they should be considered when FDA-approved medications are not available to patients due to cost issues.

TABLE 9.2 Pharmacologic Adjuvants for Smoking Cessation

Agent (Brands)	Advantages	Disadvantages
Nicotine gum (Nicorette)	OTC Flexible dosing Fast nicotine delivery May delay weight gain	Proper use required Frequent use required No food or drink 15 min before use Possible jaw pain, mouth soreness, dyspepsia, hiccups Avoid use with dental problems or temporomandibular joint syndrome
Nicotine lozenge (Commit)	OTC Flexible dosing Fast nicotine delivery	Frequent dosing required No food or drink 15 min before use Possible mouth soreness, dyspepsia
Nicotine patch (Habitrol, Nicoderm CQ, Nicotrol)	OTC Different strengths available Daily application Overnight use may reduce early morning cravings	Slow nicotine delivery Less flexible dosing Possible skin irritations Possible sleep problems if worn at night
Nicotine nasal spray (Nicotrol NS)	Fastest nicotine delivery Reduces cravings in minutes Flexible dosing	Frequent dosing required Possible nasal and eye irritation, cough Most addictive nicotine replacement therapy
Nicotine inhaler (Nicotrol inhaler)	Flexible dosing Mimics hand-to-mouth routine of smoking	Frequent dosing required Possible mouth and throat irritation
Bupropion SR (Wellbutrin SR, Zyban)	Non-nicotine Easy use May be combined with nicotine replacement therapy May delay weight gain May be effective in depression (see Chapter 13)	Possible insomnia, dry mouth, headache, tremors, nausea, anxiety Avoid use with seizure disorders, bulimia, anorexia nervosa, history of head trauma, current use of bupropion or a monoamine oxidase inhibitor

TABLE 9.2   *(Continued)*

Agent (Brands)	Advantages	Disadvantages
Varenicline tartrate (Chantrix)	Easy use May ease withdrawal symptoms May block effects of nicotine during relapse May delay weight gain May be effective in depression (see Chapter 13)	Possible headache, vomiting, flatulence, insomnia, abnormal dreams, dysgeusia (taste disturbance)
Nortriptyline (Aventyl HCl, Pamelor)	Easy use Inexpensive May be effective in depression (see Chapter 13)	Not FDA approved for smoking cessation Possible tremor, headache, dry mouth, nausea, indigestion, constipation, diarrhea, fatigue, weakness, anxiety, insomnia Avoid use with alcohol, methyprylon, or monoamine oxidase inhibitor
Clonidine, oral (Catapress)	Easy use Inexpensive	Not FDA approved for smoking cessation Possible dizziness, weight gain, drowsiness, dry mouth, constipation Avoid use with alcohol

OTC = over-the-counter; FDA = U.S. Food and Drug Administration.

Quit Lines

The use of telephone-based tobacco cessation services, commonly known as *quit lines*, has been shown to improve smoking cessation rates (20). Their effectiveness with smokers who use them is well established. In many states with comprehensive tobacco control programs, quit lines play an important role in media-based efforts to encourage smoking cessation. Depending on the state, and sometimes by insurance status within states, quit lines offer either *reactive* counseling (smokers can call as needed during their quit attempt) or the more effective *proactive* counseling (a series of counseling calls initiated by quit line personnel timed around a quit attempt) (21). Quit lines are accessible and eliminate many barriers associated with traditional smoking cessation classes or support groups. These include having to wait for sessions to be offered, needing to arrange transportation and/or childcare, and discomfort with participating in a group discussion. Patients underrepresented in traditional cessation services, such as smokers of ethnic minority backgrounds, actively seek help from quit lines (22). Every quit line serves thousands of tobacco users each year, a volume rarely achieved by other behavioral services, yet they currently reach only 1–5% of the tobacco users in their states each year.

Practices can extend their capability of providing intensive counseling by encouraging patients to utilize a quit line. One way to do this after offering brief advice to quit is simply to provide the national toll-free number (1-800-QUIT-NOW) that automatically routes callers to their state's quit line and to recommend that patients call (reactive telephone counseling). This can be done in 30 seconds. When incorporating all the 5As into busy office visits is not feasible, this "Ask, Advise, and Refer" strategy (22) is a very reasonable shortcut and far better than not addressing tobacco use at all.

In some states clinicians can send referrals directly to the quit line, whose counselors will then contact the patient directly (proactive telephone counseling). Proactive counseling, which eliminates the need for the patient to place the call and has been proved to be more effective than reactive counseling (20), is usually arranged by completing a referral form (often signed by both patient and clinician), which is then faxed to the service. Most state quit lines offer proactive counseling only to smokers ready to make a quit attempt in the next 30 days (preparation stage of the transtheoretical model, see page 132 in Chapter 5), and practices may therefore need to screen potential quit line referrals to verify their stage of readiness to change. For smokers not yet ready to quit, providing the telephone number for them to call is more appropriate. In either case, clinicians should be prepared to respond to calls from patients who are referred to quit lines and want prescription-only cessation medication options that were not discussed and arranged before their referral.

COMMON PROBLEMS AND POSSIBLE SOLUTIONS

Weight Gain

The issue of potential weight gain is important for many patients who try to stop smoking. Some patients cite weight gain as the reason for relapse after previous attempts to stop. The average amount of weight gained after cessation is approximately 5 lb. Some patients gain no weight after cessation, but a small proportion of people gain large amounts of weight.

There are several obvious recommendations that can be made to patients concerned about preventing weight gain. Attention to caloric intake can be as simple as monitoring portion size, making healthy food choices, and avoiding "rewarding" themselves for not smoking with rich foods or special meals (see Chapters 7 and 8). Recommendations for more frequent physical activity (even in short bouts) may both help prevent weight gain and support smoke-free behavior (see Chapter 6).

Multiple Relapses

Many smokers, especially adults older than 40 years, have made several serious attempts to stop smoking but have always relapsed. Nicotine is a powerfully addictive drug. These patients have frequently tried various smoking cessation products and programs, all without success. Such patients are often discouraged by their failed attempts to stop and are therefore less willing to try again.

These patients (and their clinicians) need to be aware that relapse is a typical part of the cessation process. Most smokers require several attempts to achieve permanent abstinence, and knowing this may bring encouragement to relapsing smokers. Even in a relatively short clinic visit, a clinician can help a patient benefit from past relapses rather than view them as a personal failure and a reason to avoid future quit attempts. During the visit, the clinician can help the patient to identify the circumstances that led to past relapses and to develop strategies for use in either avoiding those circumstances or responding to them in a different manner.

A simple question from the clinician—such as *"When you resumed smoking, where did your first cigarette come from?"*—or *"what was going on in your life when you started up again?"*—will start the discussion of the reason(s) for relapse. There are several common reasons offered for relapse, including withdrawal symptoms, weight gain, "stress" at work or home, alcohol intoxication, or social pressure. Once the patient has described the circumstances of the relapse, the clinician can ask, *"How do you think you would deal with that situation if it happened again?"* or *"How do you think you could avoid that situation in the future?"* The clinician can offer advice about some situations and help with withdrawal symptoms (see Table 9.3), but the patient must develop a personalized plan for responding to circumstances that have caused past relapses.

Patients commonly say that they had a relapse due to stress at their job or at home. Marital difficulties, problems with other family members, loss of a job, or increased work responsibilities are often given as reasons for relapse. Patients, with the help of their clinician, need to anticipate the difficult times that may occur while they are attempting to quit and be prepared with a response other than taking up smoking again. Simple responses to craving, such as chewing gum, taking a walk, or engaging in relaxation exercises, may be all that a patient needs to cope with a difficult personal situation. In all cases, having a concrete plan in place to address these stressful situations is critical.

TABLE 9.3 Responding to Common Concerns during Smoking Cessation

I am gaining weight

Not every person who stops smoking gains weight.

Average weight gains are small for people who do gain weight (5–10 lb).

Do not try to lose weight now—there will be time after you are an established nonsmoker.

Exercise is an effective technique to cope with withdrawal and avoid weight gain.

Avoid high-calorie snacks. Vegetables (such as carrot sticks) and fruits are good snacks.

The risks to health from smoking are far greater than the risks to health from a small weight gain.

A small increase in weight may not hurt your appearance. Smoking is unattractive, causing yellow teeth, bad breath, stale clothing odors, and, possibly, wrinkled skin.

Now that I have stopped, can I smoke a cigarette occasionally?

No. Nicotine addiction seems to be retriggered quickly in most former smokers. Do not risk getting hooked again.

What should I do when I get an urge to smoke?

Some people relieve cravings by chewing gum, sucking on a cinnamon stick, or eating a carrot stick.

Cravings for cigarettes are a normal part of withdrawal.

Most cravings last for only a few minutes and then subside.

Cravings become rare after a few weeks.

Use nicotine gum, if prescribed.

When I do not smoke, I feel restless and I cannot concentrate.

These are normal symptoms of nicotine withdrawal.

These symptoms are most acute in the first 3 days after stopping.

These symptoms will disappear after a few weeks.

What other withdrawal symptoms will I have?

Some smokers have few or no withdrawal symptoms.

Other common symptoms include anxiety, irritability, insomnia, mild headache, and gastrointestinal symptoms such as constipation.

Few smokers experience all these symptoms.

Like most other symptoms, they are only temporary.

Lack of Social Support for Stopping

Various social factors are frequently implicated in relapse, particularly when the patient is confronted by situations or friends who provide strong cues or prompts for smoking. Parties and other social gatherings are common sites of relapses, especially among patients who consume alcohol at these events.

During the time available in a brief office visit, it will not be possible for the clinician to help patients make major changes in their social skills or in their support system for behavior change. However, all patients should be encouraged to tell their family, friends, and coworkers of their decision to stop smoking in advance of their quit date and to seek their support and encouragement. Patients with little support for stopping can be referred to group cessation programs. Referral to a counselor or other health professional may also be useful.

It is often difficult for a patient to stop if his or her spouse or partner also smokes and is unwilling to stop. The unwilling spouse/partner should be encouraged to join in the quit attempt. If this is unsuccessful, that person should at least be encouraged to smoke only outside the home.

SPECIAL POPULATIONS

As discussed earlier, the advice and assistance a clinician provides should reflect an understanding of the patient's medical, social, and cultural background. By asking the patient about anticipated problems with smoking cessation and potential solutions to these problems, the clinician can help patients construct solutions that are relevant to their social and cultural setting. Clinicians should be prepared to provide factual medical information for their patients. For example, the older smoker who believes it is too late to stop and that quitting will do little good should be reminded that quitting at any age decreases the risk of future smoking-related illness and can increase both the length and quality of life.

Clinicians also need to recognize that smoking and tobacco use are viewed in different ways by different cultural groups, and that these views may influence how and why a patient stops. Self-help materials designed for special population groups are becoming more widely available. These materials address both the cultural and language issues faced by patients, and are generally available from local units of the American Cancer Society, American Lung Association, and local health departments (see "Resources" on page 250).

Young people comprise another group that can benefit from the advice and assistance of clinicians. Because most adult smokers first become addicted to nicotine during childhood and adolescence, advice from clinicians during these life stages is critical. Although any adolescent is a potential smoker, those at highest risk of becoming addicted demonstrate low self-esteem, have poor academic performance, and engage in other risky behaviors such as alcohol or drug use. It is challenging but essential to provide these young people with anticipatory guidance that is appropriate for their age and developmental stage.

Some clinicians have used cigarette advertisements to initiate discussions about smoking with adolescents, showing them the deceptive nature of the advertisements. When rapport with a young person is established, clinicians can provide reasons for avoiding tobacco use that are relevant to an adolescent and can also help the patient practice refusal skills. Adolescents who are already regular smokers should be advised and assisted in the same manner as an adult patient. However, adolescents are often much more concerned with the immediate effects of smoking, such as "smokers' breath and smell" and diminished athletic performance, and are often not influenced by information about long-term risks such as cancer and other tobacco-related diseases.

Finally, clinicians should routinely ask about vulnerable household members who might be exposed to secondhand smoke. Children of any age should be protected from exposure to environmental tobacco smoke. Parents who smoke should be advised to stop and to keep their children in smoke-free environments at home, at day care, and in other settings. Similar precautions must be taken when older adults are receiving care in the home. Even brief exposure to secondhand smoke could pose significant acute risks to ill older adults or to anyone at high risk for cardiovascular or respiratory disease. Those caring for relatives with heart or lung disease should be advised not to smoke in the presence of the sick relative. Some clinicians systematically identify passive smokers (including children) in their practices and routinely provide recommendations to reduce their exposure.

OFFICE AND CLINIC ORGANIZATION

Smoking cessation interventions cannot be delivered to patients routinely and systematically without a supportive office organization. Some simple changes in office procedures (see Chapter 21) can significantly increase the clinician's effectiveness in treating patients who smoke. The goal is to ensure that all patients who smoke are routinely and efficiently identified, consistently monitored, and appropriately treated. Evidence-based office practices shown to reduce tobacco use among patients include the following (23):

- Implementing a tobacco-user identification system (e.g., expand vital signs to include an assessment of tobacco use)
- Providing education, resources, and feedback to promote interventions by clinicians

- Dedicating staff to provide tobacco dependence treatment and then rewarding delivery of this intervention in staff performance evaluations

To act as a coordinated team, all office staff members must understand that smoking cessation is an important task for the practice, and they must know their roles. The team approach is facilitated by naming a smoking cessation coordinator, usually a nurse. With the help of the other staff members, the coordinator will incorporate the various components of the planned intervention program into the day-to-day activities of the practice. The smoking cessation coordinator also helps maintain the staff members' commitment to the program and ensures that the system is operating smoothly. Both the system itself and staff fulfillment of their roles should be reviewed periodically and adjustments made as necessary. See Chapter 21 for further background on practice system redesign.

The team approach emphasizes staff identification of each patient who uses tobacco. When patients are identified as smokers, their charts should be marked in a prominent manner. The typical identifier is a brightly colored permanent sticker or stamp, but it can also be a removable sticker that is put on the chart at each visit. Practices with paper records can revise their forms to include tobacco use as a vital sign (Figure 9.1), and those with electronic health records can go one step further and display screen prompts to staff to obtain this information (see Chapter 22). The regular use of these chart reminders, which facilitates the provision of brief cessation advice as a routine part of every office visit for patients who smoke, has been shown to significantly increase cessation rates in office practices. It is important that all staff members understand and use this kind of charting system.

There should be a specific staff member assigned to scheduling the follow-up visits and making contact with the patient just before the planned "quit date," working closely with the staff person who conducts the follow-up visits. Staff members can also review with patients their self-help materials and instructions for use of any recommended or prescribed cessation medications.

Steps for making an office or clinic itself tobacco-free include posting no-smoking signs, removing ashtrays, displaying tobacco cessation and prevention information prominently, and eliminating tobacco advertising from the office, either by subscribing to magazines that do not carry such advertising or by crossing out the tobacco advertisements with bright markers.

CONCLUSION

Clinician assistance for individual smokers can have an enormous public health impact as well as benefiting each individual patient who quits. Even with very modest expectations of cessation rates, 100,000 clinicians using effective intervention strategies could potentially assist more than 3 million smokers to quit each year. In conjunction with other tobacco-control efforts in communities, practice-based cessation intervention can lead to a marked reduction in the morbidity and mortality caused by smoking. As the former U.S. Surgeon General and author of the Foreword for the first edition of this book, C. Everett Koop, M.D., Sc.D., said "cigarette smoking is the most important public health issue of our time." And it still is.

RESOURCES — PATIENT EDUCATION MATERIALS

American Academy of Family Physicians
Links to AAFP and national resources for patients and clinicians, including patient education materials, information about the "Ask and Act" tobacco cessation program, quit lines, nicotine replacement therapy, and tips on reimbursement.
Telephone: 800-274-2237
http://www.aafp.org/online/en/home/clinical/publichealth/tobacco/
    resources.html

American Cancer Society
Online cessation guide, tools for clinicians, and information on the Great American Smokeout.
Telephone: 800-227-2345
http://www.cancer.org/docroot/PED/content/PED_10_13X_Guide_for_Quitting_
    Smoking.asp

Centers for Disease Control and Prevention
Tobacco Information and Prevention Source (TIPS) with links to free how to quit guides, education materials, TIPS for youth. Much of the information and materials are also available there in Spanish.
Telephone: 800–232–1311
http://www.cdc.gov/tobacco

National Cancer Institute
Links to tobacco information, statistics, research, and other resources
Telephone: 800–422–6237
http://www.cancer.gov/cancertopics/tobacco

Smoke Free
NCI's free online smoking cessation program
http://www.smokefree.gov

SUGGESTED READINGS

Fiore MC, Bailey WC, Cohen SJ, et al. *Treating tobacco use and dependence.* Rockville: U.S. Department of Health and Human Services, http://www.ncbi.nlm.nih .gov/books/bv.fcgi?rid=hstat2.chapter.7644, 2000.
Smoking Cessation Leadership Center. *Information on utilizing quit lines in clinical practice.* Website: http://smokingcessationleadership.ucsf.edu/30seconds.html. Accessed 2006.
U.S. Public Health Service. *Treating tobacco use and dependence—Provider's packet. A how-to guide for implementing the public health service clinical practice guideline.* U.S. Public Health Service. http://www.surgeongeneral.gov/tobacco/clinpack.html, 2003.

U.S. Surgeon General. *Patient education materials, comprehensive and abbreviated version of the clinical practice guide on smoking cessation, and links to the surgeon general reports.* Website: http://www.surgeongeneral.gov/tobacco. Accessed 2006.

References

1. Mokdad AH, Marks JS, Stroup DF, et al. Actual causes of death in the United States, 2000. *JAMA* 2004;291(10):1238–1245.

2. McGinnis JM, Foege WH. Actual causes of death in the United States. *JAMA* 1993; 270(18):2207–2212.

3. Centers for Disease Control and Prevention. Annual smoking—attributable mortality, years of potential life lost, and productivity losses—United States, 1997–2001. *MMWR* 2005;54:625–628.

4. Maciosek MV, Coffield AB, Edwards NM, et al. Priorities for improving utilization of clinical preventive services results. *Am J Prev Med* 2006;31:52–61.

5. Centers for Disease Control and Prevention. *The health consequences of smoking: a report of the surgeon general.* Atlanta: U.S. Department of Health and Human Services, CDC, 2004.

6. National Institutes of Health State-of-the-Science Conference Statement. *Tobacco use: prevention, cessation, and control.* Bethesda: National Institutes of Health, 2006.

7. U.S. Department of Health and Human Services. *The health consequences of involuntary exposure to tobacco smoke: a report of the surgeon general—executive summary.* U.S. Department of Health and Human Services, Centers for Disease Control and Prevention, Coordinating Center for Health Promotion, National Center for Chronic Disease Prevention and Health Promotion, Office on Smoking and Health, 2006:9.

8. Centers for Disease Control and Prevention. Cigarette smoking among adults—United States, 2004. *MMWR* 2005;54(44):1121–1124.

9. U.S. Department of Health and Human Services. *Healthy People 2010: Understanding and Improving Health.* 2nd ed. Washington, DC: U.S. Government Printing Office, November 2000.

10. Lancaster T, Stead LF. Physician advice for smoking cessation. *Cochrane Database Syst Rev* 2004;(4):CD000165.

11. Fiore MC, Bailey WC, Cohen SJ, et al. *Treating tobacco use and dependence.* Rockville: U.S. Department of Health and Human Services, 2000, http://www.ncbi .nlm.nih.gov/books/bv.fcgi?rid=hstat2.chapter.7644.

12. U.S. Public Health Service. *Treating tobacco use and dependence—provider's packet. A how-to guide for implementing the public health service clinical practice guideline.* U.S. Public Health Service, 2003. http://www.surgeongeneral.gov/tobacco/clinpack.html.

13. Okuyemi KS, Nollen NL, Ahluwalia JS. Interventions to facilitate smoking cessation. *Am Fam Physician* 2006;74:262–271,276.

14. Cummings SR, Coates TJ, Richard RJ, et al. Training physicians in counseling about smoking cessation. A randomized trial of the Quit for Life program. *Ann Intern Med* 1989;110(8):640–647.

15. Kenford SL, Fiore MC, Jorenby DE, et al. Predicting smoking cessation: who will quit with and without the nicotine patch. *JAMA* 1993;278(8):589–594.

16. Hollis JF, Lichtenstein E, Mount K, et al. Nurse-assisted smoking counseling in medical settings: minimizing demands on physicians. *Prev Med* 1991;20(4): 497–507.

17. Gourlay SG, Stead LF, Benowitz NL. Clonidine for smoking cessation. *Cochrane Database Syst Rev* 2004;(3):CD000058.

18. Hughes JR, Stead LF, Lancaster T. Antidepressants for smoking cessation. *Cochrane Database Syst Rev* 2004;(4):CD000031.

19. Silagy C, Lancaster T, Stead L, et al. Nicotine replacement therapy for smoking cessation. *Cochrane Database Syst Rev* 2004;(3):CDC000146.

20. Stead LF, Perera R, Lancaster T. Telephone counseling for smoking cessation. *Cochrane Database Syst Rev* 2006;(3):CD002850.

21. Keller PA, Bailey LA, Koss KJ, et al. Organization, financing, promotion, and cost of U.S. Quitlines, 2004. *Am J Prev Med* 2007;32(1):32–37.

22. Schroeder SA. What to do with a patient who smokes. *JAMA* 2005;294:482–487.

23. U.S. Public Health Service. *Treating tobacco use and dependence—a systems approach. A guide for health care administrators, insurers, managed care organizations, and purchasers.* U.S. Public Health Service, http://www.surgeongeneral.gov/tobacco/systems.htm, 2000.

CHAPTER 10

Substance Use

Randall T. Brown and Michael F. Fleming

In 2004, an estimated 22.5 million Americans aged 12 years or older met criteria for either substance abuse or dependence. In 2003, there were more than 620,000 emergency department visits related to drug or alcohol use (1). Substance use disorders (SUDs) result in significant health care and criminal justice costs as well as lost productivity. Estimates of total annual costs of these disorders exceeded $420 billion in 1995 (2), representing an almost twofold increase from estimates 3 years earlier ($240 billion in 1992).

Substance use spans a continuum starting with abstinence and continuing through at-risk use, to abuse and dependence. Individuals with *at-risk* use do not meet Diagnostic and Statistical Manual of Mental Disorders, Fourth Edition (DSM-IV) criteria for substance abuse or dependence, but they use alcohol and/or other drugs in a pattern that places them at risk for physical, psychosocial, occupational, or legal harms.

As defined by DSM-IV, *substance abuse* and *substance dependence* are formal diagnoses (3). Diagnostic criteria for these disorders appear in Tables 10.1A and B on page 254. The term *addiction* is not formally recognized in the DSM-IV, but it is often used interchangeably with substance dependence.

Adverse effects due to SUDs are numerous and can affect every organ system. The nature of the adverse effects that may be experienced by one individual depends on the type of substance, the route of use, and an individual's predisposition to such harm(s). As indicated by the definitions of abuse and dependence, these complications may be biological or psychosocial. Common complications of substance use and SUDs appear in Tables 10.2A and B.

The primary care clinician can play a critical role in the assessment and treatment of substance-related disorders and, hence, in the prevention of the individual and societal sequelae of SUDs. For most substance abusing or dependent individuals, primary care clinicians are their first point of contact with the health care system. Therefore, primary care clinicians are ideally situated to provide initial assessment, brief counseling, pharmacotherapy, and referrals to appropriate specialists and psychosocial rehabilitation. This chapter serves as a review of the risk factors, screening instruments, assessment, diagnosis, and treatment of SUDs in the primary care setting.

TABLE 10.1A   Diagnostic and Statistical Manual of Mental Disorders Fourth Edition (DSM-IV) Criteria for Substance Abuse

Repetitive harm due to use over a 12-mo period manifesting in one or more potential ways:

  Failure to fulfill major obligations

  Recurrent hazardous use

  Recurrent legal consequences

  Ongoing use despite resulting interpersonal problems

And does not meet criteria for substance dependence (see Table 10.1B)

Adapted from American Psychiatric Association. *Diagnostic and statistical manual of mental disorders*, 4th ed. Washington: American Psychiatric Association, 1994:435–436.

TABLE 10.1B   Diagnostic and Statistical Manual of Mental Disorders Fourth Edition (DSM-IV) Criteria for Substance Dependence

Repetitive harm due to use over a 12-mo period manifesting in at least three of seven potential ways:

1. Tolerance: experiencing lesser subjective effects with same amount of use; or need to use more to experience same subjective effects
2. Withdrawal: experiencing a withdrawal syndrome characteristic of the substance upon abrupt cessation that is relieved by administration of the substance; or continued use to avoid the symptoms of substance withdrawal
3. Using more over longer periods than intended
4. Repeated failed attempts or persistent desire to quit or cut down on use
5. An inordinate amount of time spent using or obtaining the substance or recovering from its effects
6. Important activities sacrificed
7. Continued use despite knowledge of harms due to use

Adapted from American Psychiatric Association. *Diagnostic and statistical manual of mental disorders*, 4th ed. Washington: American Psychiatric Association, 1994:435–436.

TABLE 10.2A Medical Complications Associated with Alcohol and/or Drug Use and Use Disorders

Alcohol

Trauma
Hypertension
Depression
Suicide
Ischemic heart disease
Stroke
Throat and esophageal cancer
Breast and colon cancer
Hepatitis
Hepatic cirrhosis
Hepatocellular carcinoma
Gastritis/gastric ulceration
Encephalopathy
Peripheral neuropathy
Cerebellar ataxia
Anemia
Thrombocytopenia

Injection Drug Use Complications

Blood-borne viruses
Hepatitis B/hepatitis C
Human immunodeficiency virus infection
Cutaneous infections
Endocarditis
Cardiomyopathy
Nephropathy
Restrictive pulmonary disease

Stimulant Use Complications

Stroke
Myocardial infarction
Cardiac arrhythmia
Seizure
Mood disorders
Psychosis

TABLE 10.2B Common Social Complications of Substance Use and Substance Use Disorders (SUDs)

Job loss

Criminal behavior

Domestic violence

Assault (victim or perpetrator)

Social isolation

Family disintegration

(See Chapter 2 for screening and exploratory questions about substance use to include in the periodic health examination [PHE] and for guidance on discussing this topic with adolescents.)

WHO SHOULD BE SCREENED?

As noted in Chapter 2, the U.S. Preventive Services Task Force, the Institute of Medicine, the American Academy of Family Physicians, and the National Institute on Alcohol Abuse and Alcoholism recommend routine screening of adults, including pregnant women, for alcohol use disorders. Screening of adolescents is also encouraged. Screening for illicit drug use and drug-related problems in PHEs is recommended by the American Academy of Pediatrics and the American Medical Association. "Illicit drugs" are virtually all of the psychoactive drugs that are illegal to sell, possess, or use (e.g., marijuana, heroin, and cocaine) and include prescription pharmaceuticals that are used on a nonprescription basis.

SCREENING INSTRUMENTS

Screening instruments for at-risk alcohol use and alcohol use disorders are much more varied and well studied than instruments for illicit drug use. Similar to screens for other clinical conditions, the clinician should keep in mind that these instruments are not diagnostic for substance abuse or dependence. A positive finding upon screening mandates further evaluation through detailed interviews and/or specialist consultation.

Screening for Alcohol

Several instruments have been developed and studied as screens for at-risk alcohol use and/or alcohol use disorders. Each has its advantages and disadvantages in terms of testing characteristics and convenience of administration. Because the diagnosis of SUDs is based on historical factors related to substance use, the gold standard used to determine the performance of screening instruments for SUDs is most frequently a clinical interview based on the DSM-IV, such as the Structured Clinical Interview for DSM-IV (4).

This section of the chapter focuses on those screens found to be most practical for use in the primary care setting. Such sophisticated screening instruments as the Michigan Alcoholism Screening Test (MAST) or the Substance Abuse Subtle Screening Inventory (SASSI) are very detailed and therefore impractical for use in a busy primary care setting. They involve complicated weighted scoring systems, are time consuming to administer, and do not provide substantially greater sensitivity, specificity, or predictive value than do instruments reviewed in this chapter. Test performance characteristics of several of the most common alcohol screening instruments targeting the general adult population are provided in Table 10.3.

An instrument familiar to most providers is the CAGE questionnaire (see Table 10.4) (8). It should be noted that the CAGE questions are time insensitive; therefore, they do not distinguish a past from a current problem. Two positive responses are most generally considered criteria for a positive screen. Reducing the cutoff for a positive screen to one positive response improves test sensitivity (from approximately 76% to 88%) but reduces test specificity (from approximately 86% to 74%).

A more detailed screening instrument, the Alcohol Use Disorders Identification Test (AUDIT, see Table 10.5), was developed by the World Health Organization as a screen for current at-risk drinking and alcohol use disorders (9). The AUDIT consists of ten questions each scored on a five-point Likert scale (0–4) yielding a possible range of 0–40. A score of 8 or greater indicates the need for further evaluation. In the outpatient clinic population, the AUDIT exhibits improved specificity (95–96%) over the CAGE at traditional cutoffs, but at the expense of sensitivity (38–63%) (10).

A single quantity question (e.g., "On any single occasion during the last 3 months, have you had more than five drinks containing alcohol?") has also been evaluated as a screen for at-risk drinking and alcohol use disorders in the outpatient clinical setting and for binge drinking. Its performance compares favorably to that of the other short screening instruments for problematic alcohol use (11).

The application and utility of the widely used screening instruments, such as CAGE, AUDIT, and variations of the MAST, have primarily been studied among men, using cutoff values and diagnostic criteria more appropriate for men. Therefore, test characteristics and the goals for alcohol screening tools may differ significantly when applied to groups other than adult males.

TABLE 10.3 Test Characteristics of Common Screening Instruments for At-Risk Alcohol Use and Alcohol Use Disorders in the General Clinic Population

Instrument and Cutoff Point	Diagnosis	Sensitivity (%)	Specificity (%)	PPV (%)	NPV (%)
CAGE score ≥2 positive responses	Abuse or dependence	74–78	76–96	32–75	95–97
CAGE score ≥1 positive response	Abuse or dependence	86–90	52–93	21–66	96–98
AUDIT score ≥8	At-risk use, abuse, or dependence	38–63	95–96	68–82	84–94
MAST score ≥5	Abuse or dependence	80	70	29	96
BMAST score ≥5	Abuse or dependence	30–78	80–99	19–92	88–97
Single quantity/frequency question (yes)[a]	Abuse or dependence	62	93	74	88

Buchsbaum DG, Buchanan RG, Welsh J, et al. Screening for drinking disorders in the elderly using the CAGE questionnaire. *J Am Geriatr Soc* 1992;40:662–665; Magruder-Habib K, Stevens HA, Alling WC. Relative performance of the MAST, VAST, and CAGE versus DSM-III-R criteria for alcohol dependence. *J Clin Epidemiol* 1993;46:435–441; Mayfield D, McLeod G, Hall P. The CAGE questionnaire: validation of a new alcoholism screening instrument. *Am J Psychiatry* 1974;131:1121–1123, (5–7).

PPV = positive predictive value; NPV = negative predictive value; AUDIT = Alcohol Use Disorders Identification Test; MAST = Michigan Alcoholism Screening test; BMAST = Brief Michigan Alcohol Screening Test.

[a]"On any single occasion during the last 3 months, have you had more than 5 drinks containing alcohol?"

TABLE 10.4 CAGE Questionnaire[a]

Have you ever felt you should **C**ut down on your drinking?

Have people **A**nnoyed you by criticizing your drinking?

Have you ever felt **G**uilty about drinking?

Have you ever had a drink in the morning (**E**ye-Opener) to steady your nerves or relieve a hangover?

Adapted from Ewing JA. Detecting alcoholism. The CAGE questionnaire. *JAMA* 1984;252: 1905–1907.
[a]Two or more positive responses is generally considered a positive screen.

Among pregnant women, for instance, dependent drinking is less common than in men and cutoffs for potentially harmful drinking patterns are lower than that for men. Studies also indicate that traditional screening instruments may not provide accurate results in the general female population and among adolescents. Screening should be modified accordingly to detect use patterns of risk in special populations.

PREGNANCY

The CAGE has been modified to yield screening questionnaires more appropriate for pregnant women. Screening in the population of pregnant women is designed to detect at-risk drinking and more severe alcohol-related behaviors. At-risk drinking for a pregnant woman has been defined as consuming 1 oz or more of alcohol daily (12). Screening instruments are therefore designed for the detection of this lower volume of consumption. Epidemiologic studies, however, indicate that fetal harm may be associated with even lower levels of consumption: three drinks per week or 0.5 oz of alcohol daily (13). Due in part to this lack of clarity in the literature, women should be counseled that no level of alcohol consumption is known to be safe during pregnancy.

T-ACE (see Table 10.6) and TWEAK (see Table 10.7) are examples of screening instruments modified for the purposes of evaluating risky drinking by pregnant women. The T-ACE replaces the "guilt" question of CAGE with a tolerance question (Table 10.6). The T-ACE was further revised to yield the TWEAK (Table 10.7) (14). The comparative performance of the more commonly used screens for risky drinking during pregnancy (1 oz or more daily) is summarized in Table 10.8.

Screening for Other Drug Use

Far fewer instruments have been investigated for screening of SUDs other than alcohol-related disorders. The evaluation of screens for which there are published results has focused on conjoint screening, or screening

TABLE 10.5 Alcohol Use Disorders Identification Test (AUDIT)[a]

	0	1	2	3	4
How often do you have a drink containing alcohol?	Never	Monthly	Two to four times a month	Two to three times a week	Four or more times a week
How many drinks containing alcohol do you have on a typical day when you are drinking?	One or two	Three or four	Five or six	Seven to nine	Ten or more
How often do you have six or more drinks on one occasion?	Never	Less than monthly	Monthly	Weekly	Daily or almost daily
How often during the last year have you found that you were not able to stop drinking once you had started?	Never	Less than monthly	Monthly	Weekly	Daily or almost daily
How often during the last year have you failed to do what was normally expected of you because of drinking?	Never	Less than monthly	Monthly	Weekly	Daily or almost daily
How often during the last year have you needed a first drink in the morning to get yourself going after a heavy drinking session?	Never	Less than monthly	Monthly	Weekly	Daily or almost daily

	Never	Less than monthly	Monthly	Weekly	Daily or almost daily
How often during the last year have you had a feeling of guilt or remorse after drinking?	Never	Less than monthly	Monthly	Weekly	Daily or almost daily
How often during the last year have you been unable to remember what happened the night before because of your drinking?	Never	Less than monthly	Monthly	Weekly	Daily or almost daily
Have you or someone else been injured because of your drinking?	No	—	Yes, but not in the last year	—	Yes, during the last year
Has a relative, friend, doctor, or other health care worker been concerned about your drinking or suggested you cut down?	No	—	Yes, but not in the last year	—	Yes, during the last year

Adapted from Saunders JB, Aasland OG, Babor TF, et al. Development of the alcohol use disorders identification test (AUDIT): WHO collaborative project on early detection of persons with harmful alcohol consumption—II. *Addiction* 1993;88:791–804.

[a]Each response is scored using the numbers at the top of each response column. Add all numbers in that column to obtain the total score. A total score of 8 or more indicates the need for further evaluation.

TABLE 10.6 T-ACE Questions[a]

1. Tolerance: "How many drinks does it take to make you feel high?" (a quantity of >2 is considered a positive response.)
2. Have people **A**nnoyed you by criticizing your drinking?
3. Have you ever felt you should **C**ut down on your drinking?
4. Have you ever had a drink in the morning (**E**ye-Opener) to steady your nerves or relieve a hangover?

Adapted from Sokol RJ, Martier SS, Ager JW. The T-ACE questions: practical prenatal detection of risk-drinking. *Am J Obstet Gynecol* 1989;160:863–868; discussion 868–870.
[a]Two or more positive responses is generally considered a positive screen warranting further evaluation.

simultaneously for alcohol and other drug use disorders. Two such instruments are the CAGE-AID (see Table 10.9) and the two-item conjoint screen (TICS). The two-item conjoint screen asks the following two questions:[1]

- In the last year, have you ever drunk or used drugs more than you meant to?
- Have you felt that you wanted or needed to cut down on your drinking or drug use in the last year?

Test performance characteristics of these instruments appear in Table 10.10.

TABLE 10.7 TWEAK Questions[a]

1. How many drinks can you hold before falling asleep or passing out? (**T**olerance: score >5 is a positive response)
2. Have close friends or relatives **W**orried or complained about your drinking in the past year?
3. Have you ever taken a drink in the morning (**E**ye-Opener) to steady your nerves or relieve a hangover?
4. Has a friend or family member ever told you about things you said or did while you were drinking that you could not remember? (**A**mnesia)
5. Have you ever felt you should "**K**ut" [sic] down on your drinking?

Adapted from Russell M, Martier SS, Sokol RJ, et al. Detecting risk drinking during pregnancy: a comparison of four screening questionnaires. *Am J Public Health* 1996;86:1435–1439.
[a]A positive response to question 1 or 2 produces a score of 2 points. Positive responses to questions 3 through 5 each produce a score of one point. A total score of 2 or more points is considered a positive screen warranting further evaluation.

[1]Adapted from Brown RL, Leonard T, Saunders LA, et al. A two-item screening test for alcohol and other drug problems. *J Fam Pract* 1997;44:151–160, (17).

TABLE 10.8 Test Performance of Screening Instruments for At-Risk Drinking During Pregnancy[a]

Instrument	Sensitivity (%)	Specificity (%)	PPV (%)	NPV (%)
CAGE score ≥2 positive responses	38	92	5–22	96–99
T-ACE score ≥2 positive responses	60–69	66–89	2–27	96–99
TWEAK score ≥2	79	85	5–24	99
AUDIT score ≥8	15	94	3–13	95–99
MAST score ≥5	36	96	9–35	96–99
SMAST ≥2	11	96	3–14	95–99

Adapted from Sokol RJ, Martier SS, Ager JW. The T-ACE questions: practical prenatal detection of risk-drinking. *Am J Obstet Gynecol* 1989;160:863–868; discussion 868–870; Windham GC, Von Behren J, Fenster L, et al. Moderate maternal alcohol consumption and risk of spontaneous abortion. *Epidemiology* 1997;8:509–514; Chang G, Wilkins-Haug L, Berman S, et al. Alcohol use and pregnancy: improving identification. *Obstet Gynecol* 1998;91:892–898, (12, 13, 15).

PPV = positive predictive value; NPV = negative predictive value; AUDIT = Alcohol Use Disorders Identification Test; MAST = Michigan Alcoholism Screening Test; SMAST = Short Michigan Alcoholism Screening Test.

[a]Greater than or equal to 1 oz of alcohol daily or greater than or equal to two drinks daily before pregnancy.

TABLE 10.9 CAGE-AID Questions[a]

Have you felt you ought to Cut down on your drinking or drug use?

Have people Annoyed you by criticizing your drinking or drug use?

Have you felt bad or Guilty about your drinking or drug use?

Have you ever had a drink or used drugs first thing in the morning to steady your nerves or to get rid of a hangover (Eye-Opener)?

Adapted from Brown RL, Rounds LA. Conjoint screening questionnaires for alcohol and other drug abuse: criterion validity in a primary care practice. *Wis Med J* 1995;94:135–140; Muntaner C, Eaton WW, Diala C, et al. Social class, assets, organizational control and the prevalence of common groups of psychiatric disorders. *Social Sci Med* 1998;47:2043–2053, (16).

[a]Greater than or equal to two positive responses is considered a positive screen warranting further evaluation.

TABLE 10.10 Testing Characteristics of Conjoint Screens for Alcohol and Other Drug Use Disorders

Instrument/Cutoff	Sensitivity (%)	Specificity (%)	PPV (%)	NPV (%)
CAGE-AID (score ≥2 positive responses)	70	85	52	92
TICS (1 positive response)	78	84	69	93

Adapted from Brown RL, Rounds LA. Conjoint screening questionnaires for alcohol and other drug abuse: criterion validity in a primary care practice. *Wis Med J* 1995;94:135–140; Brown RL, Leonard T, Saunders LA, et al. A two-item screening test for alcohol and other drug problems. *J Fam Pract* 1997;44:151–160, (16, 17).

PPV = positive predictive value; NPV = negative predictive value; TICS = two-item conjoint screen.

ADOLESCENCE

The adolescent population presents unique challenges to screening and deserves dedicated instruments for the detection of alcohol and other SUDs. Refer to Chapter 2 for a discussion of how to ask adolescents about drug and alcohol use and the sensitivities that surround these issues in this age-group (see page 36).

The "Eye-Opener" question of the CAGE questionnaire, for example, is unlikely to be appropriately targeted to the typical substance use pattern among adolescents. Factors such as self-esteem, peer acceptance, and family influence serve to predict substance use among adolescents to a greater degree than among adults.

The literature characterizing the performance of substance misuse screening instruments among adolescents, particularly adolescents not

TABLE 10.11 RAFFT Questionnaire[a]

Do you drink/drug to **R**elax, feel better about yourself, or fit in?

Do you ever drink/drug while you are **A**lone?

Do any of your closest **F**riends drink/drug?

Does a close **F**amily member have a problem with alcohol/drugs?

Have you ever gotten into **T**rouble from drinking/drugging?

Adapted from Bastiaens L, Francis G, Lewis K. The RAFFT as a screening tool for adolescent substance use disorders. *Am J Addict* 2000;9:10–16, (18).

[a] Two or more positive responses is considered a positive screen warranting further evaluation.

TABLE 10.12 CRAFFT Questions[a]

Have you ever ridden in a **C**ar driven by someone (including yourself) who was "high" or had been using alcohol or drugs?

Do you ever use alcohol or drugs to **R**elax, feel better about yourself, or fit in?

Do you ever use alcohol/drugs while you are **A**lone?

Do your family or **F**riends ever tell you that you should cut down on your drinking or drug use?

Do you ever **F**orget things you did while using alcohol or drugs?

Have you gotten into **T**rouble while you were using alcohol or drugs?

Adapted from Knight JR, Sherritt L, Shrier LA, et al. Validity of the CRAFFT substance abuse screening test among adolescent clinic patients. *Arch Pediat Adoles Med* 2002;156:607–614, (19).

[a]Two or more positive responses is considered a positive screen warranting further evaluation.

attending university, is scant. Short substance-use screening tests for adolescent populations include the RAFFT (see Table 10.11), CRAFFT (see Table 10.12), CAGE-AA (CAGE questions adapted for adolescents), the Simple Screening Instrument for Alcohol and Other Drug Abuse, and questions from the Drug and Alcohol Problem QuickScreen. Test performance characteristics of the RAFFT and CRAFFT are presented in Table 10.13.

Instruments screening for substance misuse other than alcohol have not been studied in samples of pregnant women.

TABLE 10.13 Test Performance of Alcohol/Drug Screens for Adolescents

Instrument/Cutoff	Sensitivity (%)	Specificity (%)	PPV (%)	NPV (%)
RAFFT score ≥2 positive responses	89	69	89	79
CRAFFT score ≥2 positive responses	80	86	53	96

Adapted from Bastiaens L, Francis G, Lewis K. The RAFFT as a screening tool for adolescent substance use disorders. *Am J Addict* 2000;9:10–16; Knight JR, Sherritt L, Shrier LA, et al. Validity of the CRAFFT substance abuse screening test among adolescent clinic patients. *Arch Pediat Adoles Med* 2002;156:607–614, (18,19).

PPV = positive predictive value; NPV = negative predictive value.

RISK FACTORS

Knowledge of the factors associated with the development of SUDs may help the clinician overcome some of the shortcomings of traditional screening tests. SUDs are multifactorial in their etiology. For any individual, risk is determined by an array of biological, behavioral, and environmental factors, such as family history, sex, age, ethnicity, employment status, education, and psychiatric history. The existence of such risk factors may well be revealed in the course of a general medical or social history, indicating that further evaluation for the presence of SUDs is indicated.

Family history is the most powerful and consistent risk factor for the development of SUDs. Alcohol and drug use disorders are generally more common among men than women. However, among those who consume drugs, the likelihood of developing a SUD is similar for men and women. The prevalence of alcoholism declines with age. The prevalence of the SUDs associated with the use of drugs (other than prescription drugs used on a nonprescription basis) peaks in adolescence and young adulthood (age 21–35 years) and declines thereafter. Alcohol use disorders tend to develop at a later age among African Americans than other ethnicities, and a greater proportion of African Americans tend to abstain from alcohol use. When alcohol dependence develops among African Americans and Hispanics, it tends to be more persistent and refractory than among whites. Illicit drug use disorders are more common among whites but tend to be more chronic and persistent among Hispanics and African Americans (20).

Unemployment has been linked to alcohol use disorders. Longer work hours and dropping out of high school are each associated with a greater risk of drug and alcohol use among adolescents (21), although of course excessive alcohol use can be a cause of these circumstances as well as a consequence.

The prevalence of alcohol and drug disorders has been estimated to be 20–50% respectively among individuals reporting a history of a psychiatric disorder (22). The nature of the link between specific psychiatric syndromes and SUDs is complex and beyond the scope of this chapter (23).

TREATMENT

There are a number of evidence-based methods available to treat alcohol and drug use disorders. These include brief primary care office-based interventions, motivational interviewing therapy, pharmacotherapy, cognitive behavioral therapy (CBT), Alcoholics Anonymous (AA)-based self-help groups, and traditional alcohol and drug group therapy. There is sufficient evidence to recommend each of these methods for the treatment of alcohol and drug use disorders. Other methods such as acupuncture, herbal medication, and massage therapy have insufficient evidence to recommend implementation and therefore will not be reviewed in this chapter.

Primary Care Office-Based Interventions

"Brief intervention" is a technique widely utilized by clinicians to help patients change behaviors, increase medication adherence, and improve follow-through with clinic appointments. There is compelling evidence that brief intervention can change behavior in patients who drink more than the recommended amounts (24–26); there is less information on the ability of brief intervention to change drug use habits.

There are six basic steps in the "brief intervention." The first step is for the clinician to express concern that the patient is drinking above recommended levels, or concern about the patient's drug use. The second step is to connect the patient's drinking or drug use to health, social, or family concerns of importance to that patient. Providing this objective, concrete feedback may be particularly useful in patients who are resistant to changing their alcohol or drug use behavior. The third step is to ask the patient if they have any concerns about their alcohol or drug use. The fourth step is to make a specific recommendation for the patient to reduce use or become abstinent in an effort to reduce the potential for drug-related harm. The fifth step is to negotiate with the patient a realistic change in alcohol or drug use in the next 30 days. The sixth step is to provide a self-help booklet, online references, or a list of community resources for follow-up appointments. Follow-up telephone calls and visits over the next 6–12 months can reinforce face-to-face visits.

Client-Centered Counseling

There are a number of client-centered counseling therapies available for clinician referral that are effective in helping patients reduce their substance use or to become abstinent (27): *Client-centered therapy* allows the clinician and the client to establish and prioritize a limited number of goals during a series of short counseling sessions. Included among them are Motivational Enhancement Therapy (MET), cognitive behavioral therapy, 12-step facilitation therapy, and peer self-help groups.

MET is a technique easily learned by primary care clinicians to help patients move along in the readiness-to-change paradigm (see pages 133–134). Techniques utilized in MET include rolling with patient resistance, dealing with patient ambivalence, setting up cognitive dissonance, and using behavioral change contracts. This technique can move patients from contemplating reducing their drinking or drug use to actual behavior change.

CBT provides patients with specific skills designed to deal with triggers, craving, and high-risk situations. Relapse prevention programs are based on CBT counseling strategies, which are primarily used by counselors in 1-hour sessions lasting 10–16 weeks. Clinicians can use CBT to role-play with patients on how to deal with high-risk social situations that often lead to relapse. CBT therapy is used to change a variety of behaviors and/or their results including tobacco use disorders, alcohol use problems, and obesity.

The 12-step facilitation method is another technique that can be learned by clinicians to help patients improve the ability to become abstinent. This includes having patients keep a weekly diary of their alcohol use and relapse events, read AA materials or other self-help books, and work through the 12 steps of the AA program. These techniques can be combined with pharmacotherapy. Of the AA 12 steps, completion of steps 4 and 5 is predictive of recovery and long-term abstinence. Step 4 focuses on recording how alcohol and/or drugs have damaged patients' lives and those around them. Step 5 involves sharing these events with another person. Clinicians can ask patients to complete step 4 on their own and then use a regular clinician visit to go over the items.

Self-help peer groups remain the main source of help for patients trying to deal with their alcohol and drug use. As part of the information on community resources that practices should keep on hand for patients, clinicians may want to have a list of local AA chapters and Al-Anon meetings available in the waiting room or as a handout. This list can be obtained from the local AA chapter, which is often listed in telephone directories or on websites. There is an increasing number of self-help organizations designed to address the needs of diverse groups of people trying to deal with their alcohol or drug problems. These include groups for women, gay men and women, underage drinkers, older adults, nonreligious persons, cocaine addicts, prescription drug addicts, nonsmokers, and professionals. AA meetings remain one of the most widely used options for the treatment of alcohol and drug dependence throughout the world. Unlike a patient's primary care clinician, AA is free and available after 5 PM, on weekends, and during the holidays.

Counseling Patients About Drinking and Driving

Alcohol use is a major cause of motor vehicle crashes. When counseling patients regarding drinking and driving and the risk for motor vehicle accidents and injury, it should be emphasized that, although legal blood alcohol limits promote safety to some degree, evidence indicates that impairment occurs within legal blood alcohol concentration limits. In addition to increasing the risk of injury, recent alcohol consumption also increases the probability of sustaining more severe injury with poorer clinical outcome (28). Patients should be made aware of local safe ride programs (transportation alternatives for intoxicated drivers) as a preventive measure.

Pharmacotherapy
ALCOHOL DEPENDENCE

There are two groups of medications that can be helpful in the primary treatment of alcohol dependence: aversive agents and anticraving agents (see Table 10.14). These medications are not recommended for the treatment of patients engaged in at-risk or problem drinking, pregnant women, or patients younger than 16 years.

The first class consists of aversive agents such as disulfiram and metronidazole. Patients who take the medication at least 5 days a week are likely to remain sober. Supervised medication dosing by a partner or close personal contact may facilitate compliance. Liver function tests should be monitored at baseline, 2 months after initiation, and every 6 months thereafter.

The second class of medications is the anticraving drugs. Two are currently approved by the U.S. Food and Drug Administration (FDA): naltrexone and acamprosate. An injectable formulation of naltrexone has received FDA approval for monthly administration for alcohol dependence. Acamprosate has been widely used in Europe for some years. Anticraving drugs are most effective when administered for 3–12 months. They are meant to be used in patients who are trying to become abstinent, and they are therefore less effective in patients who continue to drink intermittently while taking the medication. Liver and renal function should be checked at baseline and 2 months after initiation.

DRUG DEPENDENCE

Available pharmacotherapy for drug dependence is limited primarily to the treatment of opioid dependence. Developing effective pharmacotherapy for the treatment of cocaine, amphetamine, marijuana, and other illicit drug use is an active area of research.

Methadone and buprenorphine are the primary treatments for opioid dependence and are currently approved by the FDA. These medications reduce craving, prevent withdrawal, and often lead to abstinence from opioids and other illicit drugs, thereby preventing related complications, such as blood-borne virus transmission and cutaneous infections.

Methadone can only be prescribed for the treatment of opioid dependence at an approved methadone maintenance clinic, although any clinician with a Drug Enforcement Administration license can prescribe methadone for pain. Some states will grant clinicians who practice in rural communities permission to prescribe methadone to addicted patients living more than 50 miles from a methadone maintenance program. The effective methadone dose is 60–150 mg/day dispensed as a single morning dose. Most patients who are successfully treated receive methadone for a minimum of 5 years. Each

TABLE 10.14 Pharmacotherapy for Dependence

Diagnosis	Medication	Mechanism	Dosing	Contraindications/Cautions
Alcohol dependence	Disulfiram	Aversive agent[a]	250 mg p.o. QD	Age >65 years Liver disease[b]
	Naltrexone	Anticraving	25–100 mg p.o. QD 380 mg i.m. monthly	Liver disease[b] Active opioid dependence on opioid analgesics
	Acamprosate	Anticraving	666 mg p.o. TID	Severe renal disease[c]
Opioid dependence	Methadone[d]	Anticraving prevents withdrawal	60–150 mg p.o. QD	Severe liver disease (cirrhosis)
	Buprenorphine	Anticraving prevents withdrawal	8–32 mg s.l. QD	Initiation <24 hr after other opioid use (<48 hr after last methadone dose)

[a]Produces reaction when alcohol used concomitantly characterized by nausea, vomiting, flushing, and anxiety.
[b]Gamma-glutamyl transferase (GGT) levels greater than three times upper limit of normal.
[c]Creatinine clearance less than or equal to 30 mL/min.
[d]Only legally prescribed for dependence through appropriately licensed treatment facilities.

state has different rules that govern the dispensing of methadone for opioid dependence.

Buprenorphine is a relatively new treatment for opioid dependence. Studies have found that buprenorphine is effective in reducing injection opioid use and the frequency of hepatitis C and human immunodeficiency virus (HIV) transmission. In the United States, it is most commonly dispensed by pharmacies as a sublingual tablet combined with naloxone to prevent misuse of the medication. Primary care clinicians can obtain a license to prescribe this medication by completing an 8-hour training program. Buprenorphine has been successfully used in Europe for a number of years.

Treatment of Comorbid Mental Health Disorders

Comorbidity is a common problem seen in patients with alcohol and drug use disorders. Many patients with SUDs often have mental health disorders such as unipolar depression, anxiety, panic attacks, bipolar disorders, and post-traumatic stress disorder (PTSD). Primary care clinicians need to identify these comorbidities before developing a SUD treatment plan. Sometimes substance use is related to an underlying anxiety disorder, PTSD, or untreated chronic pain. Patients are not likely to become abstinent from alcohol and drugs if these comorbidities are not treated.

Treatment of Tobacco and Marijuana Use and Dependence

Tobacco and marijuana use are the cause of the two most common SUDs in the United States and throughout the world. The number of persons using these two substances on a regular basis far exceeds those using alcohol and all other illicit drugs combined. Continued use of these substances not only has adverse health and societal effects but these substances also interact with treatments for alcohol and other drug problems. Tobacco use is the leading cause of death in the United States and deserves special emphasis. Chapter 9 discusses the public health significance of tobacco and the important steps clinicians should take to facilitate smoking cessation. In general, however, clinicians should recommend cessation of all mood-altering drugs and then negotiate with patients as to how to proceed. Some patients will agree to try cessation of multiple drugs. Other patients prefer to start with one at a time. The key is to develop a partnership with the patient to successfully address these very challenging problems (see Chapter 5).

CHRONIC PAIN AND SUBSTANCE USE DISORDERS

Professional guidelines have advocated the use of opioid analgesics for chronic nonmalignant pain, but clinicians are also interested in preventing addiction. On the basis of the limited literature available, the prevalence of substance abuse and dependence among individuals with chronic noncancer pain (approximately 13%) appears similar to rates in the general population (29).

Clinicians often misinterpret physical dependence, an expected consequence of long-term opioid use, as opioid dependence or addiction. Withdrawal and tolerance, the manifestations of physical dependence, constitute only two of the DSM-IV criteria for a diagnosis of substance dependence (Table 10.1B). To arrive at a proper diagnosis of substance dependence, one additional criterion of the possible seven would need to be met. Additionally, the impairment must be realized on a *repetitive* basis and must *interfere with normal functioning.*

Pseudoaddiction is defined as the seeking of additional medications, appropriately or inappropriately, due to undertreatment of pain. When the pain is adequately treated, the aberrant behaviors cease (30).

Clinicians treating chronic pain should assess and monitor for signs and symptoms of substance dependence, such as aberrant behaviors surrounding medication use that might indicate a loss of control over opioid use. Clinicians should monitor the manner in which the patient is taking the medication and whether the patient complies with the recommendations of the prescribing provider. Clinicians should also determine whether the patient is taking opioid analgesics for reasons other than pain relief, such as craving, anxiety relief, insomnia, or depression.

OFFICE AND CLINIC ORGANIZATION

The development of office-based programs to deal with substance use and dependence are modeled after programs developed over the last 20 years for tobacco prevention and treatment. The model developed for tobacco use is discussed in Chapter 9, and a general systems approach for delivering preventive care in practices is discussed in Chapter 21. When applied to alcohol and drug use, the first step in such an approach is to establish a system for routinely screening for these behaviors on a regular basis. This can be accomplished by asking all new patients to complete a short set of questions on alcohol and drug use. Computer prompts can be set to remind clinicians and nurses to query all patients at some predetermined frequency and to be sure to target high-risk patients: pregnant women, patients with uncontrolled hypertension, and tobacco users (see Chapters 21 and 22 for further details on the role of electronic reminders). Some clinics assess alcohol use as a "vital sign," the process for identifying tobacco users discussed in Chapter 9 (see page 238). Toxicology screens are helpful in high-risk patients such as those receiving pain medication or sedative drugs. For further details on how to organize practices to improve the delivery of preventive services, see Chapter 21.

RESOURCES—PATIENT EDUCATION MATERIALS

Alcoholics Anonymous
The Big Book of AA, AA brochures, and AA meeting times and locations are available
    online through the AA website.
www.alcoholics-anonymous.org

American Academy of Family Physicians
www.aafp.org

FamilyDoctor.org resources
Alcohol or Drug Abuse Recovery: Your Doctor Can Help.
http://familydoctor.org/online/famdocen/home/common/addictions/alcohol/152
    .html. Accessed 2007.

Alcohol Abuse: How to Recognize Problem Drinking
http://familydoctor.org/online/famdocen/home/common/addictions/alcohol/755
    .html. Accessed 2007.

Alcohol: What To Do If It's a Problem for You
http://familydoctor.org/online/famdocen/home/common/addictions/alcohol/006
    .html. Accessed 2007.

Drinking: It Can Spin Your World Around: Facts for Teens
http://familydoctor.org/online/famdocen/home/common/addictions/alcohol/273
    .html. Accessed 2007.

Drugs: What You Should Know (Information for teens)
http://www.kidshealth.org/PageManager.jsp?dn=familydoctor&article_
    set=22660&lic=44&cat_id=20140

American Academy of Pediatrics
www.aap.org
Substance abuse information for children and teens and their parents:
    http://aap.org/healthtopics/subabuse.cfm

National Clearinghouse for Alcohol and Drug Information
Faces of Change: Do I Have a Problem with Alcohol or Drugs? Pub. No. PHD 1103
www.health.org

National Institute on Alcohol Abuse and Alcoholism (NIAAA)
Alcohol: What You Don't Know can Harm You. NIH Pub. No. 99–4323, Spanish version:
    Pub No. 99-4323-S
Make a Difference: Talk to Your Child about Alcohol. NIH Pub. No. 00–4314
Drinking and your Pregnancy. NIH Pub. No. 01–4102
www.nih.niaaa.org.

SUGGESTED READINGS

National Clearinghouse for Alcohol and Drug Information has an extensive catalog
    of research reports and information for providers on issues surrounding drug and
    alcohol use.
http://ncadistore.samhsa.gov/catalog/pubseries.aspx. Accessed 2007.

National Institute on Alcohol Abuse and Alcoholism (NIAAA)
Helping Patients Who Drink too Much: A Clinicians Guide. NIH Pub. No. 07-3769.
http://pubs.niaaa.nih.gov/publications/Practitioner/CliniciansGuide2005/guide.pdf.
   Accessed 2007.

National Institute on Drug Abuse
*InfoFacts sheets are available on substances of abuse, treatment, and prevention topics among
   many other clinical references.*
http://www.nida.nih.gov/Infofacts/Infofaxindex.html. Accessed 2007.

Websites for specific screening instruments

CAGE available at http://www.projectmainstream.net/filedownload.asp?fid=179
CAGE-AID available at http://www1.buprenorphinecme.com/PageReq?id=3030:27866
AUDIT available at http://whqlibdoc.who.int/hq/2001/WHO_MSD_MSB_01.6a.pdf
T-ACE and TWEAK available at http://www.tgorski.com/clin_mod/atp/women_at
   _risk-brief_sceening_tools.htm
CRAFFT available at http://www.projectcork.org/clinical_tools/pdf/CRAFFT.pdf
RAFFT questions are available in Table 2 of the article available at: http:
   //findarticles.com/p/articles/mi_m0978/is_4_28/ai_95765047/pg_1. Accessed 2007.
TICS available at http://www.jabfm.org/cgi/reprint/14/2/95.pdf

Additional reading for clinicians

Dackis C. O'Brien C. Neurobiology of addiction: treatment and public policy
   ramifications. *Nat Neurosci* 2005;8(11):1431–1436.
Kaye DL. Office recognition and management of adolescent substance abuse. *Curr Opin
   Pediatr* 2004;16(5):532–541
Saitz R. Clinical practice. Unhealthy alcohol use. *N Engl J Med* 2005;352(6):596–607.
U.S. Department of Health and Human Services. *The Surgeon General's Call to
   Action To Prevent and Reduce Underage Drinking.* U.S. Department of Health and
   Human Services, Office of the Surgeon General, 2007. Accessed 2007 at http://www.
   surgeongeneral.gov/topics/underagedrinking/calltoaction.pdf.
Velleman RD, Templeton LJ, Copello AG. The role of the family in preventing
   and intervening with substance use and misuse: a comprehensive review of family
   interventions, with a focus on young people. *Drug Alcohol Rev* 2005;24(2):93–109.
Volkow ND. Li TK. Drugs and alcohol: treating and preventing abuse, addiction and
   their medical consequences. *Pharmacol Ther* 2005;108(1):3–17
Williams SH. Medications for treating alcohol dependence. *Am Fam Physician* 2005;
   72(9):1775–80.

References

1. Substance Abuse and Mental Health Services Administration, Office of Applied
   Studies. *Drug abuse warning network, 2003: interim national estimates of drug-related
   emergency department visits.* DAWN Series D-26, DHHS Publication No. SMA
   04–3972. Rockville: Substance Abuse and Mental Health Services Administration,
   Office of Applied Studies, 2004.
2. Rice DP. Economic costs of substance abuse, 1995. *Proc Assoc Am Physicians* 1999;111:
   119–125.
3. American Psychiatric Association. *Diagnostic and statistical manual of mental disorders*,
   4th ed. Washington: American Psychiatric Association; 1994:435–436.

4. Michael B, Spitzer R, Gibbon M, et al. *Structured clinical interview for DSM-IV-TR axis I disorders, research version, patient edition (SCID-I/P)*. New York: Biometrics Research, New York State Psychiatric Institute, 2002.

5. Buchsbaum DG, Buchanan RG, Welsh J, et al. Screening for drinking disorders in the elderly using the CAGE questionnaire. *J Am Geriatr Soc* 1992;40:662–665.

6. Magruder-Habib K, Stevens HA, Alling WC. Relative performance of the MAST, VAST, and CAGE versus DSM-III-R criteria for alcohol dependence. *J Clin Epidemiol* 1993;46:435–441.

7. Mayfield D, McLeod G, Hall P. The CAGE questionnaire: validation of a new alcoholism screening instrument. *Am J Psychiatry* 1974;131:1121–1123.

8. Ewing JA. Detecting alcoholism. The CAGE questionnaire. *JAMA* 1984;252: 1905–1907.

9. Saunders JB, Aasland OG, Babor TF, et al. Development of the Alcohol Use Disorders Identification Test (AUDIT): WHO collaborative project on early detection of persons with harmful alcohol consumption–II. *Addiction* 1993;88:791–804.

10. Isaacson JH, Butler R, Zacharek M, et al. Screening with the Alcohol Use Disorders Identification Test (AUDIT) in an inner-city population. *J Gen Intern Med* 1994;9:550–553.

11. Canagasaby A, Vinson DC. Screening for hazardous or harmful drinking using one or two quantity-frequency questions. *Alcohol Alcohol* 2005;40:208–213.

12. Sokol RJ, Martier SS, Ager JW. The T-ACE questions: practical prenatal detection of risk-drinking. *Am J Obstet Gynecol* 1989;160:863–868; discussion 868–870.

13. Windham GC, Von Behren J, Fenster L, et al. Moderate maternal alcohol consumption and risk of spontaneous abortion. *Epidemiology* 1997;8:509–514.

14. Russell M, Martier SS, Sokol RJ, et al. Detecting risk drinking during pregnancy: a comparison of four screening questionnaires. *Am J Public Health* 1996;86:1435–1439.

15. Chang G, Wilkins-Haug L, Berman S, et al. Alcohol use and pregnancy: improving identification. *Obstet Gynecol* 1998;91:892–898.

16. Brown RL, Rounds LA. Conjoint screening questionnaires for alcohol and other drug abuse: criterion validity in a primary care practice. *Wis Med J* 1995;94:135–140.

17. Brown RL, Leonard T, Saunders LA, et al. A two-item screening test for alcohol and other drug problems. *J Fam Pract* 1997;44:151–160.

18. Bastiaens L, Francis G, Lewis K. The RAFFT as a screening tool for adolescent substance use disorders. *Am J Addict* 2000;9:10–16.

19. Knight JR, Sherritt L, Shrier LA, et al. Validity of the CRAFFT substance abuse screening test among adolescent clinic patients. *Arch Pediatr Adolesc Med* 2002;156:607–614.

20. Turner RJ, Gil AG. Psychiatric and substance use disorders in South Florida: racial/ethnic and gender contrasts in a young adult cohort. *Arch Gen Psychiatry* 2002;59:43–50.

21. Muntaner C, Eaton WW, Diala C, et al. Social class, assets, organizational control and the prevalence of common groups of psychiatric disorders. *Soc Sci Med* 1998;47: 2043–2053.

22. Armstrong TD, Costello EJ. Community studies on adolescent substance use, abuse, or dependence and psychiatric comorbidity. *J Consult Clin Psychol* 2002;70:1224–1239.

23. Brady KT, Myrick H, Sonne SC. Co-occurring addictive and affective disorders. In: Graham A, Schultz T, Mayo-Smith M, et al. eds. *Principles of addiction medicine*, 3rd ed. Chevy Chase: American Society of Addiction Medicine, 2003.

24. Whitlock EP, Polen MR, Green CA, et al. Behavioral counseling interventions in primary care to reduce risky/harmful alcohol use by adults: a summary of the evidence for the U.S. Preventive Services Task Force. *Ann Intern Med* 2004;140:557–568.

25. Cuijpers P, Riper H, Lemmers L. The effects on mortality of brief interventions for problem drinking: a meta-analysis. *Addiction* 2004;99:839–845.

26. Fleming M, Mundt M, French M, et al. Brief physician advice for problem drinkers: long-term efficacy and benefit-cost analysis. *Alcohol Clin Exp Res* 2002;26:36–43.

27. Anonymous. Matching alcoholism treatments to client heterogeneity: project MATCH posttreatment drinking outcomes. *J Stud Alcohol*. 1997;58:7–29.

28. Ogden EJ, Moskowitz H. Effects of alcohol and other drugs on driver performance. *Traffic Inj Prev* 2004;5:185–198.

29. Fleming M, Balousek S, Klessig C, et al. *Chronic pain, addiction, and opioids in a primary care sample*. Madison: University of Wisconsin, 2005.

30. Weissman DE, Haddox JD. Opioid pseudoaddiction—an iatrogenic syndrome. *Pain* 1989;36:363–366.

CHAPTER 11

Family Planning

Karen T. Feisullin and Carolyn L. Westhoff

Contraception is among the most effective forms of preventive care. The ratio between the number of women who use contraception and the number of pregnancies prevented is essentially one or even less. Despite this, approximately one half of the 6.3 million pregnancies in the United States every year are unplanned (1). Of these unplanned pregnancies, approximately half the number of women used a contraceptive method imperfectly and half used no method at all. Exceedingly few pregnancies are due to the failure of correctly used contraceptive methods.

Women are sometimes reluctant to use contraceptives because of perceived health risks, but most women are unaware that pregnancy itself carries far greater risks. The latter is especially true for women with coexisting medical problems that make pregnancy more complicated and dangerous. Among women with medical problems, highly effective contraception must be provided for those who are using teratogenic medications.

Throughout the world, family planning also improves certain nonreproductive health outcomes; ovarian and endometrial cancer risk reduction in oral contraceptive (OC) users is the paramount example of such effects. Maternal deaths are common in developing countries, with maternal mortality rates 20–100 times higher than those in the United States. The largest health impact of family planning in such settings is the reduction of maternal mortality through a decrease in unwanted and potentially dangerous pregnancies. Contraceptive use also leads to a decrease in infant mortality through increased spacing between pregnancies. Spacing pregnancies more than 2 years apart decreases infant mortality by 50% (2). In addition to these health benefits, allowing women to control their fertility can give them opportunities to pursue education and employment outside the home.

CONTRACEPTIVE COUNSELING

For an individual, the best contraceptive method is the one she chooses for herself and will use. Patients can make this decision only with excellent access to information and timely access to the full spectrum of methods. The primary care clinician can help reduce unintended pregnancy by proactively asking each patient about her contraceptive needs and experience (see Chapter 2, page 34). Chapter 12 (pages 296–297) discusses general principles for discussing sexual practices with patients. Appropriate counseling about contraception requires presentation of a range of options with expected effectiveness rates and side effects (see Table 11.1). The discussion should both elicit the patient's concerns and debunk any contraceptive myths (e.g., hormonal contraceptives cause weight gain). Many women avoid effective methods because they or their partners hold mistaken beliefs. Clinicians who correct these misconceptions can improve continuation rates and adherence (3). Clinicians can also refer patients to community resources, such as Planned Parenthood (www.plannedparenthood.org), for further counseling about family planning options.

TABLE 11.1 Contraceptive Methods by Effectiveness

Highly Effective

Injectable contraceptives
Intrauterine devices
Subdermal progestin implants

Effective

Oral contraceptives
Transdermal contraceptive patches
Vaginal rings

Less Effective

Condoms
Diaphragms
Cervical caps
Spermicides
Microbicides
Sponges
Periodic abstinence
Anovulation during lactational amenorrhea

Informational counseling is especially important for adolescents. Approximately 1 million adolescent pregnancies occur each year in the United States, and about half of adolescents use no contraception during the first episode of sexual intercourse. Clinicians should counsel adolescents in private, with the assurance that all discussions will remain confidential (see Chapter 17, page 452). Many adolescents will not raise the issue of contraception, so a clinician needs to start this discussion on a routine basis, perhaps by inquiring what the patient has heard from her friends (see page 35). Early puberty is a good time to give a young patient notice that contraception is an acceptable topic for discussion. Assurance must be given that the discussion will remain private and that parents will not be notified without the patient's consent. Although the advantages of abstinence merit discussion, as discussed in Chapter 12, clinicians should also discuss contraception because most adolescents become sexually active sooner rather than later.

All adolescents starting to use a method should receive an explicit invitation to make additional visits or telephone calls to discuss contraceptive concerns; this may prevent premature discontinuation. In adolescents and adults continuation rates may be improved by reviewing how contraceptives work and their expected side effects, by giving oral and written instructions, and by providing samples at the initial visit (4).

A pelvic examination is useful to screen for sexually transmitted infection and to carry out a Pap test (see Chapter 4), but it is unnecessary before initiating most contraceptives. Requiring a pelvic examination introduces a barrier to the initiation of hormonal contraception, although it is clearly necessary to initiate use of an intrauterine device (IUD) or a diaphragm.

As compared with "no method," use of contraception by adolescents or adults leads to medical care cost savings. Male condom use along with a female-based method, and advance provision of emergency contraception (EC), provide additional savings (5). There is little definitive evidence to determine the effectiveness of counseling *per se* on decreasing unintended pregnancies (6).

CONTRACEPTIVE METHODS

Highly Effective Reversible Methods: Injectable Contraceptives, Intrauterine Devices, and Implants

Long-acting reversible methods have an efficacy rate of at least 99%. They provide continuous contraception and either cannot be passively discontinued (IUDs and implants) or are only slowly reversible (injections). None of these methods contain estrogen, and they are generally a first choice for women who cannot take estrogen and for those women in whom pregnancy is medically contraindicated.

INJECTABLE CONTRACEPTIVES

Depot medroxyprogesterone acetate (DMPA), or Depo Provera, is the most commonly used injectable contraceptive. It is available as a deep intramuscular injection of 150 mg every 12 weeks, or as a subcutaneous injection of 104 mg every 12 weeks. The failure rate under ideal conditions is 0.3% but the failure rate with typical use is 3%. Failure rates with typical use occur because of delays in scheduled reinjection every 12 weeks. Noncontraceptive benefits of DMPA include diminished menstrual bleeding and dysmenorrhea, decreased risk of pelvic inflammatory disease and of endometrial and ovarian cancers, and fewer sickle cell crises (7). After their third injection, almost half of DMPA users become amenorrheic. Amenorrhea occurs in 70% of women after 2 years of use and 80% of women after 5 years. Data from prospective studies of DMPA do not support a causal relationship between its use and either depression or marked weight gain (8–12).

Bone loss during use is comparable to that seen during breastfeeding, and studies indicate that bone is regained after discontinuing this method (13). DMPA is contraindicated in women who may be pregnant because it would offer no benefit and because its use may delay the diagnosis of pregnancy. The contraceptive effect of DMPA is very slowly reversible. Although continued reliable contraceptive protection requires a reinjection every 3 months, the average time for return to ovulation is 6 months, and for some women longer than 1 year. Therefore, DMPA is not a good method for women who are planning pregnancy in the near future.

Norethindrone enanthate is a bimonthly progestin-only injection used mainly in sub-Saharan Africa. It has clinical characteristics similar to DMPA. *Lunelle* is a monthly combined estrogen and progestin injection that is unavailable in the United States but is used in other countries. Women using the monthly injection typically have regular menses.

INTRAUTERINE DEVICES

The ParaGard Copper T 380A IUD is a highly effective low-maintenance method. It has greater than 99% efficacy, which is comparable to sterilization, and it may remain in place for up to 10 years. The mechanism of action of the Copper T is impairment of sperm function, rendering sperm unable to fertilize ova. It is recommended for women who desire long-term contraception. Due to the immediate return of fertility after removal, it is also suitable for women who are spacing pregnancies. The clinician can easily insert the IUD during an office visit at any time during the menstrual cycle (see Fig. 11.1). The copper IUD typically causes longer or heavier menstrual bleeding, especially in the first few months after insertion. The risk of involuntary expulsion is approximately 5% in the first year after insertion. In order to ensure that the device is still in place, women should be advised to feel the strings of the IUD after every menses.

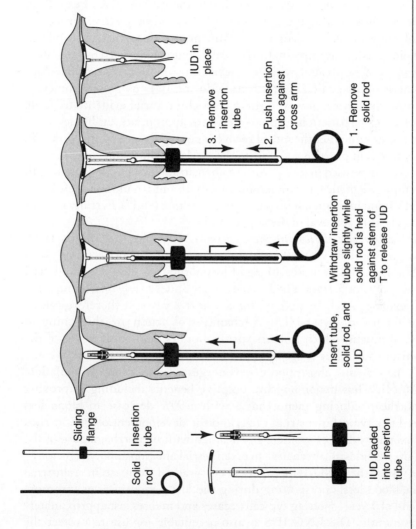

Figure 11.1 • Insertion technique for Copper T380A intrauterine device. High fundal placement is achieved by using a withdrawal technique. IUD = intrauterine device. (Reproduced with permission from Beckmann CRB, Ling FW, Laube DW, et al. *Obstetrics and gynecology*, 4th ed. Baltimore: Lippincott Williams & Wilkins, 2002.)

The initial cost of the IUD is higher than that of many other contraceptives, but IUDs become the most cost-effective method when utilized for 2 years or longer (14). The IUD can also be used for EC (see section on "Emergency Contraception," page 291) as well as immediately postpartum (see section on "Contraception after Pregnancy," pages 291–292).

Contraindications to IUD insertion are current pelvic infection and anomalies of the uterine cavity, as these might increase the risk of expulsion of the device. Insertion should not occur in the presence of active cervical or pelvic infection, but it can occur after treatment of both partners. If, while an IUD is being used, an asymptomatic cervical infection is detected by screening, the woman can be treated with the device *in situ*. If a woman develops symptomatic upper genital tract infection during IUD use, many clinicians will remove the device; however, there is no clinical trial evidence to guide this practice. If the patient is being treated with appropriate antibiotics, IUD removal increases neither the rate of recovery nor recurrence of infection (15). Contrary to recent practice and within the guidance of product labeling, the copper IUD can be used in nulliparous women, in adolescents, in women with a past ectopic pregnancy, in women infected with human immunodeficiency virus (HIV), and in women with past pelvic infection (16,17). Fertility returns immediately after removal of the copper IUD.

The *Levonorgestrel Intrauterine System* (LNG-IUS), the Mirena IUD, also has greater than 99% efficacy and may remain in place for up to 5 years. The LNG-IUS releases 20 μg of levonorgestrel into the endometrial cavity every day for 5 years. The LNG-IUS continues to release a therapeutic dose of levonorgestrel, 14 μg/day, for the next 2 years. It therefore can be effective for up to 7 years. The mechanisms of action are thickening of the cervical mucus, which impairs sperm motility, and suppression of the endometrium such that it becomes hostile to the ascent of sperm. In some women, the systemic absorption of levonorgestrel may suppress ovulation. The LNG-IUS has major noncontraceptive benefits including improving dysmenorrhea, reducing menorrhagia with a 90% decrease in blood loss compared to a typical menstrual cycle, and the development of amenorrhea in approximately 20% of women. For women with menorrhagia, use of the LNG-IUS provides an alternative to endometrial ablation and hysterectomy. Women using the LNG-IUS experience a gradual decrease in menstrual duration, blood loss, and spotting during the first 6 months after insertion. By the end of 1 year, spotting typically ceases and menses last approximately 1–2 days/month. The LNG-IUS is also acceptable for use to protect the endometrium in menopausal women using estrogen therapy (18).

There are many other IUD designs in use throughout the world. Most of these products contain copper and may be effective for at least 3 years or even longer, depending on the amount of copper. These devices are less effective than the Copper T380A and the levonorgestrel-containing IUDs.

SUBDERMAL PROGESTIN IMPLANTS

Implanon is a reversible single-rod implant that has been used outside of the United States and was approved by the U.S. Food and Drug Administration (FDA) in 2006. The rod, a flexible device measuring 40 mm by 2 mm, is impregnated with 68 mg of etonogestrel, a progestin. The implant releases approximately 40 μg of etonogestrel daily, providing continuous contraception for up to 3 years (19). With typical use, it has a failure rate of 0.1% (20). It is inserted subcutaneously in the upper arm during an office procedure performed by a trained clinician. Noncontraceptive benefits include dimunition of dysmenorrhea. The main side effect of this implant is irregular, unpredictable bleeding throughout use. Implanon does not adversely affect bone mineral density (21). Removal by a trained clinician entails a quick and simple office procedure. Fertility returns immediately after removal. The effectiveness of Implanon has not been evaluated in women with liver disease or those who take concomitant medications that might accelerate metabolism of the hormone.

No longer in use in the United States, *Norplant* was a reversible 6-rod implant system designed for 5 years of continuous use. The silastic implants contain levonorgestrel. In 2000, the manufacturer discontinued distribution of the product in the United States following adverse publicity regarding problems of unsubstantiated clinical importance. The single-rod system, Implanon, is easier to insert and to remove than was Norplant.

Effective Reversible Methods: Pills, Patch, and Vaginal Ring

Combined ethinyl estradiol and progestin methods (pills, transdermal patch, and vaginal ring) and the progestin-only pills (POPs) have "perfect-use" failure rates of 1–2%, and typical use failure rates of approximately 5%. Failure rates quoted with perfect use are achieved when the method is used exactly as directed. These hormonal methods all require active decision making and a regular routine for successful use. These are generally cyclic methods designed to produce a regular withdrawal bleeding episode, but they have the potential for continuous rather than cyclic use.

ORAL CONTRACEPTIVES

OCs are the most popular reversible method of contraception in the United States. There are combined estrogen and progestin formulations and POPs. The estrogen in combined OCs is ethinyl estradiol. To decrease the risk of thromboembolic events, the estrogen dose has been steadily reduced since the first introduction of the pill in the 1960s. Currently, low-dose pills contain 20–35 μg of ethinyl estradiol per tablet, compared to 100–150 μg of ethinyl estradiol in the 1960s. The amount of progestin in the pill has been lowered even more than the amount of estrogen. There are at least six different progestins used in current pills. Many believe that the choice of progestin can influence the tolerability of the pill, with different women preferring different products.

Traditional cyclic use of combined OCs involves following the routine prescribed by the monthly pill pack for 28 days, taking 21 active pills followed by 7 placebo pills. The predictable withdrawal bleeding occurs during the week in which the placebo pills are taken. A new pill pack is to be started the day after finishing the placebo pills regardless of the bleeding pattern. The most recently approved 28-day OC regimens typically contain more days of active pills and fewer days of placebo; the rationale is to minimize cyclic symptoms that may be related to fluctuations in hormone levels. These regimens may also yield fewer days of withdrawal bleeding.

Continuous use of combined OCs is achieved in two FDA-approved products by daily use of active pills for 84 consecutive days followed by 7 days of placebo (or low estrogen-dose) tablets. The benefit of this approach is less frequent withdrawal bleeding. Another product contains active pills only, which is intended to avoid any scheduled withdrawal bleeding. Comparison of continuous and cyclic use of combined OCs demonstrates that continuous use is safe, effective, and well tolerated. Breakthrough bleeding and spotting decrease with successive cycles (22).

Conventional approaches to the initiation of oral contraception require waiting until the next menstrual period to take the first pill. Following this approach, up to 25% of women for whom an OC is prescribed never begin taking the pills; an alternative encourages patients to swallow the first tablet (preferably with direct observation) immediately upon prescription, regardless of menstrual cycle day. This approach, called *Quick Start*, has been shown to increase OC use. The Quick Start approach is safe, acceptable, and useful for initiation of pills as well as for DMPA and other hormonal contraceptives (23).

Despite dose reductions, there remain some risks in the use of OCs. Some women should not take estrogen-containing contraception due to an increased risk of myocardial infarction or stroke; this contraindication applies to all women aged 35 years or older who smoke or have diabetes, hypertension, or migraine headaches (24). A family history of adverse effects from OCs does not raise the risk of adverse events. In younger women with these conditions, the underlying probability of cardiovascular events is so low that the possible risks of OC use are substantially smaller than the risks of pregnancy itself. Regardless of age, the use of an estrogen-containing OC is contraindicated in the presence of known ischemic heart disease, a personal history of stoke, migraine headaches with aura, diabetes with vascular changes, or uncontrolled hypertension. Such women need other forms of highly effective contraception due to the risks of major complications during pregnancy.

The increased risk of venous thromboembolism (VTE) generally contraindicates the use of OCs (or patch or ring) in women with a personal history of VTE, those with a known high-risk thrombogenic mutation, those with morbid obesity (body mass index greater than 40 kg/m^2), and postpartum women within 14 days of giving birth. An exception is that certain women currently receiving anticoagulant therapy will benefit from OC use. For example, ovulation may be catastrophic in an anticoagulated woman if a hemorrhagic cyst were to rupture. Also, certain anticoagulants (e.g., warfarin) are teratogenic. The risk of VTE does vary among the estrogen-containing contraceptives. However, because the baseline risk of adverse effects is so low, because there is occasional diagnostic misclassification of the events, and because risk factors are not equal across the users of different products, even very large studies have not been able to precisely define VTE risk on a product-specific basis. Most studies agree that the greatest risk of VTE occurs in the first 1–2 years of OC use. The risk of VTE in young women is greatest during pregnancy, particularly during the puerperium; the risk of VTE associated with OC use is substantially lower than the VTE risk attributable to pregnancy itself.

Use of combined OCs is appropriate in breastfeeding women once milk flow is well established (approximately 4 weeks postpartum), in women with benign breast disease or a family history of breast cancer, and in women with lupus who do not have antiphospholipid antibodies.

Despite widely held beliefs that the use of OC leads to weight gain, a systematic review of 44 randomized controlled trials found no evidence of a causal relationship between combination contraceptives and weight gain (25). Data indicating higher failure rates in obese women are inconsistent.

POPs or "minipills" contain 0.35 mg of norethindrone, in Micronor or 0.075 of norgesterel, in Ovrette. They are to be taken every day with no hormone-free interval. Although the failure rate with perfect use is 0.3% in the first year, with typical use the rate is 8%. This makes them slightly less effective in preventing pregnancy than are combined OCs.

POPs may be most appropriate in women who should not take estrogen-containing contraceptives. Noncontraceptive benefits of POPs include reduced menstrual bleeding (and in some cases amenorrhea), anemia, dysmenorrhea, and premenstrual symptoms such as bloating and breast tenderness. As with combined OCs there is decreased risk of endometrial and ovarian cancer. Like the combined OCs, the contraceptive effect of POPs is immediately reversible. Disadvantages of POPs include the need to take the pills on a very regular schedule. Missing pills or taking them at irregular intervals greatly reduces effectiveness. Back-up methods such as condoms or other barrier methods (see "Barrier and Related Methods" section, pages 287–291) are generally recommended for 48 hours if a pill is taken more than 3 hours late. Drugs that increase hepatic enzyme levels probably decrease the efficacy of POPs. Menstrual irregularities are a reason that many women discontinue use of this particular type of OC; adequate counseling on this side effect may reduce discontinuation rates.

TRANSDERMAL CONTRACEPTIVE PATCH

Ortho Evra is a combined hormonal contraceptive patch. Each patch contains 0.75 mg ethinyl estradiol and 6.0 mg norelgestromin. As with OCs, the main mechanism of action is the prevention of ovulation. Each patch is worn for 7 days and replaced each week, for 3 weeks out of every four. A withdrawal bleed occurs during the fourth week, when no patch is worn. Once-a-week dosing is convenient and may enhance the chances of correct use, compared to OCs. The benefits of the patch are similar to combined OCs, including usefulness in the management of both menorrhagia and dysmenorrhea. Disadvantages include lack of privacy when the patch is worn on a visible area, and possible skin irritation and pigment change at the site of application. Like the OC, the patch does not protect against sexually transmitted infections. Women who have contraindications to using estrogen may not use the patch. In a clinical trial, Ortho Evra had a higher failure rate in women weighing more than 198 lb compared to lighter women.

VAGINAL RING

NuvaRing is a monthly vaginal contraceptive that is inserted by the patient and remains in place for 3 weeks. It is a soft flexible ring made of ethylene vinyl acetate (see Fig. 11.2). Its outer diameter is 5.4 cm and it is 4 mm thick. It contains ethinyl estradiol and etonogestrel which is dispersed evenly throughout the ring. It releases 15 μg of ethinyl estradiol and 120 μg of

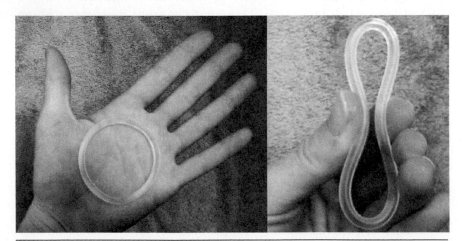

Figure 11.2 • NuvaRing (Organon Pharmaceuticals USA Inc, Roseland, NJ), a monthly vaginal contraceptive that is inserted by the patient and remains in place for 3 weeks.

etonogestrel each 24-hour period. The vaginal ring has the advantage of once-a-month dosing and its use is completely discreet (26).

The vaginal ring may be used in a cyclic or continuous manner, both of which are acceptable to patients and well tolerated (27). If used in a cyclic manner, the ring is removed after the third week and there is a withdrawal bleed. A new ring is placed 1 week later. For continuous use mode, a new ring is inserted immediately after the ring that has been in place for 3 weeks is removed. The continuous method may reduce cyclic symptoms such as premenstrual syndrome. It yields fewer total bleeding days but results in more spotting. Comparison of the pharmacokinetics of the vaginal ring, transdermal patch, and combined OCs demonstrated significantly lower and less varied ethinyl estradiol serum levels among ring users compared to women using the other methods (28).

Less Effective Methods: Condoms, Diaphragms, Sponges, and Spermicides

When less effective contraceptive methods are used, outcomes are widely variable with typical use. These methods must be in use at the time of coitus. Annual failure rates range from 10–25%. Parous women experience higher failure rates.

BARRIER AND RELATED METHODS

Condoms

Condoms are widely available and are the method most frequently used at first intercourse. The most recent National Survey of Family Growth (NSFG) showed an increase in condom use among adolescents and an increase in use at first intercourse (29). Male condoms are available in latex; for latex-sensitive or allergic users, condoms manufactured with natural membrane from animal skin or with polyurethane and synthetic elastomers are available. The animal membrane material has a larger pore size that prevents transmission of sperm but may allow passage of infectious organisms. As noted in Chapter 12, this type of condom is not recommended for prevention of sexually transmitted infections.

A Cochrane review of all randomized controlled trials evaluated male nonlatex condoms made of polyurethane film or synthetic elastomers as compared with latex condoms. Nonlatex condoms had higher rates of breakage than latex condoms but are still an acceptable alternative (30).

Typical users of condoms report approximately 10 pregnancies per 100 couples in the first year of condom use. Actual per-use failure rates experienced by condom users vary greatly depending upon the correctness and consistency of use. There are several reasons for the occurrence of unplanned pregnancy among condom users, for example: slippage and breakage; failure to use condoms during an imperfectly calculated "safe period;" and nonuse of the condom during the early minutes of intercourse, leading to insemination by the pre-ejaculatory fluid. Any of these occurrences can be remedied by the use of EC.

The key noncontraceptive benefit of synthetic condoms is that they are the only contraceptive method proved to reduce the risk of sexually transmitted infections, including infection with HIV and human papilloma virus (15,31) (see Chapter 12). *Dual method use* refers to the simultaneous use of condoms and an additional effective or highly effective pharmaceutical contraceptive to provide optimal protection against both infection and pregnancy. Women who rely on effective pharmaceutical contraceptives but who do not use condoms consistently have a higher risk of acquiring sexually transmitted infections. Consistent dual method use is uncommon, however.

Female Condoms

FC, the first-generation FC female condom formerly called *Reality*, is made of polyurethane. It is inserted into the vagina before sexual intercourse. FC2 is a second-generation female condom made of synthetic latex, which is less expensive than polyurethane. Female condoms are 17 cm long and contain two flexible polyurethane rings, one at each end. The ring at the closed end is inserted into the vagina, and the open ring remains outside the vagina after insertion. Female condoms provide protection against both pregnancy and sexually transmitted infections, and they can be inserted up to 8 hours before intercourse. Female and male condoms should not be used together; they can adhere to each other, causing slippage or displacement of one or both devices. Female condom 6-month failure rates can be as high as 9.5% (32).

Diaphragm and Cervical Cap

The diaphragm is a dome-shaped latex rubber cup that was much more popular decades ago before the introduction of more highly effective pharmaceutical methods. The diaphragm is now used by less than 1% of women in the United States. It has a flexible rim available with diameters from 60–100 mm. It is inserted into the vagina before intercourse, covering the cervix (see Fig. 11.3). The Prentif cavity rim cervical cap fits more tightly over the cervix than does the diaphragm, with diameters of 18–25 mm. Both the diaphragm and cap must be individually fitted. They are both designed for use with a spermicide. After intercourse, the diaphragm must remain in place for 6 hours to maximize spermicidal action. The spermicide must be reapplied with an applicator with the diaphragm in place before subsequent intercourse. The cap can provide continuous contraception for 48 hours without the need to reapply spermicide.

Prolonged use of either device for greater than 24 consecutive hours is associated with an increased risk of toxic shock syndrome (4),

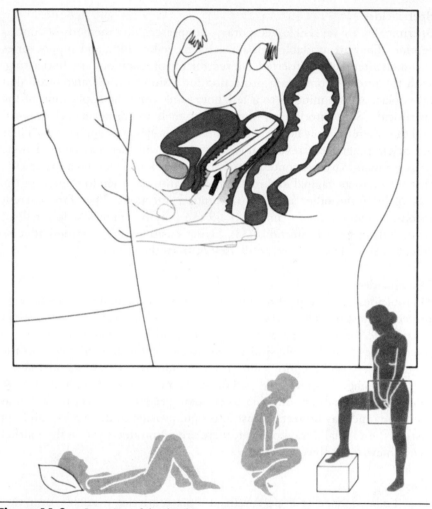

Figure 11.3 • Insertion of the diaphragm. Proximal edge fits in posterior fornix and distal edge behind symphysis. (Reproduced with permission from Speroff L, Darney PD. *A clinical guide for contraception*. Baltimore: Williams & Wilkins, 1992.)

which is a systemic infection with *Staphylococcus aureus*. Both caps and diaphragms protect against upper genital tract infections that ordinarily gain entry through the cervical mucosa, including gonorrhea and chlamydia. Contraceptive failure rates with these devices are approximately 16% per year, with a wide range depending upon the correctness and consistency of use. Diaphragm use carries an increased risk of urinary tract infection. If a woman has prolapse of the uterus or relaxation of the introitus or is immediately postpartum, it may not be possible to fit a diaphragm or cap successfully. Users should be refitted after childbirth or substantial changes in weight.

Spermicides

Spermicides are reversible, temporary, nonprescription methods of contra-ception. They are available as foams, creams, jellies, film, and suppositories that melt after they are inserted. All spermicide preparations are short acting, with the intent of providing protection for a single act of intercourse that takes place within minutes to a few hours following the application of the spermicide. Suppositories and films need to melt and disperse in the vagina, and they therefore may not be active until 20 minutes after application. Their efficacy in pregnancy prevention is 70–85%. Spermicides may be used alone or as adjuncts to barrier contraceptive methods. Nonoxynol-9 is a spermicide that may irritate vaginal and rectal mucosa and may therefore increase the risk of HIV and other sexually transmitted infections. Therefore, current recommendations are for nonoxynol-9 use only by couples at low risk of sexually transmitted infections (33). Hypersensitivity is a common adverse reaction, either from nonoxynol-9 itself or from the vehicle.

Microbicides

Microbicides are compounds that can be used vaginally or rectally to protect against sexually transmitted infections. Contraceptive microbicides are intended to prevent pregnancy as well as kill bacteria and viruses. Some microbicides provide a physical barrier to prevent exposure of cells in the vagina, cervix, and rectum; some help maintain the natural vaginal acidic pH; and some kill or disable pathogens or prevent viral replication (34). Many phase 3 trials are ongoing to evaluate products in this group that at the same time may protect against infection, provide contraception, and not disrupt the vaginal flora; however, there are no products yet on the market that achieve these objectives.

Sponges

The Today sponge is a polyurethane sperm barrier available over-the-counter. It contains 1 g of nonoxynol-9 spermicide. There is a dimple on one side that is designed to fit over the cervix, and a loop on the other side for removal. The sponge provides continuous contraception for 24 hours and must be left in place for 6 hours after intercourse. Wearing the sponge for greater than 30 hours may increase the risk of toxic shock syndrome.

Periodic Abstinence

Periodic abstinence techniques (rhythm method) are designed to work by avoiding coitus during the fertile days of the menstrual cycle. All variations of this method rely on assumptions about the timing of ovulation. Examples of periodic abstinence techniques include the calendar method, which estimates fertile days based on cycle length; the temperature method, which relies on recording the basal body temperature to detect ovulation;

and the symptothermal method, which relies on temperature and cervical mucus changes. Advantages of periodic abstinence methods include no cost and no direct medical risks. Disadvantages include long training periods, unreliability in predicting fertility, poor adherence and continuation rates, and resulting high failure rates. This method is not suitable for women who are recently postpregnancy, older than 35 years, or having irregular cycles.

Anovulation during Lactational Amenorrhea

Anovulation during lactational amenorrhea can be exploited as a contraceptive method. Natural postpartum infertility occurs when a woman is amenorrheic and fully breastfeeding. To rely on this method, women must be exclusively breastfeeding at least six times a day or 85% breastfeeding, have not had menses since delivery, and be less than 6 months postpartum (2). Done correctly, this temporary method is highly effective (up to 98%). It does not, of course, protect against sexually transmitted infections (35).

EMERGENCY CONTRACEPTION

EC is intended for use after unprotected intercourse or recognized contraceptive failure. It can reduce the risk of pregnancy by more than 75%. Research shows that EC prevents fertilization by delaying ovulation until viable sperm no longer reside in the upper female genital tract. Plan B is a progestin-only formulation with two tablets containing 0.75 mg of levonorgestrel that may be taken in two divided doses 12 hours apart or once in a single dose (15). EC is more effective the sooner it is used, but it has been shown to decrease the incidence of pregnancy when taken up to 5 days later.

Some have hypothesized that EC has some effect postfertilization, but direct supporting evidence is lacking. EC will not end an established pregnancy. If EC is inadvertently used after a pregnancy is already established, teratogenic risk is thought to be unlikely because teratogenicity under these circumstances has not been seen with daily combined OCs (36). Women using EC after unprotected intercourse should start an effective form of contraception immediately. Apparent EC failure occurs due to additional unprotected acts of intercourse following treatment. Plan B is available over the counter for women older than 18 years, but a prescription is required for minors. Providing a prescription in advance increases the likelihood of use. IUDs may also be used as an EC for up to 5 days after unprotected intercourse in women who desire long-term contraception (37). All methods of EC are cost effective except for the IUD, which becomes more cost effective only with extended use (see page 282) (14).

CONTRACEPTION AFTER PREGNANCY

Discussion of contraceptive methods with parturient patients should begin during prenatal care. Sterilization may be performed immediately after delivery, and occurs following approximately 10% of all births in the United

States. DMPA, implants, and POPs may be initiated immediately after delivery without increasing VTE risk or affecting breast milk production (4). The use of combined OCs may be initiated 2 weeks after delivery without increasing the risk of VTE. Breastfeeding women can initiate combined oral contraceptives 6 weeks postpartum without decreasing breast milk production enough to limit infant weight gain, but some guidelines discourage the use of combined OCs when breastfeeding. IUDs, diaphragm fitting, and laparoscopic or hysteroscopic tubal sterilization must wait until 4–6 weeks postpartum. Patients should use condoms if they are sexually active before their postpartum visit because ovulation can occur as soon as 20 days postpartum except when the mother is breastfeeding exclusively. The copper IUD may be inserted immediately after delivery of the placenta. If not inserted within 10 minutes of delivery of the placenta, insertion cannot be performed until involution of the uterus occurs, at approximately 4 weeks postpartum. The LNG-IUS should not be inserted immediately postpartum because the hormonal effects of levonorgestrel on uterine involution are unknown (15).

CONTRACEPTION AFTER ABORTION

The unwanted pregnancies that lead to induced abortions often occur because women did not receive sufficient information about family planning before becoming pregnant. In a nationwide survey, 46% of women undergoing abortion had not used contraception in the month they conceived. The main reasons cited were the perceived low risk of pregnancy and concerns about contraception (38). Women undergoing abortion should be counseled that pregnancy can occur again almost immediately. Delaying the initiation of contraception postabortion only increases the probability of a repeat unintended pregnancy. Patients interested in hormonal methods of contraception can initiate any of these methods on the same day or within 7 days of an abortion procedure. If patients say that they will never be sexually active again and refuse contraception, they should nevertheless be provided with information on a variety of contraceptive methods and how to obtain them should circumstances change (39).

MALE HORMONAL CONTRACEPTION

Methods to suppress sperm production are under evaluation in phase 3 trials, but none are yet routinely available. A promising combination of testosterone and a progestin for use by men has been studied in pill, patch, injection, and implant forms (40).

OFFICE AND CLINIC ORGANIZATION

Practices that care for women of childbearing age should maintain supplies of relevant patient education materials (or listings of pertinent websites), such as those listed in the subsequent text, to help women learn more about contraceptive options. As noted earlier, stocking samples of contraceptive preparations can help women begin use immediately. Clinicians who perform contraceptive procedures (e.g., hormone injections, insertion of IUDs) should maintain necessary supplies and an appropriate setting in the clinic for doing so.

RESOURCES — PATIENT EDUCATION MATERIALS

American College of Obstetricians and Gynecologists
www.acog.org

> ACOG Patient Information Pamphlets
> *Birth Control* (brochure # AP005; Spanish SP005)
> *The Intrauterine Device* (brochure # AP014; Spanish SP014)
> *Birth Control Pills* (brochure #AP021)
> *Barrier Methods of Contraception* (brochure # AP022; Spanish SP022)
> *Natural Family Planning* (brochure #AP024; Spanish SP024)
> *Emergency Contraception* (brochure # AP114)
> *Hormonal Contraception-Injections, Rings, and Patches* (brochure # AP159 Spanish SP159)
> *Birth Control-Especially for Teens* (brochure # AP114)
> *Your First Gyn Visit-Especially for Teens* (brochure # AP150 Spanish SP150)
> http://www.acog.org/publications/patient_education/

Association of Repoductive Health Professionals
www.arhp.org

Planned Parenthood
http://www.plannedparenthood.org/

not-2-late
http://www.not-2-late.com

SUGGESTED READINGS

American College of Obstetricians and Gynecologists. ACOG Committee Opinion #337. *Noncontraceptive uses of the levonorgestrel intrauterine system.* Washington, DC: American College of Obstetricians and Gynecologists, June 2006.

American College of Obstetricians and Gynecologists. ACOG Practice Bulletin #59. *Intrauterine device.* Washington, DC: American College of Obstetricians and Gynecologists, January 2005.

American College of Obstetricians and Gynecologists. ACOG Practice Bulletin #69. *Emergency contraception.* Washington, DC: American College of Obstetricians and Gynecologists, December 2005.

American College of Obstetricians and Gynecologists. ACOG Practice Bulletin #73. *Use of hormonal contraception in women with coexisting medical conditions.* Washington, DC: American College of Obstetricians and Gynecologists, June 2006.

Hatcher RA, Trussel J, Stewart F, et al. *Contraceptive technology*, 18th rev. ed. New York: Ardent Media Inc, 2004.

World Health Organization. *Medical eligibility criteria for contraceptive use*, 3rd ed. 2004.

References

1. Henshaw SK. Unintended pregnancy in the United States. *Fam Plann Perspect* 1998;30:24–29, 46.
2. Upadhyay UD, Robey B. *Why Family Planning Matters. Population Reports*, Series J, No. 49. Baltimore: Johns Hopkins University School of Public Health, Population Information Program, July 1999.
3. De Cetina T, Canto P, Luna M. Effect of counseling to improve compliance in Mexican women receiving depot-medroxyprogesterone acetate. *Contraception* 2001;63: 143–146.
4. Hatcher RA, Trussel J, Stewart FH, et al. *Contraceptive technology*, 18th rev. ed. New York: Ardent Media Inc, 2004.
5. Trussell J, Koenig J, Stewart F, et al. Medical care cost savings for adolescent contraceptive use. *Fam Plann Perspect* 1997;29:248–255, 295.
6. Moos M-K, Bartholomew NE, Lohr KN. Counseling in a clinical setting to prevent unintended pregnancy: an evidence-based research agenda. *Contraception* 2003;67: 115–132.
7. deAbood M, de Castillo Z, Guerrero F, et al. Effect of Depo-Provera or Microgynon on the painful crises of sickle cell anemia patients. *Contraception* 1997;56:313.
8. Westhoff C, Truman C, Kalmuss D, et al. Depressive symptoms and depo-provera. *Contraception* 1998;57:237–240.
9. Westhoff C, Wieland D, Tiezzi L. Depression in users of depo-medroxyprogesterone acetate. *Contraception* 1995;51:351–354.
10. Westhoff C. Depot medroxyprogesterone acetate contraception: metabolic parameters and mood changes. *J Reprod Med* 1996;41:401–406.
11. Pelkman C. Hormones and weight change. *J Reprod Med* 2002;47:791–794.
12. Pelkman C, Chow M, Heinbach R, et al. Short-term effects of a progestational contraceptive drug on food intake, resting energy expenditure, and body weight in young women. *Am J Clin Nutr* 2001;73:19–26.
13. Scholes D, LaCroix AZ, Ichikawa LE, et al. Injectable hormone contraception and bone density: results from a prospective study. Epidemiology. 2002;13(5):581–7. Erratum in: Epidemiology 2002;13(6):749.
14. Trussell J, Koenig J, Ellertson C, et al. Preventing unintended pregnancy: the cost-effectiveness of three methods of emergency contraception. *Am J Public Health* 1997;87:932–937.
15. The INFO Project. *World Health Organization updates guidance on how to use contraceptives*. Baltimore: Johns Hopkins University. INFO Reports April 2005, Issue 4.
16. Hubacher D, Lara-Ricalde R, Taylor D, et al. Use of copper intrauterine devices and the risk of tubal infertility among nulligravid women. *N Engl J Med* 2001;345:561–567.
17. Paragard website, Duramed Pharmaceuticals. http://www.paragard.com/paragard/index.php. Accessed 2007.
18. American College of Obstetricians and Gynecologists. ACOG Committee opinion #337. *Noncontraceptive uses of the levonorgestrel intrauterine system*. Washington, DC: American College of Obstetricians and Gynecologists. June 2006.
19. Creinin M, Clark B. The latest contraceptive option: the single-rod implant. *Contemp Ob Gyn* 2005;50:54–59.
20. Harrison-Woolrych M, Hill R. Unintended pregnancies with the etonogestrel implant (Implanon): a case series from postmarketing experience in Australia. *Contraception* 2005;71:306–308.

21. Beerthuizen R, van Beek A, Massai R, et al. Bone mineral density during long-term use of the progestagen contraceptive implant Implanon compared to a non-hormonal method of contraception. *Hum Reprod* 2000;15:118–122.

22. Anderson F, Hait H. Seasonale-301 Study Group. A multicenter, randomized study of an extended cycle oral contraceptive. *Contraception* 2003;68:89–96.

23. Westhoff C, Kerns J, Morroni C, et al. Quick start: novel oral contraceptive initiation method. *Contraception* 2002;66:141–145.

24. American College of Obstetricians and Gynecologists. ACOG Practice Bulletin #73. *Use of hormonal contraception in women with coexisting medical conditions*. Washington, DC: American College of Obstetricians and Gynecologists. June 2006.

25. Gallo MF, Lopez LM, Grimes DA, et al. Combination contraceptives. *Cochrane Database Syst Rev* 2006;(1):CD003987.

26. Organon International website: http://www.organon.com/news/. Access year 2007.

27. Miller L, Verhoeven CHJ. Results of a randomized, multicenter trial comparing extended contraceptive ring regimens. *Obstet Gynecol* 2005;105:6S.

28. van den Heuvel M, van Brigt A, Alnabawy A, et al. Comparison of ethinyl estradiol pharmacokinetics in three hormonal contraceptive formulations: the vaginal ring, the transdermal patch and an oral contraceptive. *Contraception* 2005;72:168–174.

29. Abma JC, Martinez, GM, Mosher, WD, et al. *Teenagers in the United States: Sexual activity, contraceptive use, and childbearing, 2002*. Hyattsville, MD: National Center for Health Statistics. Vital Health Stat 2004;23(24). http://www.cdc.gov/nchs/data/series/sr_23/sr23_024.pdf. Accessed 2007.

30. Gallo MF, Grimes DA, Lopez LM, et al. Non-latex versus latex condoms for contraception. *Cochrane Database Syst Rev* 2006;1.

31. Winer RL, Hughes JP, Feng Q, et al. Condom use and the risk of genital human papillomavirus infection in young women. *N Engl J Med* 2006;354:2645–2654.

32. The Female Health Company. FC and FC2 female condom website: http://www.femalehealth.com/theproduct.html.

33. Planned Parenthood. Nonoxynol-9: benefits and risks. http://www.plannedparenthood.org/news-articles-press/politics-policy-issues/birth-control-access-prevention/nonoxynol-9-6546.htm.

34. World Health Organization. Microbicides. http://www.who.int/hiv/topics/microbicides/microbicides/en/

35. Family Health International. Frequently asked questions on contraception. http://www.fhi.org/en/RH/FAQs/index.htm.

36. Bracken MB. Oral contraception and congenital malformations in offspring: a review and meta-analysis of the prospective studies. *Obstet Gynecol* 1990;76:552–558.

37. Westhoff C. Emergency contraception. *N Engl J Med* 2003;349:1830–1835.

38. Jones RK, Darroch JE, Henshaw SK. Contraceptive use among US women having abortions in 2000–2001. *Perspect Sex Reprod Health* 2002;34(6):294–303.

39. Upadhyay UD. *Informed choice in family planning: Helping people decide*. Population Reports, Series J, No. 50. Baltimore: Johns Hopkins University School of Public Health, Population Information Program, 2001. http://www.infoforhealth.org/pr/j50/j50.pdf.

40. Upadhyay UD. *Population reports-new contraceptive choices*. Baltimore: Johns Hopkins University School of Public Health, Population Information Program, Series M, Number 19, April 2005.

CHAPTER 12

Sexually Transmitted Infections

Charles M. Kodner

INTRODUCTION

Described in 1997 by the Institute of Medicine as the "hidden epidemic," (1) sexually transmitted infections (STIs) remain a public health problem of major proportions and with far-reaching consequences. Beyond the spectrum of clinically evident STIs that are encountered frequently in practice, the much larger burden of asymptomatic infection highlights the magnitude of the problem confronting both clinicians and health policy planners. The clinical outcomes of such infections include not only short-term symptomatic states but also "ascending infections" such as pelvic inflammatory disease (PID). STIs also act as cofactors that increase the risk of human immunodeficiency virus (HIV) transmission. They are also a major cause of chronic pelvic pain, infertility, and adverse outcomes of pregnancy such as ectopic pregnancy, low birthweight and fetal loss, prematurity, and vertically transmitted neonatal infections (2). As noted in Chapter 4, human papilloma virus (HPV) infection is a risk factor for cervical and genital cancer that at present cannot be effectively identified or cured.

The prevention of STIs and their long-term consequences remains an important clinical and public health goal. According to Centers for Disease Control and Prevention (CDC) guidelines (3), STI prevention and control are based on five key principles:

1. Education and counseling of persons at risk on ways to adopt safe sexual practices.
2. Identification of asymptomatic infected persons and of symptomatic persons unlikely to seek diagnostic and treatment services.
3. Effective diagnosis and treatment of infected persons.
4. Evaluation, treatment, and counseling of sex partners of persons who are infected with a STI.
5. Preexposure vaccination of persons at risk for vaccine-preventable STIs.

A number of factors must work in conjunction to achieve the best prevention outcomes based on these principles:

1. Clinicians should remain aware of current screening, diagnostic, and treatment protocols that most effectively prevent and identify STIs, and they should find practice opportunities for implementing them.
2. Clinical practice and counseling should respect individual needs as well as evolving societal norms for sexual and health behaviors.
3. Health systems should facilitate counseling, diagnosis, and treatment through appropriate office systems, health insurance coverage, and community resources.

The goals of this chapter are to describe effective strategies for clinicians to foster STI prevention and to review briefly current recommendations for STI screening, diagnosis, treatment, and reporting with a focus on prevention strategies. The emphasis is on STIs, resources, and clinical practice in the United States. The spectrum and severity of disease burden, as well as the range of available and effective management options, differ widely in other countries where STIs remain an overwhelming public health problem. Sexual practices to prevent unwanted pregnancy are discussed in Chapter 11.

Epidemiology

Chlamydia trachomatis infection is the most prevalent of all STIs (4), and it accounts for many of the observed complications of STIs, such as PID, infertility, ectopic pregnancy, and chronic pelvic pain. Approximately 70% of chlamydia infections are asymptomatic. In 2004, a total of 929,462 chlamydia cases were reported to the CDC in the United States. This corresponds to a rate of 319.6 cases per 100,000 population, a 5.9% increase since 2003. The continued rise in the case rate reflects increased screening, the use of more sensitive diagnostic tests, and improved efforts to ensure case reporting, as well as a real increase in incidence. During the same year, 330,132 cases of gonorrhea infection were reported. Gonorrhea, the second most commonly reported notifiable disease in the United States, also increases the risk of a variety of complications. Gonococcal infection also facilitates HIV infection. In 2004, the rate of gonorrhea was 113.5 cases per 100,000 population, the lowest rate of gonorrhea ever reported in the United States. Approximately 50% of gonococcal infections are asymptomatic.

PID represents one of the most visible adverse outcomes of STIs. If not adequately treated, 20–40% of women with chlamydia and 10–40% of women with gonorrhea will develop PID (4). Among women with PID, 20% will develop infertility, 9% will experience an ectopic pregnancy, and 18% will experience chronic pelvic pain.

Young age (younger than 25 years) is an important risk factor for the acquisition of a STI. It is frequently used as a criterion for offering screening (see Chapter 4, page 108). Other demographic characteristics such as race and ethnicity, marital status, urban location, and low income have been less consistently associated with infection.

STRATEGIES FOR THE PREVENTION OF SEXUALLY TRANSMITTED INFECTIONS

Education and Counseling

As discussed in Chapter 5, counseling for any behavioral change is challenging. Counseling people at risk for STIs to change their sexual behaviors is a special challenge for clinicians, who strive to communicate effectively with their patients. For many clinicians and patients, sexual activity is an especially difficult matter to discuss. Counseling to change sexual behaviors must be conducted with an extra measure of sensitivity, in a way that respects individuals' health needs, privacy, and motivation to prevent illness.

A number of techniques can be used to approach the general sexual history, as described elsewhere (5). The key features include the following:

1. Approach the sexual history in a matter-of-fact yet sensitive manner.
2. Ask the patient's permission to discuss sexual behavior and health issues.
3. Acknowledge and provide support for positive steps already made; previous risk reduction attempts, whether successful or not, or even efforts to get tested for STIs or HIV, should be recognized.
4. Avoid assumptions about the patient's sexual orientation or activity—initially use the term *partner* rather than *boyfriend, girlfriend, husband, or wife.*
5. Communicate clearly, gently teaching patients the correct terminology regarding sexual behaviors. Use appropriate language and terminology: avoid compromising professionalism by using slang terms.
6. Avoid moral or religious judgment of patients' behaviors. Provide information that is directed at emotional and psychological as well as physical health.
7. Correct misinformation and dispel myths, but provide factual information in limited amounts so that patients can ask for further details if desired. Clarify specific misconceptions rather than correcting "common" or general misinformation; focus on patients' personal risk factors and clarify misinformation about their own behaviors.
8. Keep the discussion focused on personal STI/HIV risk reduction.
   - Avoid emphasizing delivery of predetermined didactic information.
   - Use open-ended questions that keep the patient focused on personal STI/HIV risks.
   - Discuss specific STI/HIV risks and risk reduction in depth.

9. Negotiate a concrete, achievable behavioral change step that will reduce STI or HIV risk.
   - Small behavioral changes are significant, and counseling should emphasize realistic, specific, achievable steps, at the outset possibly targeted to just one of many high-risk behaviors (see Chapter 5).
   - Behavioral change steps should be acceptable to patients and relevant to their specific behaviors.
   - Identifying and resolving barriers to achieving this goal, possibly through role-playing or discussion, can increase the likelihood of success.
   - Writing down the goal, for the patient and/or in the chart, may be helpful for later reinforcement.
   - Be flexible in the prevention approach and counseling process.
10. Provide skill-building opportunities.

Once the topic of sexual health has been broached and a general sexual history obtained, more detailed steps can be taken to promote sexual behavioral changes that prevent STIs. A counseling model developed by the CDC (6) typically involves two counseling sessions, each approximately 15–20 minutes long. The model for such sessions, which was developed primarily with respect to HIV prevention, devotes the first visit to testing and counseling and the second to test result follow-up and counseling. This model can easily be adapted for generic sexual behavior counseling. Patients with a lower risk of HIV infection or STIs may require less time. The critical features are the use of the patient-centered approach, focusing initial counseling on behavior change with a follow-up discussion to assess the impact of counseling on patient behavior.

The use of open-ended questions in STI counseling is consistent with general techniques for behavioral change counseling (see Chapter 5). It differs from traditional, prescriptive STI counseling styles to which physicians may have been exposed during their training. Table 12.1 shows examples of questions that are more patient focused and may be more likely to result in meaningful behavioral change (see also Chapter 2, pages 34–35); Table 12.2 illustrates the difference between global, or general, risk-reduction recommendations, which patients are not likely to follow, and more specific, patient-focused recommendations that may be more likely to induce a change in sexual behavior. Although it may require special effort to identify such patient-specific behaviors during clinical encounters, tailoring counseling in this way may be more effective at ultimately preventing STIs.

Both direct education by clinicians as well as general education in public health campaigns must take into account the reading level and baseline health beliefs and misunderstandings of the population. The cultural context affects sexual and health behaviors and beliefs. Misconceptions are common,

TABLE 12.1   Closed-Ended versus Open-Ended Questions to Assess Behaviors That Increase the Risk of Sexually Transmitted Infection/Human Immunodeficiency Virus (STI/HIV) Infection

Closed-Ended Questions, Which Might Interfere with Patient-Centered STI/HIV Counseling	Open-Ended Questions Which Promote Patient-Centered STI/HIV Counseling
Have you ever injected drugs? *For a male patient:* Have you ever had sex with a man? *For a female patient:* Have you ever had sex with a bisexual man?	What are you doing that you think might be putting yourself at risk for STI or HIV infection? What are the riskiest things that you are doing? *If counseling during STI/HIV testing:* If your test comes back positive, how do you think you may have become infected?
Have you ever had sex when you were under the influence of alcohol or drugs?	When was the last time you put yourself at risk for STIs or HIV? What was happening then? How often do you use drugs or alcohol? How do you think drugs or alcohol influence your STI or HIV risk?
Do you always use condoms when you have sex? Can you always use condoms when you have sex?	How often do you use condoms when you have sex? When (or with whom) do you have sex without a condom and when with a condom? What are you currently doing to protect yourself from STIs or HIV? How is that working? Tell me about specific situations when you have reduced your STI or HIV risk. What was going on that made that possible?

Adapted from Centers for Disease Control and Prevention. Revised guidelines for HIV counseling, testing, and referral. Technical expert panel review of CDC HIV counseling, testing, and referral guidelines. *MMWR* 2001;50(RR-19):1–10.

especially among adolescents and young adult women. Often, people believe that it is not possible to have more than one STI at a time; that people with STIs will always have symptoms; that it is not possible to have a STI and HIV infection at the same time; that traditional healers have medicines that can cure STIs (this is a special problem among patients from some regions in Africa and the Indian subcontinent); or that washing the genitals after

TABLE 12.2 Global versus Specific Sexually Transmitted Infection (STI) Risk-Reduction Steps

Global Risk-Reduction Steps That Are Unlikely to Be Effective in Changing Behavior	Specific Risk-Reduction Steps That Are More Likely to Be Effective in Changing Behavior
Always use condoms	• Buy a condom tomorrow and try it on • Carry a condom the next time I go out (e.g., to a bar, nightclub) • Starting today, put condoms on the nightstand beside the bed • Starting tonight, require my partner to use a condom, or I will not have vaginal (or anal) sex
Have fewer or less risky partners	• Stop seeing (specific partner) who is seeing other people • Break up with (specific partner) before getting together with someone new
Have safer sex	• Talk honestly with (specific partner) about my STI or HIV status and ask about his/her STI or HIV status • Next time I am out with friends and may have sex, avoid getting "high" on drugs or alcohol • Only kissing, etc. with (specific partner) until we both are tested for STI and/or HIV • Tomorrow, ask (specific partner) if he/she has had a recent HIV test and has been tested for other STIs
Stop injecting drugs	• Obtain clean works (i.e., needles, syringes, cottons, or cookers[a]) tomorrow so I have them before I use next time • Contact drug treatment center and make an appointment

Adapted from Centers for Disease Control and Prevention. Revised guidelines for HIV counseling, testing, and referral. Technical expert panel review of CDC HIV counseling, testing, and referral guidelines. *MMWR* 2001;50(RR-19):1–10.

HIV = human immunodeficiency virus.

[a]Cottons are filters used to draw up the drug solution. Cookers include bottle caps, spoons, or other containers used to dissolve drugs.

sex, use of oral contraceptives, or urinating or douching after sex protects against STIs (7).

The potential role of the Internet in increasing high-risk sexual activity is constantly evolving, possibly necessitating new approaches to STI prevention. Adolescents, men who have sex with men, and other demographic groups may meet sexual partners online, with an attendant increased risk of STIs. The Internet is an increasingly important venue for the acquisition of new sexual contacts with little knowledge of their sexual health status. Online and offline approaches to targeting prevention messages to such individuals are in their infancy (8).

COUNSELING FOR SAFER SEXUAL PRACTICES

Updated CDC guidelines from 2006 (9) provide specific information regarding the efficacy of various "safer" sexual practices. They include detailed instructions for male condom use that can be shared with patients. Table 12.3 summarizes these recommendations. While these counseling guidelines apply to all patient populations, some specific recommendations for STI risk reduction counseling pertain to particular patient groups or situations.

Counseling Adolescents

Adolescent patients present with specific risk factors, barriers to effective treatment, and other issues that impact effective STI prevention (10). In 2003, 28% of girls in the 9th grade and 62% of girls in the 12th grade reported having sexual intercourse. See Chapter 2 (page 35) for suggestions on how to approach the discussion of sexual practices with teenage patients. Adolescents have a number of risk factors for acquiring STIs, including lack of emotional development to recognize the consequences of risky behavior; use of alcohol or other substances that increase the risk of intercourse without a condom, with multiple partners, or with high-risk partners; and in women, biologic factors such as exposed cervical columnar epithelium that constitutes the primary site of invasion for chlamydia and gonococcal infection.

Statutory, ethical, and financial issues also complicate STI prevention and treatment in the adolescent population. Despite statutes in all states allowing minors to receive STI testing and treatment without parental consent, concerns about confidentiality and fears of parental discovery limit the willingness of many adolescents to seek effective health care for STIs. Although discussions with adolescent patients can emphasize the parameters for confidentiality, it is also important that clinicians encourage and possibly facilitate open communication of sexual health matters between minors and their parents. This is especially important if insurance billing for these services may come to parental attention despite the best efforts of the clinician to prevent disclosure. Out-of-pocket expenditures for office visits, testing, and

TABLE 12.3   Recommendations for Safer Sexual Practices to Reduce Transmission of Sexually Transmitted Infection/Human Immunodeficiency Virus (STI/HIV) and Unintended Pregnancy

Measure	Information to Share with Patients
Abstinence	• Counsel patients (especially those being treated for STIs, or whose partners are being treated) that abstinence from sexual activity, or being in a mutually monogamous relationship with an uninfected partner, is the most reliable way to avoid transmission of STIs
Male condoms	• When used consistently and correctly, male latex condoms are highly effective at reducing the transmission of HIV and other STIs • Polyurethane condoms provide similar protection against STIs and unintended pregnancy as do latex condoms, and can be used for patients with latex allergy • Natural membrane or "natural" condoms prevent passage of sperm, but they have pores that allow transmission of HIV and HBV and are not recommended for STI prevention
Female condoms	• When male condoms cannot be used properly, patients should be counseled to consider using female condoms (see page 288), which can substantially reduce the risk for STIs
Vaginal spermicides and diaphragms	• Nonoxynol-9 vaginal spermicides are not effective in preventing most common STIs and HIV transmission, and they should not be recommended for this purpose • Diaphragms may provide some protection against STI transmission, but they should not be relied upon as the sole means of protection • Diaphragm and spermicide use have been associated with an increased risk of bacterial urinary tract infections in women • Condoms lubricated with spermicide are no more effective than other lubricated condoms in preventing STI transmission, may have a shorter shelf life than other condoms, and should not be recommended to reduce STIs

Adapted from Centers for Disease Control and Prevention. Sexually transmitted diseases treatment guidelines 2006. *MMWR* 2006;55(RR-11):1–9.

treatment may be prohibitive for adolescents. Clinicians should be flexible about providing effective and affordable care while maintaining adolescents' confidentiality. Referral to a publicly funded clinic may be appropriate in some cases.

Modern societal norms and circumstances have introduced new risk factors for STIs that need to be frankly and openly addressed and considered during patient counseling. Children and adolescents spend an increasing amount of time without parental supervision, which increases the risk of experimentation with sexual activity and with alcohol and drug use (11). Clinicians should encourage opportunities for supervised activities as well as traditional approaches to prevention, such as abstinence and safer sex. For female adolescents, sexually active relationships with individuals who were first "friends" before becoming sexual partners are more likely to include discussions of STIs and consistent birth control (12).

Other potential barriers that are more pronounced among adolescents include lack of awareness of what constitutes abnormal physical symptoms of STIs; fears of physical examination or embarrassment about pelvic examination; concerns about the discovery of sexual activity or sexual abuse by others; or reluctance to confront the reality of a STI that may raise questions about the fidelity or stability of their relationship with their partner (10).

Patient education regarding abstinence, safer sexual practices, and health beliefs and behaviors is especially important for adolescent patients. These topics are difficult for many clinicians to discuss with teenagers. Such discussions are also limited by the misconception of clinicians that their patients are not sexually active or that the prevalence of STIs is low in their patient population.

Recommendations on the subject from the American College of Obstetricians and Gynecologists suggest a number of other specific interventions that may be appropriate for adolescent patients, although not all are supported by firm evidence of efficacy in reducing STI rates:

- Include reproductive health care counseling, screening, and preventive care beginning at age 13–15 years.
- Screen sexually active adolescent patients for STIs (see Chapter 4).
- Begin Pap testing approximately 3 years after first intercourse (see page 104).
- Ascertain if adolescents are in a new sexual relationship, because this is an important risk factor for acquiring STIs.
- Consider urine-based testing for gonorrhea or chlamydia (see page 109) if pelvic examination is not feasible or otherwise declined by adolescent patients.
- Counsel adolescent patients specifically about the role of abstinence from sexual activity to prevent STIs or unwanted pregnancy.

Even for adults and adolescents who are not currently sexually active, reminders about the benefits of abstinence may be helpful, especially for adolescents who are ambivalent about whether to become sexually active. It is also potentially important in this age-group to identify factors that would place the patient at risk for unsafe sexual activity and subsequent STIs. These factors include substance abuse, social settings that would create pressure for unwanted sexual activity, or a new partner who might apply pressure to become sexually active.

Secondary prevention in patients who already have STIs should emphasize education along the lines described, with an emphasis on specific behaviors that can be modified in order to reduce the risk of STIs, as in Table 12.2.

Screening for Sexually Transmitted Infections

Screening asymptomatic patients for early detection of asymptomatic STIs remains one of the most important measures to reduce disease transmission, prevent the development of symptoms or complications in the individual patient, and reduce the overall prevalence of common STIs. See Chapter 4 and Appendix A to this book for details on screening guidelines issued by clinical and professional organizations for various patient groups. Individual practices may wish to modify their STI screening policies based on local disease prevalence rates. Clinicians should therefore be aware of local STI rates, which are available from the local or state public health department. There is very little evidence available to guide the determination of the proper frequency of STI screening. Most screening interventions are assumed to take place during routine health maintenance or prenatal care visits.

Identification of asymptomatic HPV infection in women through routine Pap testing may help prevent HPV-related illness, including genital cancers, but such screening is not universally recommended (see page 104) (13). CDC guidelines recommend testing patients with genital ulcers for herpes and syphilis, and possibly for *Haemophilus ducreyi* in settings where chancroid is prevalent to help reduce the transmission of HIV (9). Table 12.4 summarizes clinical scenarios and opportunities for testing and prevention of STIs.

Effective Diagnosis and Treatment of Sexually Transmitted Infections

The diagnosis and treatment of symptomatic STIs in community clinics, primary care offices, emergency rooms, and other settings is generally straightforward. In addition to improving short-term STI-related symptoms, prompt diagnosis and treatment of STIs play a key role in preventing coinfection, complications, and transmission of STIs to others. Empiric treatment recommendations for urethritis/cervicitis are summarized in Table 12.5. See standard texts for guidance on treatment of genital ulcerative illness, genital warts, herpes, and other STIs.

TABLE 12.4 Interventions to Prevent Sexually Transmitted Infections (STIs)

Clinical Scenario	Intervention	Outcomes
Asymptomatic patient: adolescent, young adult, or high-risk patient	• Screen for STI risk factors • Screen for STIs (see Chapter 4)	• Reduces adverse health outcomes (PID, etc.) • Possibly decreases STI prevalence rates
Patient with symptomatic urethritis or cervicitis	• Use appropriate diagnostic tests to rapidly diagnose STIs • Treat empirically for STIs if clinical suspicion is high • Consider providing treatment for partners • Consider retesting for cure • Consider rescreening in 3–4 mo • Notify public health department of reportable diseases	—
Patient with symptomatic or asymptomatic genital ulcer	• Test specifically for herpes simplex virus and syphilis • Consider testing for *Haemophilus ducreyi* • Test for HIV • Consider biopsy if not responding to treatment	• Reduces transmission of HIV, syphilis, and HSV-related disease
Patient with genital herpes	• Test for herpes simplex virus • Treat acute episode • Counsel to prevent HSV transmission • Provide maintenance suppressive treatment if recurrent	• Reduces HSV transmission • Reduces HIV transmission

PID = pelvic inflammatory disease; HIV = human immunodeficiency virus; HSV = herpes simplex virus.

TABLE 12.5 Summary of Treatment Guidelines for Urethritis and Cervicitis

Clinical Scenario	Recommended Treatment	Alternative Regimens
Urethritis or cervicitis[a]	• *For nongonococcal urethritis:* azithromycin 1 g orally one dose, OR doxycycline 100 mg orally twice a day for 7 d • *For gonorrhea:* ceftriaxone 125 mg i.m. in a single dose OR cefixime 400 mg orally in a single dose OR ciprofloxacin 500 mg orally in a single dose OR ofloxacin 400 mg orally in a single dose OR levofloxacin 250 mg orally in a single dose[b]	• *For nongonococcal urethritis:* erythromycin base 500 mg orally four times a day for 7 d OR erythromycin ethylsuccinate 800 mg orally four times a day for 7 d OR ofloxacin 300 mg orally twice a day for 7 d OR levofloxacin 500 mg orally once daily for 7 d
Recurrent or persistent urethritis	• Metronidazole 2 g orally in a single dose OR tinidazole 2 g orally in a single dose PLUS azithromycin 1 g orally in a single dose (if not used for initial episode)	• N/A

Adapted from Centers for Disease Control and Prevention. Sexually transmitted diseases treatment guidelines 2006. *MMWR* 2006;55(RR-11):1–9, 35–40.

[a] Treatment should be based on confirmed urethritis or cervicitis; empiric treatment without testing is recommended only for high-risk patients who are not likely to return for follow-up; cotreatment for gonorrhea and nongonococcal urethritis (NGU; frequently *Chlamydia trachomatis*) is generally recommended.

[b] Due to possible quinolone-resistant *Neisseria gonorrhea* (QRNG), quinolones should not be used to treat men who have sex with men, patients in areas known to have a high prevalence of QRNG, or patients who acquired their infection outside the United States.

Preventing Transmission of Sexually Transmitted Infections

An important way to prevent transmission of STIs from the patient to sexual contacts is through required reporting of selected illnesses to local and/or state public health departments with subsequent contact tracing. The list of reportable STIs varies somewhat from state to state, and different infections have different reporting requirements in terms of the time permitted between diagnosis and reporting.

All persons diagnosed with STIs should be counseled to notify their sex partners and urge them to seek medical evaluation and treatment. An important question for clinical management is whether the primary sexual contact of a patient diagnosed with an STI should be offered treatment, particularly if they are not an established patient of the index patient's clinician, and are not present at the time of the index patient's visit. "Partner services," which raise important ethical and clinical considerations, commonly take the form of "patient-delivered therapy" (a prescription written in the sexual partner's name, or by giving a sufficient quantity of antibiotics prescribed to the index patient to allow treatment of the partner as well). Further details about the benefits and risks of this practice are described elsewhere (14,15).

Vaccination to Prevent Sexually Transmitted Infections

Patients undergoing evaluation or treatment for STIs should be vaccinated against hepatitis A and B. This practice is discussed in more detail in Chapter 16 (see pages 397 and 400). That chapter also discusses the role of HPV vaccination as a strategy to prevent cervical cancer (see page 417).

OFFICE AND CLINIC ORGANIZATION

At the level of the individual practice, a number of systems interventions can help expand effective provision of services for preventing STIs:

- On the basis of local STI rates, determine which subset of patients should be screened for STIs during routine health maintenance examinations (focusing on higher risk populations, such as women aged 18–24 years). The practice should adopt a protocol as discussed in Chapter 20.
- Incorporate reminder systems (see Chapters 21 and 22), ideally through the use of electronic health records that will prompt clinicians when STI screening is indicated.
- Consider dedicating physical space and/or personnel to providing behavioral counseling focused on STI prevention.
- Consider posting flyers or handouts with STI prevention information, and listings of helpful websites, in places where patients can access this information privately and discretely.
- Consider providing male condoms, and instructions for their use, in settings where the risk of STIs is especially high.

STI screening, counseling, and other prevention measures have not been implemented with the frequency and effectiveness that are warranted by the high prevalence of STIs in many communities. This occurs because effective

STI prevention involves the larger health care system, including not only the individual practice but also community-based and national resources and a policy environment involving insurers and local, regional, and national institutions. Each of these entities influences the effectiveness with which clinicians can prevent the transmission of STIs and HIV infection. With STI prevention as with other aspects of medical care, a systems approach is as important as individual patient management. Community resources and community-based STI prevention measures are therefore increasingly important to address these widespread diseases.

RESOURCES—PATIENT EDUCATION MATERIALS

Medline Plus
Sexually Transmitted Diseases
http://www.nlm.nih.gov/medlineplus/sexuallytransmitteddiseases.html.

TeensHealth
About Sexually Transmitted Diseases
http://www.kidshealth.org/teen/sexual_health/stds/std.html

eMedicineHealth
Sexually Transmitted Diseases
http://www.emedicinehealth.com/sexually_transmitted_diseases/article_em.htm.

womenshealth.gov
Sexually Transmitted Diseases Overview
http://www.4woman.gov/faq/stdsgen.htm

HealthAtoZ
Sexually Transmitted Diseases
http://www.healthatoz.com/healthatoz/Atoz/common/standard/transform.jsp?
     requestURI=/healthatoz/Atoz/dc/caz/repr/stds/stds_gen_ovw.jsp

SUGGESTED READINGS

ACOG Committee on Adolescent Health Care. Sexually transmitted diseases in adolescents. *ACOG Comm Opin No. 301* 2004;104(4):891–898.
Centers for Disease Control and Prevention. Sexually transmitted diseases treatment guidelines 2006. *MMWR* 2006;55(RR-11):1–9. Available at http://www.cdc.gov/std/
Golden MR. Effect of expedited treatment of sex partners on recurrent or persistent gonorrhea or chlamydia infection. *New Engl J Med* 2005;352(7):676–685.

References

1. Eng TR, Butler WT, eds. *The hidden epidemic: confronting sexually transmitted diseases. Institute of Medicine. Committee on Prevention and Control of Sexually Transmitted Diseases*. Washington, DC: National Academy Press, 1997:1–432.
2. Workowski KA. U.S. Centers for Disease Control and Prevention guidelines for the treatment of sexually transmitted diseases: an opportunity to unify clinical and public health practice. *Ann Intern Med* 2002;137(4):255–262.

3. Centers for Disease Control and Prevention. Sexually transmitted diseases treatment guidelines 2002. *MMWR* 2002;51(RR-6):1–7.

4. Centers for Disease Control and Prevention. *STD surveillance 2004: national profile.* http://www.cdc.gov/std/stats/natprointro.htm, accessed September 28, 2006.

5. Nusbaum MRH. The proactive sexual health history. *Am Fam Phys* 2002; 66(9):1705–1712.

6. Centers for Disease Control and Prevention. Revised guidelines for HIV counseling, testing, and referral. Technical expert panel review of CDC HIV counseling, testing, and referral guidelines. *MMWR* 2001;50(RR-19):1–10.

7. Crosby RA. Project RESPECT Study Group. Misconceptions about STD-protective behavior. *Am J Prev Med* 2000;19(3):167–173.

8. Bull SS. The process of seeking sex partners online and implications for STD/HIV prevention. *AIDS Care* 2004;16(8):1012–1020.

9. Centers for Disease Control and Prevention. Sexually transmitted diseases treatment guidelines 2006. *MMWR* 2006;55(RR-11):1–9.

10. ACOG Committee on Adolescent Health Care. Sexually transmitted diseases in adolescents. *ACOG Comm Opin No. 301* 2004;104(4):891–898.

11. Cohen DA. Where and when do youths have sex? The potential role of adult supervision. *Pediatrics* 2002;110(6):e66.

12. Kaestle CE. Sexual activity among adolescents in romantic relationships with friends, acquaintances, or strangers. *Arch Pediatr Adolesc Med* 2005;159(9):849–853.

13. U.S. Preventive Services Task Force Guide to Clinical Preventive Services. http://www.ahrq.gov/clinic/cps3dix.htm#infectious, accessed September 28, 2006.

14. Golden MR. Effect of expedited treatment of sex partners on recurrent or persistent gonorrhea or chlamydia infection. *New Engl J Med* 2005;352(7):676–685.

15. Klausner JD. Patient-delivered therapy for chlamydia: putting research into practice. *Sex Transm Dis* 2003;30(6):509–511.

16. Mao C. Efficacy of human papillomavirus-16 vaccine to prevent cervical intraepithelial neoplasia: a randomized controlled trial. *Obstet Gynecol* 2006;107(1): 18–27.

17. Family Health International AIDSCAP Project. *Behavioral change communication for STD prevention and treatment handbook.* http://www.fhi.org/en/HIVAIDS/pub/ guide/BCC+Handbooks/BCC+for+STD+Treatment+and+Prevention.htm, accessed September 28, 2006.

18. Campos-Outcalt D. Clarifying the U.S. Preventive Services Task Force's 2005 recommendations. *J Fam Pract* 2005;55(5):425–428.

19. Bolu OO. Is HIV/sexually transmitted disease prevention counseling effective among vulnerable populations?: a subset analysis of data collected for a randomized, controlled trial evaluating counseling efficacy (Project RESPECT). *Sex Transm Dis* 2004;31(8):469–474.

20. Kamb ML. Efficacy of risk-reduction counseling to prevent human immunodeficiency virus and sexually transmitted diseases (Project RESPECT). *JAMA* 1998;280(13):1161–1167.

21. Henderson Z. Sexually transmitted disease care in managed care organizations. *Infect Dis Clin N Am* 2005;19:491–511.

22. Nelson HD. Screening for Chlamydia infection: a summary of the evidence. *Am J Prev Med* 2001;20(3S):95–107.

23. Handsfield HH. Hepatitis A and B immunization in persons being evaluated for sexually transmitted diseases. *Am J Med* 2005;118(10A):69S–74S.

CHAPTER 13

Depression, Mood Disorders, and Cognitive Impairment

Daniel E. Ford

Clinicians now acknowledge what the population has known for many years. Health is more than just the absence of physical disease. In 1948, the World Health Organization defined health as "a state of complete physical, mental, and social well-being and not merely the absence of disease or infirmity" (1). Research makes it clear that it is very difficult to maintain a perfect state in any of these areas without nurturing strengths in the others. The availability of social support and social integration is associated with a better prognosis for many chronic illnesses. Poor physical health is a predictor of poor mental health, and poor mental health, particularly depression and cognitive impairment, leads to poor physical health, through multiple pathways. Patients also benefit from positive mental health—not just the absence of depression or negative symptoms, but the presence of positive well-being including vitality, satisfaction, creativity, productivity, and high self-esteem. Attention to mental health is therefore central to health promotion and disease prevention in clinical practice.

This chapter examines the assessment and treatment of depression, mood disorders, and cognitive impairment. Its predominant focus is on depression, the treatment of which is supported by the strongest evidence of benefit. The presentation and treatment of depression in the clinical setting are the subject of an extensive literature. This chapter does not discuss the assessment and treatment of patients with other mental or behavioral concerns (e.g., anger, loneliness, and general unhappiness). The evidence base for both the accuracy and clinical utility of such assessment is limited, and the public is even more ambivalent about discussing these topics in the primary care setting than it is about discussing depression. For depression, outcomes can be greatly improved by closing the gap between the ideal and current treatment practices. Doing so should be their first priority, before clinicians turn to dealing with less well-identified mental conditions.

Mental health relates to many of the topics discussed in this book. Depression is a risk factor for many of the conditions that are targeted by clinical preventive services. For example, depression approximately doubles the risk of a new myocardial infarction or an ischemic stroke. Individuals

311

with depression are less likely to be adherent to taking medications, such as aspirin chemoprophylaxis for heart disease (see Chapter 15), or to successfully adopt new health behaviors. Patients with depression are more likely to smoke cigarettes, less likely to try quitting, and less successful at quitting than those without depression (see Chapter 9). Adolescents with depression are more likely to start smoking than are their peers. Alcohol and substance abuse are also more common among those with depression (see Chapter 10). Individuals with depression may be more likely to be sedentary and obese. Given the low levels of self-efficacy and the undervaluing of the future that characterize depression, it is not surprising that behavior change is particularly difficult for this group of patients. Anxiety and cognitive impairment also affect the ability of patients to pursue health-promoting behavior change, to obtain recommended clinical preventive services, and to adhere to follow-up regimens.

DEPRESSION

Screening and Clinical Assessment

The first step in the appropriate management of depression is accurate detection. The prevention program of a practice should include a plan for identifying patients with depression, both to accurately assess risk for new health conditions and to offer effective options for treatment or management. Depression is present in approximately 5–15% of patients who present for primary care, with higher prevalence rates observed among women and young adults. Although depression presents clinically in heterogeneous forms, particularly in primary care, two major syndromes are recognized by the *Diagnostic and Statistical Manual Fourth Edition* (DSM-IV) (2). The diagnosis of *major depression* requires the presence of at least five symptoms, with one being depressed mood or lack of joy for a duration of at least 2 weeks. *Dysthymia* requires depressed mood or lack of joy lasting at least 2 years with fewer depression symptoms than are required for major depression. See "Suggested Readings" (page 331) for more details on diagnostic criteria.

A variety of questionnaire instruments is available to screen for depression. Instruments that have been used for many years include the Zung Self-Rating Depression Scale, the Center for Epidemiological Studies Depression Scale, and the Beck Depression Inventory. In its 2002 review of depression screening, the U.S. Preventive Services Task Force provided details about instruments available at the time (3). It concluded that the accuracy of most depression questionnaires for the primary care setting was comparable. The decision about which depression instrument to use in practice is guided less by the accuracy of the questionnaire and more by the number of questions, the ease of formatting, the associated costs, and the symptom domains the questionnaire covers.

The Patient Health Questionnaire (PHQ-9) is a recently developed depression assessment instrument that is becoming the most commonly used standard (4,5). Its advantages include its relative brevity—it has only nine questions (see Fig. 13.1)—and its sensitivity (85%) and specificity (75%) compared with structured clinical interviews by mental health specialists. The questions in the PHQ-9 are very similar to those used in the most common psychiatric diagnostic interviews and reflect the criteria for major

PATIENT HEALTH QUESTIONNAIRE (PHQ-9)

NAME:_____ DATE:_____

Over the *last 2 weeks,* how often have you been bothered by any of the following problems? (use "✓" to indicate your answer)	Not at all	Several days	More than half the days	Nearly every day
1. Little interest or pleasure in doing things	0	1	2	3
2. Feeling down, depressed, or hopeless	0	1	2	3
3. Trouble falling or staying asleep, or sleeping too much	0	1	2	3
4. Feeling tired or having little energy	0	1	2	3
5. Poor appetite or overeating	0	1	2	3
6. Feeling bad about yourself—or that you are a failure or have let yourself or your family down	0	1	2	3
7. Trouble concentrating on things, such as reading the newspaper or watching television	0	1	2	3
8. Moving or speaking so slowly that other people could have noticed. Or the opposite—being so fidgety or restless that you have been moving around a lot more than usual	0	1	2	3
9. Thoughts that you would be better off dead, or of hurting yourself in some way	0	1	2	3

add columns: [ ] + [ ] + [ ]

(Healthcare professional: For interpretation of TOTAL, **TOTAL:** [ ]
please refer to accompanying scoring card.)

10. If you checked off *any* problems, how *difficult* have these problems made it for you to do your work, take care of things at home, or get along with other people?	**Not difficult at all** _____
	Somewhat difficult _____
	Very difficult _____
	Extremely difficult _____

PHQ-9 is adapted from PRIME MD TODAY, developed by Drs Robert L. Spitzer, Janet B.W. Williams, Kurt Kroenke, and colleagues, with an educational grant from Pfizer Inc. For research information, contact Dr Spitzer at rls8@columbia.edu. Use of the PHQ-9 may only be made in accordance with the Terms of Use available at *http://www.pfizer.com.* Copyright ©1999 Pfizer Inc. All rights reserved. PRIME MD TODAY is a trademark of Pfizer Inc.

Figure 13.1 • Patient Health Questionnaire (PHQ). (Courtesy of Pfizer.)

Fold back this page before administering this questionnaire

INSTRUCTIONS FOR USE

for doctor or healthcare professional use only

PHQ-9 QUICK DEPRESSION ASSESSMENT

For initial diagnosis:

1. Patient completes PHQ-9 Quick Depression Assessment on accompanying tear-off pad.
2. If there are at least 4✓s in the shaded section (including Questions #1 and #2), consider a depressive disorder. Add score to determine severity.
3. **Consider Major Depressive Disorder**
   –if there are at least 5✓s in the shaded section (one of which corresponds to Question #1 or #2)
   Consider Other Depressive Disorder
   –if there are 2 to 4✓s in the shaded section (one of which corresponds to Question #1 or #2)

Note: Since the questionnaire relies on patient self-report, all responses should be verified by the clinician and a definitive diagnosis made on clinical grounds, taking into account how well the patient understood the questionnaire, as well as other relevant information from the patient. Diagnoses of Major Depressive Disorder or Other Depressive Disorder also require impairment of social,occupational, or other important areas of functioning (Question #10) and ruling out normal bereavement, a history of a Manic Episode (Bipolar Disorder), and a physical disorder, medication, or other drug as the biological cause of the depressive symptoms.

To monitor severity over time for newly diagnosed patients or patients in current treatment for depression:

1. Patients may complete questionnaires at baseline and at regular intervals (eg, every 2 weeks) at home and bring them in at their next appointment for scoring or they may complete the questionnaire during each scheduled appointment.
2. Add up ✓s by column. For every✓: Several days = 1   More than half the days = 2   Nearly every day = 3
3. Add together column scores to get a TOTAL score.
4. Refer to the subsequent PHQ-9 Scoring Card to interpret the TOTAL score.
5. Results may be included in patients' files to assist you in setting up a treatment goal, determining degree of response, as well as guiding treatment intervention.

PHQ-9 SCORING CARD FOR SEVERITY DETERMINATION
for healthcare professional use only
Scoring–add up all checked boxes on PHQ-9
For every✓ : Not at all = 0; Several days = 1;
More than half the days = 2; Nearly every day = 3
Interpretation of Total Score
Total Score Depression Severity
      0-4   None
      5-9   Mild depression
    10-14 Moderate depression
    15-19 Moderately severe depression
    20-27 Severe depression

Figure 13.1 • *(Continued).*

depression presented in the DSM-IV. Perhaps the most important advantage of the PHQ-9 is that it can serve not only to help make the diagnosis but also to help the clinician to follow the course and severity of the depression. A PHQ-9 score below 5 indicates resolution of depression, 10–14 indicates moderate depression, and 15 or more indicates severe depression. A 5-point reduction in the PHQ-9 score is considered a significant clinical improvement in depression even if complete resolution is not achieved.

The PHQ-9, like other depression questionnaires, has its limitations. For example, the PHQ-9 score does not by itself establish the primary diagnosis. When patients present with both a high PHQ-9 score and substantial medical comorbidity, substance abuse, or severe mental illness, clinicians must use their clinical judgment to identify the primary treatment target. Further, the PHQ-9 does not measure anxiety, pain, hopelessness, or loneliness. Functional status, a very important factor in assessing the need for treatment, is addressed by only one question (question 10) appended to the PHQ-9. The PHQ-9 does include a question on suicidal ideation (question 9); clinicians who use the instrument must therefore institute a plan to examine the patient's response in a timely manner.

Although the level of attention to depression in primary care has improved in recent years—clinicians know more about depression than they did formerly, and rates of detection and treatment have increased—a substantial gap in the detection of depression persists. Closing the gap requires not only greater diligence in detecting the disease and assessing its severity but also the adoption of system solutions to ensure that those identified with the disease receive proper care. In its last review of the topic, the U.S. Preventive Services Task Force recommended screening for depression only if the practice has a comprehensive program to care for screen-detected cases. Studies that have evaluated isolated depression screening without standardized follow-up have not reported improved outcomes. The elements of a comprehensive practice system for depression care are reviewed in the subsequent text (see "Comprehensive Programs" on page 322). Greater resources are required to improve outcomes for screen-detected cases not previously recognized by the patient or clinician, because these individuals are less likely to accept usual forms of depression treatment and may have more associated comorbidities.

Treatment

Most individuals with depression do not respond to the first treatment that is provided. Success depends on careful monitoring for the persistence or progression of symptoms and developing a relationship where both clinicians and patients are willing to work together until the best treatment plan is identified. Some patients who appear to have acute symptoms of depression can resolve their illness within weeks without any specific treatment. In patients presenting with signs of depression and who do not require urgent treatment, clinicians can reasonably initiate a "watchful waiting" protocol. This protocol involves a brief diagnostic assessment, including a determination of the level of functioning, education about the natural history and consequences of depression, presentation of depression treatment options, and agreement on the criteria for initiating treatment. For example, the patient and clinician might agree that the patient will return in 4 weeks to meet with the practice's depression care manager (see page 324), who will administer the PHQ-9 and initiate treatment if the score is abnormal or the patient has missed more than 3 days of work in the last month.

The two general approaches to treating depression—both supported by strong evidence of effectiveness—are counseling/psychotherapy and pharmacotherapy. Patients should be offered a choice between these options.

COUNSELING/PSYCHOTHERAPY

At least 50% of patients diagnosed with depression prefer to begin with the counseling/psychotherapy approach. Patients should be informed that counseling/psychotherapy is generally effective only if they complete six to eight sessions at a periodicity of every 1–2 weeks under the care of a competent therapist. Cognitive-behavioral, interpersonal, and problem-solving therapy have all been demonstrated to be more effective than unfocused talk therapy. Access to competent therapists who do not charge high out-of-pocket copayments is limited under many health plans, but locating such therapists to whom their patients can be referred should be a priority for primary care clinicians. This is particularly true for those practices serving a large number of African American and Hispanic patients, who tend to prefer counseling over pharmacotherapy (6).

Current knowledge is incomplete regarding the quality of counseling provided in the community. In general, licensed professionals such as psychologists, social workers, or Masters-level counselors are thought to consistently provide the highest level of quality. Although primary care physicians can provide supplemental counseling that may increase the effectiveness of pharmacotherapy, most do not have the time or skills to provide intensive counseling for those patients who elect a counseling-only approach. Increasingly, psychiatrists are focusing on diagnosis and medication management and for the most part no longer provide intensive counseling services.

PHARMACOTHERAPY

Currently available antidepressant medications are listed in Table 13.1. The foundation for successful pharmacotherapy is the creation of a relationship and understanding with patients that will allow the dose and choice of medications to be modified without dousing optimism that an effective antidepressant with acceptable side effects will be identified. As of this writing (2006), current research has not yet determined which patients are most likely to respond to a specific class of antidepressants. Certainly it is worthwhile to take a history of previous use of antidepressant medications to assess past experience with effectiveness and side effects. Knowing whether close family members with depression have responded to certain medications or experienced side effects may also be helpful.

Selective serotonin reuptake inhibitors (SSRIs) remain the first choice for antidepressant pharmacotherapy because of their effectiveness, once-a-day dosing, and relatively low incidence of side effects. At this time, there is

TABLE 13.1 Commonly Used Antidepressant Medications

Antidepressant[a]	Daily Therapeutic Dose Range	Initial Suggested Dose	Advantages	Disadvantages
		Serotonin Reuptake Inhibitors (SSRIs)[b]		
Citalopram (Celexa)	20–40 mg	20 mg in morning with food (10 mg in elderly or those with panic disorder)	Possibly fewer cytochrome P-450 interactions; generic available	Need lower dose in presence of hepatic failure
Escitalopram (Lexapro)	10–20 mg	10 mg	S-enantiomer more potent than racemic; 10 mg dose usually effective for most patients	—
Fluoxetine (Prozac)	10–80 mg	20 mg in morning with food (10 mg in elderly and those with comorbid panic disorder)	Indicated for obsessive compulsive disorder; long half-life good for poor adherence and missed doses; generic available; less frequent discontinuation symptoms	Slower to reach steady state; sometimes too stimulating; possibly more cytochrome P-450 interactions

(continued)

TABLE 13.1 (Continued)

Antidepressant[a]	Therapeutic Dose Range (mg/d)	Initial Suggested Dose	Advantages	Disadvantages
Paroxetine (Paxil)	10–50 mg (40 mg in elderly)	20 mg once daily, usually in morning with food (10 mg in elderly and those with comorbid panic disorder)	FDA approved for most anxiety disorders; generic available	Sometimes sedating; occasionally more anticholinergic-like effects; possibly more cytochrome P-450 interactions; may have more frequent discontinuation symptoms
(Paxil CR)	25–62.5 mg (50 mg in elderly)	25 mg daily (12.5 mg in elderly and those with panic disorder)	May cause less nausea and GI distress	May have greater risk of major congenital malformations than other SSRIs
Sertraline (Zoloft)	25–200 mg	50 mg once daily, usually in morning with food (25 mg for elderly)	FDA approved for anxiety disorders; safety shown post myocardial infarction; generic available	Slightly more GI side effects

Serotonin and Norepinephrine Antagonists

Mirtazapine (Remeron)	15–45 mg	15 mg at bedtime (7.5 mg for those in need of sedation/hypnotic)	Few drug interactions; less or no adverse effects on sexual function; less sedation as dose increased; may stimulate appetite	Sedation at low dose only; may initially stimulate appetite

Norepinephrine and Dopamine-Reuptake Inhibitors

Bupropion[c] (Wellbutrin, Wellbutrin SR, Wellbutrin XL)	300–400 mg	150 mg in morning	Stimulating; less or no adverse effects on sexual function	At higher dose, may induce seizures in persons with seizure disorder; no effect on anxiety disorders

Serotonin and Norepinephrine-Reuptake Inhibitor

Venlafaxine (Effexor, Effexor XR)	75–375 mg	75 mg with food; if anxious or debilitated, 37.5 mg	XR version can be taken QD; helpful for anxiety disorders; possibly fewer cytochrome P-450 interactions	May increase blood pressure at higher doses; overdose may be more serious than for SSRIs
Duloxetine (Cymbalta)	30–60 mg	20–30 mg	May be better at relieving pain; may have lower sexual side effects	GI side effects more common; expensive

(continued)

319

TABLE 13.1 (Continued)

Antidepressant[a]	Therapeutic Dose Range (mg/d)	Initial Suggested Dose	Advantages	Disadvantages
		Primarily Norepinephrine Reuptake Inhibitor		
Desipramine[d] (Norpramin, Pertofrane)	100–300 mg (25–100 mg in elderly)	50 mg in the morning	More effect on norepinephrine than serotonin; less sedating; generic available	Anticholinergic effects of TCAs; caution with BPH; can exacerbate cardiac conduction problems or CHF
Nortriptyline[d] (Aventyl, Pamelor)	25–150 mg	25 mg (10 mg in frail elderly) in the evening	Availability of reliable, valid blood levels; less likely than other TCAs to induce orthostatic hypotension; generic available	Anticholinergic effects of TCAs; caution with BPH; can exacerbate cardiac conduction problems or CHF

FDA = U.S. Food and Drug Administration; GI = gastrointestinal; TCA = tricyclic antidepressants; BPH = benign prostatic hyperplasia; CHF = congestive heart failure.

[a]There are more antidepressants than those listed in this table; however, this list provides a reasonable variety of drugs that have different side effects and act by different neurotransmitter mechanisms. Monoamine oxidase (MAO) inhibitors are not included.

[b]For SSRIs, generally start at the beginning of the therapeutic range. If side effects are bothersome, reduce the dose and increase more slowly. In debilitated patients or those sensitive to medications, start at a lower dose. For all antidepressants, allow 4 weeks at a therapeutic dose and assess for a response. If the response is only partially effective, then increase the dose. If there is no response or symptoms worsen, then consider switching drugs.

[c]Generally avoid bupropion in patients with a history of seizures or anorexia nervosa.

[d]Tricyclic antidepressants (TCAs) have lower costs but somewhat higher discontinuation rates compared to SSRIs due to side effects, and they are more lethal in an overdose.

very little evidence that any one SSRI is substantially better than another. Citalopram and sertraline may produce fewer drug–drug interactions. As more of the SSRIs become available in generic form, wider variability in costs may also influence the selection of agents.

Starting treatment with bupropion is also a reasonable choice, particularly because approximately 50% of patients with depression may be current smokers. Chapter 9 discusses the effectiveness and use of bupropion to assist patients with smoking cessation (see page 241). Bupropion is more likely than SSRI medications to increase motivation and physical activity, but this may be difficult for patients who had high levels of anxiety and insomnia before starting treatment.

Effective management of antidepressant medications extends beyond the initial prescription, as patients usually require subsequent adjustments. Initial rates of adherence to antidepressants are relatively low. Many patients require an adjustment in the medication schedule to address either the occurrence of side effects or an inadequate therapeutic response. Patients started on an antidepressant should be given a return appointment in 1–2 weeks. If this is not possible, they should be contacted by telephone during this time. Clinicians should be prepared to increase the dose of the medication to the accepted limit in an effort to achieve resolution, and they should not be satisfied with partial treatment of the depression.

By 6 weeks of treatment, if there has not been at least some improvement in the level of clinical depression, a change in therapy and more careful monitoring are warranted. More than half of patients with depression will require either a switch from or augmentation of their first antidepressant medication. In the Sequenced Treatment Alternatives to Relieve Depression (STAR*D) study (7), approximately one-third of the patients who did not respond to citalopram as the initial therapy did respond to a second SSRI. Therefore, if a patient does not respond to one SSRI and experiences minimal or no side effects, switching to a second SSRI is a reasonable choice. Switching to a serotonin and norepinephrine dual agent, such as venlafaxine or duloxetine, is also a good choice. Clinicians should be aware that venlafaxine can raise blood pressure, a potential concern for patients at high risk of cardiovascular disease.

Tricyclic antidepressants are also effective, but they carry a higher risk of anticholinergic side effects (e.g., orthostatic hypotension, dry mouth, urinary retention). Managing these side effects is particularly challenging with older adults. Tricyclic antidepressants with fewer anticholinergic effects, such as nortriptyline or desipramine, are preferred over amitryptyline.

As with hypertension, treatment of depression frequently requires the use of multiple medications to reach target goals. It is difficult to determine who will respond to which antidepressant. Both the clinician and the patient must be prepared for multiple assessments and have patience until goals are reached. As with hypertension, it usually makes sense to combine medications that utilize different mechanisms of action. When augmenting with a second agent, such as adding bupropion to an SSRI, the clinician should first prescribe a low dose.

It is important to regularly monitor patients on antidepressant medication. The primary care clinician must be conscientious about intervening when therapy is proving to be unsatisfactory (i.e., inadequate resolution of the depression). Clinicians should keep trying different medication regimens—there is no one correct choice in this realm. Most primary care clinicians are capable of managing complex antidepressant medication schedules. However, if the clinician feels that referral to a psychiatrist is necessary, it is better to make such a referral sooner rather than later.

Comprehensive Programs

The elements of a comprehensive approach to the care of depression in primary care are captured in the Chronic Care Model synthesized by Edward Wagner et al. (8). This model emphasizes six elements that are necessary for a prepared patient and health care delivery system: (a) organizational support, (b) enhancing self-management, (c) practice design, (d) decision support, (e) information technology, and (f) community linkages. These elements are reviewed further in the subsequent text. Furthermore, studies of depression care indicate that successful comprehensive depression programs apply more than one practice intervention (including more than one clinician in the team) and are supported by a long-term commitment by the practice (9).

ORGANIZATIONAL SUPPORT

The extensive changes required to support the Chronic Care Model in primary care call upon practices and systems of care to provide organizational support to provide the necessary resources and to keep the staff engaged when the inevitable bumps in the road arise. Leaders need to communicate their vision for the new program, invest the resources for requisite information technology (see page 324), provide time off for staff to plan and be trained, and be willing to reward those staff who adopt the new model of care. Although the requisite organizational leadership is most easily identified in larger practices, even smaller practices can ensure that senior management will support implementation of the new model of care. High quality care for depression will often require practices to consider new relationships with behavioral health organizations. Practice managers and health systems need to provide support and take initiative in working through the funding and care coordination issues that are part of forging new relationships between primary care and behavioral health providers.

ENHANCING SELF-MANAGEMENT

Patients with depression spend a tiny portion of their lives with clinicians. Each day, patients with depression and other chronic diseases must decide whether and how to manage their conditions and respond to symptoms. The goal of each patient visit should be to prepare patients for this work. The support of self-management can begin by asking patients exactly what they do when they have a bad day and feel depressed, or how they typically respond when someone invites them to go shopping or see a movie. Knowing this, the clinician can discuss constructive alternatives that are more likely to mitigate their depression.

The objective during the patient visit should be to identify a specific measurable self-management goal that the patient feels can be successfully achieved. For example, a patient might respond that she tends to stay home and eat more when she feels blue. A constructive goal to be achieved before the next visit might be to not eat and instead walk to her sister's house at least half the days she feels depressed. Other self-management goals might include taking antidepressant medication 6 out of 7 days, making an appointment at an employment agency, reading a book on depression, visiting a depression Internet support group, or leaving the house everyday for at least 1 hour. By having this discussion, clinicians acknowledge the day-to-day struggles of their patients, help their patients identify specific problems, assess potential coping strategies, deconstruct problems into smaller pieces, respect patients' choices, and ultimately enhance their self-efficacy.

DECISION SUPPORT

Primary care clinicians should have ready access to treatment protocols for patients with depression. Practice guidelines on the topic are listed on page 331 under "Suggested Readings." Most primary care practices will benefit from developing a close working relationship with a mental health specialist who can provide overall decision support for a comprehensive depression detection and treatment program. The mental health specialist can help the practice develop strategies/protocols for diagnosing and monitoring depression, assessing psychiatric comorbidity, developing complex psychopharmacology protocols, and establishing criteria for referral to mental health specialists. This consultant may also be able to outline clearer pathways for referring patients to specialty mental health providers as well.

Aside from this general consultative role, clinicians should also engage mental health specialists for consultations concerning difficult cases, patients who will not accept referrals to mental health specialists, or those lacking insurance coverage. Some practices hire part-time mental health specialists or forge new relationships with behavioral health centers to enhance this level of decision support. Mental health specialists are often identified to supervise and provide decision support to the depression care coordinators of a practice (see subsequent text). Decision support for patients is also important. Clinicians should provide patients with information about best practices for treatment of depression and how depression is treated at the practice. See "Resources—Patient Education Materials" at the end of the chapter.

PRACTICE DESIGN

Several elements of practice design are necessary for quality depression care. The first is to utilize a standard for both diagnosing and monitoring depression treatment within the practice. A depression assessment instrument, such as the PHQ-9 discussed on page 313, should be adopted. If optimal outcomes are to be achieved for patients with depression, in most primary care practices it will be necessary to utilize the services of a mental health care manager. The care manager may have several roles, including performing the follow-up for patients who do not return for their appointments, assessing the severity of depression symptoms, educating patients about depression treatment options, reinforcing treatment plans, monitoring self-management goals and patients' efforts to achieve them, and providing emotional support.

If resources are available to support a dedicated individual to work exclusively as a depression care manager, there is a high probability that depression outcomes will improve. If such resources are lacking, quite often the best alternative is to divide the work of the care manager among multiple personnel in the office such as the primary care clinicians, nurses, or extant behavioral health specialists. Personnel with limited professional education can undergo training to provide a limited but very useful service of following up and monitoring patients with depression.

Although it is ideal to have the care manager based within the primary care practice, this is often not feasible nor financially viable. Telephone-based care management from a central location, such as that offered through health plans and employers, has been shown to be effective. When the care management services are not based within the practice, however, clinicians may take longer to acquire confidence in the care managers and the depression protocols.

CLINICAL INFORMATION SYSTEMS

Effective monitoring of depression to establish whether remission is partial or complete is best accomplished by using some type of clinical information system. The optimal clinical information system is electronic. See Chapter 22 for further details about automated systems. Although direct entry of data by patients is ideal, the most common systems require data entry by staff. Finding an efficient way to accomplish data entry is essential to the long-term success of a comprehensive depression treatment program.

The clinical information system should also provide prompts for staff when processes of care and outcomes are not reaching goals. In the trials that demonstrated the effectiveness of multicomponent collaborative care, an essential element was the existence of procedures to make certain that clinicians received reminders when a patient had not undergone a reassessment of their depression within 4 weeks of starting treatment. Finally, a clinical information system can help measure overall performance in relation to depression care. Performance measures might include the proportion of patients with depression that make contact with the health care system 1–3 weeks after starting treatment, that are adherent to the depression treatment plan, and that meet criteria for resolution of depression by 6 months.

Measuring these process and outcome measures serves several purposes. First, performance is usually less than what the practice might predict, and documenting the discrepancy can act as a catalyst for change. Primary care practices with established systems for quality improvement and "benchmarking" can motivate individual clinicians to improve the quality of their care by demonstrating how their performance compares to that of their peers. Second, tracking the process and outcome measures over time can guide strategic planning on where to most efficiently target resources to improve outcomes. For example, performance data might persuade a practice that its depression care manager should emphasize recontact with patients for the first depression reassessment (1–3 weeks after initiating treatment) and that additional follow-up will not be cost effective.

Third, performance data are increasingly being requested from quality assessment organizations as a measure of the quality of care in a practice. With these data a practice can negotiate with funders for additional resources, and performance data are essential for "pay-for-performance" arrangements (see page 579). Primary care practices are better positioned to obtain payment for additional resources when they can provide data to substantiate a need and underscore the potential improvement in outcomes that would be achieved by more rational funding of depression care.

LINKAGES WITH COMMUNITY RESOURCES

Primary care clinicians sometimes believe that they must provide all of the services required by patients in their care. Patients with depression, however, often face a complex array of challenges including financial difficulties, inadequate housing, lack of health insurance, unstable employment, disrupted relationships and living arrangements, and lack of social support. For women presenting with depression in primary care, the exposure to interpersonal violence is substantial. Primary care clinicians should engage community resource support organizations informally, and when possible, under more formal arrangements. These organizations commonly include community mental health centers, domestic violence shelters, the local Young Men's Christian Association (YMCA), and vocational rehabilitation centers. Community resource organizations may be willing to trade easier access to their services in exchange for primary care for their clients. Through these partnerships, clinicians can help ensure that their patients receive the highest quality of care and level of support for their depression.

SCREENING AND MANAGEMENT OF OTHER MENTAL DISORDERS

There is limited evidence that screening for other mental disorders, such as anxiety and cognitive impairment, is effective in improving patient outcomes even when accompanied by a comprehensive treatment program. However, many primary care practices find it inefficient to implement a new program for mental disorders that only addresses depression. Expanding the focus to include screening for anxiety and cognitive disorders in certain circumstances may be more efficient and more consistent with the comprehensive philosophy of primary care.

Anxiety Disorders

Common anxiety disorders in the primary care population include generalized anxiety disorder, panic disorder, phobias, and posttraumatic stress disorder. An evidence-based argument to support screening for these conditions would require evidence that screening methods (beyond the usual clinical interview) would identify individuals with previously undetected anxiety disorders and that treatment at this earlier stage would produce better outcomes than usual care. For several reasons, this is a difficult threshold to meet.

First, there is wide variation in usual care. Some clinicians are much better at detection and treatment of anxiety disorders than others. The best performing clinicians would have the least to gain from new screening programs. Second, there are multiple anxiety disorders and specific questions that are required to screen for each disorder. Third, failure to recognize a mental disorder is less common with anxiety disorders than with depression, creating less of a need for screening. Fourth, there is a large overlap between depression and the more severe anxiety disorders. Screening programs for depression can also detect a large percentage of patients with severe anxiety disorders.

Although there is currently little evidence that an active program to screen for anxiety disorders is effective, randomized trials have demonstrated improved outcomes and reasonable costs when primary care practices adopt comprehensive treatment programs for anxiety disorders that come to clinical attention under usual care. For example, in one trial the comprehensive intervention consisted of cognitive behavioral therapy and pharmacotherapy, delivered by a mental health therapist and primary care physician over six sessions with up to six follow-up telephone calls during 1 year (10). In another trial, the practices adopted a telephone-based care management program for patients with panic and generalized anxiety disorder (11).

With a comprehensive treatment program in place, a primary care practice might find it reasonable to look for anxiety disorders in patients with atypical presentations or anxiety symptoms that are too subtle to normally trigger treatment. Validated screening instruments for anxiety disorders are lacking, but one option is the Generalized Anxiety Disorder Severity Scale (12).

Cognitive Impairment or Dementia

Dementia is defined as an acquired syndrome of decline in memory and at least one other cognitive domain such as language, visual-spatial, or executive function sufficient to interfere with social and occupational functioning in an alert person (2). Dementia is most frequently due to Alzheimer's disease or multiple infarcts from cerebrovascular disease.

Interest in cognitive impairment has heightened in recent years with the growth in the number of seniors and of patients with dementia, and the availability of new medications that have at least a modest impact on the decline of cognitive function.

SCREENING

Screening for cognitive impairment could be considered for patients aged 65 years and older, especially those with a family history of dementia or with a high risk of cardiovascular disease. Potential approaches include directly testing cognitive function, assessing functional deficits, or asking for reports of cognition and function from proxy informants.

The U.S. Preventive Services Task Force, the American Academy of Neurology, and the American Academy of Family Physicians have each concluded that evidence is lacking to recommend routine screening for dementia (13). Available data do not permit the magnitude of benefit from early detection and treatment to be accurately gauged. Screening could be of potential benefit by finding a reversible cause of dementia (e.g., hypothyroidism, vitamin B_{12} deficiency), but such causes explain only 1–2% of cases and are often detected in other ways. Cognitive function screening could identify individuals who cannot safely drive a motor vehicle, but evidence that such screening is of practical utility is limited (14). Nor has control of cardiovascular risk factors (e.g., with blood pressure control or aspirin chemoprophylaxis) been shown to reduce the progression of dementia due to cerebrovascular disease.

Standardized instruments for evaluating cognitive function are available but unfortunately have limited diagnostic precision. The Mini-Mental Status Examination (MMSE, see Table 13.2) has been studied the most (15). The MMSE takes approximately 7 minutes to administer. Its scores are affected

TABLE 13.2 Mini-Mental Status Examination

Orientation
1. What is the
   Year? (1 point)
   Season? (1 point)
   Date? (1 point)
   Day? (1 point)
   Month? (1 point)
2. Where are we?
   State? (1 point)
   County? (1 point)
   Town/city? (1 point)
   Floor? (I point)
   Address/name of building? (1 point)

Registration
3. Name three objects, taking one second to say each. Then ask the patient all three after you have said them. Repeat the answers until the patient learns all three. (3 points)

Attention and Calculation
4. Serial sevens: give one point for each correct answer. Stop after five answers.
   (Alternative: spell *world* backward.) (5 points)

Recall
5. Ask for names of three objects learned in question 3. Give one point for each correct answer. (3 points)

Language
6. Point to a pencil and a watch. Have the patient name them as you point. (2 points)
7. Have the patient repeat "No ifs, ands, or buts." (1 point)
8. Have the patient follow a three-stage command: "Take the paper in your right hand. Fold the paper in half. Put the paper on the floor." (3 points)
9. Have the patient read and obey the following: "Close your eyes." (1 point)
10. Have the patient write a sentence of his or her own choice. (The sentence should contain a subject and an object and should make sense. Ignore spelling errors when scoring.) (1 point)
11. Show the patient a picture of two overlapping pentagrams. Ask the patient to copy it.(Give one point if all the sides and angles are preserved and if the intersecting sides form a quadrangle.) (1 point)

Adapted from Crum RM, Anthony JC, Bassett SS, et al. Population-based norms for the mini-mental state examination by age and educational level. *JAMA* 1993;269:2386–2391.
A total score of less than 24 out of 30 points is generally considered abnormal.

by the patient's level of educational attainment. Depending on the cutoff utilized for scoring, the MMSE has a sensitivity of 70–92% and a specificity of 56–96%. The poor specificity leads to a relatively low positive predictive value and the need for clinicians to sort out positive screening results. Rather than reflecting a deterioration in cognition, the MMSE score may be falsely low because of other medical conditions, such as hearing impairment or failure to complete the questions.

There are other tests that show promise. They include the Modified MMSE, Short Portable Mental Status Questionnaire, and the Mini-Cog (16). The Mini-Cog consists of a clock drawing task and the recall of three unrelated words (17). Some questionnaires ask the patient to rate their problems with memory across a range of activities. Finding more severe cases of cognitive impairment is possible by administering informant-based functional tests (completed by relatives or caregivers) such as the Functional Activities Questionnaire, the Informant Questionnaire on Cognitive Decline in the Elderly, and the Instrumental Activities of Daily Living questionnaire.

TREATMENT

If cognitive impairment is detected, use of cholinesterase inhibitors (see Table 13.3) has been shown to reduce progression of dementia, but their benefits are modest. Randomized controlled trials indicate that the medication effect is equivalent to delaying progression by up to 7 months in those with mild dementia and 2–5 months in those with moderate dementia. Cholinesterase inhibitors have had no demonstrable effect on maintaining function. Memantine, an N-methyl D-aspartate receptor antagonist, may be neuroprotective. It is generally well tolerated and appears to modestly reduce progression of dementia. It has also not been demonstrated to preserve function. Consistent evidence of effectiveness is also lacking for supplements to improve cognition, such as *Ginkgo biloba*, selegiline, and vitamin E.

Nonpharmacologic interventions such as mental exercises, behavioral training, and caregiver education have been proposed, but in rigorous trials, no improvements in functional status have been demonstrated. Observational studies suggest that integrated social networks, physical activity, and nonphysical activities that require mental work may reduce the risk of dementia (18).

CONCLUSION

Although further research will be required to establish supporting evidence to justify routine screening for mental disorders other than

TABLE 13.3 Medications for Dementia

Drug	Therapeutic Dose Range	Starting Dose	Advantages	Disadvantages
			Acetylcholinesterase Inhibitors	
Tacrine (Cogrex)	20–40 mg QID	10 mg QID	First in class	Rarely used; needs frequent dosing; must be avoided in the presence of liver disease; substantial GI side effects
Donepezil (Aricept)	5–10 mg QD	5 mg QD	Once-a-day dosing	Abnormal dreams; insomnia possible; avoid if a history of arrhythmia is present
Galantamine (Razadyne)	BID 8–12 mg	4 mg BID	Cognitive benefits sustained for 3 yr	Avoid if history of seizures; may have more GI side effects than donepezil
Rivastigmine (Exelon)	4–6 mg BID	1.5 mg BID	Useful for Parkinson's associated dementia	Slow titration recommended; possibly more GI side effects than donepezil; avoid if a history of arrhythmias is present
			N-methyl-D-aspartate (NMDA) Blockers	
Memantine (Namenda)	10 mg BID	5 mg QD	Very low side effect rate	Dizziness; do not use with sodium bicarbonate or acetazolamide (Diamox)

GI = gastrointestinal

depression—dementia, anxiety, and other conditions—clinicians should remain alert for these disorders as they interview patients, family members, and caregivers. As noted in Chapter 2, concerns raised by relatives and friends and subtle clues in the behavior and comments of patients can help the astute clinician recognize findings that require further diagnostic evaluation. Depression and other conditions often coexist with substance abuse. See Chapter 10 for further details about the assessment of alcohol and drug use in the primary care setting.

Although clinicians do need to improve their assessment skills, more complete detection and treatment of depression and other mental disorders will most likely also require greater public education. Patient attitudes regarding the need for depression treatment play an important role in their acceptance of and adherence to treatment.

As noted at the outset of this chapter, mental health involves more than the absence of pathology. The mental well-being of patients often suffers because of emotional difficulties, stress-related illness, personality disorders, and dysfunctional relationships. Such patients often benefit from individual counseling and/or family therapy. The amelioration of these conditions can play an important preventive role in averting secondary health and social consequences.

Finally, clinicians caring for children and adolescents should be conscientious about recognizing the presenting features of depression and other mental illnesses at these life stages. They should also recognize parents in need of emotional support, training in parenting skills, or reporting to protective service agencies for investigation of potential child abuse or neglect.

RESOURCES—PATIENT EDUCATION MATERIALS

National Institute of Mental Health
Depression
www.nimh.nih.gov/healthinformation/depressionmenu.cfm. Accessed 2007.

AetnaInteliHealth
Interactive tools: are you depressed? Depression screening with CES-D including feedback.
www.intelihealth.com/IH/ihtIH/WSIHWOOD/23722/9025.html. Accessed 2007.

SUGGESTED READINGS

American Academy of Neurology. *Detection, Diagnosis and Management of Dementia.*
www.aan.com/professionals/practice/pdfs/dementia_guideline.pdf.
Adelman AM, Daly MP. Initial evaluation of the patient with suspected dementia. *Am Fam Physician* 2005;71(9):1745–50. www.aafp.org/afp/20050501/1745.html.
Canadian Task Force Statement on Depression Screening. www.guideline.gov/summary/summary.aspx?doc_id=6524. 2005.
MacArthur Depression Primary Care Resources. www.depression-primarycare.org.
STAR*D Website on Sequenced Treatment of Depression. http://www.nimh.nih.gov/healthinformation/stard.cfm.

References

1. World Health Organization Constitution. *Basic documents*. Geneva: World Health Organization, 1948.
2. American Psychiatric Association. *Diagnostic and statistical manual of mental disorders*, 4th ed. Washington, DC: American Psychiatric Association, 1994.
3. U.S. Preventive Services Task Force. *Screening for depression: Recommendations and rationale*. May 2002. Agency for Healthcare Research and Quality, Rockville, MD. http://www.ahrq.gov/clinic/3rduspstf/depression/depressrr.htm. Accessed 2007.
4. Spitzer RL, Kroenke K, Williams JB. Validation and utility of a self-report version of the PRIME-MD: the PHQ primary care study. Primary care evaluation of mental disorders. Patient health questionnaire. *JAMA* 1999;282:1737–1744.
5. Lowe B, Unutzer J, Callahan CM, et al. Monitoring depression treatment outcomes with the patient health questionnaire. *Med Care* 2004;42:1194–2001.
6. Cooper LA, Gonzales JJ, Gallo JJ, et al. The acceptability of treatment for depression among African American, Hispanic and white primary care patients. *Med Care* 2003; 41:479–489.
7. Rush AJ, Trivedi MH, Wisniewski SR, et al. Acute and longer-term outcomes in depressed patients requiring one or several treatment steps: a STAR*D report. *Am J Psychiatry* 2006;163:1905–1917.
8. Bodenheimer T, Wagner EH, Grumbach K. Improving primary care for patients with chronic illness. *JAMA* 2002;288:1775–1779.
9. Gilbody S, Bower P, Fletcher J, et al. Collaborative care for depression: a cumulative meta-analysis and review of longer-term outcomes. *Arch Intern Med* 2006; 166:2314–2321.
10. Katon W, Russo J, Sherbourne C, et al. Incremental cost-effectiveness of a collaborative care intervention for panic disorder. *Psychol Med* 2006;36(3):353–363.
11. Rollman BL, Belnap BH, Mazumdar S, et al. A randomized trial to improve the quality of treatment for panic and generalized anxiety disorders in primary care. *Arch Gen Psychiatry* 2005;62:1332–1341.
12. Shear K, Belnap BH, Mazumdar S, et al. Generalized anxiety disorder severity scale (GADSS): a preliminary validation study. *Depress Anxiety* 2006;23:77–82.
13. U.S. Preventive Services Task Force. *Screening for dementia: Recommendations and rationale*. June 2003. Agency for Healthcare Research and Quality, Rockville, MD. http://www.ahrq.gov/clinic/3rduspstf/dementia/dementrr.htm. Accessed 2007.
14. Molnar FJ, Patel A, Marshall SC, et al. Clinical utility of office-based cognitive predictors of fitness to drive in persons with dementia: a systematic review. *J Am Geriatr Soc* 2006;54:1943–1944.
15. McDowell I, Kristjansson B, Hill GB, et al. Community screening for dementia: the Mini Mental State Exam (MMSE) and Modified Mini-Mental State Exam (3 MS) compared. *J Clin Epidemiol* 1997;50:377–383.
16. Borson S, Scanlon JM, Watanabe J, et al. Improving identification of cognitive impairment in primary care. *Int J Geriatr Psychiatry* 2006;21:349–355.
17. Borson S, Scanlan JM, Chen P, et al. The mini-cog: a cognitive 'vital signs' measure for dementia screening in multi-lingual elderly. *Int J Geriatr Psychiatry* 2000;15:1021–1024.
18. Fratiglioni L, Paillard-Borg S, Winblad B. An active and socially integrated lifestyle in late life might protect against dementia. *Lancet Neurol* 2004;3:343–353.

CHAPTER 14

Self-examination of the Breasts, Testes, and Skin

Steven H. Woolf

When diagnosed at an early stage, cancers of the breast, skin (e.g., malignant melanoma), and testes have relatively good prognoses. In addition to obtaining periodic cancer screening by clinicians, which is discussed in Chapters 3–4, the public has been advised for many years to perform monthly self-examinations at home to help detect malignant or premalignant conditions at a curable stage. Clinicians have been encouraged to devote time during clinical encounters to train and remind patients how to correctly perform self-examination.

The appropriateness of these recommendations is not universally accepted, however. As is discussed in more detail on pages 334–338, performing and teaching self-examination have not been shown in prospective studies to reduce morbidity or mortality. They may have unintended adverse effects. For example, abnormalities detected by patients on self-examination, most of which are false positives, often generate office visits to clinicians, biopsies, and other procedures. During the period of time while they await their follow-up appointments and biopsy results, patients may experience anxiety over the possibility of having cancer.

In 2002, the U.S. Preventive Services Task Force echoed the findings of its prior reviews when it concluded that the extant evidence was insufficient to recommend for or against teaching or performing routine breast self-examination (BSE) (1). Its 2003 review of skin cancer screening found "little evidence to determine the effects of counseling on other preventive behaviors . . . such as practicing skin self-examination." (2). Its 2004 review of screening for testicular cancer recommended against routine screening and reported that there was "no new evidence that screening with clinical examination or testicular self-examination is effective in reducing mortality from testicular cancer." (3). The American Academy of Family Physicians has adopted similar positions (4).

Recognizing this weak supporting evidence, the American Cancer Society—which for two decades had recommended that all women older than 20 years and all postpubertal males should perform monthly breast or testicular self-examinations, respectively—has softened its position on the topic. In 2003, the American Cancer Society reclassified BSE as optional and advised clinicians to educate women about the benefits and limitations of the practice (5). It now no longer recommends taking time during the periodic health examination to systematically teach patients how to perform self-examination of the breast, skin, or testicles. Its 2006 guidelines for clinicians state only that, "self-examination techniques or increased awareness about signs and symptoms of skin cancer, breast cancer, or testicular cancer can be discussed" (6).

Other groups, however, continue to advocate self-examination practices. For example, the American College of Obstetricians and Gynecologists states that "[d]espite a lack of definitive data for or against breast self-examination, breast self-examination has the potential to detect palpable breast cancer and can be recommended" (7).

This chapter examines both sides of the controversy. For those clinicians interested in teaching self-examination to their patients, the chapter discusses current methods for teaching it and for promoting adherence among patients who have been taught the techniques. The inclusion of these sections by the editors, however, is offered as an information resource for readers but does not necessarily imply an endorsement of self-examination.

The chapter focuses on the examination of three organs—breasts, testes, and skin—for which self-examination is most commonly recommended. Self-examination of the oral cavity, eyes, and other parts of the body is recommended less frequently, is supported by even weaker scientific evidence, and is therefore not discussed in this chapter. Screening for cancer through clinical examinations and laboratory screening tests (e.g., mammography) is discussed in Chapters 3 and 4.

THE CONTROVERSY OVER SELF-EXAMINATION

The primary debate over self-examination concerns the question of whether it reduces morbidity or mortality. There is currently no direct evidence from controlled prospective studies that persons who practice self-examination have longer survival from cancer than those who do not. There is some indirect supporting evidence for that outcome, however, primarily related to self-detection of breast cancer. Most breast cancers are first discovered by patients, not by their clinicians (8). Observational studies suggest that breast cancers detected through self-examination are likely to be smaller and less advanced than those first discovered by clinicians, to have less axillary node involvement, and to be associated with higher survival rates than cancers detected by other means. Similarly, a thin malignant melanoma (less than 0.76 mm thickness) carries little risk of metastatic spread to other sites. Five-year survival for patients with melanomas between 1.5–4 mm is approximately 70%, and survival for those with melanomas thicker than 4 mm is approximately 45% (9).

Skeptics cite several problems with this evidence. First, some observational studies found no benefit from self-examination (although many of these studies suffered from design limitations themselves). Second, although some observational studies have reported a benefit—for example, a case–control study reporting lower incidence and mortality associated with self-examination of melanomas (10)—the higher survival rates may reflect statistical artifacts (e.g., lead-time, length, or selection biases) rather than an actual reduction in mortality. In *lead-time bias,* survival appears to be longer simply because the cancer was diagnosed at an earlier age and not because death was postponed. In *length bias,* self-examination preferentially detects slowly growing tumors rather than aggressive malignancies, producing an artificially higher estimate of survival rates. *Selection bias* reflects the tendency of persons who practice self-examination to come from a more health-conscious population than the general public, making it unclear whether health-promoting practices other than self-examination (e.g., low dietary fat or alcohol intake) are more directly responsible for the observed benefits.

A third limitation relating to BSE data is that many, if not most, women engaging in this practice also undergo screening by clinicians and routine mammography, making it difficult to isolate the benefits attributable to self-examination. Fourth, in the case of testicular cancer, survival is good even without screening. Approximately 60% of testicular seminomas are diagnosed at stage I without screening, and current survival rates approach 100% for early-stage disease (11). According to the National Cancer Institute, "[t]esticular cancer is so curable even at advanced stages and there are so few cases that it would be virtually impossible to document a decrease in mortality associated with screening" (12). Given these potential biases, the only type of study that can convincingly demonstrate the effectiveness of self-examination is one that is both controlled and prospective, comparing morbidity and mortality rates in persons who do and do not perform self-examination.

Such studies—conducted in China (13), Russia (14), and the United Kingdom (15)—did evaluate the effect of teaching BSE on mortality and other outcomes. The three trials, which involved a total of approximately 400,000 women, each demonstrated that self-examination produced no reduction in breast cancer mortality or significant improvements in the number or stage of cancers detected. The Chinese trial, which involved 266,064 female textile workers, concluded that intensive instruction in BSE not only had no effect on mortality, but it also increased the chances of having a benign breast biopsy, due to the high proportion of false-positive results. In a good-quality nested case–control analysis from a Canadian screening study, the overall practice of

BSE was not associated with a reduction in mortality (16). Meta-analyses and systematic reviews by the Cochrane Collaboration also reported no benefit from BSE in terms of mortality and near doubling in the performance of biopsies (17). Although none of these studies provides support for BSE, these studies do not entirely exclude the possibility of benefit due to their limited duration of follow-up and questions about whether results from other countries are generalizable to women in North America (18).

Proponents of self-examination cite other benefits of the practice beyond lowering mortality. Introducing self-examination at an early age may make patients more familiar with the appearance and texture of their breasts, skin, and testes, thereby enabling more accurate and prompt detection of malignant changes later in life. Self-examination is inexpensive and empowers patients to take a more active role in the care of their body. In rural areas or other regions of the country with limited access to clinicians or imaging centers (e.g., facilities for mammography or scrotal ultrasonography), self-examination may provide the only available means of early cancer detection. However, these potential benefits have remained unproven.

The seeming harmlessness and low cost of self-examination are also debated. The examination skills of patients are often less sensitive and specific than those of clinicians trained in physical examination techniques and familiar with the physical characteristics of suspicious lesions. For example, although breast examination by physicians has a reported sensitivity of 40–69%, the reported sensitivity of BSE is only 26–41% (19). The sensitivity of skin and testicular self-examination in detecting cancer is unknown. Reports indicate that the sensitivity of skin self-examination in detecting large nevi or those with new changes is approximately 70% (20), suggesting that there is an even lower sensitivity in detecting more subtle, malignant lesions.

Self-examination is thought to have a low positive predictive value: a large proportion of abnormalities found by the patient are likely to be benign conditions or normal tissue. For statistical reasons outlined in Chapter 4 (see page 90), the chances of false-positive results are even greater when the target condition is rare. For example, the incidence of testicular cancer is extremely low (less than 3:100,000) (21). Therefore, it is far more likely that abnormal findings on testicular self-examination will be for benign conditions (e.g., epididymitis, spermatocele, and hydrocele) than cancer. The low positive predictive value of self-examination has led some to worry that it may lead to an overdetection of harmless findings and to the unnecessary anxiety, discomfort, and cost of follow-up office visits and biopsies for benign lesions. A Dutch study reported that women who were at increased risk of breast cancer and examined their breasts twice a week had higher scores for psychological distress (22). As noted earlier, BSE is also associated with an increased risk of breast biopsies generated by false-positive results.

Other potential harms of self-examination have also been discussed. For example, it has been proposed that persons who perform self-examination may mistakenly conclude that, if they do not find an abnormality, routine examinations by clinicians are unnecessary. A particular concern for women is that this misunderstanding about BSE might lead to poorer adherence in obtaining routine examinations by clinicians and mammography screening. Another concern is that a negative workup for an abnormality detected through self-examination might be misjudged by the patient as a reason to discontinue further screening. However, there is little evidence to support these concerns or to suggest that they could not be remedied by proper patient education. In fact, some studies suggest that women who perform BSE are more health conscious and therefore more likely than other women to comply with screening examinations by clinicians.

Another focus of controversy is whether standardized self-examination is more sensitive or specific than incidental detection. Many lesions detected by patients are discovered during bathing, dressing, and other routine activities. It is unclear whether the detection rate that occurs with these normal activities differs appreciably from that of self-examination performed according to a schedule (e.g., monthly) or to the step-by-step techniques recommended by experts.

Recommendations that clinicians incorporate self-examination instructions into routine visits have also drawn criticism. Many practitioners lack enthusiasm for teaching self-examination. In one survey, for example, 82% of physicians were unfamiliar with how to teach testicular self-examination or had not thought about it (23). A national survey of family physicians in 2002 found that only 24% recommended skin self-examinations in average-risk patients. Lack of time and training, along with patient reluctance to engage in the practice, were cited as the most significant barriers to teaching skin self-examination (24).

There are several key objections to teaching self-examination. First, a thorough demonstration of self-examination technique is time consuming; busy clinicians often lack the time for such counseling or do so at the expense of other forms of health education. A second concern is the lack of evidence that teaching is effective. Although some studies suggest that teaching self-examination improves patient knowledge levels and self-reported performance of self-examination, other studies have shown no effect. There is evidence that certain techniques do improve the accuracy of skin self-examination. For example, partner interventions and mole-mapping diagrams show promise. Third, self-reports of performance may not correlate with either actual performance or improved detection; knowing how to perform the examination does not necessarily mean that the patient will adhere to the technique.

In a national survey, 88% of women aged 18 years or older reported that they knew how to perform BSE, but only 43% of the same sample reported performing the procedure at least 12 times each year (25). Among respondents to the Women Physicians' Health Study, only 21% reported performing monthly BSE (26) (and the patients in that study were *physicians*). A fourth concern, as discussed on page 341, is recidivism: patients who begin practicing self-examination on the advice of their clinician often abandon the practice over time, or perform the technique incorrectly.

Nevertheless, these concerns aside, self-examination clearly has the *potential* to reduce morbidity and mortality through early detection. In the case of breast cancer, for example, between 50 and 90% of tumors are first detected by patients and not clinicians. Studies of women undergoing regular breast cancer screening with clinical breast examinations and mammography report that 13–17% of cancers are detected by patients, between screenings. Some evidence suggests that breast cancers detected on self-examination are more virulent than those detected on mammography (27). Although, as noted earlier, theoretic harms from self-examination have been raised, the risks and costs of this simple practice are certainly far less than those of expensive or invasive clinical procedures that are routinely used in patient care despite similarly inadequate supporting evidence. Whether the benefits of self-examination outweigh its harms therefore remains uncertain.

PROPER TECHNIQUE

Clinicians should consider these issues in deciding whether to devote time to teaching patients how to perform self-examination. For those interested in doing so, Tables 14.1–14.3 summarize the key instructions that patients are generally given. The editors of this book include this information for clinicians who wish to teach self-examination, but the inclusion does not necessarily indicate an endorsement of the practice.

Unfortunately, the absence of conclusive scientific evidence makes it difficult to know whether each of the steps outlined in Tables 14.1–14.3 is necessary. Few self-examination protocols have been validated in studies that measured clinical outcomes. Studies using intermediate outcomes have often produced conflicting results regarding the importance of specific self-examination procedures.

The lack of evidence of an optimal self-examination protocol should be kept in mind in interpreting the recommendations of some experts that patients perform a series of specific self-examination procedures in special positions, using certain equipment, and sometimes with the assistance of

TABLE 14.1 Instructions for Breast Self-examination

Do not check your breasts during your period. The best time is 3–7 d after your period ends.

How to Examine Your Breasts

- Lie down and place your right arm behind your head. The examination is done while lying down, and not standing up. This is because when lying down the breast tissue spreads evenly over the chest wall and it is as thin as possible, making it much easier to feel all the breast tissue.
- Use the finger pads of the three middle fingers on your left hand to feel for lumps in the right breast. Use overlapping dime-sized circular motions of the finger pads to feel the breast tissue.
- Use three different levels of pressure to feel all the breast tissue. Light pressure is needed to feel the tissue closest to the skin; medium pressure to feel a little deeper; and firm pressure to feel the tissue closest to the chest and ribs. A firm ridge in the lower curve of each breast is normal. If you are not sure how hard to press, talk with your doctor or nurse. Use each pressure level to feel the breast tissue before moving on to the next spot.
- Move around the breast in an up and down pattern starting at an imaginary line drawn straight down your side from the underarm and moving across the breast to the middle of the chest bone (sternum or breastbone). Be sure to check the entire breast area going down until you feel only ribs and up to the neck or collarbone (clavicle).
- There is some evidence to suggest that the up and down pattern (sometimes called the *vertical pattern*) is the most effective pattern for covering the entire breast without missing any breast tissue.
- Repeat the examination on your left breast, using the finger pads of the right hand.
- While standing in front of a mirror with your hands pressing firmly down on your hips, look at your breasts for any changes of size, shape, contour, dimpling, pulling, or redness or scaliness of the nipple or breast skin. (The pressing down on the hips position contracts the chest wall muscles and enhances any breast changes.) Continue to look for changes with your arms down at your sides and then with your arms raised up over your head with your palms pressed together.
- Examine each underarm while sitting up or standing and with your arm only slightly raised so you can easily feel in this area. Raising your arm straight up tightens the tissue in this area and makes it difficult to examine.

If there are lumps, knots, nipple discharge, or other suspicious changes, contact your doctor.

Adapted from American Cancer Society. *How to perform a breast self examination.* http://www.cancer.org/docroot/CRI/content/CRI_2_6x_How_to_perform_a_breast_self_exam_5.asp. Accessed 2007.

TABLE 14.2 Instructions for Skin Self-examination

Your doctor or nurse may suggest that you do a regular skin self-examination to check for skin cancer, including *melanoma*.

The best time to do this examination is after a shower or bath. You should check your skin in a room with plenty of light. You should use a full-length mirror and a handheld mirror. It is best to begin by learning where your birthmarks, moles, and other marks are and their usual look and feel.

Check for anything new:
- New mole (that looks different from your other moles)
- New red or darker color flaky patch that may be a little raised
- New flesh-colored firm bump
- Change in the size, shape, color, or feel of a mole
- Sore that does not heal

Check yourself from head to toe. Do not forget to check your back, scalp, genital area, and between your buttocks.
- Look at your face, neck, ears, and scalp. You may want to use a comb or a blow dryer to move your hair so that you can see better. You also may want to have a relative or friend check through your hair. It may be hard to check your scalp by yourself.
- Look at the front and back of your body in the mirror. Then, raise your arms and look at your left and right sides.
- Bend your elbows. Look carefully at your fingernails, palms, forearms (including the undersides), and upper arms.

Contact your doctor if you notice a change in a mole or other skin marking or if you have a new unexplained mole, skin lump, ulcer, or unhealed sore that has appeared since your last examination.

Adapted from: National Cancer Institute. *How to do a skin self examination.* http://www.cancer.gov/cancertopics/wyntk/skin/page13. Accessed 2007.

spouses or friends. For example, some instructions for skin self-examination specify multiple examination positions and the need for a full-length or hand-held mirror, blow dryer, two chairs, or an examination partner. Although common sense suggests that following these instructions would help patients examine themselves more carefully, there is no evidence that they achieve higher detection rates than more limited self-examinations. Quite the contrary, routines that are so complex may discourage patients from performing self-examination. Finally, there is no evidence to support the common advice to perform self-examination every month; no studies have determined whether monthly self-checks achieve higher detection rates than less frequent examinations.

TABLE 14.3 Instructions for Testicular Self-examination

- Perform the examination after a warm bath or shower, while your hands are still warm.
- Examine each testicle gently with both hands. The index and middle fingers should be placed underneath the testicle, while the thumbs are placed on top. Roll the testicle gently between the thumbs and fingers.
- Your testicles should feel smooth, rubbery, and slightly tender. Surfaces should be smooth and without lumps. It is common for one testicle to be larger than the other.
- Feel for any abnormal hard lumps, nodules, or swelling on the front or side of the testicle.
- The epididymis is a cord-like structure on the top and back of the testicle. Do not confuse the epididymis with an abnormal lump.

If you find a lump, nodule, swelling, or dull ache, or if you notice another change, contact your doctor.

Adapted from National Cancer Institute. *Testicular self-examination NIH publication No. 94–2636.* Bethesda: National Cancer Institute, 1994.

ADHERENCE

Most persons who are advised to perform monthly self-examinations do not do so, and a large proportion of persons who receive counseling or training to perform self-examination do not maintain the habit over time. Persons are more likely to perform self-examination if they fear cancer and believe that they are susceptible, believe that self-examination is an effective screening tool, understand how to perform the procedure, and have confidence in their examination skills (self-efficacy).

The principal barriers to performance include the absence of these beliefs, as well as fears of finding an abnormality, embarrassment, lack of time, and forgetting to do so. Poor adherence is also sometimes due to misconceptions, such as believing that cancer can be detected early by simply paying attention to symptoms or that a healthy lifestyle is fully protective against cancer. Some barriers are related to age. BSE and the recognition of suspicious lesions by older women can be impaired by poor visual acuity, tactile sensation, and range of motion. Testicular examination and BSE by adolescent boys and girls, respectively, can be influenced by embarrassment and uncomfortable feelings about body image.

Teaching patients how to perform self-examination, by itself, is unlikely to be effective if the clinician does not also address these concerns. Therefore, clinicians who have decided, despite the caveats mentioned earlier, to teach self-examination must do more than teach the technique to achieve the desired ends. That is, the likelihood of adherence is increased if clinicians take time to assess the patient's understanding of the underlying rationale, attitudes, and beliefs about cancer and early detection, perceived self-efficacy, and relevant fears and anxieties about detecting cancer. Practical constraints, such as lack of time, privacy, and the need for reminders to perform self-examination, should also be addressed. The physical and cognitive limitations of older adults should receive special attention. Once this information has been gathered, the clinician's counseling about self-examination should be tailored to the patient's concerns. This may include correcting misconceptions about cancer, reassuring the patient that his or her self-examination technique is correct, suggesting reminder systems, and altering instructions for patients with physical limitations.

Many physicians lack the time, skills, or interest to properly teach self-examination. Trained nurses, physician assistants, and other counselors in the office or clinic are often better prepared and more capable than physicians of ensuring that patients fully understand examination techniques and of reevaluating self-examination skills at future visits. Delegating the task to these personnel may be advisable.

Patient education materials are often useful to help patients remember when to perform self-examination and to remind them of the proper technique. Although pamphlets and websites (see "Resources—Patient Education Materials" at the end of this chapter) are often used to supplement counseling, videotapes and films are sometimes more effective in demonstrating examination techniques. Self-examination can be taught in group settings, but the evidence is equivocal regarding the relative superiority of individual versus group counseling. Finally, patients need reminders and reinforcements to continue performing self-examination. Studies have shown that reassessment and retraining in BSE may achieve higher breast lump detection rates. Therefore, after teaching patients how to perform self-examination, clinicians may find it useful to reassess their performance and proficiency at a later date.

OFFICE AND CLINIC ORGANIZATION

Offices and clinics in which self-examination is taught should have private examination rooms in which the technique can be demonstrated. Some practices use models, diagrams, and illustrations as teaching aids. Patient education materials that reinforce and explain further the technique of self-examination and that define abnormal results (see examples listed on page 343) should be easily accessible to hand to the patient, or a list of useful websites should be provided. Photographs of malignant and premalignant skin lesions, included either in office teaching aids or patient education resources, may help the patient identify important skin findings.

RESOURCES—PATIENT EDUCATION MATERIALS

Breast Self-Examination

American Cancer Society
How to perform a breast self examination
http://www.cancer.org/docroot/CRI/content/CRI_2_6x_How_to_perform_a_breast_self_
    exam_5.asp. Accessed 2007.

Skin Self-Examination

American Cancer Society
Overview: skin cancer—melanoma. How is melanoma skin cancer found?
http://www.cancer.org/docroot/CRI/content/CRI_2_2_3X_How_is_melanoma_skin_
    cancer_found_50.asp?sitearea=. Accessed 2007.

National Cancer Institute
What you need to know about skin cancer
http://www.cancer.gov/cancertopics/wyntk/skin/page1. Accessed 2007.

National Cancer Institute
How to do a skin self examination
http://www.cancer.gov/cancertopics/wyntk/skin/page13.

Testicular Self-Examination

American Cancer Society
Detailed guide: testicular cancer. Can testicular cancer be found early?
http://www.cancer.org/docroot/CRI/content/CRI_2_4_3X_Can_Testicular_Cancer_Be_
    Found_Early_41.asp?sitearea=. Accessed 2007.

SUGGESTED READINGS

American Academy of Family Physicians. *Clinical preventive services.* http://www
    .aafp.org/online/en/home/clinical/exam.html. 2007.
American College of Obstetricians and Gynecologists. Breast cancer screening. ACOG
    Practice Bulletin No. 42. *Obstet Gynecol* 2003;101:821–832.
Smith RA, Cokkinides V, Eyre HJ. American Cancer Society guidelines for the early
    detection of cancer, 2006. *CA Cancer J Clin* 2006;56:11–25.
U.S. Preventive Services Task Force. *Screening for breast cancer: recommendations and
    rationale.* Rockville: Agency for Healthcare Research and Quality, http://www.ahrq
    .gov/clinic/3rduspstf/breastcancer/brcanrr.htm, February 2002.
U.S. Preventive Services Task Force. *Counseling to prevent skin cancer: recommendations
    and rationale.* Rockville: Agency for Healthcare Research and Quality, http://www
    .ahrq.gov/clinic/3rduspstf/skcacoun/skcarr.htm, October 2003.
U.S. Preventive Services Task Force. *Screening for testicular cancer: recommendation
    statement.* Rockville: Agency for Healthcare Research and Quality, http://www
    .ahrq.gov/clinic/3rduspstf/testicular/testiculrs.htm, February 2004.

References

1. U.S. Preventive Services Task Force. *Screening for breast cancer: recommendations and rationale*. Rockville: Agency for Healthcare Research and Quality, http://www.ahrq.gov/clinic/3rduspstf/breastcancer/brcanrr.htm, February 2002.
2. U.S. Preventive Services Task Force. *Counseling to prevent skin cancer: recommendations and rationale*. Rockville: Agency for Healthcare Research and Quality, http://www.ahrq.gov/clinic/3rduspstf/skcacoun/skcarr.htm, October 2003.
3. U.S. Preventive Services Task Force. *Screening for testicular cancer: recommendation statement*. Rockville: Agency for Healthcare Research and Quality, http://www.ahrq.gov/clinic/3rduspstf/testicular/testiculrs.htm, February 2004.
4. American Academy of Family Physicians. *Clinical preventive services*. http://www.aafp.org/online/en/home/clinical/exam.html. 2007.
5. American Cancer Society. *Chronological history of ACS recommendations on early detection of cancer*. http://www.cancer.org/docroot/PED/content/PED_2_3X_Chronological_History_of_ACS_Recommendations_on_Early_Detection_of_Cancer.asp?sitearea=PED. 2007.
6. Smith RA, Cokkinides V, Eyre HJ. American Cancer Society guidelines for the early detection of cancer, 2006. *CA Cancer J Clin* 2006;56:11–25.
7. American College of Obstetricians and Gynecologists. Breast cancer screening. ACOG Practice Bulletin No. 42. *Obstet Gynecol* 2003;101:821–832.
8. Foster RS Jr, Worden JK, Costanza MC, et al. Clinical breast examination and breast self-examination. *Cancer* 1992;69:1992–1998.
9. Agency for Healthcare Research and Quality. Screening for skin cancer: summary of the evidence. *Am J Prev Med* 2001;20(3S):47–58; Rockville: Agency for Healthcare Research and Quality, Article originally in http://www.ahrq.gov/clinic/ajpmsuppl/helfand1.htm.
10. Berwick M, Begg CB, Fine JA, et al. Screening for cutaneous melanoma by skin self-examination [see comments]. *J Natl Cancer Inst* 1996;88(1):17–23.
11. American Cancer Society. *Testicular cancer*. http://www.cancer.org/downloads/PRO/TesticularCancer.pdf. 2007.
12. National Cancer Institute. *Testicular cancer (PDQ®): screening*. http://www.cancer.gov/cancertopics/pdq/screening/testicular/HealthProfessional/page2. 2007.
13. Thomas DB, Gao DL, Ray RM, et al. Randomized trial of breast self-examination in Shanghai: final results. *J Natl Cancer Inst* 2002;94:1445–1457.
14. Semiglazov VF, Moiseenko VM, Manikhas AG, et al. Role of breast self-examination in early detection of breast cancer: Russia/WHO prospective randomized trial in St. Petersburg. *Cancer Strategy* 1999;1:145–151.
15. UK Breast Cancer Detection Working Group. 16-year mortality from breast cancer in the UK trial of early detection of breast cancer. *Lancet* 1999;353(9168):1909–1914.
16. Harvey BJ, Miller AB, Baines CJ, et al. Effect of breast self-examination techniques on the risk of death from breast cancer. *CMAJ* 1997;157(9):1205–1212.
17. Kosters JP, Gotzsche PC. Regular self-examination or clinical examination for early detection of breast cancer. *Cochrane Database Syst Rev* 2003;(2):CD003373.
18. Kearney AJ, Murray M. Evidence against breast self examination is not conclusive: what policymakers and health professionals need to know. *J Public Health Policy* 2006;27:282–292.
19. Humphrey LL, Chan BKS, Detlefsen S, et al. *Screening for breast cancer*. Systematic Evidence Review No. 15, (Prepared by the Oregon Health & Science University

Evidence-based Practice Center under Contract No. 290-97-0018). Rockville: Agency for Healthcare Research and Quality, (Available on the AHRQ Web site at: www.ahrq.gov/clinic/serfiles.htm). September 2002.

20. Oliveria SA, Chau D, Christos PJ, et al. Diagnostic accuracy of patients in performing skin self-examination and the impact of photography. *Arch Dermatol* 2004;140:57–62.

21. National Cancer Institute. *AGE-adjusted SEER incidence and U.S. death rates and 5-year relative survival rates.* http://seer.cancer.gov/csr/1975_2003/results_single/sect_01 _table.04_2pgs.pdf, 2000–2003.

22. van Dooren S, Rijnsburger AJ, Seynaeve C, et al. Psychological distress and breast self-examination frequency in women at increased risk for hereditary or familial breast cancer. *Community Genet* 2003;6:235–241.

23. Sayger SA, Fortenberry JD, Beckman RJ. Practice patterns of teaching testicular self-examination to adolescent patients. *J Adolesc Health Care* 1988;9:441–442.

24. Geller AC, O'Riordan DL, Oliveria SA, et al. Overcoming obstacles to skin cancer examinations and prevention counseling for high-risk patients: results of a national survey of primary care physicians. *J Am Board Fam Pract* 2004;17:416–423.

25. Piani A, Schoenborn C. National Center for Health Statistics. Health promotion and disease prevention: United States, 1990. *Vital Health Stat* 1993;10(185):59.

26. Frank E, Rimer BK, Brogan D, et al. U.S. women physicians' personal and clinical breast cancer screening practices. *J Womens Health Gend Based Med* 2000;9:791–801.

27. Kaplan HG, Malmgren JA. Disease-specific survival in patient-detected breast cancer. *Clin Breast Cancer* 2006;7:133–140.

CHAPTER 15

Chemoprophylaxis

Linda S. Kinsinger, Michael Pignone, and Heidi D. Nelson

Chemoprophylaxis (or chemoprevention) in preventive medicine is the use of drugs, nutritional and mineral supplements, or other natural substances by asymptomatic persons to prevent future disease. It does not include using such agents to treat symptomatic illnesses or in persons with a prior history of the disorder. This chapter examines the use of medications for chemoprophylaxis. (Examples of other agents used for chemoprophylaxis are iron supplements in menstruating or pregnant women or in young children to decrease the risk of iron-deficiency anemia, fluoride supplements to decrease the risk of dental caries, folic acid supplements to decrease women's risk of giving birth to children with neural tube defects, and multivitamins to reduce the risk of cancer and heart disease. Only some of these practices are fully supported by current evidence.) Chemoprophylactic agents are used in people without the condition for which they are taking the medication; therefore great care must be taken to be certain that the benefits of the agents substantially outweigh their harms.

This chapter examines three common situations in which drugs (or classes of drugs) may (or may not) be recommended for chemoprophylaxis: selective estrogen receptor modulators to prevent breast cancer; aspirin to prevent heart disease, stroke, and possibly cancer; and postmenopausal hormone therapy to prevent chronic conditions, such as heart disease. The chapter examines the role of these drugs in primary prevention (i.e., for asymptomatic persons). It does not focus on the use of tamoxifen to treat breast cancer, the use of aspirin in patients with known cardiovascular disease, and the use of estrogen to control postmenopausal symptoms.

CHEMOPREVENTION OF BREAST CANCER

Despite improvements in the rates of screening and early detection and advances in treatment, breast cancer remains the most commonly diagnosed non–skin cancer among women in the United States. It is not possible to modify the strongest risk factors for breast cancer—increasing age and a family history. Therefore, other preventive strategies must be considered. Evidence that drugs might be able to prevent breast cancer was first recognized in trials testing tamoxifen as adjuvant chemotherapy in women with breast cancer. Tamoxifen is a member of a class of drugs called *selective estrogen receptor modulators*, compounds with both estrogen-like and antiestrogen properties. In a meta-analysis of 55 studies of adjuvant tamoxifen chemotherapy, the drug was found to reduce the risk of new cancer in the opposite breast by 47% (p <0.001) among women who took tamoxifen for 5 years (1).

Breast cancer prevention with tamoxifen in women at increased risk of breast cancer has been studied in four randomized clinical trials; raloxifene, another selective estrogen receptor modulator, has been studied in three trials. A meta-analysis of the tamoxifen trials showed a 38% reduction (95% confidence interval [CI] 28–46%) in breast cancer incidence after 5 years of therapy (2). Raloxifene was found to reduce incidence by 72% (95% CI 54–83%) after 4 years in a trial of postmenopausal women with osteoporosis (3) and by 44% (95%, CI 17–62%) in a trial of postmenopausal women with coronary heart disease (CHD) or risk factors for CHD (4). Both drugs reduce the incidence of estrogen receptor–positive tumors only. In the Study of Tamoxifen and Raloxifene (STAR) trial, a direct comparison of the two drugs in postmenopausal women at increased risk of breast cancer, the drugs were found to be equally effective and reduced expected cancers by 50% (5). No benefit in terms of breast cancer mortality has yet been seen in any trial. Aromatase inhibitors, useful in the treatment of breast cancer, are also under consideration as chemoprophylactic agents. Tamoxifen is the only agent currently approved by the U.S. Food and Drug Administration (FDA) for primary breast cancer risk reduction (chemoprevention) in high-risk women; approval for raloxifene to be used for this indication is under review at this writing.

The use of these drugs, however, carries an increased risk of harms, a significant concern given that the women who take them do not have invasive cancer. Both tamoxifen and raloxifene are associated with a threefold higher risk for venous thromboembolic disease, especially pulmonary embolism, although the actual number of events in the studies was small (6). Increases in stroke and deep venous thrombosis were also noted but not found to be statistically significant (except for the risk of fatal stroke in one study [4]). Tamoxifen, but not raloxifene, has been shown to increase the risk of stage I endometrial cancer and uterine sarcoma. These serious side effects occur mostly in women aged 50 years and older. In the STAR trial, however, postmenopausal women taking raloxifene not only had 36% fewer uterine cancers but also 29% fewer blood clots than the women who were assigned to take tamoxifen. Both tamoxifen and raloxifene are associated with an increased incidence of hot flashes, and tamoxifen is associated with an increased incidence of bothersome vaginal discharge. Raloxifene is also effective in reducing the risk of osteoporotic fractures in older women.

Official Recommendations

The U.S. Preventive Services Task Force (USPSTF) recommends against the routine use of tamoxifen or raloxifene for the primary prevention of breast cancer in women at low or average risk of breast cancer (7). The USPSTF recommends that clinicians discuss chemoprevention with women at high risk of breast cancer and at low risk of adverse effects from chemoprevention. The American Society of Clinical Oncology recommends offering tamoxifen (at 20 mg/day for 5 years) to women with a defined 5-year projected breast cancer risk of greater than or equal to 1.66% (8). The group does not recommend the use of raloxifene, any aromatase inhibitor, or fenretinide to lower the risk of developing breast cancer outside of a clinical trial setting.

Essentials of Counseling

Clinicians should discuss the pros and cons of breast cancer prevention with women for whom benefits would likely be greater than harms. Women with higher breast cancer risk are more likely to benefit from chemoprevention than women with lower risk, and younger women are less likely to suffer harms than older women; therefore, the group of women for whom benefits are most likely to exceed harms is younger women at higher risk of breast cancer. There is no definitive cutoff to indicate low versus high risk for breast cancer. Women are considered at high risk of breast cancer if their risk factors include a family history of breast cancer in a first-degree relative (mother, sister or daughter), previous breast biopsy showing atypical hyperplasia, early age of menarche, or late age at first pregnancy or no pregnancy.

An estimated 5-year risk can be calculated from the Gail risk model calculator (see page 22 in Chapter 1 and "Office and Clinic Organization" on page 354). The Gail model was developed from a large study of breast cancer screening and has been shown to be accurate in follow-up studies. Other risk assessment models, such as one developed by Claus et al., are also available; each has advantages and disadvantages. A risk level of greater than 1.66% in 5 years has been used in one of the major breast cancer chemoprevention trials as an indication of increased risk (but that level was chosen for statistical analysis reasons, not because it carried biologic significance). This approach to breast cancer chemoprevention does not apply to women with genetic abnormalities, such as *BRCA1* or *BRCA2* abnormalities, who have a much higher risk of breast cancer and require testing and preventive measures as discussed in Chapter 4 (see pages 115–116).

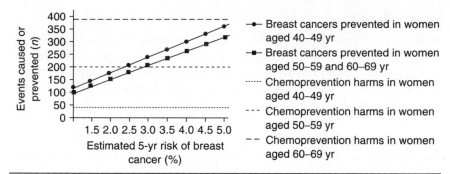

Figure 15.1 • Benefits and harms of chemoprevention with tamoxifen per 10,000 women in three age-groups. Harms include endometrial cancer, stroke, and pulmonary embolism combined. (Adapted from Gail MH, Constantino JP, Bryant J, et al. Weighing the risks and benefits of tamoxifen treatment for prevention. *J Natl Cancer Inst* 1999;91:1829–1846.)

An approximation of the balance between benefits and harms is shown in Figure 15.1. The benefits (sloped lines) increase with increasing breast cancer risk, whereas the harms (flat horizontal lines) are age-dependent and not related to breast cancer risk. Keep in mind, however, that women may weigh the importance of these outcomes differently. The possible benefit of reducing the risk of breast cancer may have more value for some women than does an increased risk of early-stage endometrial cancer (or vice versa). These estimates of benefits and harms should be applied only to white women, as the chemoprevention trials included few women of color. The trade-off between benefits and harms will likely be less favorable for African American women, who have a lower risk of breast cancer and higher background rates of adverse events. The proportion of women aged 35–70 years who are potentially eligible for tamoxifen chemoprevention has been estimated to be 15.5% (18.7% of white women, 5.7% of African American women, and 2.9% of Hispanic women) (9). Only a small percentage of eligible women are likely to have a positive benefit/risk index. Studies in clinical settings have found, so far, that few women are willing to take chemoprevention, citing concerns about potential adverse effects as the main limiting factor (10).

The current recommended dose of tamoxifen is 20 mg/day for 5 years. Benefits appear to last longer than 5 years but the total duration of effect is not known. Because the detrimental effect of tamoxifen on the endometrium is dose dependent and the drug has a long half-life, a lower dose has been suggested as a possible way to reduce side effects, but studies to determine the optimal dose have not yet been completed. The dose of raloxifene used in studies of breast cancer prevention was 60 mg/day. The optimal duration of therapy is not known.

Contraindications

Women at increased risk of adverse effects from tamoxifen or raloxifene should carefully consider taking breast cancer chemoprevention. Women with a uterus should report any vaginal bleeding when taking tamoxifen. Women should report symptoms of chest pain, shortness of breath, or leg pain and swelling when taking either tamoxifen or raloxifene.

ASPIRIN PROPHYLAXIS

This section examines the use of low-dose aspirin (50–325 mg/day) for primary prevention of heart disease, stroke, and possibly cancer. Aspirin has been shown to reduce the risk of mortality and subsequent vascular events for patients with known cardiovascular disease (secondary prevention) and is highly recommended in that setting. The use of aspirin for primary prevention, however, is more controversial: the benefits and adverse effects in patients at lower risk are more closely balanced, and decisions about who should or should not take aspirin require careful consideration of risks and of patient preferences and values.

At this writing (2006), the effectiveness of aspirin for the primary prevention of cardiovascular events has been examined in six large randomized trials. A meta-analysis of five of these studies found that men who take aspirin daily can reduce their relative odds of coronary events by 28% (11). The five studies included in this meta-analysis were 4–7 years in duration and compared doses of aspirin ranging from 75–500 mg/day. Three of the five trials included only men; two others included mixed populations of men and women. The results for women are discussed in the subsequent text.

In addition to its effect on total coronary events, evidence from these five trials also suggested that aspirin may reduce the risk of fatal CHD events by 13%, although the summary result did not reach statistical significance. The effect on total mortality was smaller (7% reduction) and also statistically nonsignificant, reflecting the fact that few participants died over the 4- to 7-year duration of these trials. The effect of aspirin on the development of angina is unclear—the trials that measured this outcome produced mixed results. In these five trials, aspirin did not reduce the risk of ischemic stroke, although the ascertainment of the nature of strokes in these trials (some of which predate the widespread routine use of neuroimaging for acute stroke) was suboptimal. In terms of adverse effects, aspirin increased the incidence of major gastrointestinal bleeding and hemorrhagic stroke (odds ratios of 1.7 and 1.4, respectively) (12).

Effectiveness in Women

The effectiveness of aspirin prophylaxis in women has been examined in three trials. In two, women were included in mixed populations of patients.

Although the total number of women enrolled in these two studies was large, the relatively small number of cardiovascular events occurring in these women made estimates of the effects of aspirin imprecise (9). Relevant data were published in 2005 by the large Women's Health Study, a 10-year trial of more than 39,000 women health professionals aged 45 years and older who were randomized to aspirin 100 mg every other day versus placebo (13). The Women's Health Study found that aspirin reduced the risk of ischemic stroke by 24% but had no effect on myocardial infarction overall. The risk of adverse effects was similar to previous trials: aspirin increased the risk of major gastrointestinal bleeding and hemorrhagic stroke. In subgroup analysis, older women (aged 65 years and older) derived greater benefit: in addition to a reduction in stroke, aspirin also reduced the risk of myocardial infarction.

The overall results of the Women's Health Study stand in contrast to previous evidence regarding aspirin prophylaxis in men (for whom myocardial infarction but not stroke was reduced) and evidence from secondary prevention (where the effects in men and women have been similar). It is currently unclear whether the observed differences are true biological differences or whether they may result from the low dosage of aspirin tested in the Women's Health Study or from the simple effects of chance (14).

Other Effects

Beyond its effect on cardiovascular events, evidence from some observational studies suggests that aspirin may reduce the risk of colorectal cancer (15). Aspirin also reduces headaches and can have other pain-relieving effects; on the other hand, aspirin can also cause dyspepsia and increase the risk of minor bleeding and bruising.

Official Recommendations

The USPSTF recommends that clinicians discuss aspirin with patients when the 10-year risk of CHD events is 6% or greater (16). These discussions should include information about potential benefits and harms, and the final decision about whether to take aspirin should be informed by the relative chances of beneficial and adverse outcomes. The American Heart Association recommends aspirin prophylaxis when the 10-year risk of CHD events is greater than 10% (17).

Essentials of Counseling

Clinicians should discuss the potential benefits and harms of routine aspirin use with men and women older than 40 years. In order to do so effectively, clinicians should estimate the patient's 10-year risk of cardiovascular events, using an appropriate (e.g., Framingham) risk calculator (see page 22 in Chapter 1) (18). Patients at low risk (men with a 10-year CHD risk less than

5% or women with a 10-year stroke risk less than 2%) should be counseled against aspirin use, as the benefits in these populations may not exceed the harms. For patients at increased CHD risk (men with a 10-year CHD risk greater than 10% or women older than 65 years with a stroke risk of 3% or greater) who are not at increased risk of adverse effects, aspirin can generally be recommended.

For patients between these risk levels, the decision about whether to take aspirin will depend on how the patient feels about the relative chances and impact of the potential benefits and harms, the extent to which taking a daily pill is onerous, and alternative means of reducing cardiovascular risk. Patients who choose to begin aspirin prophylaxis should take 75–325 mg daily, based on the dosages tested in most trials.

Contraindications

Routine aspirin use may not be appropriate for patients with a history of peptic ulcer disease, gastrointestinal bleeding, cerebral hemorrhage, history of uncontrolled hypertension, a bleeding diathesis, allergy to aspirin, liver or kidney disease, or diabetic retinopathy.

POSTMENOPAUSAL HORMONE THERAPY

Postmenopausal use of estrogen with or without concomitant use of progestin in healthy women for the prevention of chronic conditions, such as heart disease, is no longer recommended. Results of the WHI indicated that use of conjugated equine estrogen and medroxyprogesterone acetate resulted in increased risks of breast cancer, myocardial infarction, stroke, and deep vein thrombosis and reduced risks of colorectal cancer and fractures compared to placebo (see Table 15.1) (19). In addition, estrogen and progestin did not protect against mild cognitive impairment, and they increased the risk of dementia in women aged 65 years and older (20). In a second WHI study of more than 10,000 women with prior hysterectomies, use of estrogen alone compared to placebo resulted in increased risks of stroke and deep vein thrombosis, reduced risk of fracture, and no significant effect on breast cancer, colorectal cancer, and myocardial infarction (Table 15.1) (21). Both trials were discontinued early because of lack of benefit and concern for harms. Findings from the two studies cannot be compared directly because women in the estrogen-alone study were more likely to have CHD risk factors at baseline, such as hypertension, high blood cholesterol, diabetes, and obesity.

Results of the WHI confirmed and refuted prior evidence about the effects of postmenopausal hormone therapy on multiple health outcomes (22). Its unanticipated adverse effect on cardiovascular disease, in particular, shifted

TABLE 15.1   Estimates of Main Benefits and Harms from the Women's Health Initiative (WHI) trials. Number of events per 10,000 women per year.

	Combined Therapy Trial		Estrogen-Alone Trial	
	Estrogen + Progestin	Placebo	Estrogen	Placebo
Cases of breast cancer	38	30	26[a]	33
Myocardial infarction	37	30	49[a]	54
Stroke	29	21	44	32
Deep vein thrombosis	26	13	21	15
Hip fracture	10	15	11	17
Colorectal cancer	10	16	17[a]	16
Death	52[a]	53	81[a]	78

Adapted from Writing Group for the Women's Health Initiative Investigators. Risks and benefits of estrogen plus progestin in healthy postmenopausal women: principal results from the Women's Health Initiative randomized controlled trial. *JAMA* 2002;288:321–333 and Writing Group for the Women's Health Initiative Investigators. Effects of conjugated equine estrogen in postmenopausal women with hysterectomy. *JAMA* 2004;291:1701–1712.
[a] Differences between treatment and placebo are not statistically significant using unadjusted hazard ratios.

the balance of benefits and harms. As a result, recommendations changed and the FDA placed safety warnings on estrogen products and altered indications for use. Estrogen is currently approved for relief of moderate to severe hot flashes and symptoms of vulvar and vaginal atrophy, and it should be used at the lowest dose for the shortest duration needed to achieve treatment goals. Estrogen is also approved for the prevention of postmenopausal osteoporosis, but it is not considered a first-line agent. Estrogen therapy should not be taken to prevent heart disease or other chronic conditions.

Official Recommendations

The USPSTF recommends against the routine use of either combined estrogen and progestin or estrogen alone for the prevention of chronic conditions in postmenopausal women (23). After review of the evidence, including results of the WHI, the USPSTF concluded that the harmful effects of either combined estrogen and progestin or estrogen alone are likely to exceed the chronic disease prevention benefits in most women. Professional societies, such as the American College of Physicians, American Academy of Obstetricians and Gynecologists (24), American Academy of Family Physicians, and the North American Menopause Society (25), have taken similar positions.

Essentials of Counseling

Women who use or are considering using postmenopausal hormone therapy should discuss the possible benefits and harms with their clinicians. Women should initiate postmenopausal hormone therapy only for the currently approved indications and only if potential benefits outweigh potential harms. Hormone therapy to treat hot flashes and vulvovaginal atrophy is most often initiated in women at least 10 years younger than women enrolled in the WHI trials (26) and the generalizability of the WHI findings to guide their care is therefore unclear. Subgroup analyses of women in the WHI aged 50–59 years and those with menopausal symptoms are limited by small numbers of subjects and adverse events. Potential harms could be reduced by using the smallest effective dose for the shortest duration necessary.

As noted, estrogen is effective for the prevention of osteoporosis and fractures (27,28), although other FDA-approved agents, such as bisphosphonates, are also available. Women with substantial risks for osteoporosis and fractures and who are intolerant of other medications may be appropriate candidates for estrogen. Risk estimates from the WHI may be applicable in weighing potential benefits and harms of long-term therapy depending on the candidate's age.

Women who have been taking postmenopausal hormones for a long while based on outdated information about the benefits should discontinue use. Although many women are able to discontinue estrogen easily, many others experience hot flashes and other ill effects, such as pain or stiffness, after stopping use (29). Reducing doses in a stepwise taper may minimize symptoms. This can be done by decreasing the daily dose, reducing the numbers of days per week that estrogen is taken, or a combination of these approaches. Some women may require several weeks or months at each step. As with all patients changing or discontinuing a therapy, a woman discontinuing estrogen should follow up periodically with her clinician to assess response, monitor adverse effects, reexamine needs, and make adjustments.

Contraindications

Women considering hormone therapy for approved indications should not be prescribed estrogen if they have prior or current breast cancer, are pregnant, or have thrombophlebitis, endometrial cancer, or unevaluated abnormal vaginal bleeding.

OFFICE AND CLINIC ORGANIZATION

Offices or clinics should develop plans to routinely assess the breast cancer risk of women aged 40 years and older. Younger women (those younger than 55 years) who do not have a family history of breast cancer and who have not had a breast biopsy are not likely to be at increased risk of breast cancer, so further risk assessment is generally not necessary (30). Women in their late 50s and older do benefit from risk assessment, however, and practices should have access to a 5-year breast cancer risk calculator, which can be used on a handheld device or online (http://www.cancer.gov/bcrisktool/). Patient education materials on breast cancer risk and use of chemoprevention should be available for patients.

Offices and clinics should also develop plans to routinely assess the cardiovascular risk of all men and women aged 40 years and older, as well as younger persons with other cardiovascular risk factors. Framingham risk calculators are available online at http://hp2010.nhlbihin.net/atpiii/calculator.asp?usertype=prof, as discussed further in Chapter 1 (see page 22). Patients' cardiovascular risk assessments should be made available to clinicians so that appropriate counseling about chemoprophylaxis can be provided and other cardiovascular interventions considered (see page 469). The office should offer relevant decision aid materials in the waiting area and in the examining room, so that the clinician can hand the brochures or website listings directly to the patient after counseling.

Patient education materials about postmenopausal hormone therapy should also be readily available, especially for women who have been taking these drugs and may have questions about why and how to discontinue them.

RESOURCES—PATIENT EDUCATION MATERIALS

Breast Cancer Chemoprevention

American Cancer Society
Clifton Road
Atlanta, GA
Medicines to Reduce Breast Cancer Risk
http://www.cancer.org/docroot/CRI/content/CRI_2_6X_Tamoxifen_and_Raloxifene_
    Questions_and_Answers_5.asp

National Cancer Institute
Bethesda, MD
1-800-4-CANCER (1-800-422-6237), 9:00 a.m. to 4:30 p.m. local time, Monday through
    Friday
Breast Cancer (PDQ): Prevention
http://www.cancer.gov/cancertopics/pdq/prevention/breast/patient

U.S. Preventive Services Task Force
Breast Cancer Chemoprevention
http://www.ahrq.gov/clinic/uspstf/uspsbrpv.htm

Aspirin Prophylaxis

American Heart Association
Office of Scientific Affairs
7272 Greenville Avenue

Dallas, TX 75231-4596
800-242-8721
Aspirin as a Therapeutic Agent in Cardiovascular Disease

UpToDate
Patient information: Aspirin and cardiovascular disease
http://patients.uptodate.com/topic.asp?file=hrt_dis/2908

U.S. Preventive Services Task Force
Aspirin Chemoprevention
http://www.ahrq.gov/clinic/uspstf/uspsasmi.htm

Postmenopausal Hormone Therapy

Agency for Healthcare Research and Quality
Rockville, MD
Postmenopausal Hormone Replacement Therapy for Primary Prevention of Chronic Conditions
http://www.ahrq.gov/clinic/3rduspstf/hrt/hrtwh.htm

Food and Drug Administration
Estrogen and Estrogen with Progestin Therapies for Postmenopausal Women
http://www.fda.gov/cder/drug/infopage/estrogens progestins/default.htm

National Heart, Lung, and Blood Institute
Bethesda, MD
Facts about Menopausal Hormone Therapy
http://www.nhlbi.nih.gov/health/women/pht_facts.htm

National Institute on Aging
Bethesda, MD
Hormones after Menopause
http://www.niapublications.org/agepages/hormonesafter.asp

U.S. Preventive Services Task Force
Postmenopausal Hormone Therapy
http://www.ahrq.gov/clinic/uspstf/uspspmho.htm

Women's Health Initiative
http://www.nhlbi.nih.gov/whi/index.html

SUGGESTED READINGS

Cusick J, Powles T, Veronesi U, et al. Overview of the main outcomes in breast-cancer prevention trials. *Lancet* 2003;361:296–300.

Peto R, Gray R, Collins R, et al. Randomized trial of prophylactic daily aspirin in British male doctors. *Br Med J* 1988;296:313–316.

Steering Committee of the Physicians' Health Study Research Group. Final report on the aspirin components of the ongoing Physicians' Health Study. *N Engl J Med* 1989;321:129–135.

U.S. Preventive Services Task Force. Aspirin for the primary prevention of cardiovascular events: recommendation and rationale. *Ann Intern Med* 2002;136:157–60.

U.S. Preventive Services Task Force. Chemoprevention of breast cancer: recomendations and rationale. *Ann Intern Med* 2002;137:56–58.

U.S. Preventive Services Task Force. Hormone therapy for the prevention of chronic conditions in postmenopausal women. *Ann Intern Med* 2005;142:855–60.

Writing Group for the Women's Health Initiative Investigators. Risks and benefits of estrogen plus progestin in healthy postmenopausal women. *JAMA* 2002;288: 321–333.

Writing Group for the Women's Health Initiative Investigators. Effects of conjugated equine estrogen in postmenopausal women with hysterectomy. *JAMA* 2004;291: 1701–1712.

References

1. Early Breast Cancer Trialists' Collaborative Group. Tamoxifen for early breast cancer: an overview of the randomized trials. *Lancet* 1998;351:1451–1467.
2. Cusick J, Powles T, Veronesi U, et al. Overview of the main outcomes in breast-cancer prevention trials. *Lancet* 2003;361:296–300.
3. Cauley JA, Norton L, Lippman ME, et al. Continued breast cancer risk reduction in postmenopausal women treated with raloxifene: 4-year results from the MORE trial. Multiple outcomes of raloxifene evaluation. *Breast Cancer Res Treat* 2001;65: 125–134.
4. Barrett-Conner E, Mosca L, Collins P, et al. Effects of raloxifene on cardiovascular events and breast cancer in postmenopausal women. *N Engl J Med* 2006;355: 125–137.
5. Vogel GV, Costantino JP, Wickerham DL, et al. Effects of tamoxifen vs. raloxifene on the risk of developing invasive breast cancer and other disease outcomes. The NSABP Study of Tamoxifen and Raloxifne (STAR) P-2 Trial. *JAMA* 2006;295:2727–2741.
6. Kinsinger LS, Harris R, Woolf SW, et al. Chemoprevention of breast cancer: a summary of the evidence for the U.S. Preventive Services Task Force. *Ann Intern Med* 2002;137:59–67.
7. U.S. Preventive Services Task Force. Chemoprevention of breast cancer: recommendations and rationale. *Ann Intern Med* 2002;137:56–58.
8. Chlebowski RT, Collyar DSE, Somerfield MR, et al. American Society of Clinical Oncology technology assessment on breast cancer risk reduction strategies: tamoxifen and raloxifene. *J Clin Oncol* 1999;17:1939–1955.
9. Freedman AN, Graubard BI, Rao AR, et al. Estimates of the number of US women who could benefit from tamoxifen for breast cancer chemoprevention. *J Natl Cancer Inst* 2003;95:526–532.
10. Melnikow J, Paternitit D, Azari R, et al. Preferences of women evaluating risks of tamoxifen (POWER) study of preferences for tamoxifen for breast cancer risk reduction. *Cancer* 2005;103:1996–2005.
11. Hayden M, Pignone M, Phillips C, et al. Aspirin for the primary prevention of cardiovascular events: a summary of the evidence for the U.S. Preventive Services Task Force. *Ann Intern Med* 2002;136:161–172.
12. Sudlow C. Anthithrombotic treatment. In: *Clinical evidence*, 5th ed. London: BMJ Publishing Group, 2001.
13. Ridker PM, Cook NR, Lee IM, et al. A randomized trial of low-dose aspirin in the primary prevention of cardiovascular disease in women. *N Engl J Med* 2005;352: 1293–1304.
14. Mulrow C, Pignone M. An editorial update: should she take aspirin? *Ann Intern Med* 2005;142:942–943.

15. Chan AT, Giovannucci EL, Meyerhardt JA, et al. Long-term use of aspirin and nonsteroidal anti-inflammatory drugs and risk of colorectal cancer. *JAMA* 2005;294: 914–923.

16. U.S. Preventive Services Task Force. Aspirin for the primary prevention of cardiovascular events: recommendation and rationale. *Ann Intern Med* 2002;136: 157–160.

17. Pearson TA, Blair SN, Daniels SR, et al. AHA guidelines for primary prevention of cardiovascular disease and stroke: 2002 update: consensus panel guide to comprehensive risk reduction for adult patients without coronary or other atherosclerotic vascular diseases American Heart Association Science Advisory and Coordinating Committee. *Circulation* 2002;106:388–391.

18. Sheridan S, Pignone M, Mulrow C. Framingham-based tools to calculate the global risk of coronary heart disease: a systematic review of tools for clinicians. *J Gen Intern Med* 2003;18:1039–1052.

19. Writing Group for the Women's Health Initiative Investigators. Risks and benefits of estrogen plus progestin in healthy postmenopausal women. *JAMA* 2002;288:321–333.

20. Shumaker S, Legault C, Thal L, et al. Estrogen plus progestin and the incidence of dementia and mild cognitive impairment in postmenopausal women: the Women's Health Initiative memory study: a randomized controlled trial. *JAMA* 2003;289:2651–2662.

21. Writing Group for the Women's Health Initiative Investigators. Effects of conjugated equine estrogen in postmenopausal women with hysterectomy. *JAMA* 2004;291:1701–1712.

22. Nelson HD, Humphrey LL, Nygren P, et al. Postmenopausal hormone replacement therapy: scientific review. *JAMA* 2002;288:872–881.

23. U.S. Preventive Services Task Force. Hormone therapy for the prevention of chronic conditions in postmenopausal women. *Ann Intern Med* 2005;142:855–860.

24. ACOG Task Force on Hormone Therapy. Hormone therapy. *Obstet Gynecol* 2004;104(4 Suppl):1S–131S.

25. The North American Menopause Society. Recommendations for estrogen and progestogen use in peri- and postmenopausal women: October 2004 position statement of the North American Menopause Society. *Menopause* 2004;11(6):589–600.

26. Nelson HD. Commonly used types of postmenopausal estrogen for treatment of hot flashes: scientific review. *JAMA* 2004;291:1610–1620.

27. Torgerson DJ, Bell-Syer SE. Hormone replacement therapy and prevention of nonvertebral fractures: a meta-analysis of randomized trials. *JAMA* 2001;285(22): 2891–2897.

28. Cauley JA, Robbins J, Chen Z, et al. Effects of estrogen plus progestin on risk of fracture and bone mineral density. *JAMA* 2003;290:1729–1738.

29. Ockene JK, Barad JH, Cochrane BB, et al. Symptom experience after discontinuing use of estrogen plus progestin. *JAMA* 2005;294:183–193.

30. Lewis CL, Kinsinger LS, Harris RP, et al. Breast cancer risk in primary care: implications for chemoprevention. *Arch Intern Med* 2004;164:1897–1903.

CHAPTER 16

Immunizations

Robert M. Wolfe

Immunization is one of the most successful examples of primary prevention. Infectious diseases that were, at the turn of the 20th century, the leading causes of childhood death and disability are now relatively rare in the United States. Vaccination programs are responsible for the global eradication of smallpox and are close to eliminating other diseases (e.g., poliomyelitis) hopefully in the near future. Decades of organized efforts to vaccinate children in the United States have very significantly reduced the incidence of diseases such as pertussis and measles. Nevertheless, incidence rates of some vaccine-preventable diseases are now rising, due to a variety of barriers to immunization, including cost, accessibility, the increasing complexity of vaccination schedules, and a rising focus on the potential adverse effects of vaccines leading to fear in the public (1).

This chapter reviews the indications and contraindications for routine childhood and adult vaccinations. It focuses on commonly used vaccines in the primary care setting and those that offer the greatest protective public health benefits among asymptomatic persons. Vaccines for selected population groups (e.g., rabies vaccine), for international travelers, and for postexposure prophylaxis are not emphasized. Patients with altered immune competence (e.g., patients with cancer, acquired immunodeficiency syndrome [AIDS]) require special immunization protocols (2,3) and are therefore beyond the scope of this chapter.

Until the 1990s, inadequate immunization coverage among preschool children had been a particular problem in the United States, which had lower early childhood immunization rates than many other industrialized and developed countries (4,5). A nine-city survey in 1991 found that only 10–38% of 2-year-old children were properly immunized (6). However, recent surveys have shown higher coverage, perhaps in response to the national Healthy People 2010 initiative to increase preschool immunization. In July 2005, the Centers for Disease Control and Prevention (CDC) announced that the nation's childhood immunization coverage rates had reached record high levels, with approximately 81% of the nation's 19- to 35-month-old children receiving all the vaccinations in the recommended series (7). Recent World

359

Health Organization (WHO) data indicate that immunization rates in the United States are comparable to those in most developed countries (8). Unfortunately, problems still exist, especially regarding delayed vaccination. A study in 2005 found that while more than 85% of U.S. children aged 19–35 months had received a recommended set of six vaccines, more than one in three children were undervaccinated for more than 6 months during the first 24 months of life and one in four children had lapses in at least four vaccines (9).

Inadequate immunization coverage is not limited to children, however. The current burden of suffering from vaccine-preventable diseases may even be higher among adults. An estimated 50,000–70,000 adults die each year in the United States from vaccine-preventable diseases such as pneumococcal infection, influenza, and hepatitis B whereas it is rare that more than 200 children die annually in the United States from the vaccine-preventable diseases of childhood.

The causes of inadequate immunization are multifactorial. They include systems barriers (e.g., those involving the organization/financing of the health care system), clinician barriers (e.g., inadequate clinician knowledge about vaccines and contraindications), and parent/patient barriers (e.g., fear of immunization-related adverse events) (1).

Problems with the supply and distribution of vaccines are among the most noticeable systems barriers. The supply of some vaccines, such as influenza vaccine, has been inadequate during recent years. Vaccine manufacturers face a variety of difficulties, including research costs, regulatory stringencies, and liability issues (10). Maldistribution is also a problem, particularly in the United States, where many adults and children are uninsured or underinsured (1).

Clinician misconceptions and lack of knowledge of proper indications and contraindications to vaccine administration are surprisingly widespread. The increase in the number of vaccines now indicated for routine administration has made it difficult for clinicians to keep up with new recommendations. For example, the introduction of many new vaccines in the last four decades has quadrupled the number of immunizations that should be administered before a child's second birthday. On the basis of current recommendations, a child would receive as many as six vaccine injections in a single visit (11). Several studies have revealed significant knowledge deficits among clinicians regarding immunization schedules, vaccine contraindications, and vaccine side effects (12–14).

"Missed opportunities," or the failure to use acute care visits for immunizations, are often cited as a common cause of a clinician failing to properly vaccinate patients. Although most clinicians will give needed vaccinations at well child visits, the use of vaccines is much lower at acute visits. According to one study of adolescent immunization practices, only 43%

of clinicians reported checking immunization status, and only 23% reported providing necessary immunizations during acute visits (15). However, the notion that a policy of providing vaccines during acute visits actually increases immunization rates has been challenged by the results of other studies (16,17).

Parent/patient barriers can arise from problems of logistics (lack of access to transportation), finance (inadequate insurance), or knowledge and attitude issues, such as concerns about vaccine safety issues (see "Parental Education and Counseling" on page 375).

The recommendations in this chapter are consistent with guidelines issued by the Advisory Committee on Immunization Practices (ACIP) of the CDC, a committee of 15 experts in immunization-related fields, appointed by the Secretary of the U.S. Department of Health and Human Services (HHS). Recommendations of the ACIP become CDC policy when they are accepted by the director of the CDC and are published in the CDC's *Morbidity and Mortality Weekly Report* (MMWR).

Since 1994, the ACIP, American Academy of Pediatrics (AAP), and American Academy of Family Physicians (AAFP) have produced a harmonized childhood and adolescent immunization schedule (see Fig. 16.1), and the ACIP and AAFP produce a harmonized adult immunization schedule. The American College of Physicians (ACP) has not participated in the harmonized schedule, partly because ACP believes that ACIP recommendations are not sufficiently evidence based. To address this issue, the ACIP recently established an Evidence-Based Working Group, which is examining how the ACIP evaluates evidence and seeking a more consistent evidence-based approach for each ACIP recommendation. The American College of Obstetricians and Gynecologists (ACOG) has a liaison representative on the ACIP. Although its recommendations are not harmonized with the ACIP, AAFP, and AAP, ACOG has generally supported ACIP recommendations regarding adolescent and adult vaccinations for females.

Vaccine products and recommendations are frequently updated; therefore readers are encouraged to consult up-to-date resources for current guidelines (see "Suggested Readings" at the end of this chapter).

GENERAL PRINCIPLES

Administration of a vaccine is generally recommended for those individuals at risk of the disease at the youngest age at which the patient will develop an adequate postvaccination antibody response. Suggested ages for childhood immunizations (see Fig. 16.1 and Table 1 in Appendix B) have some flexibility (e.g., many immunizations recommended for infants at 2 months of age can be given at 6 weeks of age). Nonetheless, immunizations should generally

Childhood Schedule

Age (Yrs)	Birth	1	2	4	6	12	15	18	19–23	2–3	4–6
HepB		HepB	①		HepB				HepB series		
Rota											
DTaP						DTaP					DTaP
Hib				②	Hib		Hib				
PCV/PPV					PCV					PCV ③ / PPV	
IPV					IPV						IPV
Flu					Influenza (yearly)						
MMR						MMR ④					MMR
Var						Var					Var
HepA						HepA (two doses)				HepA Ser.	
Men											MPSV4

Legend:
- Range of recommended ages
- Catch-up vaccination
- Certain high-risk groups

1. 4-mo dose of **HepB**: It is permissible to administer four doses of **HepB** when combination vaccines are given after the birth dose. If monovalent **HepB** is used for doses after the birth dose, a dose at age 4 mo is not needed

2. If **PRP-OMP (PedvaxHIB** or **Comvax** [Merck]) is adminstered at ages 2 and 4 mo, a dose at age 6 mo is not required

3. Administer **PCV** at ages 24–59 mo in certain high-risk groups. **PCV** is not generally recommended for children ≥5 yr, Administer PPV to children aged ≥2 yr in certain high-risk groups. (see Table 1 for high risk indication for **PCV** and **PPV**)

4. **MMRV (ProQuad®** [Merck]) is preferred over giving MMR and varicella vaccine separately

Adolescent Schedule

Age (Yrs)	7–10	11–12	13–14	15	16–18
Tdap	Note 1	Tdap	Tdap		
HPV	Note 2	HPV three doses	HPV series		
Men	MPSV4	MCV4	MCV4 [3] / MCV4		
PPV	PPV				
Flu	Flu (yearly)				
HepA	HepA series				
HepB	HepB series				
IPV	IPV series				
MMR	MMR series				
Var	Varicella series				

1. Minimum age for **Tdap**: 10 yr for **BOOSTRIX** and 11 yr for **ADACEL**

2. Minimum age for **HPV**: 9 yr

3. Administer **MCV4** at age 11–12 yr and to previously unvaccinated adolescents at high school entry (appproximately 15 yr of age)

Figure 16.1 • Immunization recommendations from the Advisory Committee on Immunization Practices (ACIP). Figure used with permission from SHOTS 2007, developed by the Group on Immunization Education of the Society of Teachers of Family Medicine (see page 425 for further details). See ACIP website for current versions and footnotes. See the following websites for updates of the harmonized immunization schedules: http://www.cdc.gov/nip/recs/child-schedule.htm and http://www.cdc.gov/nip/recs/adult-schedule.htm.

Adult Schedule

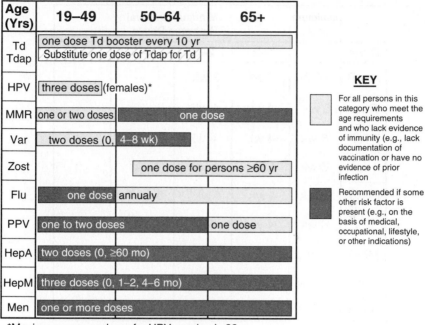

Age (Yrs)	19–49	50–64	65+
Td Tdap	one dose Td booster every 10 yr		
	Substitute one dose of Tdap for Td		
HPV	three doses (females)*		
MMR	one or two doses	one dose	
Var	two doses (0, 4–8 wk)		
Zost		one dose for persons ≥60 yr	
Flu	one dose annualy		
PPV	one to two doses	one dose	
HepA	two doses (0, ≥60 mo)		
HepM	three doses (0, 1–2, 4–6 mo)		
Men	one or more doses		

KEY

☐ For all persons in this category who meet the age requirements and who lack evidence of immunity (e.g., lack documentation of vaccination or have no evidence of prior infection

■ Recommended if some other risk factor is present (e.g., on the basis of medical, occupational, lifestyle, or other indications)

*Maximum approved age for HPV vaccine is 26 yr

Medical Schedule

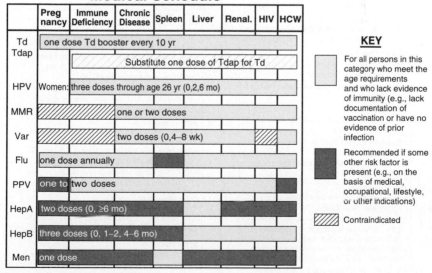

	Pregnancy	Immune Deficiency	Chronic Disease	Spleen	Liver	Renal.	HIV	HCW
Td Tdap	one dose Td booster every 10 yr							
		Substitute one dose of Tdap for Td						
HPV	Women: three doses through age 26 yr (0,2,6 mo)							
MMR		one or two doses						
Var		two doses (0,4–8 wk)						
Flu	one dose annually							
PPV	one to two doses							
HepA	two doses (0, ≥6 mo)							
HepB	three doses (0, 1–2, 4–6 mo)							
Men	one dose							

KEY

☐ For all persons in this category who meet the age requirements and who lack evidence of immunity (e.g., lack documentation of vaccination or have no evidence of prior infection

■ Recommended if some other risk factor is present (e.g., on the basis of medical, occupational, lifestyle, or other indications)

▨ Contraindicated

Figure 16.1 • *(Continued)*.

4-Month to 6-Year Catch-Up Schedule

Dose	Minimum Age	Minimum Interval between Doses			
		1–2	2–3	3–4	4–5
HepB	Birth	4 wk	8 wk^1		
Rota	6 wk^2	4 wk	4 wk^3		
DTaP	6 wk	4 wk	4 wk	6 mo	6 mo^4
Hib^5	6 wk	4 wk^6	4 wk^7	8 wk^8	
PCV^5	6 wk	4 wk^9	4 wk^{10}	8 wk^{11}	
IPV	6 wk	4 wk	4 wk	4 wk^{12}	
MMR	12 mo	4 wk			
Var	12 mo	3 mo			
HepA	12 mo	6 mo			

1. **HepB** - Dose three
   Give at least 8 wk after the second dose and at least 16 wk after the first dose.

2. Do not start **Rotavirus** series later than age 12 wk.

3. Administer final **Rotavirus** dose by age 32 wk
   Do not administer a dose later than age 32 wk.

4. **DTaP** - Dose five
   The fifth dose is not necessary if the fourth dose was administered at age ≥4 yr.

5. **Hib** and **PCV** are not generally recommended for children ≥5 yr.

6. **Hib** - Dose two
   • 4 wk after the first dose if the first dose was given at age <12 mo.
   • 8 wk after the first dose (as final dose) if the first dose was given at age 12–14 mo.
   • No further doses are needed if previous dose given at age ≥15 mo.

7. **Hib** - Dose three
   • 4 wk after the second dose^a if the child's current age is <12 mo.
   • 8 wk after the second dose (as final dose)* if the child's current age is ≥12 mo and the second dose was given at age <15 mo.
   • No further doses are needed if the previous dose was given at age ≥15 mo.
   • If current age <12 mo and the first 2 doses were **PRP-OMP** (**PedvaxHIB** or **Comvax** [Merck]), the third (and final) dose should be given at age 12–15 mo and at least 8 wk after the second dose.

8. **Hib** - Dose four
   8 wk after dose three (as final dose). This dose is only necessary for children aged 12 mo–5 yr who received three doses before age 12 mo.

9. **PCV** - Dose two
   • 4 wk after the first dose if the first dose was given at age <12 mo and the child's current age is <24 mo.
   • 8 wk after the first dose (as final dose) if the first dose was given at age ≥12 mo or the child's current age is 24–59 mo.
   • No further doses are needed for healthy children if the first dose was given at age 24 mo or older.

10. **PCV** - Dose three
    • 4 wk after dose two if the child's current age is <12 mo.
    • 8 wk after dose two (as final dose) if the child's current age is ≥12 mo.
    • No further doses are needed for healthy children if the previous dose was given at age ≥24 mo.

11. **PCV** - Dose four
    8 wk after dose three (as final dose). This dose is only necessary for children aged 12 mo –5 yr who received three doses before age 12 mo.

12. **IPV** - Dose four
    • For children who received an all-**IPV** or all-oral poliovirus (**OPV**) series, a fourth dose is not necessary if third dose was administered at age ≥4 yr.
    • If both **OPV** and **IPV** were administered as part of a series, a total of four doses should be given, regardless of the child's current age.

Figure 16.1 • *(Continued).*

7-Year to 18-Year Catch-Up Schedule

Dose	Minimum Age	Minimum Interval between Doses		
		1–2	2–3	3–4
Td/Tdap	7 yr[13]	4 wk	8 wk[14]	6 mo[15]
HPV[16]	9 yr	4 wk	12 wk	
HepA	12 mo	6 mo		
HepB	Birth	4 wk[17]	8 wk[18]	
IPV	6 wk	4 wk	4 wk	4 wk[19]
MMR	12 mo	4 wk		
Var	12 mo	4 wk[20]		

13.	Minimum ages: 7 yr for **Td**, 10 yr for **BOOSTRIX** and 11 yr for **ADACEL**
14.	**Td/Tdap** - Dose three • 8 wk if first dose given at age <12 mo. • 6 mo if first dose given at age ≥12 mo.
15.	**Td/Tdap** Dose four • Adolescents aged 11–18 yr should receive a single dose of **Tdap**. instead of **Td** for booster immunization. • For children age 7–10 yr, the interval (6 mo) between the third and booster (fourth) dose is determined by the age when the first dose was given. For adolescents aged 11–18 yr, the interval (5 or 10 yr) is determined by the age when the third dose was given. The minimum interval follows: • 6 mo if the first dose was given at age <12 mo and the child's current age is <11 yr. • 5 yr if the first dose was given at age ≥12 mo and third dose given at age <7 yr and current age ≥11 yr. • 10 yr if the third dose was given at age ≥7 yr.
16.	**HPV** vaccine is not approved for females <9 yr or ≥27 yr, nor for males.

17.	An alternative two-dose schedule for unvaccinated adolescents ages 11 through 15 yr: give two doses **Recombivax HB** 1.0 mL (adult formulation, 10 µg) spaced 4–6 mo apart. (**Engerix-B** is not licensed for a two dose schedule)
18.	**HepB** - Dose three Give at least 8 wk after the second dose and at least 16 wk after the first dose.
19.	**IPV** - Dose four • For children who received an all-**IPV** or all-oral poliovirus (**OPV**) series, a fourth dose is not necessary if third dose was administered at age ≥4 yr. • If both **OPV** and **IPV** were administered as part of a series, a total of four doses should be given, regardless of the child's current age.
20.	**Varicella** - Minimum interval for dose two • 4 wk if first dose given at age ≥13 yr. • 3 mo if first dose given at age <13 yr.

Figure 16.1 • (*Continued*).

be given at the earliest recommended age at which the child presents to the clinician. Partial doses or doses given too soon may dampen the antibody response and should not be counted as part of a primary series. Doses administered 5 or more days earlier than the minimum interval or age for any vaccine should not be counted as valid doses and should be repeated as is appropriate for the age. The repeat dose should be spaced after the invalid dose by the recommended minimum interval (2). It is unnecessary to restart an interrupted series of a vaccine or toxoid or to add extra doses. Table 1 in Appendix B provides catch-up schedules and minimum intervals between doses for children whose vaccinations have been delayed. The current schedule for adult immunization is shown in Figure 16.1 and Table 2 in Appendix B.

Intramuscular injections are generally administered in the anterolateral aspect of the thigh in infants and in the deltoid muscle in older children and adults; they should not be administered in the gluteal muscles at any age because of risk of injury to the sciatic nerve (see Fig. 16.2) (2). Further details about vaccine handling and injection technique are provided in the references at the end of this chapter.

For most vaccines, simultaneous administration does not impair antibody responses or increase rates of adverse reactions (18). In fact, simultaneous administration is an important public health strategy, decreasing the number of visits needed and the potential for missed doses as well as enabling earlier protection (19). With the increasing number of vaccinations that are recommended for administration before the age of 18 months, combination vaccines offer many practical advantages: the avoidance of deferred immunizations due to clinician or parental concern over multiple shots with the attendant risks of missed opportunities, an increase in adherence and improved vaccination coverage rates, reduced pain, and potentially lower costs from reduced vaccine charges and reduced office visits (20,21). The ACIP, AAFP, and AAP have issued a joint statement endorsing the use of combination vaccines whenever any component of the combination is indicated and its other components are not contraindicated, provided they are approved by the U.S. Food and Drug Administration (FDA) for use in children at the recommended ages (22). Vaccines that prevent the same disease but are from different manufacturers may be interchanged when a particular antibody is known to protect against disease (called the *serologic correlate of immunity*) and when using vaccines from different manufacturers results in sufficient antibody titers (22,23).

Immune globulin may interfere with viral replication and the antibody response to certain live virus vaccines. Administration of measles-mumps-rubella-varicella (MMRV) vaccine or its component vaccines should therefore be delayed for 3–11 months after the administration of antibody-containing

Vaccines	Dose	Route
Diphtheria, tetanus, pertussis (DTaP, DT, Tdap, Td)	0.5 mL	i.m.
Haemophilus influenzae type b(Hib)	0.5 mL	i.m.
Hepatitis A (HepA)	≤18 yr: 0.5 mL ≥19 yr: 1.0 mL	i.m.
Hepatitis B (HepB) *Persons 11-15 yr may be given Recomnivax HP 1.0 mL adult formulation on a two-dose schedule.*	≤19 yr: 0.5 mL[a] ≥20 yr: 1.0 mL	i.m.
Human papillomavirus (HPV)	0.5 mL	i.m.
Influenza, live attenuated (LAIV)	0.5 mL	Intranasal spray
Influenza, trivalent inactivated (TIV)	6-35 mo: 0.25 mL ≥3 yr : 0.5 mL	i.m.
Measles, mumps, rubella (MMR)	0.5 mL	s.c.
Meningococcal, conjugated (MCV4)	0.5 mL	i.m.
Meningococcal, polysaccharide (MPSV4)	0.5 mL	i.m.
Pneumococcal conjugate (PCV)	0.5 mL	i.m.
Pneumococcal polysaccharide (PPV)	0.5 mL	i.m. or s.c.
Polio, inactivated (IPV)	0.5 mL	i.m. or s.c.
Rotavirus (Rv)	2.0 mL	Oral
Varicella (Var)	0.5 mL	s.c.
Zoster (Zos)	0.65 mL	s.c.
Combination Vaccines DTaP+HepB+IPV (Pediarix) DTaP+Hib (Trihibit) Hib+HepB (Comvax)	0.5 mL	i.m.
MMR+Var (ProQuad)	≤12 yr: 0.5 mL	s.c.
HepA+HepB (Twinrix)	≥18 yr: 1.0 mL	i.m.

Injection Site and Needle Size

Subcutaneous (sc) Injection
Use a 23–25 gauge needle. Choose the injection site that is appropriate to the person's age and body mass.

Age	Needle Length	Injection Site
Infants (1–12 mo)	5/8″	Fatty tissue over anterolateral thigh muscle
Children (≥12 mo), adolescents, & adults	5/8″	Fatty tissue over anterolateral thigh muscle or fatty tissue over triceps

Intramuscular (im) Injection
Use a 22–25 gauge needle. Choose the injection site and needle length appropriate to the person's age and body mass.

Age	Needle Length	Injection Site
Newborn (1st 28 days)	5/8″[b]	Anterolateral thigh muscle
Infant (1–12 mo)	7/8″–1″	Anterolateral thigh muscle
Toddler (1–2 yr)	1″–1 1/4″ 5/8″[b]–1″	Anterolateral thigh muscle or deltoid muscle of arm
Children 3–18 yr	5/8″[b]–1″ 1″–1 1/4″	Deltoid muscle of arm or anterolateral thigh muscle
≥19 yr (Sex/Weight)		
Male/Female less than 130 lb	5/8″[b]–1″	Deltoid muscle of arm
Female (130–200 lb) Male (130–260 lb)	1″–1 1/2″	Deltoid muscle of arm
Female (200+ lb) Male (260+ lb)	1 1/2″	Deltoid muscle of arm

[b]*If skin is stretched tight and subcutaneous tissue is not bunched.*

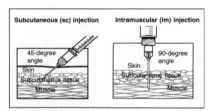

[a]Always refer to the package insert included with each biologic for complete vaccine administration information. CDC's advisory committee on immunization practices (ACIP) recommendations for the particular vaccine should be reviewed as well.

Figure 16.2 • Administering vaccines: dose, route, site, and needle size. Used with permission of the Immunization Action Coalition, St. Paul, MN. www.immunize.org/catg.d/p3085.pdf.

blood products (such as immune globulins), depending on the type of preparation and its dose (see Tables 16.1 and 16.2). If vaccination with MMRV or its component vaccines precedes immune globulin administration, it need not be readministered if the interval between the two products is longer than 14 days. Some live virus vaccines can theoretically interfere with viral replication and the antibody response to other live virus vaccines if not administered as recommended. Measles-mumps-rubella (MMR) vaccine and varicella vaccine may be given simultaneously; otherwise their administration should be separated by at least 4 weeks. Specific guidelines for spacing administration are provided elsewhere (2).

TABLE 16.1 Combination Vaccines

Combination Vaccine (manufacturer)	Components	Advantages	Recommended Schedule
Comvax (Merck) (IM)	Hib (PedvaxHIB) + HepB (Recombivax)	Combines Hib and hepatitis B shots; only three shots needed for Hib immunity, avoiding 6-mo Hib shot	Infants born to HbsAg-negative mothers should be vaccinated with three 0.5 mL doses of Comvax, ideally at 2, 4, and 12–15 mo of age. If the recommended schedule cannot be followed, interval between the first two doses should be at least 2 mo and the interval between the second and third dose should be as close as possible to 8 to 11 mo. COMVAX is approved for use in infants aged 6 weeks to 15 months.
Twinrix (GlaxoSmithKline) (IM)	HepA (Havrix) + HepB (Engerix B)	Two less shots to achieve full immunity to hepatitis A and B by combining the two-dose HepA series with the three shots of the HepB series	Indicated in the United States for persons 18 yr and older. Each 1-mL dose contains 720 EL.U. of inactivated hepatitis A virus and 20 µg of hepatitis B surface antigen. Primary immunization for adults consists of three doses, given on a 0-, 1-, and 6-mo schedule. The first and second doses should be separated by at least 4 wk, and the second and third doses should be separated by at least 5 mo, with at least 6 mo between the first and third doses. Alternatively, a four-dose schedule, given on days 0, 7, and 21 to 30 followed by a booster dose at 12 mo may be used.

| TriHIBit (sanofi pasteur) (IM) | **DTaP** (Tripedia) **+ Hib** (ActHIB) | One less shot at 15–18 mo checkup by combining DTaP and Hib boosters. Not recommended for primary series because of evidence of decreased immunogenicity of the Hib component when combined with DTaP | TriHIBit is licensed for use in children aged 15–18 mo as a fourth dose in the schedule for DTP/DTaP and Hib. TriHIBit can be used if the child is 12 mo or older and has received at least one prior dose of Hib vaccine 2 or more mo earlier and TriHIBit will be the last dose in the Hib series. Infants who received TriHIBit before age 12 mo should be age-appropriately reimmunized with another Hib vaccine as if they have never received a dose.

Note: the vaccines are provided in separate vials, and the DTaP component (Tripedia) is used to reconstitute the Hib component (ActHIB). Supplied this way, there is a single lot number for both. Clinicians may combine Tripedia and ActHIB that have been supplied separately (i.e., not packaged as TriHIBit); if this is done, the lot numbers of both vaccines must be recorded in the child's chart. |
| Pediarix (GlaxoSmithKline) (IM) | **DTaP** (Infanrix) **+ HepB** (Engerix-B) **+ IPV**[a] | Combines the DTaP, HepB, and IPV series in three shots by age 6 mo, reducing by as many as six fewer the total number of shots needed by age 2 years. Child still needs another DTaP and Hib booster at age 15–18 mo (Pediarix is not approved for this use). | Recommended schedule: The primary immunization series for Pediarix is three doses of 0.5 mL, given intramuscularly, at 6- to 8-wk intervals (preferably 8 wk), typically at 2, 4, and 6 mo of age. The customary age for the first dose is 2 mo, but it may be given starting at 6 wk. Pediarix should not be administered to any infant before the age of 6 wk. Pediarix is licensed for children aged 6 weeks through 6 years, and may be used to complete a 3-dose primary series that was begun with individual DTaP, hepatitis B, and IPV vaccines, even if from a different manufacturer. |

(continued)

369

TABLE 16.1 (*Continued*)

Combination Vaccine (manufacturer)	Components	Advantage	Recommended Schedule
ProQuad (Merck) (IM)	MMR (M-M-RII) + Varicella (Varivax)	Combines MMR due at 12–15 mo with varicella vaccine due at 12–18 mo. May also be used for MMR and varicella boosters due at 4–6 yr.	ProQuad is indicated for simultaneous vaccination against measles, mumps, rubella, and varicella in children 12 mo to 12 years of age; it may be used in children 12 mo to 12 years of age if a second dose of measles, mumps, and rubella vaccine is to be administered. Dose: a single 0.5-mL dose of ProQuad administered subcutaneously. At least 1 mo should elapse between a dose of a measles-containing vaccine such as M-M-RII, and a dose of ProQuad. If for any reason a second dose of varicella-containing vaccine is required, at least 3 mo should elapse between administration of the two doses.

Hib = haemophilus influenzae type b; EL.U. = ELISA units; DTaP = diphtheria-tetanus-acellular pertussis; DTP = diphtheria-tetanus-pertussis; IPV = inactivated poliovirus vaccine; MMR = measles-mumps-rubella.

Note: Principles for use of combination vaccines:

1. The use of licensed combination vaccines is preferred over separate injection of their equivalent component vaccines.

2. Only combinations approved by the U.S. Food and Drug Administration (FDA) should be used.

3. When administering combination vaccines, the minimum age for administration is the oldest age for any of the individual components; the minimum interval between doses is equal to the greatest interval of any of the individual antigens.

[a]The IPV component is derived from a vaccine that has been used in other countries since 1996. It has not been used previously in the United States, but contains the same three poliovirus types, strains, and antigen content as the currently licensed U.S. vaccine.

(CDC. Combination vaccines for childhood immunization: recommendations of the Advisory Committee on Immunization Practices (ACIP), the American Academy of Pediatrics (AAP), and the American Academy of Family Physicians (AAFP). *MMWR* 1999;48(RR-5:5. See also http://www.immunize.org/resources/pharmac.asp#packetinserts.)

TABLE 16.2 Scheduling Strategies for Using the Current Combination Vaccines for Children (HepB, Hib, DTaP, Polio only)[a]

	Birth		2 mo		4 mo		6 mo		12-18 mo		Number of Shots Required through 2 yr
	Vaccine	Brandname	Vaccine	Brandname	Vaccine	Brandname	Vaccine	Brandname	Vaccine	Brandname	
Option 1	Hep B	Engerix B Recombivax HB	Hep B,	Engerix B Recombivax HB			HepB	Engerix B Recombivax HB			14
			Hib	HibTITER ActHIB	Hib	HibTITER ActHIB	Hib	HibTITER ActHIB	Hib	HibTITER ActHIB Tripedia[b]	
			DTaP	Tripedia DAPTACEL Infanrix	DTaP	Tripedia DAPTACEL Infanrix	DTaP	Tripedia DAPTACEL Infanrix	DTaP	DAPTACEL[c] Infanrix	
			IPV	IPOL	IPV	IPOL	IPV	IPOL			
Option 2			Hep B	Engerix B Recombivax HB	HepB	Engerix B Recombivax HB	HepB	Engerix B Recombivax HB			14
			Hib	HibTITER ActHIB	Hib	HibTITER ActHIB	Hib	HibTITER ActHIB	Hib	HibTITER ActHIB[b] Tripedia[b]	
			DTaP	Tripedia DAPTACEL Infanrix	DTaP	Tripedia DAPTACEL Infanrix	DTaP	Tripedia DAPTACEL Infanrix	DTaP	DAPTACEL[c] Infanrix	
			IPV	IPOL	IPV	IPOL	IPV	IPOL			
Option 3	Hep B	Engerix B Fecombivax HB	HepB	Engerix B Recombivax HB	HepB	Engerix B Recombivax HB	HepB	Engerix B Recombivax HB			13
			Hib	PedvaxHIB[d]	Hib	PedvaxHIB[d]			Hib	PedvaxHIB[d]	
			DTaP	Tripedia DAPTACEL Infanrix	DTaP	Tripedia DAPTACEL Infanrix	DTaP	Tripedia DAPTACEL Infanrix	DTaP	Tripedia DAPTACEL Infanrix	
			IPV	IPOL	IPV	IPOL	IPV	IPOL			
Option 4			HepB	Engerix B Recombivax HB	HepB	Engerix B Recombivax HB	HepB	Engerix B Recombivax HB			13
			Hib	PedvaxHIB[d]	Hib	PedvaxHIB[d]			Hib	PedvaxHIB[d]	
			DTaP	Tripedia DAPTACEL Infanrix	DTaP	Tripedia DAPTACEL Infanrix	DTaP	Tripedia DAPTACEL Infanrix	DTaP	Tripedia DAPTACEL Infanrix	
			IPV	IPOL	IPV	IPOL	IPV	IPOL	IPV	IPOL	

TABLE 16.2 (Continued)

		Birth		2 mo		4 mo		6 mo		12-18 mo		Number of Shots Required through 2 yr
		Vaccine	Brandname	Vaccine	Brandname	Vaccine	Brandname	Vaccine	Brandname	Vaccine	Brandname	
Option 5	C o m v a x	HepB	Engerix B Recombivax HB	HepB/Hib	COMVAX	HepB/Hib	COMVAX			HepB/Hib or Hib	COMVAX^f PedvaxHIB^f HibTITER ActHIB	11
				DTaP	Tripedia DAPTACEL Infanrix	DTaP	Tripedia DAPTACEL Infanrix	DTaP	Tripedia DAPTACEL Infanrix	DTaP	Tripedia DAPTACEL	
				IPV	IPOL	IPV	IPOL	IPV	IPOL			
Option 6				HepB/Hib	COMVAX	HepB/Hib	COMVAX			HepB/Hib	COMVAX	10
				DTaP	Tripedia DAPTACEL Infanrix	DTaP	Tripedia DAPTACEL Infanrix	DTaP	Tripedia DAPTACEL Infanrix	DTaP	Tripedia DAPTACEL Infanrix	
				IPV	IPOL	IPV	IPOL	IPV	IPOL			
Option 7	P e d i a r i x	HepB	Engerix B Recombivax HB	HepB/IPV/DTaP	Pediarix	HepB/IPV/DTaP	Pediarix	HepB/IPV/DTaP	Pediarix	DTaP	Infanrix^g	9
				Hib	HibTiter ActHib	Hb	HibTiter ActHib	Hib	HibTiter ActHib	Hib	HibTiter ActHib	
Option 8				HepB/IPV/DTaP	Pediarix	HepB/IPV/DTaP	Pediarix	HepB/IPV/DTaP	Pediarix	DTaP	Infanrix^g	8
				Hib	HibTITER ActHIB	Hb	HibTITER ActHIB	Hib	HibTITER ActHIB	Hib	HibTITER ActHIB	
Option 9		HepB	Engerix B Recombivax HB	HepB/IPV/DTaP	Pediarix	HepB/IPV/DTaP	Pediarix	HepB/IPV/DTaP	Pediarix	DTaP	Infanrix^g	8
				Hib	PedvaxHIB*	Hb	PedvaxHIB*			Hib	PedvaxHIB^d	
Option 10				HepB/IPV/DTaP	Pediarix	HepB/IPV/DTaP	Pediarix	HepB/IPV/DTaP	Pediarix	DTaP	Infanrix^g	7
				Hib	PedvaxHIB*	Hb	PedvaxHIB*			Hib	PedvaxHIB^d	

(Adapted from the State of New Mexico Immunization Program. http://www.health.state.nm.us/immunize/provider.html#anchor-prov-3. Pdf of table can be found at: http://www.health.state.nm.us/immunize/Forms/UseofCombVaccines.pdf.)

Hib = Haemophilus influenzae type b; DTaP = diphtheria – tetanus-acellular pertussis; IPV = inactivated poliovirus vaccine; MMR = measles – mumps-rubella.

[a] See ACIP recommendations. In addition to these series, by age 2 years the ACIP also recommends a dose of MMR at 12–15 months, a dose of Varicella at 12–18 months, four doses of PCV-7 at 2, 4, 6 and 12–15 months, two doses of hepatitis A vaccine starting at 12 months (doses should be at least 6 months apart), and annual influenza vaccine for all children starting at 6 months. Do not mix Comvax and Pediarix in the same child—Use one or the other.

[b] If ActHIB and Tripedia are used here, they can be reconstituted together (or as the combination vaccine TriHIBit), reducing the number of shots by one.

[c] Only sanofi pasteur DTaP-Tripedia or the diluent shipped with the product may be used to reconstitute the sanofi pasteur ACTHIB product. sanofi pasteur DAPTACEL is not licensed for use in reconstitution of ActHIB.

[d] For Hib: PedvaxHIB (PRP-OMP) is approved for a three-dose schedule; HibTITER (HbOC) and ActHIB (PRP-T) require a four-dose schedule.

[e] ACIP states that licensed combination vaccines may used whenever any component of the combination is indicated and the vaccine's other components are not contraindicated.

See: http://www.cdc.gov/nip/faqs/hib-faqs.htm for details about mixing Comvax with other vaccine combinations

[f] In this option, any Hib vaccine may be used here instead of Comvax or PedvaxHIB. Comvax contains PedvaxHIB; the primary series of PedvaxHIB consist of two primary doses at 2 and 4 months followed by a booster dose at 12–15 months. Therefore, in this option the primary HIB series is complete, and any brand of Hib vaccine can be used for a booster dose.

[g] Whenever feasible, the ACIP recommends that the same brand of DTaP should be used for all doses of the primary series. Therefore, Infanrix, which is the DTaP component of Pediarix, is preferred when the series was begun using Pediarix. However, if this isn't possible, use a different manufacturer's product rather than defer vaccination.

Appropriate indications, contraindications, and precautions for vaccination are listed in Tables 1 and 2 in Appendix B. According to the CDC's *Epidemiology and Prevention of Vaccine-Preventable Diseases* (*"The Pink Book"*) a *contraindication* to immunization is a condition in a recipient that increases the chance of a serious adverse reaction, such as an allergy to one of the vaccine components (24). A vaccine should generally not be given when a contraindication is present. A *precaution* is a condition in a recipient that *might* increase the chance or severity of a serious adverse reaction, or compromise the ability of the vaccine to produce immunity (such as administering measles vaccine to a person with passive immunity to measles from a blood transfusion). The clinician may consider giving a vaccine in some conditions where a precaution applies, but the benefits of giving the vaccine should outweigh the risks. It is important for the clinician to recognize that mild illnesses, low-grade fever, penicillin allergy, a history of preterm birth, family history of allergies, and current antibiotic therapy are generally *unfounded reasons for deferring vaccination* (24).

Rare anaphylactic reactions to certain vaccines or vaccine components have been reported. A study of four health maintenance organizations found five cases of potential vaccine-related anaphylaxis among children and adolescents following administration of 7,644,049 vaccine doses, for a risk of 0.65 cases per million doses, with no deaths reported (25). Hypersensitivity to vaccines can occur in reaction to antigen, animal proteins, antibiotics (e.g., neomycin), preservatives, or stabilizers contained in the vaccine. The most common animal protein allergen is egg protein, which is found in the influenza and yellow fever vaccines because they are prepared using embryonated chicken eggs. Ordinarily, patients who are able to eat eggs safely may receive these vaccines. They are, however, contraindicated in most persons with a history of anaphylactic reactions to egg products: a history of hives, swelling of the mouth or throat, difficulty breathing, hypotension, or shock; protocols have been developed for the vaccination of such persons against influenza (26). Although measles and mumps vaccine viruses are grown in chick embryo fibroblast tissue culture, persons with a serious egg allergy can receive measles- or mumps-containing vaccines without skin testing or desensitization to egg protein because the quantity of egg proteins found in these vaccines is not sufficient to induce immediate-type hypersensitivity reactions (27).

Neomycin-containing antibiotics are contraindicated in persons with a history of anaphylactic reactions to neomycin. The most common allergic response to neomycin, delayed-type hypersensitivity manifested as contact dermatitis, is not a contraindication to receiving these vaccines.

Thimerosal is a preservative, containing approximately 50% ethylmercury by weight, used in some multidose vials of vaccines since the 1930s. Preservatives are not required in single-dose vials, but they were added to multidose vials because of some illness and deaths in the early 20th century caused by bacterial contamination of biologicals. Until 1999, vaccines given to infants to protect them against diphtheria, tetanus, pertussis, *Haemophilus influenzae* type b (Hib), and hepatitis B contained thimerosal as a preservative. As a result of theoretic concerns about toxicity, the U.S. Public Health Service (PHS) agencies, the AAP, and vaccine manufacturers agreed in 1999 that thimerosal levels in vaccines should be reduced or eliminated as a precautionary measure (28). This agreement was reaffirmed in 2000 in a joint statement of the AAFP, AAP, ACIP, and PHS (29). Currently, thimerosal has been removed from or reduced to trace levels in all vaccines routinely recommended for children 6 years of age and younger. Although some inactivated influenza vaccines still contain thimerosal, several brands are thimerosal-free (30). Some groups of concerned parents and antivaccination groups have claimed that thimerosal might cause neurologic problems, particularly autism, in children. The Institute of Medicine (IOM) studied this question and concluded in 2004 that there was insufficient evidence to link neurologic injury to thimerosal (31). A number of other studies reached similar conclusions (32–34).

PARENTAL EDUCATION AND COUNSELING

Many children do not receive vaccines because their parents or guardians do not appreciate the importance of immunizations, timely administration, or maintaining complete personal immunization records. It is therefore important for clinicians to explain the purpose of immunizations, the diseases that they prevent, and the rationale for the recommended immunization schedules. They should be counseled about the importance of obtaining immunizations at the recommended ages and should be urged to bring the child's immunization record to each visit.

In recent years, a growing minority of parents have begun to question the safety and efficacy of childhood immunizations. The extent of the problem was shown by a national survey of parental attitudes that found that although most parents supported vaccination, 25% believed that too many vaccinations could weaken a child's immune system and 23% believed that children get too many immunizations (35). According to a periodic survey of fellows of the AAP, seven of ten pediatricians reported that they had a parent refuse an immunization on behalf of a child in the 12 months preceding the survey (36). A study of pediatricians in 2002 found that 39% reported that they would dismiss a family for refusing all vaccinations, and 28% reported that they would dismiss a family for refusing certain vaccines (37).

A number of factors may account for the increasing level of parental refusals. In part they reflect vaccine successes; the diseases that vaccines prevent are no longer present to serve as a reminder of the need for immunization (35). Parents are also influenced by publicized controversies about vaccine safety. These concerns have been fueled by an aggressive antivaccination presence on the Internet (38,39), and by highly publicized controversies in the media that allege links between vaccinations and various illnesses such as autism.

All states have legal requirements that children be properly immunized before attending school. However, in addition to medical exemptions offered in every state, 48 states allow for religious exemptions and 19 states permit philosophic or personal exemptions. (The vaccine requirements for school entry for each state, as well as information about state vaccine exemptions, can be found online at http://www.cdc.gov/nip/vaccine/state-reqs.htm) Increasing vaccine refusals for "philosophic" reasons can have a significant public health impact. A study of vaccine-preventable diseases among children who have philosophic and religious exemptions from immunization mandated by law in Colorado found that exempted children were 22.2 times more likely to acquire measles and 5.9 times more likely to acquire pertussis than were vaccinated children; furthermore, during measles outbreaks an estimated 11% of vaccinated children acquired infection through contact with an exempted child (40).

How should a clinician approach parents who refuse vaccinations for their children? The AAP has published guidelines for counseling such parents (41). The list of recommendations includes the following:

- Listen carefully and respectfully to the parent's concerns.
- Share honestly what is and is not known about the risks and benefits of the vaccine in question, attempt to understand the parent's concerns about immunization, and attempt to correct any misperceptions and misinformation.
- Refer parents to one of several reputable and evidence-based websites for additional information.
- Be flexible; some parents have concerns about giving multiple vaccines at a single visit and may be willing to permit a modified schedule with more visits and fewer shots at each visit.
- Explore the possibility that cost is a reason for refusing immunization.
- Revisit the immunization discussion at each subsequent appointment.
- Clinician concerns about liability should be addressed by good documentation of the discussion of the benefits of immunization and the risks associated with remaining unimmunized; clinicians may also wish to consider having the parents sign a refusal waiver.

As with other forms of patient education, counseling about immunizations should be culturally sensitive.

Websites for parents with vaccine safety concerns:
- *CDC/National Immunization Program:*
  http://www.cdc.gov/nip/
  See sections: "Vaccine Safety" and "Why Immunize?"
- *Immunization Action Coalition:*
  http://www.vaccineinformation.org/concern.asp
- *National Network for Immunization Information:*
  http://www.immunizationinfo.org/
  See section: "Parents"

Children with inadequate immunization coverage often come from families of low socioeconomic status; their parents may have low educational levels or may not understand the clinician's language. Clinicians should take special measures under these circumstances (e.g., obtaining assistance from translators) to ensure that parents obtain accurate information. Parental counseling is critically important in order to maximize immunization efforts. A CDC study found that perceived lack of information by parents was associated with negative attitudes about immunizations and toward clinicians. Basic information about the benefits and risks of vaccines presented by a trusted clinician can help maintain and/or improve confidence in the immunization process (42).

VACCINE INFORMATION STATEMENTS

In addition to being prepared to answer patients' or parents' questions about common as well as alleged vaccine-related adverse events, clinicians must utilize "Vaccine Information Statements" (VISs) for vaccines covered under the National Vaccine Injury Compensation Program (43). Federal legislation passed in 1986, the National Childhood Vaccine Injury Act, requires that adult vaccinees or the parent/legal representative of child vaccinees receive a copy of a specially prepared VIS developed by the CDC. VISs are required for any vaccine containing diphtheria, tetanus, pertussis, measles, mumps, rubella, polio, hepatitis A, hepatitis B, Hib, varicella, influenza, or pneumococcal conjugate vaccine. Further details are available at the CDC website at http://www.cdc.gov/nip/publications/VIS/vis-facts.htm. The mandated one-page, two-sided information sheets provide patients with information about the disease, the benefits and harms of the vaccine, the recommended immunization schedule, indications for delaying or not administering the vaccine, potential postimmunization complications and ways to reduce them, along with addresses and telephone numbers for reporting adverse events (if the clinician fails to do so) and for obtaining federal compensation under the National Vaccine Injury Compensation

Program. The pamphlets have been translated into 30 different languages. Copies are also available on the CDC website at http://www.cdc.gov/nip/publications/VIS, or from the Immunization Action Coalition (IAC) website at http://www.immunize.org/vis/.

VISs are also available for other vaccines including human papillomavirus (HPV), meningococcal, pneumococcal polysaccharide, and rotavirus vaccines, as well as for various nonroutine vaccines such as anthrax, rabies, yellow fever, typhoid, smallpox, and Japanese encephalitis vaccines. Using the VISs for these vaccines is strongly encouraged but not required by law, although they must be used when giving vaccines purchased through a CDC contract. Physician requirements regarding VISs are provided at the CDC website.

VACCINES FOR DIPHTHERIA, TETANUS, AND ACELLULAR PERTUSSIS

Diphtheria-tetanus-pertussis (DTP) vaccine, made from a formalin-treated suspension of whole *Bordetella pertussis* cells, was introduced in the mid-1940s. Owing to concerns about possible neurologic adverse effects, a safer acellular pertussis vaccine was introduced in 1991 that used cell fragments of the pertussis bacterium. Since 1999 only formulations with acellular pertussis (diphtheria-tetanus-acellular pertussis [DTaP] and tetanus-diphtheria-acellular pertussis [Tdap]) have been used in the United States.

Tetanus and diphtheria have become rare in the United States. In 2003, there were 20 reported cases of tetanus and 1 reported case of diphtheria (44). Most cases occurred in adults who had not completed a primary immunization series. Both tetanus and diphtheria carry high case-fatality rates: 25–30% and 5–10%, respectively. Booster doses of the vaccines given every 10 years are recommended to maintain antibody levels.

Pertussis is also considerably less common in the United States than it was before the advent of the pertussis vaccine. Still, more than 25,000 cases were reported in the United States during 2004, the highest annual total since 1959 (45). Pertussis therefore remains an endemic disease, with the true number of cases estimated to be between 800,000 and 3.3 million annually in the United States. One explanation for the rise in the number of cases is that the newer, acellular form of pertussis vaccine may be less efficacious than the older whole-cell formulation. In addition, immunity to pertussis from either natural infection or vaccination wanes more rapidly than for other vaccine-preventable diseases (46).

In recent years, adolescents and adults have accounted for an increasing proportion of cases; in 2004 and 2005, approximately 60% of cases were among those 11 years and older (47). This older group of individuals is becoming a

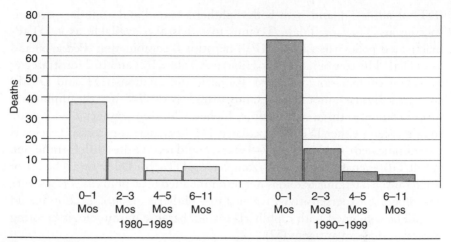

Figure 16.3 • Infant pertussis deaths by decade (1980–1989 vs. 1990–1999). From Vitek CR, Pascual FB, Baughman AL, et al. Increase in deaths from pertussis among young infants in the United States in the 1990s. *Pediatr Infect Dis J* 2003;22(7):628–634.

reservoir of infection that can spread disease to other age-groups, especially unimmunized infants who are at the highest risk of severe complications and death from pertussis infection (48). Particularly troubling has been the fact that in the 1990s, the incidence of reported pertussis among infants in the United States increased by almost 50% compared with the 1980s, with the increase occurring almost exclusively among infants too young to have received three doses of pertussis-containing vaccine (see Fig. 16.3) (49,50).

　　To attempt to reduce endemic disease in the adolescent and adult population, and thereby reduce morbidity and mortality in unimmunized infants, two new tetanus toxoids, reduced diphtheria toxoid and acellular pertussis absorbed vaccines (Tdap), were released in 2005. Boostrix (GlaxoSmithKline Biologicals, Rixensart, Belgium) was licensed for use in persons aged 10–18 years, and Adacel (sanofi pasteur, Toronto, Ontario, Canada) was licensed for use in persons aged 11–64 years. These agents, rather than the older tetanus-diphtheria (Td) vaccine, are recommended for use in those 11 years and older. The pertussis component of the vaccine delivers approximately one-third the antigenic dose of infant DTaP, but it produces antibody titers at least as strong, with an efficacy of 92% (51).

Indications

DTaP vaccination is indicated in all children, except those with the contraindications listed in Table 1 in Appendix B, beginning at age 6 weeks to 2 months. Pertussis immunization is not currently recommended for children from age 7–9 years. Tetanus toxoid is available as a single-antigen preparation, combined with diphtheria toxoid as pediatric diphtheria-tetanus

(DT) or adult Td, and with both diphtheria toxoid and acellular pertussis vaccine as DTaP or Tdap. Tetanus toxoid is also available as a DTaP-inactivated poliovirus vaccine (IPV)-hepatitis B combination (Pediarix) and as a DTaP-Hib combination (TriHibit) (see Tables 16.1 and 16.2 for strategies for using combination vaccines). Pediatric formulations (DT and DTaP) contain a similar amount of tetanus toxoid as do Td, but the diphtheria toxoid content is three to four times higher. Children younger than 7 years should receive either DTaP or pediatric DT (the latter if pertussis vaccine is contraindicated). Persons aged 7–9 years should receive the adult formulation (adult Td), even if they have not completed a DTaP or DT series. The use of single-antigen tetanus toxoid is not recommended (except in cases of a severe neurologic or hypersensitivity reaction to diphtheria toxoid). Tetanus toxoid should be combined with diphtheria toxoid, because immunologic boosting is needed for both antigens (52).

The ACIP recommends Tdap for children aged 11–12 years who have completed the recommended DTP/DTaP vaccination series and have not received a Td booster dose (53). Adolescents aged 13–18 years who missed the age 11- to 12-year Td/Tdap booster dose should also receive a single dose of Tdap if they have completed the recommended childhood DTP/DTaP vaccination series. It is recommended that subsequent Td or tetanus toxoid boosters be administered every 10 years.

The following ACIP recommendations for a single dose of Tdap (Adacel) apply to adults 19–64 years of age who have not yet received Tdap.

- **Routine** Adults should receive a single dose of Tdap to replace a single dose of Td for booster immunization against tetanus, diphtheria, and pertussis if they received their most recent tetanus toxoid–containing vaccine (e.g., Td) 10 years before or earlier.
- **Prevention of pertussis among infants younger than 12 months by vaccinating adult contacts.** Adults who have or who anticipate having close contact with an infant younger than 12 months (e.g., parents, clinicians, childcare providers) should receive a single dose of Tdap. Also, health care personnel who work in hospitals or ambulatory care settings and have direct patient contact should receive a single dose of Tdap as soon as feasible if they have not previously received Tdap. An interval of 2 years or more since the most recent tetanus toxoid–containing vaccine is suggested; shorter intervals may be used. Ideally, Tdap should be given at least 1 month before beginning close contact with the infant. Women should receive a dose of Tdap in the immediate postpartum period if they have not previously received Tdap. Any woman who might become pregnant is encouraged to receive a single dose of Tdap. To prevent neonatal tetanus, pregnant women who have received their last tetanus-containing vaccine 10 years before or earlier should receive Td during

TABLE 16.3 Tetanus Wound Prophylaxis

	Previous Immunization History		
	Uncertain or < Three Doses		**Three or More Doses**[a]
	Give Tdap		**Give Tdap or Td?**
Type of Wound	**or Td?**	**Give TIG?**	**(No TIG Needed)**
Clean, minor	Yes	No	No, unless >10 years since previous dose
Contaminated with dirt, feces, or saliva	Yes	Yes	No unless >5 years since previous dose
Puncture or missile	Yes	Yes	No unless >5 years since previous dose
Burns, frostbite, or crush injury	Yes	Yes	No, unless >5 years since previous dose

Reproduced with permission from Red Book: 2006 Report of the Committee on Infectious Diseases. Elk Grove Village, Ill: American Academy of Pediatrics: 2006. Available at: http://www.jfponline .com/uploadedFiles/Journal_Site_Files/Journal_of_Family_Practice/supplement_archive/ JFPSupp_Vaccines07_0207.pdf
Tdap = diphtheria and tetanus toxoids and acellular pertussis; Td = adult tetanus and diphtheria toxoids; TIG = tetanus immune globulin.
[a] If the individual has received only three doses of the nonadsorbed (fluid) tetanus toxoid, administer a fourth dose of Td, Tdap, or tetanus toxoid. Nonadsorbed (fluid) vaccine was only available as single antigen tetanus toxoid; diphtheria and tetanus toxoids and pertussis vaccine (DTP), Td, and pediatric diphtheria and tetanus toxoids (DT) all use adsorbed preparations.

pregnancy in preference to Tdap. Although Tdap is not contraindicated, there is some concern that antibodies acquired during pregnancy might reduce the response to DTaP vaccine in the infant at routine vaccination.

Guidelines for tetanus prophylaxis for wounds are listed in Table 16.3.

Administration

The full DTaP series consists of four doses, the first three doses given at 4- to 8-week intervals and the fourth dose given 6–12 months after the third dose (preferably at age 15 months) to maintain adequate immunity during the preschool years. The booster (fifth) dose, which is normally given at age 4–6 years, is unnecessary if the fourth dose in the primary series is given after age 4 years. The recommended childhood immunization schedule for ages 0–6 years is presented in Figure 16.1.

For adolescents, routine immunization with Tdap is recommended at a preadolescent health care visit for all 11- and 12-year olds, replacing the Td vaccine (Fig. 16.1). Children who are behind on immunizations should be vaccinated according to the schedules in Table 1 in Appendix B depending on their age. Adults should be immunized according to the schedule in Figure 16.1.

Once the primary DTaP series is started, interruptions in the recommended schedule or delays in administering subsequent doses do not require restarting the series. Therefore, persons who received a partial series in the past need only complete the schedule. Premature infants should be vaccinated at their chronologic age from birth.

Children 6 years or younger for whom pertussis vaccination is contraindicated should complete the primary series with DT vaccine. Because no pertussis vaccine has been approved for children aged 7–9 years, primary immunization at this age should be with adult Td, even if they have not completed a series of DTaP or pediatric DT. The first two doses should be given at least 4 weeks apart, and the third dose should be given 6 months after the second dose (see Fig. 16.1 and Table 1 in Appendix B).

Adverse Effects

Local reactions (e.g., erythema, induration) and mild systemic reactions (e.g., fever, drowsiness, irritability, and anorexia) were common after the administration of DTP or its component antigens but are less common after the administration of DTaP. Anaphylactic reactions to DTaP vaccine are rare. Arthus-type reactions to tetanus toxoid can occur, especially in adults who have received frequent tetanus toxoid boosters. Therefore, Td boosters should be avoided in patients who have completed a primary series or have received a booster dose within the previous 5 years. They should also be avoided in patients who have experienced Arthus reactions and received a dose within the last 10 years.

Moderate or severe systemic events (such as a temperature of 105°F [40.5°C] or higher, febrile seizures, persistent crying lasting 3 hours or more, and hypotonic hyporesponsive episodes) have been reported after administration of DTaP but occur less frequently among children receiving DTaP than among children receiving whole-cell DTP (estimated occurrence is less than 1 per 10,000 doses). However, occurrence of one of these adverse reactions following DTaP vaccination in childhood is neither a contraindication nor a precaution to administration of Tdap to an adolescent or adult.

Swelling of the injection site is more common after the fourth or fifth dose of DTaP. There have been reports of swelling of the entire thigh or upper arm, sometimes accompanied by erythema, pain, and fever. Parents should be informed of the increase in reactogenicity that has been reported following the fourth and fifth doses of DTaP. The ACIP, because of the risk of pertussis in this age-group, recommends that a history of extensive swelling after the fourth dose should *not* be considered a contraindication to receipt of a fifth dose at school entry.

The most common reactions reported after Tdap vaccination are local redness or swelling at the injection site. Low-grade fever and nonspecific systemic symptoms such as headache and fatigue have also been reported. Adverse reactions occur at a similar rate in recipients of Tdap and Td. A history of extensive limb swelling following DTaP is not a contraindication to Tdap vaccination.

Precautions and Contraindications

Precautions and contraindications to DTaP, DT, Tdap, and Td vaccine are listed in Tables in Appendix B. In general, pertussis vaccine should not be given to patients with unstable neurologic conditions, such as uncontrolled seizure disorders or progressive encephalopathy. Stable neurologic conditions, such as cerebral palsy and well-controlled seizures, are not contraindications. A history of a single seizure that was not temporally related to DTaP administration does not contraindicate vaccination, especially if the seizure can be explained by other factors. A family history of seizures or other neurologic diseases, or stable or resolved neurologic conditions (e.g., controlled idiopathic epilepsy, cerebral palsy, and developmental delay) are not contraindications to pertussis vaccination. To reduce the likelihood of postvaccination fever among children with such histories, acetaminophen or ibuprofen may be provided at the time of vaccination and every 4–6 hours for 24 hours.

Moderate or severe acute illness is a precaution to vaccination, but children with mild illness, such as an upper respiratory infection or otitis media, should be vaccinated.

Children who have recovered from documented pertussis do not need further doses of pertussis vaccine until adolescence, when one dose of Tdap should be given (because pertussis immunity is not permanent, even from natural infection). Satisfactory documentation of pertussis infection includes recovery of *B. pertussis* on culture or typical symptoms and clinical course when these are linked epidemiologically to a culture-confirmed case. When confirmation of diagnosis is lacking, vaccination should be completed because cough may be caused by other species of *Bordetella*, or by other bacteria or viruses (47).

The only contraindications to Td/DT are a history of a severe neurologic or hypersensitivity reaction following a previous dose, and moderate to severe illness.

VACCINES FOR MEASLES, MUMPS, AND RUBELLA

Measles, mumps, and rubella are all human viral diseases with no known animal reservoir. Measles can cause severe illness, often complicated by middle ear infection or bronchopneumonia. Measles is still a common and often fatal disease in developing countries. The WHO estimates that more than

20 million cases occur annually, with an estimated 345,000 deaths from measles occurring in 2005 (54). The incidence of measles has fallen dramatically since 1963, when the vaccine was first licensed and routine childhood vaccination instituted. Nevertheless, a resurgence in the incidence of measles occurred in the United States between 1989 and 1991. During these 3 years, there were 55,622 cases of measles, 11,251 hospitalizations, and 132 deaths (55). Although this epidemic occurred primarily among unvaccinated preschool children, a substantial number of school-aged children (most of whom had been vaccinated) and adults were affected. Data suggested that measles could indeed spread among highly vaccinated school-age populations, largely because 2–5% of vaccine recipients remained susceptible after receiving only a single dose. In 1989, this information prompted a national effort to expand childhood immunization coverage and the addition of a second dose of measles vaccine to the childhood immunization schedule, given either at preschool or on entry to middle or junior high school (Fig. 16.1). As a result of this vaccination effort, reported cases of measles declined rapidly after the 1989–1991 resurgence. Since then the incidence of measles has declined steadily, with a record low annual total of 37 cases reported in 2004. Available epidemiologic and laboratory data indicate that measles transmission in the United States has been interrupted. Most cases are now imported from other countries, chiefly originating in Asia and Europe, both among Americans traveling abroad and persons visiting the United States from elsewhere (56).

Mumps is a viral disease spread by respiratory droplets. It usually begins with swelling and tenderness of one or more of the salivary glands, with 30–40% of persons developing unilateral or bilateral parotitis. Complications can include orchitis (20–50% of postpubertal males infected), brain involvement including aseptic meningitis (15% of cases), and inflammation of the pancreas (2–5% of cases) and ovaries (5% of postpubertal females). Permanent deafness occurs in 1 out of 20,000 cases. Mumps vaccine was introduced in 1967, following which the incidence of the disease declined from 212,000 cases in 1964 to approximately 3,000 cases per year by 1985. There was a surge in the number of cases in 1986 and 1987 with almost 13,000 cases reported in 1987, which correlated with a lack of state immunization requirements and apparent incomplete immunity conferred by the original single-dose protocol. Since the two-shot MMR series was introduced, the number of reported cases has fallen steadily in the United States, with an average of 265 mumps cases reported per year between 2001 and 2005 (57). However, in 2006 a multistate outbreak of mumps occurred, with 5,783 cases of mumps reported between January and October in 45 states. The highest incidence of cases was among persons aged 18–24 years (58). Multiple factors were implicated, including a lower rate of two-dose MMR vaccine coverage among college students compared with younger ages, and waning immunity in this age range (59). This led to updated ACIP recommendations for the control of mumps, including the recommendation that two doses of live mumps virus vaccine be required for all students in post–high school educational institutions and for all health care workers born after 1957 (one dose is suggested for those born before 1957, or two doses during outbreaks).

Rubella is spread by droplet infection. Although approximately half of the cases are subclinical, rubella infection may be associated with significant morbidity in adults; the greatest risk is when infection occurs in pregnant women, in whom vertical transmission to the fetus can produce congenital rubella syndrome (CRS). A rubella epidemic in the United States in 1964–1965 resulted in 12.5 million cases of rubella infection and approximately 20,000 newborns with CRS. Rubella vaccination of children was introduced in 1969, after which the incidence of new cases fell from 30 per 100,000 to less than 0.5 per 100,000 by 1983. In 2003, a record low annual total of seven cases were reported. In October 2004, a CDC panel concluded that endemic rubella transmission in the United States had ceased by 2000, with all subsequent reported cases having been imported from other countries. The conquest of rubella and CRS in the United States is one of the great public health victories of the modern era. Nonetheless, it is essential that all persons, especially women of childbearing age, continue to be vaccinated or show proof of immunity to prevent a resurgence of disease.

Indications

In the United States, single-antigen live virus vaccine preparations are available for measles (Attenuvax; Merck), mumps (Mumpsvax; Merck) and rubella (Meruvax II; Merck), and as combination vaccines for measles-mumps (M-M-Vax: Merck), measles-mumps-rubella (M-M-R II; Merck), and measles-mumps-rubella-varicella (ProQuad; Merck). The ACIP recommends that a combination vaccine (MMR or MMRV) be used when any of the individual components is indicated (for MMRV, the vaccinee must be 12 months through 12 years of age). Use of single-antigen vaccines is not recommended.

All children (at least 12 months of age) and nonpregnant adults, with the exception of those with the contraindications listed in Table 1 in Appendix B, should receive MMR vaccine if they are susceptible to measles, mumps, or rubella infection. Acceptable presumptive evidence of immunity to measles, rubella, and mumps varies by vaccine (57) but in general such evidence requires documentation of administration, laboratory evidence of immunity, birth before 1957, or physician-diagnosed disease. Owing to the 2006 mumps outbreak in the United States, the ACIP recommends the following vaccination measures for mumps outbreak settings:

• Children aged 1–4 years and adults who have received one dose of mumps vaccine: if affected by the outbreak, consider a second dose (the minimum interval between doses being 28 days [60]) of live mumps virus vaccine.

- Health care workers born before 1957 without other evidence of immunity: strongly consider two doses of live mumps virus vaccine.

Because many rashes may mimic rubella infection and many rubella infections are unrecognized, the clinical diagnosis of rubella is unreliable and should not be considered in assessing immune status. The ACIP recommends that, unless susceptible women are certain to return for vaccination, women who may be immune to rubella but lack adequate documentation of immunity should be vaccinated, rather than first performing serologic testing for rubella antibodies (27). Serologic testing need not be done before vaccinating for measles and rubella unless the facility considers it cost effective.

Administration

The recommended primary immunization schedule for MMR is presented in Figure 16.1. Children who are behind on immunizations should be vaccinated according to the schedule in Table 1 in Appendix B. As noted on page 367, MMR should be administered at least 14 days before, or deferred for 3–11 months after, administration of immune globulin because passively acquired antibodies may interfere with the response to the vaccine; guidelines for spacing the immunizations based on the type and dose of immune globulin are provided elsewhere (2). MMR is the preferred vaccine for individuals who are susceptible to measles, mumps, or rubella and who lack contraindications.

A combination vaccine, combining MMR with varicella vaccine (MMRV), is now available (ProQuad [Merck]). ProQuad is indicated for simultaneous vaccination against measles, mumps, rubella, and varicella in children aged 12 months to 12 years and may be used whenever any components of the combination vaccine are indicated and the other components are not contraindicated (Table 16.1). ProQuad appears to stimulate the same antibody levels as M-M-R II and varicella vaccine (Varivax; Merck) when given separately (61,62), and concomitant administration of MMRV, Hib/HepB and DTaP is well tolerated (63). Because varicella vaccine is recommended to be given at the same age as MMR vaccine, MMRV is preferred over a separate injection of equivalent component vaccines (22).

Adverse Effects

Primary vaccination with measles vaccine may be associated with mild fever and a transient rash, beginning 7–12 days after vaccination and usually lasting several days. Approximately 5–15% of patients develop a temperature greater than 103°F (39.4°C). Neurologic complications, including encephalitis and encephalopathy, reportedly occur in less than one case per million doses administered (an incidence rate lower than the rate for encephalitis of unknown etiology). Mild, self-limited thrombocytopenia may occur in 1 out of 30,000–40,000 doses of MMR vaccine. However, the risk of thrombocytopenia during rubella or measles infection is much greater than the risk after vaccination. On rare occasions, mumps vaccination can produce parotitis and lymphadenopathy. Allergic reactions such as rash and pruritus, which are usually brief, are reported occasionally. Very rarely, manifestations of central nervous system involvement (e.g., febrile seizures, aseptic meningitis, unilateral nerve deafness, and encephalitis) occur; almost all of these cases resolve uneventfully, and none have been linked conclusively to vaccines used in the United States. Recipients of rubella vaccine can develop low-grade fever, a rash lasting 1–2 days, and lymphadenopathy that may persist 1–2 months after vaccination. Arthralgias and transient arthritis are more common in susceptible adults than in children, and women are more prone to this than men. Approximately 25% of women who receive the vaccine report arthralgias, and approximately 10% of recipients can develop acute arthritis-like signs and symptoms. When acute joint symptoms occur, they generally begin 1–3 weeks after vaccination, persist for 1 day to 3 weeks, and rarely recur. Rarely, transient peripheral neuritis is reported following rubella vaccination.

Precautions and Contraindications

Precautions and contraindications to MMR are listed in Tables in Appendix B. MMR vaccines should not be given to females known to be pregnant or who might become pregnant within 4 weeks of vaccination. No cases of congenital rubella syndrome have been documented among infants born to women who inadvertently received rubella vaccine during pregnancy. Therefore, although rubella vaccination should be avoided during pregnancy, there is insufficient evidence of risk to justify termination of pregnancy if a pregnant woman inadvertently receives the vaccine. Children of pregnant women can safely receive MMR vaccine without risk to the mother or fetus. Although MMR vaccination of persons with moderate or severe illness should be postponed, minor illnesses such as upper respiratory infection, with or without a low-grade fever, do not preclude vaccination.

Hypersensitivity reactions to MMR vaccine are rare. They generally consist of wheal-and-flare or urticarial reactions at the injection site. Although measles and mumps vaccines (but not rubella vaccine) are propagated in chick embryo fibroblast cells in culture, the quantity of egg proteins found in these vaccines is not sufficient to induce immediate-type hypersensitivity reactions, and these vaccines can safely be administered to children with severe egg allergies (64). Persons who have experienced a severe allergic reaction (i.e., hives, angioedema, difficulty breathing, and hypotension) after receiving a prior dose of MMR vaccine or a vaccine component (e.g., gelatin, neomycin) should generally not be vaccinated with MMR.

Because MMR is a live attenuated viral vaccine, it is contraindicated in persons with known severe immunodeficiency (e.g., those with hematologic and solid tumors who are receiving chemotherapy, with congenital immunodeficiency, or with human immunodeficiency virus [HIV] infection who are severely immunocompromised). However, MMR can be given safely to persons with HIV infection who are asymptomatic or mildly symptomatic with age-specific $CD4^+$ counts equal to or greater than 15%. MMR is contraindicated in persons on long-term immunosuppressive therapy (a significant immunosuppressive steroid dose is considered to be daily receipt of at least 20 mg/day [at least 2 mg/day/kg of body weight] of prednisone or its equivalent for 14 days or more).

Certain antibody-containing blood products can interfere with the immune response to live attenuated viral vaccines. HIV patients receiving immune globulin intravenously may receive MMR if given 2 weeks before the next scheduled dose of immune globulin (if it is not otherwise contraindicated) (2).

POLIO VACCINE

Poliomyelitis, a disease that once crippled or killed millions of persons, has become a rare disease in industrialized nations because of routine polio vaccination. In the United States, the number of cases of polio peaked in 1952 with more than 21,000 cases of paralytic polio. The last episode of the spread of wild poliovirus in this country occurred in 1979; all current U.S. cases are due to vaccine-associated paralytic poliomyelitis (VAPP). No new cases of wild-type virus have been reported in the Western Hemisphere since 1991, and global eradication of the disease may be possible.

Two forms of trivalent polio vaccines are available for use: inactivated poliovirus vaccine or IPV (introduced by Jonas Salk in 1954) and live attenuated oral poliovirus vaccine or OPV (introduced by Albert Sabin in 1961). Use of live attenuated virus vaccine can lead to mutation during viral replication in the intestine, causing VAPP. It occurs approximately once per every 6.2 million OPV doses administered to immunologically competent recipients. The risk of VAPP is 7 to 21 times higher after the first dose than after other doses in the series. To eliminate the risk for VAPP, exclusive use of IPV has been recommended for routine vaccination in the United States since 1999. OPV remains the vaccine of choice for areas where wild poliovirus is still present because it stimulates more potent intestinal immunity against wild poliovirus. Ongoing vaccination of the U.S. population against poliovirus will be required until wild poliovirus infection is eradicated worldwide (2).

Indications

Polio vaccine should be administered to all children. Although routine immunization of adults (18 years or older) living in the United States is not recommended, some adults at higher risk of infection should be immunized (see subsequent text).

Administration

Only enhanced-potency IPV vaccine is now available for routine use in the United States. The recommended childhood immunization schedule for IPV is presented in Figure 16.1, and contraindications are listed in Table 1 in Appendix B. Children who are behind on immunizations should be vaccinated according to the schedule in Table 1 in Appendix B. A polio vaccination schedule begun with OPV should be completed with IPV. If a child receives both types of vaccines, four doses of any combination of IPV or OPV by age 4–6 years is considered a complete poliovirus vaccination series. However, for children who receive an all-IPV or all-OPV series, a fourth dose is not necessary if the third dose was given at 4 years or older. A minimum interval of 4 weeks should separate all doses of the series.

Routine vaccination with IPV is not recommended for adults (aged 18 years or older) in the United States because most adults are already immune and have little risk of acquiring poliovirus infection. However, immunization is recommended for certain adults at higher risk, such as travelers to areas where poliomyelitis is endemic or epidemic, laboratory workers handling specimens that may contain wild-type polioviruses, and health care workers in close contact with patients who may be excreting wild poliovirus. Unimmunized adults exposed to high-risk environments should receive three doses of IPV. The first two doses should be given 1–2 months apart, with a third dose 6–12 months after the second dose. An incompletely immunized adult who started the series with OPV should receive the remaining doses using IPV; there is no need to restart the series if the schedule was interrupted. Fully immunized adults entering a high-risk situation should get one booster dose of IPV.

Adverse Effects

The administration of IPV can cause tenderness at the injection site. No serious adverse reactions to IPV have been documented. Allergic reactions may occur in persons sensitive to streptomycin, polymyxin B, and neomycin, which are present in trace amounts in IPV.

Precautions and Contraindications

Moderate or severe acute illness, or pregnancy, is a precaution in the use of IPV. However, breastfeeding is not a contraindication to the use of this vaccine. IPV is contraindicated in persons with a previous anaphylactic or neurologic reaction to the vaccine or to any of its components.

HAEMOPHILUS INFLUENZAE TYPE B VACCINE

Hib is the cause of a wide variety of serious bacterial diseases among children, such as meningitis, pneumonia, septic arthritis, epiglottitis, and sepsis. Before the development of the vaccines, Hib meningitis accounted for 50–65% of Hib cases. Even with the availability of antibiotic therapy, the case fatality rate was 2–5%, and neurologic sequelae, such as hearing impairment, occurred in 15–30% of survivors.

These illnesses occur primarily among children younger than 5 years. Although severe disease is most common in children aged 6–12 months, approximately 20–35% of cases of severe disease occur in children aged 18 months or older. In the United States during the 1980–1990 decade, the incidence of Hib disease was 40–100 per 100,000 among children younger than 5 years. With the routine use of Hib conjugate vaccine since 1990, the incidence of invasive Hib disease has decreased to 1.3 per 100,000 children. However, in developing countries where the vaccines are not widely used, Hib remains a major cause of lower respiratory tract infections in infants and children: the bacterium is estimated to cause at least 3 million cases of serious disease and 400,000–700,000 deaths each year.

Indications

A complete Hib vaccination series is indicated in all infants and children, starting at age 2 months. Certain older children and adults are at higher risk of invasive Hib disease than is the general population. Such persons should receive a single dose of any pediatric Hib vaccine. This group includes persons with functional or anatomic asplenia (e.g., sickle cell disease, postsplenectomy patients), immunodeficiency (in particular, persons with immunoglobulin [IgG2] subclass deficiency), immunosuppression from cancer chemotherapy, HIV infection, and past receipt of a hematopoietic stem cell transplant (56). Children who have had Hib disease when they were younger than 24 months should still receive Hib vaccine, because most fail to mount an immune response to clinical disease. Children aged 24 months or older who have had reliably diagnosed invasive disease do not need vaccination. Household contacts of patients with Hib disease (regardless of the contacts' age) should receive rifampin postexposure prophylaxis if one of the contacts is a child younger than 1 year who has not received the primary Hib series or a child aged 12–48 months who has not been fully vaccinated. Postexposure prophylaxis should also be given to all household contacts, regardless of age, if one of the child contacts (any age) is immunocompromised (65).

Administration

Three single-antigen Hib conjugate vaccines and two combination vaccines that contain Hib conjugate are available in the United States. HbOC (HibTITER, Wyeth) links Hib polysaccharide to a diphtheria protein; PRP-T (ActHIB, sanofi pasteur) uses tetanus toxoid; and PRP-OMP (PedvaxHIB, Merck) uses a group B meningococcal protein. HbOC and PRP-T require three doses for a primary series at ages 2, 4, and 6 months followed by a single booster at age 12–15 months. PRP-OMP only requires two doses for the primary series, at ages 2 and 4 months, with a booster at age 12–15 months.

Two combination vaccines are available that contain Hib: Comvax (Merck) contains PRP-OMP (PedvaxHIB, Merck) as the Hib component plus hepatitis B vaccine (Recombivax, Merck). TriHIBit (sanofi pasteur) contains PRP-T (ActHIB, sanofi pasteur) as the Hib component, which is reconstituted with DTaP (Tripedia, sanofi pasteur) from a second vial (66). Alternatively, ActHIB and Tripedia from separate lots can be reconstituted together to make a combined Hib/DTaP vaccine. In such cases, the lot numbers of ActHIB and Tripedia vaccines used must be registered separately in the child's medical record. TriHIBit is supplied with a single lot number for the two components. TriHIBit may be administered to children 12 months or older who have received at least one prior dose of Hib vaccine 2 or more months earlier and TriHIBit will be the last dose in the Hib series. Infants who received TriHIBit before age 12 months should be age-appropriately reimmunized with another Hib vaccine as if they had never received a dose (Table 16.1). All three Hib vaccines licensed for use in the United States are interchangeable; any combination may be used to complete a primary series, except for the restrictions for TriHIBit noted in the preceding text.

The recommended immunization schedule for Hib vaccination is presented in Table 1 in Appendix B. Children who are behind on Hib immunizations (and are younger than 5 years) should be vaccinated according to the schedule in Table 1 in Appendix B. Adults and older children at high risk (see "Indications" on page 390) should receive a single dose of any pediatric Hib vaccine.

Adverse Effects

Serious complications from Hib vaccine are unusual. Erythema, swelling, or pain at the injection site has been reported in 5–30% of recipients. They usually resolve within 24 hours. A temperature of 101.3°F (38.5°C) or greater occurs in approximately 1% of recipients. Severe hypersensitivity reactions are rare.

Precautions and Contraindications

Vaccination with Hib conjugate vaccine is contraindicated for persons known to have experienced an anaphylactic allergic reaction following a prior dose of that vaccine. Vaccination should be delayed for children with moderate or severe acute illnesses. Minor illnesses (e.g., mild upper respiratory infection) are not contraindications to vaccination. Hib conjugate vaccines are contraindicated for children younger than 6 weeks because of the potential for development of immunologic tolerance. Contraindications and precautions for the use of TriHIBit and Comvax are the same as those for its individual component vaccines.

PNEUMOCOCCAL VACCINES

Pneumococcal disease is still a major cause of morbidity and mortality in the United States, especially in infants and the elderly. In the United States, before the introduction of pneumococcal conjugate and polysaccharide vaccines, pneumococcal disease caused an estimated 3,000 cases of meningitis, 50,000 cases of bacteremia, 500,000 cases of pneumonia, and 7 million cases of otitis media each year (67). *Streptococcus pneumoniae* is the most common cause of invasive bacterial disease in U.S. children, with the peak incidence occurring between 6 and 23 months of age. Since the disappearance of invasive Hib disease secondary to Hib vaccination, *S. pneumoniae* has now become the leading cause of bacterial meningitis in the United States. Pneumococcal disease also takes a great toll on the elderly, causing half of adult hospitalizations for pneumonia. Of those with pneumococcal pneumonia, bacteremia occurs in 25–30% of cases. The overall fatality rate for pneumococcal bacteremia is 20% but rises to as high as 60% in the elderly population (older than 65 years).

There are two vaccines against pneumococcal disease: pneumococcal polysaccharide vaccine (PPV) and pneumococcal conjugate vaccine (PCV). PPV was originally licensed in 1977 as a 14-valent vaccine against pneumococcal polysaccharide bacterial antigens. In 1983, a 23-valent polysaccharide vaccine (PPV23) was licensed. Pneumovax 23 (Merck) contains antigens against strains that account for 88% of bacteremia-causing pneumococci.

PPV stimulates B cells to produce antibody immunity, but it does not produce T-cell immunity. This results in temporary immunity from antibody production, but immune memory is lacking, and repeated doses do not produce a boost in antibody titers. PPV is effective in older children and adults, but children younger than 2 years do not produce reliable immune responses to polysaccharide antigens. PCV, by contrast, stimulates long-term T-cell immunity, which is necessary to reduce nasal carriage and produce herd immunity. Also, in children younger than 2 years, only PCV is effective against bacteria with polysaccharide capsules, including pneumococcus, meningococcus, and Hib.

Prevnar (Wyeth) was the first pneumococcal conjugate vaccine (PCV7) licensed in the United States, in 2000. It contains purified capsular polysaccharides of seven *S. pneumoniae* serotypes (conjugated to a nontoxic diphtheria protein). Between 1978 and 1994 in the United States, among children younger than 6 years, these seven types accounted for 86% of bacteremia, 83% of meningitis, and 65% of acute otitis media (68). A CDC study of data from 1998–2003 showed dramatic results from universal immunization of children with PCV7. In the United States, after the introduction of PCV7 immunization, in children younger than 5 years, invasive pneumococcal disease (IPD) caused by one of the seven PCV7 pneumococcal serotypes declined by 94% between 1997–1998 and 2003, and IPD from all serotypes declined by 75% (69). In Canadian children younger than 2 years, there was a decline of 93% in PCV7 serotype IPD between 1998 and 2004, and a decline of 82% for all serotypes (70). In both countries, there were also significant declines in IPD from these pneumococcal serotypes in persons older than 65 years, indicating an indirect effect from childhood vaccination with PCV7.

To date (2007), the effect of PPV23 vaccination in the elderly has not produced results as dramatic as has the use of PCV7 vaccine in children. One study showed a reduction in pneumococcal bacteremia, but not a reduction in pneumonia, in elderly vaccinees (71). A systematic review by the Cochrane Collaboration did not show that PPV23 vaccination lowers the incidence of pneumonia or death in persons older than 55 years or in high-risk subjects (72). However, one study showed definite additive effects of combined pneumococcal and influenza vaccination in elderly persons, with some independent benefit of PPV23 vaccination (73), and two studies published in 2006 showed clear benefits from the vaccine. A U.S. study of almost 63,000 patients admitted to hospitals for pneumonia found that prior immunization with PPV23 was associated with a 40–70% reduction in deaths in-hospital, as well as decreased risk of complications and a shorter length of stay (74). A prospective cohort study from Spain of more than 11,000 persons 65 years or older who had received PPV23 showed significant reductions in the incidence of pneumococcal pneumonia and in hospitalization and death due to pneumonia (75). Continued efforts to improve PPV23 vaccination rates in the elderly are recommended by the ACIP and have been particularly encouraged for immunocompromised patients (76).

Indications

PPV is indicated for the following:

- All patients 65 years or older (in Alaska, PPV-23 is recommended for all adults 55 years or older due to a high rate of invasive disease among Alaskan Natives [77])
- Patients aged 2 years or older with a normal immune system who have a chronic illness, including cardiovascular disease, pulmonary disease, diabetes, alcoholism, cirrhosis, or cerebrospinal fluid leakage
- Immunocompromised patients 2 years or older at increased risk of pneumococcal disease or its complications; this includes patients with asplenia (either from disease or surgical removal), lymphoma (including Hodgkin's disease), multiple myeloma, chronic renal failure, nephrotic syndrome, or conditions such as organ transplantation associated with immunosuppression. Patients who are immunosuppressed secondary to

chemotherapy or high-dose corticosteroid therapy (see earlier definition) should be vaccinated

• Patients 2 years or older with asymptomatic or symptomatic HIV infection

PPV23 should also be considered for patients living in special environments or social settings with an identified increased risk of pneumococcal disease, such as certain Native American populations (i.e., Alaska Native, Navajo, and Apache) (68).

PCV7 is indicated for all children younger than 2 years and children aged 24–59 months with a high-risk medical condition (sickle cell disease; anatomic/functional asplenia; chronic cardiac, pulmonary, or renal disease; diabetes; cerebrospinal fluid leakage; HIV infection; or immunosuppression).

Administration

PPV23 can be administered either intramuscularly or subcutaneously. A one-time revaccination is recommended for patients aged 65 years or older if the first dose was given before age 65 years and if 5 years or more have elapsed since the previous dose. Revaccination is also recommended 5 years later for persons at highest risk of fatal pneumococcal infection or rapid antibody loss (e.g., renal disease). In Alaska, where PPV vaccination is given at 55 years or older, revaccination is recommended every 6 years.

Children aged 2 years or older who have immunocompromising conditions, HIV infection, sickle cell disease, or functional or anatomic asplenia, should receive a second dose of PPV at least 3–5 years after the previous PPV if they are 10 years or younger; if they are older than 10 years, the two doses of PPV should be separated by 5 or more years.

The primary PCV series beginning in infancy consists of three doses routinely given at 2, 4, and 6 months of age. The vaccine is administered intramuscularly. A fourth (booster) dose is recommended at age 12–15 months (see Fig. 16.1 for routine indications and Table 1 in Appendix B for catch-up schedule). Unvaccinated healthy children aged 24–59 months should receive one dose of PCV7. Unvaccinated children aged 24–59 months with sickle cell disease, asplenia, HIV infection, chronic illness, or immunocompromised conditions should receive two doses of PCV7 separated by at least 8 weeks. PCV7 is not routinely recommended for those older than 59 months.

Adverse Effects

The most common reactions after pneumococcal vaccination are local erythema and swelling, seen in 30–50% of PPV recipients and 10–20% of PCV recipients. Local reactions are seen more commonly after a second dose of PPV. Fever and myalgia have occurred in less than 1% of PPV recipients, and in 15–24% of PCV recipients; in the latter, a temperature higher than 102.2°F (39°C) is uncommon. Severe adverse events are rare with either vaccine.

Precautions and Contraindications

Previous anaphylactic reaction to this vaccine or to any of its components is a contraindication. Moderate or severe acute illness is a precaution.

MENINGOCOCCAL VACCINE

Neisseria meningitidis spreads through exposure to aerosol droplets or contact with respiratory tract secretions. The bacterium is carried transiently in the nasopharynx of up to 10% of adolescents and adults; carriage rates in children younger than 10 years are much lower. Invasive disease occurs when the bacterium penetrates the nasal mucosa and invades the bloodstream. This occurs in less than 1% of colonized persons. The incidence of invasive disease peaks between the ages of 6 months and 2 years, with a second, lower peak occurring during adolescence. *N. meningitidis* causes approximately 2,000 to 3,000 cases of invasive disease in the United States each year, with an annual incidence of 0.8 to 1.5 cases per 100,000 persons. Meningitis occurs in up to 50% of cases of invasive disease, with a 3–10% fatality rate. A more serious form of invasive disease is meningococcemia, which occurs in 5–20% of cases and can have a fatality rate of up to 40%. Even with antibiotic treatment, up to 20% of survivors can have permanent sequelae, such as hearing loss, neurologic damage, or loss of a limb. *N. meningitidis* has become the leading cause of bacterial meningitis in persons aged 2–18 years as a result of the success of Hib and pneumococcal conjugate vaccines in controlling those pathogens.

Certain groups are at higher risk of invasive disease. Host risk factors include functional or anatomic asplenia and terminal complement pathway deficiency. HIV disease is probably also a risk factor. Environmental risk factors include upper respiratory tract infection, household crowding, and both active and passive smoking. College freshmen living in dormitories have a modest increase in their risk of invasive disease.

Five serogroups (A, B, C, W-135, and Y) account for virtually all meningococcal disease. Two vaccines are available for use. Meningococcal tetravalent polysaccharide vaccine (MPSV4 [Menomune, sanofi pasteur]) was licensed in 1981 for use in children older than 2 years as well as adults. Each dose consists of purified bacterial capsular polysaccharides from serogroups A, C, Y, and W-135. However, MPSV4 has serious limitations: it stimulates temporary protective antibody production but, like other polysaccharide vaccines, produces poor immunogenicity in children younger than 2 years. In addition, it does not eliminate nasopharyngeal carriage of the bacterium and it produces no boost in antibody titer with repeated doses. Meningococcal tetravalent conjugate vaccine (MCV4 [Menactra, sanofi pasteur]) was licensed for use in the United States in 2005 for use in those aged 11–55 years. Each dose contains capsular polysaccharide from serogroups A, C, Y, and W-135 conjugated to diphtheria toxoid. The wide use of MCV4 is expected to reduce nasopharyngeal carriage of *N. meningitidis* and produce herd immunity. As an example of its potential effectiveness, after universal vaccination of children was instituted in the United Kingdom in 1999 with a monovalent group C conjugate vaccine, within 2 years the incidence rate of group C disease had decreased by more than 80% (78).

Indications

- MCV4 should be given to all children at age 11–12 years.
- Adolescents not previously vaccinated should receive MCV4 before entering high school (or at approximately age 15 years).
- Other adolescents who wish to reduce their risk of meningococcal disease may receive the vaccine.

The ACIP also recommends that MCV4 should be given to the following high-risk groups:

- College freshmen living in dormitories
- Microbiologists who are routinely exposed to *N. meningitidis*
- Military recruits
- Persons who travel to or reside in countries in which *N. meningitidis* is hyperendemic or epidemic, especially travelers to sub-Saharan Africa and particularly if contact with the local population will be prolonged; vaccination is required by the government of Saudi Arabia for all travelers on the annual Hajj to Mecca.
- Persons who have terminal complement component deficiencies
- Persons who have anatomic or functional asplenia

MCV4 is preferred for persons aged 11–55 years, whereas MPSV4 is used in persons at increased risk who are aged 2–10 years or older than 55 years; its routine use is not recommended in these age-groups in the absence of increased risk. Routine vaccination with MPSV4 is not recommended for children younger than 2 years because it is relatively ineffective in this age-group and offers limited duration of immunity (79).

Both MPSV4 and MCV4 are recommended for use in the control of meningococcal outbreaks caused by vaccine-preventable meningococcal serogroups (A, C, W-135, and Y). Both MCV4 and MPSV4 can be used for this purpose, but MCV4 is preferred if the population targeted for vaccination includes age-groups for which MCV4 is licensed. Revaccination with MPSV4, when necessary (e.g., persons residing in an epidemic region), should occur after 2–3 years in children initially vaccinated between ages 2 and 4 years, and after 5 years in older children or adults (79). When a case of meningococcal disease occurs, close contacts should be given chemoprophylaxis, preferably within 24 hours of the identification of the infection. Antibiotic chemo-prophylaxis guidelines are available online at http://www.cdc.gov/mmwr/

preview/mmwrhtml/rr5407a1.htm (79). Contact with individual cases is not an indication for immunization.

Administration

For persons aged 11–55 years, MCV4 is administered intramuscularly as a single 0.5-mL dose. MPSV4 is administered subcutaneously as a single 0.5-mL dose to persons aged 2 years or older. MCV4 and MPSV4 can be administered at the same time as other vaccines, but they should be given at a different anatomic site. Protective levels of antibodies are usually achieved within 7–10 days of vaccination (79).

Adverse Effects

Adverse reactions to MPSV4 and MCV4 are similar and are generally mild. Local reactions, such as pain and erythema at the injection site, can last for 1–2 days. They occur in up to 48% of recipients of MPSV4, and up to 59% of recipients of MCV4. A temperature of 100–103°F within 7 days of vaccination is reported for up to 3% of recipients of MPSV4, and for up to 5% of recipients of MCV4. Systemic reactions, such as headache and malaise, within a week of vaccination are reported for up to 60% of recipients. Fewer than 3% of recipients characterized these systemic reactions as severe.

Precautions and Contraindications

Vaccination with MCV4 or MPSV4 is contraindicated among persons known to have a severe allergic reaction to any component of the vaccine, including dipththeria toxoid (for MCV4), or to latex (the vaccine vial stopper of MPSV4 and MCV4 contains dry natural rubber latex). Moderate or severe acute illness is a precaution for vaccination.

As of 2006, 17 cases of Guillain-Barré syndrome (GBS) that had an onset within 6 weeks of MCV4 administration had been reported to the CDC and FDA (80,81). The number of GBS cases is similar to what might have been expected to occur by chance alone (one to two cases per 100,000 population). Although the manufacturer has inserted a warning in the package insert, the CDC has not altered its recommendations for administering MCV4 (80,81).

HEPATITIS B VACCINE

Hepatitis B virus (HBV) is a serious global health problem; one-third of the world's population has evidence of present or past infection and 200 million persons are chronically infected. There are more than 250,000 deaths each year from HBV-associated acute and chronic liver disease. Approximately 1 million Americans are thought to be infectious carriers, with 78,000 new infections per year resulting in 22,000 new cases of HBV and 5,000 deaths annually from HBV-related liver disease. HBV causes approximately 80%

of cases of hepatocellular carcinoma, which makes it second only to tobacco among known human carcinogens (82).

HBV infections occur through contact with infected secretions, most commonly through sexual contact, or through inoculation from infected needles. Perinatal transmission from mother to fetus is also a common route of infection. If the mother is positive for the hepatitis B surface antigen marker (HBsAg), the likelihood of transmission to the infant at birth is 10%. However, the rate rises to 70–90% if the mother is positive for both HBsAg and the highly infective HBeAg. Chronic HBV infection develops in 90% of infected infants, 30–50% of those infected between age 1 and 5 years, and 6–10% of those infected as adults. In Western countries, only 0.1-0.5% of the population are chronic HBV carriers. However, in Southeast Asia and China, most of Africa, most Pacific Islands, parts of the Middle East, and the Amazon Basin, 8–15% of the population carry the virus. The lifetime risk of HBV infection in these countries is greater than 60%. Most infections are acquired at birth or during early childhood, when the risk of developing chronic infection is highest (82).

In 1990, because of the failure of selective vaccination to reduce the burden of illness in persons who lack identifiable risk factors, the U.S. PHS modified its high-risk strategy and recommended universal infant vaccination and more intensive screening of adults (including universal screening of pregnant women). Following these measures, the overall incidence of reported acute HBV declined 75%, from 8.5 to 2.1 per 100,000 persons between 1990 and 2004. The most dramatic declines occurred in the cohort of children to whom recommendations for routine infant and adolescent vaccination were applied (83).

Indications

The ACIP recommends vaccinating all newborns soon after birth and before hospital discharge in addition to universal HBV screening of pregnant women. Routine vaccination is also recommended for all children and adolescents through age 18 years. Children not previously vaccinated with hepatitis B vaccine should be vaccinated at age 11–12 years with the age-appropriate dose of vaccine.

Vaccination is also recommended for adults in high-risk groups. In general, persons at markedly increased risk of acquiring HBV include injection drug users; homosexual and heterosexual persons with multiple partners; health care workers and others with potential exposure to blood products; hemodialysis and hemophilia patients; recipients of certain blood products; household contacts or sexual partners of HBV carriers; inmates of long-term correctional institutions; immigrants from certain countries (e.g., China, Southeast Asian countries, African countries, the Philippines, Haiti, eastern European countries); other population groups (e.g., Alaskan Natives,

Pacific Islanders) in which HBV is common; and international travelers to these regions for whom sexual contact, exposure to blood, or residence longer than 6 months is likely. The ACIP now recommends hepatitis B vaccination for all adults in settings in which a high proportion of persons are likely to be at risk of HBV infection. The ACIP also recommends that standing orders in primary care and specialty settings should promote the vaccination of adults at risk of HBV infection (84).

Administration

The recommended immunization schedule for hepatitis B vaccine is presented in Figure 16.1; the pediatric catch-up schedule is in Table 1 in Appendix B. The recommended dose of the vaccine varies between 5 and 40 μg, depending on the patient's age and immune status and the manufacturer (see "Suggested Readings" on page 426 for more details).

Two formulations of recombinant vaccines are available in the United States: Recombivax HB (Hep-B; Merck) and Engerix-B (Hep-B; GlaxoSmithKline). As shown in Table 16.1, three combination vaccines containing hepatitis B vaccine are also available: Comvax (Merck), Twinrix (GlaxoSmithKline), and Pediarix (GlaxoSmithKline). In March 2007 the FDA approved an accelerated dosing schedule for Twinrix, which consists of three doses given within 3 weeks followed by a booster dose at 12 months (at 0, 7, and 21–30 days, and at 12 months). The accelerated schedule can benefit individuals needing rapid protection, such as travelers to high-risk areas, or emergency responders, especially those being deployed to disaster areas.

Although postvaccination testing is not routinely recommended, it should be considered for certain persons, such as health care workers in dialysis units, or infants born to HBsAg-positive or HBsAg-unknown mothers. When indicated, postvaccination testing should be performed 1–2 months after completion of the vaccine series. All infants born to HBsAg-positive or HBsAg-unknown women should be tested 3–12 months after their final (third or fourth) dose of hepatitis B vaccine (i.e., at age 9–18 months). Occasionally, vaccinated individuals will not have a detectable antibody response. Persons who do not respond to the first series of hepatitis B vaccine should complete a second three-dose series. Fewer than 5% of persons receiving six doses of hepatitis B vaccine administered in the deltoid muscle following the appropriate schedule fail to develop detectable anti-HBs antibody. An individual who remains seronegative after six doses of vaccine should be managed as a nonresponder (in such individuals HBV infection should be ruled out; details are available in the "*Pink Book*," which can be accessed online at http://www.cdc.gov/vaccines/pubs/pinkbook/default.htm) (82).

In certain cases, persons exposed to HBV require administration of hepatitis B immune globulin (HBIG) which contains a high concentration of hepatitis B antibody. Rules for various vaccination and exposure scenarios, including the management of infants born to women who are HBsAg-positive, are complex. Detailed information can be found in the CDC's *"Pink Book"* (82) and in the "Suggested Readings" (page 426).

Adverse Effects

The most common side effects of hepatitis B vaccination are pain at the injection site (reported in 13–29% of adults and 3–9% of children) and mild fever (less than 1%). Some mild systemic symptoms, such as headache or fatigue, may also occur. The principal side effects of HBIG are pain and swelling at the injection site. Urticaria, angioedema, and anaphylaxis have been reported but their occurrence is rare.

Precautions and Contraindications

A severe allergic reaction to a vaccine component or following a prior dose of hepatitis B vaccine is a contraindication to further doses, although as noted such reactions are rare.

Moderate or severe acute illness is a precaution against vaccination, but minor illness is not a contraindication to vaccination. Studies to date indicate that hepatitis B vaccine is probably safe for pregnant women. Since acquiring an HBV infection during pregnancy can cause severe disease for both mother and infant, hepatitis B vaccine may be administered to a pregnant woman who is otherwise eligible for it.

HEPATITIS A VACCINE

Hepatitis A viral (HAV) infection is caused by a nonenveloped RNA picornavirus. It is spread by fecal–oral transmission. After an incubation period averaging 28 days, it causes a clinical course characterized by fever, jaundice, anorexia, and malaise. In children younger than 6 years, 70% of infections are asymptomatic, but in older children and adults more than 70% develop jaundice. In the prevaccine era, HAV epidemics occurred in 10- to 15-year cycles. Between 1980 and 1995 the attack rate in the United States was approximately 10 cases per 100,000 population, and 31% of the U.S. population had evidence of prior HAV infection. Since 1995 the total number of cases has been declining, probably due to increasing use of HAV vaccine. A record low annual total of 5,970 cases was reported in 2004 (rate: 1.9 cases per 100,000 population) (85).

HAV causes significant morbidity. Rates of hospitalization are approximately 11–22%. Infected adults usually miss almost a month of work. Fulminant HAV infection causes approximately 100 deaths per year in the United States.

Two inactivated whole-virus hepatitis A vaccines are available: Havrix (GlaxoSmithKline) and Vaqta (Merck). Both vaccines are manufactured in both pediatric and adult formulations, and both produce excellent immunity. In clinical trials, all vaccinees had protective levels of antibody after receiving two doses (86).

After the vaccine was released in 1995 it was first used chiefly in individuals at high risk of acquiring disease. In 1999 the ACIP recommended routine vaccination of children aged 24 months and older in high-risk communities (attack rate more than double the national average). Success in reducing rates of HAV in these communities led the ACIP in 2005 to recommend universal vaccination at ages 12–23 months.

Indications

All children should be vaccinated at age 12–23 months. Those not vaccinated by age 2 years can be vaccinated at later visits. Vaccination is also recommended for other groups, including those older than 12 months who will be traveling to areas of increased risk, men who have sex with men, injection drug users, persons with clotting factor disorders, and persons with occupational risk of infection. Persons with chronic liver disease who are susceptible should be vaccinated. The ACIP does not recommend routine vaccination of all health care workers or food service workers.

Administration

Vaqta is quantified in antigen units (U). Children and adolescents aged 1–18 years should receive one dose of the pediatric formulation (25 U per dose; 0.5-mL volume) with a booster 6–12 months later. Adults aged 19 years or older should receive one dose of adult formulation (50 U per dose; 1 mL volume) with a booster dose 6–12 months later.

Havrix is quantified in ELISA units (EL.U.) per 0.5-mL dose. Children aged 1–18 years should receive a single dose of the pediatric formulation (720 EL.U. per 0.5 mL dose) followed by a booster dose 6–12 months later. Adults aged 19 years or older should receive one dose of the adult formulation (1,440 EL.U. per 1.0-mL dose) followed by a booster dose 6–12 months later.

Since 2001 one combination vaccine, Twinrix (GlaxoSmithKline), has been available. It is approved for persons aged 18 years or older. A 1.0-mL dose of vaccine contains 720 EL.U. of inactivated HAV (equivalent to a single pediatric dose of Havrix) and 20 μg of recombinant HBsAg protein (equivalent to a single adult dose of Engerix-B). The vaccine is administered in a three-dose series at 0, 1, and 6 months. The first and second doses should be separated by at least 4 weeks, and the second and third doses should be separated by at least 5 months, with at least 6 months between the first and third doses. It is not necessary to restart the series or add doses if the interval between doses is longer than the recommended interval. In March 2007, the FDA approved an accelerated dosing schedule that consists of three doses given within 3 weeks followed by a booster dose at 12 months (at 0,

7, and 21–30 days and at 12 months). The accelerated schedule can benefit individuals needing rapid protection, such as travelers to high-risk areas or emergency responders, especially those being deployed to disaster areas.

All hepatitis A vaccines should be administered intramuscularly into the deltoid muscle. Those vaccinated can be assumed to be immune 4 weeks after receiving the first dose of vaccine.

Prevaccination testing is not recommended for children who are expected to be susceptible. However, because HAV infection produces life-long immunity, prevaccination testing may be indicated in certain groups at high risk of prior HAV infection, such as adults born in Africa, Asia, or South America.

Persons exposed to HAV who have not had at least one dose of hepatitis A vaccine at least 1 month before exposure may benefit from the administration of standard IG. IG is more than 85% effective in preventing hepatitis A if given within 2 weeks of exposure. A single intramuscular dose of 0.02 mL/kg of IG confers protection for less than 3 months; 0.06 mL/kg protects for 5 months. Detailed information about this can be found in the CDC "*Pink Book*" or in the AAP "*Red Book*" (86) (see "Suggested Readings" section at the end of this chapter).

Adverse Effects

The most common adverse effects are pain, erythema, or swelling at the injection site, reported by 20–50% of recipients. These events are generally mild and self-limited. Mild systemic complaints, such as malaise, fatigue, or low-grade fever, are reported by less than 10% of recipients. No serious adverse reactions have been reported.

Precautions and Contraindications

A history of a severe allergic reaction to a vaccine component, a reaction following a prior dose of hepatitis A vaccine, hypersensitivity to alum or, in the case of Havrix, to the preservative 2-phenoxyethanol, are all contraindications to further vaccine administration. Vaccination of persons with moderate or severe acute illnesses should be deferred until recovery occurs. Because hepatitis A vaccines are inactivated, theoretically the risk of a serious adverse event in pregnant women is low. Possible risks of vaccination should be weighed against the risk of HAV infection. The vaccine is considered safe for immunocompromised persons.

INFLUENZA VACCINE

Influenza is characterized by sudden onset of fever, headache and muscle aches, fatigue, dry painful cough, and coryza. Intestinal symptoms, such as nausea and vomiting, can also occur. Influenza viruses are spread from person to person, primarily through respiratory droplet transmission, although aerosol transmission may also play a role (87). Hand-to-mouth transmission may occur through fomites, but is less important. The typical incubation period for influenza is 1–4 days. Adults can be infectious from 1 day before to approximately 5 days after the onset of illness; the infectious period in children may be 10 days or more, and they can shed virus before the onset of their illness. Severely immunocompromised persons can shed virus for weeks or months.

In temperate climates, seasonal influenza activity peaks between late December and early March. Deaths occur not only from influenza itself, but also from complications in patients with respiratory and cardiovascular diseases. In the United States, approximately 19,000 influenza-associated pulmonary and circulatory deaths per influenza season occurred during 1976–1990, compared with approximately 36,000 deaths per season during 1990–1999 (88). The highest rates of serious illness and death occur in persons aged 65 years or older and in children younger than 2 years, as well as in persons with certain medical conditions that are exacerbated by influenza. Pregnant women are also at increased risk of complications, especially in the second and third trimesters, when the risk of hospitalization from influenza is more than four times higher than for nonpregnant women.

Three antigenic types cause human influenza: types A, B, and C, with epidemics caused by types A and B. Type A influenza causes the most severe disease in all ages, and also affects certain wild and domesticated birds. The three subtypes of influenza type A that are responsible for most epidemics are characterized by their different surface antigens: hemagglutinin (H_1, H_2, and H_3) and neuraminidase (N_1 and N_2). Influenza type B occurs only in humans and is a milder disease that chiefly affects children. Influenza C is not a disease of humans.

Influenza vaccine is prepared each year in an attempt to anticipate antigenic variation among influenza viruses. Only three subtypes are currently circulating among humans: H_1N_1, H_1N_2, and H_3N_2. The choice of strains to be used by vaccine manufacturers is determined by the FDA based on recommendations from the WHO. Three strains are selected each year: a type A (H_1N_1), a type A (H_3N_2), and a type B.

Two types of influenza vaccines are currently available in the United States. Trivalent inactivated influenza vaccine (TIV) is administered by the intramuscular route. The vaccine is available in both pediatric (0.25-mL dose) and adult (0.5-mL dose) formulations. Thimerosal-free vaccine is available in individual doses. TIV is 70–90% effective in healthy persons younger than 65 years and 30–40% effective in the frail elderly. Among older residents of nursing homes, the vaccine reportedly reduces hospitalizations by 50–60% and reduces influenza-related deaths by 80% (89). At least one reviewer has questioned the quality of the studies of inactivated influenza vaccine effectiveness and has called for careful randomized trials to study this question more accurately (90).

Live attenuated influenza vaccine (LAIV) is administered intranasally and contains the same influenza viruses as TIV. The live viruses in LAIV are temperature sensitive. They do not replicate effectively at human core body temperature and cannot produce disease. However, the viruses are also cold adapted, so that they can replicate in nasopharyngeal mucosa and produce immunity. Because LAIV contains live, attenuated viruses it has the potential to produce mild signs or symptoms related to influenza virus infection, and it is therefore not approved for use in persons with weakened immunity. The vaccine is packaged in a single-dose sprayer unit; half of the dose is sprayed into each nostril. Although vaccinated children can shed vaccine viruses in nasopharyngeal secretions for up to 3 weeks, any transmitted virus retains its temperature-sensitive and cold-adapted properties. The reported effectiveness of LAIV and TIV are similar.

In 2007, the FDA approved a change from the frozen formulation of LAIV (stored at temperature equal to or less than $-15°C$) to a refrigerated formulation called *cold-adapted influenza vaccine trivalent* (CAIV-T; stored at $2–8°C$). Both products contain the same types and quantity of virus. The dose of CAIV-T is 0.2 mL (0.1 mL per nostril). CAIV-T was expected to be available for the 2007–2008 influenza season (91).

In 2003 and early 2004, outbreaks of highly pathogenic avian H_5N_1 influenza occurred among poultry in Asia, causing the death or destruction of tens of millions of birds. The strain, known as *bird flu*, is not very contagious among humans. However, it has an apparent 50% fatality rate in humans who receive a high viral dose from contact with infected poultry (consumption of raw duck blood, "mouth-to-beak" resuscitation at cockfights, and handling infected birds or cleaning their feces) (92). While reports of human-to-human transmission are very rare at this writing, concern exists that the H_5N_1 strain might acquire the capacity for sustained human-to-human transmission and thereby set off serious pandemics (93). The development of human vaccines against the H_5N_1 strain (and other possible strains) and capacity building for a potential pandemic were under way at the time of publication. The first H_5N_1 vaccine for use in the United States was approved by the FDA in April 2007 (94).

Indications
INDICATIONS FOR INACTIVATED INFLUENZA VACCINE
- Children aged 6–59 months
- Women who will be or expect to be pregnant during the influenza season (TIV may be given safely in any trimester)
- Persons older than 50 years

- Children and adolescents (aged 6 months–18 years) who are receiving long-term aspirin therapy and, therefore, might be at risk for experiencing Reye's syndrome after influenza infection
- Adults and children who have chronic disorders of the pulmonary or cardiovascular systems, including asthma (hypertension is not considered a high-risk condition)
- Adults and children who have required regular medical follow-up or hospitalization during the preceding year because of chronic metabolic diseases (including diabetes), renal dysfunction, hemoglobinopathies, or immunodeficiency (including immunodeficiency caused by medications or by HIV)
- Adults and children who have any condition (e.g., cognitive dysfunction, spinal cord injury, seizure disorder, or another neuromuscular disorder) that can compromise respiratory function or the handling of respiratory secretions, or that can increase the risk of aspiration
- Residents of nursing homes and other chronic-care facilities that house persons of any age who have chronic medical conditions
- Persons who live with or care for persons at high risk of influenza-related complications, including healthy household contacts and caregivers of children aged 0–59 months
- Health care workers

INDICATIONS FOR LIVE, ATTENUATED INFLUENZA VACCINE

- Healthy, nonpregnant females aged 5–49 years who want to avoid contracting influenza, and those who might be in close contact with persons at high risk of severe complications, including health care workers.

It should be noted that if a health care worker receives LAIV, that worker should refrain from contact with severely immunocompromised patients for 7 days after receiving the vaccine (but can still care for other patients). Hospital visitors who have received LAIV should refrain from contact with severely immunocompromised persons for 7 days after vaccination; however, such persons may visit patients who are not severely immunocompromised (89).

Administration

Resources listed in the "Suggested Readings" detail the types and dosages of available influenza vaccines. Influenza vaccine should be offered beginning in September during routine patient visits. Persons at high risk of complications from influenza can still be vaccinated after an influenza outbreak has begun in a community. When influenza vaccine is administered during an influenza epidemic, chemoprophylaxis (see subsequent text) should be considered for persons at high risk during the time from vaccination until immunity has developed, which is 2 weeks after vaccination for most adults. Children younger than 9 years who receive influenza vaccine for the first time can require 6 weeks of prophylaxis (i.e., prophylaxis for 4 weeks after the first dose of vaccine and prophylaxis for an additional 2 weeks after the second dose) (89). Because TIV only contains viral subunits, there is no risk in administering influenza antivirals and TIV simultaneously. However, because influenza antiviral drugs interfere with the replication of active or attenuated influenza virus, LAIV should not be administered until 48 hours after finishing influenza antiviral therapy; influenza antiviral medications should not be administered for 2 weeks after LAIV is administered.

Certain antiviral drugs have been used for treatment or chemoprophylaxis against influenza strains. The four drugs available in the United States are amantadine, rimantadine, oseltamivir, and zanamivir. Amantadine and rimantadine, which were highly effective for prophylaxis or treatment of type A influenza, could no longer be used during the 2005–2006 influenza season due to more than 90% resistance among the viral strains. The resistance is believed to have developed because of the widespread veterinary use of these drugs to prevent the spread of avian influenza in poultry in China and Southeast Asia, leading to drug resistance in both human and the H_5N_1 avian influenza strains.

The neuraminidase inhibitors oseltamivir (Tamiflu; Roche) and zanamivir (Relenza; GlaxoSmithKline) are both effective against influenza types A and B if given within 48 hours of the onset of symptoms; they can reduce the length of illness by 1 day. Both are also approved for chemoprophylaxis of influenza. A review of studies of both drugs found an efficacy of 61% for oseltamivir and 62% for zanamivir in preventing symptomatic influenza. The efficacy of oseltamivir for postexposure prophylaxis was 59% for households and 68–89% for contacts of index cases. Both drugs reduced, but did not eliminate, viral shedding when given to persons with influenza. Neither drug showed any benefit when given for treatment of influenza-like illness (a syndrome in which patients present to a clinician with influenza-like symptoms when laboratory or epidemiologic evidence of influenza is not available). The authors of this review concluded that, because of their low effectiveness and the risk of promoting drug-resistant strains, "neuraminidase inhibitors should not be used in seasonal influenza control and should only be used in a serious epidemic or pandemic alongside other public-health measures." (95)

The CDC recommends chemoprophylaxis in the following circumstances (89):

- **Persons at high risk who are vaccinated after influenza activity has begun.** When influenza vaccine is administered while influenza viruses are circulating, chemoprophylaxis should be considered for persons at high risk during the time from vaccination until immunity has developed. As noted earlier, children younger than 9 years who receive influenza vaccine for the first time can require 6 weeks of chemoprophylaxis.

- **Persons who provide care to those at high risk.** Chemoprophylaxis during peak influenza activity can be considered for unvaccinated persons who have frequent contact with persons at high risk. If an outbreak is caused by a strain of influenza that might not be covered by the vaccine, chemoprophylaxis should be considered for all such persons, regardless of their vaccination status.
- **Persons who have immune deficiencies.** Chemoprophylaxis can be considered for persons at high risk who are expected to have an inadequate antibody response to influenza vaccine. This category includes persons infected with HIV, chiefly those with advanced HIV disease.
- **Other persons.** Chemoprophylaxis throughout the influenza season or during peak influenza activity might be appropriate for persons at high risk who should not be vaccinated. Chemoprophylaxis can also be offered to persons who wish to avoid influenza illness. Clinicians and patients should make this decision on an individual basis.

Control of Influenza Outbreaks in Institutions

When outbreaks occur in institutions, chemoprophylaxis should be administered to all residents, regardless of whether they received influenza vaccinations during the previous Fall, and should continue for a minimum of 2 weeks. If surveillance indicates that new cases continue to occur, chemoprophylaxis should be continued until approximately 1 week after the end of the outbreak. The dosage for each resident should be determined individually. Chemoprophylaxis can also be offered to unvaccinated staff members who provide care to persons at high risk.

Chemoprophylaxis should be considered for all employees in such institutions, regardless of their vaccination status, if the outbreak is suspected to be caused by a strain of influenza virus that is not well matched to the vaccine. If cases continue to occur despite chemoprophylaxis, it is probably ineffective and may need to be discontinued.

In addition to nursing homes, chemoprophylaxis can also be considered for controlling influenza outbreaks in other closed or semiclosed settings (e.g., dormitories or other settings in which persons live in close proximity).

Because these antiviral agents reduce replication of influenza viruses, LAIV should not be administered until 48 hours after cessation of influenza antiviral therapy, and influenza antiviral medications should not be administered for 2 weeks after receipt of LAIV (96).

Details about current recommendations for influenza vaccination and antiviral drugs can be found online at http://www.cdc.gov/flu/.

Adverse Effects
TRIVALENT INACTIVATED INFLUENZA VACCINE

Adverse reactions to TIV are generally mild, consisting of discomfort at the injection site for up to 2 days. Immediate allergic reactions (e.g., urticaria, angioedema) are rare and are usually related to allergies to egg proteins. Fever, malaise, and myalgia, usually lasting 6 to 48 hours, have been infrequently reported. Although GBS was associated with the use of the "swine flu" vaccine in 1976, annual surveillance in subsequent years has not demonstrated a clear association between influenza vaccination and neurologic complications. The estimated risk of GBS is approximately one additional case per 1 million persons vaccinated (if GBS was found to be associated with influenza vaccine). This risk is, in any case, much less than the health risk of severe influenza, which is vaccine preventable.

LIVE ATTENUATED INFLUENZA VACCINE

In children, LAIV is not associated with a significant increase in upper respiratory tract infection symptoms, fever, or other systemic symptoms. Data from an unpublished study suggested a significantly increased risk of asthma or reactive airway disease among children aged 12–59 months who received LAIV. Accordingly, LAIV is not approved for use in children younger than 60 months, and it should not be used in persons with asthma, reactive airway disease, or other chronic pulmonary diseases.

In adults, LAIV is associated with a slightly increased risk of cough, runny nose, nasal congestion, sore throat, and chills (3–10% higher than reported for placebo recipients) but no increase in the occurrence of fever. No serious adverse reactions or cases of GBS have been identified in LAIV recipients, either children or adults.

Precautions and Contraindications

Contraindications and precautions to vaccination with influenza vaccines are listed in Tables in Appendix B.

VARICELLA VACCINE

Varicella is a highly contagious disease caused by the varicella zoster virus (VZV). It usually lasts 4–5 days and is characterized by fever, malaise, and a generalized vesicular rash typically consisting of 250–500 lesions. Secondary attack rates among close contacts may be as high as 90%.

Complications of varicella infection include secondary bacterial infections of the skin, pneumonia, and complications involving the central nervous system, especially meningitis and encephalitis. The complication rate increases with age: adults account for only 5% of cases of varicella but

35% of deaths. Immunocompromised persons have a particularly high rate of varicella complications and disseminated disease. A late complication of VZV infection, herpes zoster (HZ) (shingles), carries a lifetime risk of 10–20% and can cause serious illness in elderly persons (see page 413). Other high-risk groups include pregnant women who develop varicella from 5 days before to 2 days after delivery, which can result in serious infection in the neonate and a fatality rate of up to 30%. Maternal varicella infection in the first 20 weeks of pregnancy can also cause congenital varicella syndrome in up to 2% of exposed fetuses, characterized by segmental areas of skin loss or scarring, limb hypoplasia, and reduced birth weight. No cases of congenital varicella syndrome have been reported from the use of varicella vaccine.

Because of the high rate of infectivity, and because communicability through aerosol droplets begins 1–2 days before the appearance of the rash, a universal vaccination program is necessary to prevent the spread of VZV. Varicella vaccine was first licensed for use in the United States in 1995. The current vaccine (Varivax; Merck) is a live attenuated vaccine derived from the Oka strain of VZV and is approved for vaccination of children aged 12 months or older. A combined MMR and varicella vaccine (MMRV;[ProQuad; Merck]) was approved for use in 2005 for children aged 12 months to 12 years in cases when both MMR and varicella vaccine are due.

After one dose of Varivax, detectable antibody titers develop in 97% of children aged 1–12 years. More than 90% of responders maintain antibody for at least 6 years. In Japanese studies, 97% of children maintained antibody 7–10 years after vaccination. Postlicensure studies have shown that vaccine efficacy is usually 80–85% against infection (range of 44–100%), and more than 95% effective against moderate or severe disease (97). An average of 78% of adolescents and adults develop antibody after one dose, and 99% develop antibody after a second dose given 4–8 weeks later. Antibody has persisted for at least 1 year in 97% of vaccinees who received the second dose (4–8 weeks after the first dose) (98). ProQuad (MMRV) appears to stimulate the same antibody levels as M-M-RII and Varivax when given separately (61,62), and concomitant administration of MMRV, Hib/HepB and DTaP is well tolerated (63).

Before the widespread use of varicella vaccine, there were approximately 4 million cases of VZV infection in the United States every year, causing approximately 11,000 hospitalizations (rate of 5 cases per 1,000), and 100 deaths each year (approximately 1 in 60,000 cases) (99). Since the varicella vaccine was introduced in the United States, varicella cases, hospital admissions, and deaths have been reduced by more than 80% in children, with lesser reductions in infants and adults from indirect effects (herd immunity) (97). There is a theoretic concern that a decline in wild-type varicella infections from vaccination could lead to a rise in the incidence of HZ. This is because exposure to wild VZV is thought to boost cell-mediated immunity to VZV, preventing reactivation of latent VZV infections. As widespread childhood vaccination against varicella reduces exposure to wild VZV, the incidence of HZ might rise. At present, no rise in HZ has been found, but continued monitoring will be needed (100). A mild form of varicella can occur in 1–4% of vaccinees per year following exposure to wild-type VZV. Such illness is usually shorter and less severe than naturally occurring varicella (less than 50 lesions with minimal or no fever).

Initially, the ACIP recommended one dose for children younger than 13 years and two doses for those aged 13 years and older. However, subsequent studies have found that 15–20% of children who have received one dose of the vaccine were not fully protected and were susceptible to develop chickenpox after exposure to VZV. Also, there was concern that one dose of the vaccine might not provide protection into adulthood when chickenpox is more severe. As noted, in 2006 the ACIP recommended a two-dose schedule for all children in the United States.

Indications

Routine immunization with varicella vaccine is recommended for all susceptible children and adolescents without a contraindication. As noted, in 2006 the ACIP recommended that the vaccine be administered to all children and to all other people aged 13 years or older without evidence of immunity. See Table 2 in Appendix B for revised criteria of evidence of immunity to varicella in adults.

Administration

Two doses of varicella virus vaccine are administered at an interval of at least 3 months for patients aged 12 months to 12 years and at an interval of 4–8 weeks for people aged 13 years or older. In children, the first dose should be administered at age 12–15 months and the second dose at age 4–6 years (i.e., before entering kindergarten or first grade). The second dose can be administered at an earlier age provided the interval between the first and second dose is at least 3 months. However, if the second dose is administered at least 28 days following the first dose, the second dose need not be repeated. Because it is recommended that varicella vaccine be given at the same age as MMR vaccine, MMRV is preferred over a separate injection of equivalent component vaccines, unless contraindicated.

A second-dose, catch-up varicella vaccination is recommended for children, adolescents, and adults who previously had received one dose, to improve individual protection against varicella and for more rapid impact on school outbreaks. Catch-up vaccination can be implemented during routine visits to the clinician and through school and college entry requirements. The catch-up second dose can be administered at any interval longer than 3 months after the first dose.

HIV-infected children aged 12 months or older in CDC clinical class N, A, or B with CD4$^+$ T-lymphocyte counts of 15% or greater and without evidence of varicella immunity should receive two doses of single-antigen varicella vaccine at a minimum interval of 3 months. Because data are not available on safety, immunogenicity, or efficacy of MMRV vaccine in HIV-infected children, MMRV vaccine should not be administered as a substitute for the component vaccines when vaccinating HIV infected children.

The ACIP recommends assessing pregnant women for evidence of varicella immunity. Clinicians should not vaccinate women who are pregnant or might become pregnant within 4 weeks of receiving the vaccine. Women who do not have evidence of immunity should receive the first dose of varicella vaccine upon completion or termination of pregnancy and before discharge from the health care facility. The second dose should be given 4–8 weeks after the first dose.

A dose of varicella vaccine used as postexposure prophylaxis is 70–100% effective at preventing or reducing the severity of varicella if given within 3 days of exposure. It may also be effective up to 5 days after exposure. The ACIP also recommends a second dose of varicella vaccine during outbreaks: persons who have received one dose of varicella vaccine should receive a second dose (resources permitting), provided the appropriate vaccination interval has elapsed since the first dose.

Oral acyclovir is recommended by some experts for postexposure prophylaxis and should be started between day 7 and 10 after exposure for a total of 7 days of therapy. Other antiviral agents, such as valacyclovir and famciclovir, can be used for prophylaxis in susceptible adults who have been exposed.

Varicella immune globulin contains high titers of VZV antibody and is recommended for postexposure prophylaxis in certain high-risk individuals, such as immunosuppressed patients, susceptible pregnant women exposed in early pregnancy, infants of mothers who develop chickenpox from 5 days before to 2 days after delivery, and certain premature infants exposed during the neonatal period (98). It is most effective when administered within 96 hours of exposure. The only available varicella immune globulin (as of early 2007) is VariZIG (Cangene Corporation, Winnipeg, Canada), which is a purified lyophilized human immune globulin preparation made from plasma containing high levels of antivaricella antibodies (immunoglobulin class G). VariZIG became available under an investigational new drug application submitted to the FDA in 2006. This product can be requested from the sole authorized U.S. distributor, FFF Enterprises (Temecula, CA; tel: 800-843-7477), for patients who have been exposed to varicella and who are at increased risk of severe disease and complications (101).

For the management of uncomplicated cases of varicella in healthy children the AAP does not recommend routine use of oral acyclovir therapy.

However, certain groups at increased risk of complicated disease should be considered for oral acyclovir therapy, including healthy, nonpregnant persons aged 13 years and older; children older than 12 months with chronic cutaneous or respiratory disorders and those receiving long-term salicylate therapy; and children receiving short, intermittent, or aerosolized courses of corticosteroids. Some experts advise using oral acyclovir for secondary cases within a household. For maximum benefit, oral acyclovir therapy should be started within 24 hours of the appearance of the rash. Intravenous acyclovir therapy is recommended for the treatment of immunocompromised children with primary varicella or recurrent HZ and for otherwise healthy individuals suffering from viral-mediated complications of varicella (e.g., pneumonia).

Adverse Effects

The most common adverse reactions following varicella vaccine are usually mild and self-limited: injection site irritation, such as pain, erythema, and swelling. Such local reactions are reported by approximately 20% of vaccinated persons. A varicella-like rash (usually several maculopapular lesions) at the injection site is reported by 3% of children, and by 1% of adolescents and adults, following the second dose. A generalized varicella-like rash, which is usually maculopapular rather than vesicular, is reported by 4–6% of recipients of varicella vaccine (1% after the second dose in adolescents and adults). Fever within 6 weeks of vaccination is reported by 15% of children and 10% of adolescents and adults; however, fever occurs in a similar percentage of persons receiving placebo and may be due to other infections rather than the vaccine.

Varicella vaccine, containing a live virus, can theoretically cause a mild latent infection. The rate of HZ after vaccination appears to be less than the rate after wild-virus infection. Unpublished CDC data indicate a rate of 2.6 cases of HZ per 100,000 varicella vaccine doses administered versus a rate of 68 cases per 100,000 person-years in healthy persons aged 20 years or older. Not all these cases have been confirmed as having been caused by the vaccine virus, and many may in fact be due to wild virus. Cases of zoster after vaccination appear to be milder than after natural infection, with fewer sequelae such as postherpetic neuralgia (98).

Transmission of vaccine-borne virus appears to be a rare event. Cases of suspected secondary transmission of vaccine virus have been reported, and in studies of household contacts, several instances of asymptomatic seroconversion have been observed. It appears that transmission occurs mainly, and perhaps only, when the vaccinated patient develops a rash. If a vaccinated child develops a rash, close contact should be avoided with persons who do not have evidence of varicella immunity and who are at high risk of complications of varicella, such as immunocompromised persons, until the rash in the vaccinated patient has resolved (98).

Serious adverse events, such as encephalitis, ataxia, erythema multiforme, Stevens-Johnson syndrome, pneumonia, thrombocytopenia, seizures, neuropathy, and death have been reported rarely in temporal association with varicella vaccine. In some cases, wild-type VZV or another causal agent has been identified. In most cases, data are insufficient to determine a causal association.

Precautions and Contraindications

Contraindications and precautions to varicella vaccine can be found in Tables in Appendix B.

HERPES ZOSTER VACCINE

HZ, or shingles, is caused by reactivation of VZV, which remains latent in the dorsal root (sensory) ganglia after a primary chickenpox infection. HZ is characterized by a vesicular rash and radicular pain, usually along a single dermatome. Pain usually occurs 2–3 days before the rash appears. Vesicles from HZ typically crust over in 7–10 days but may take up to a month to heal. VZV infection can be spread by contact with uncrusted lesions.

Persons at higher risk of HZ include the elderly and immunosuppressed persons, apparently because they experience a decline in cell-mediated immunity. The overall incidence of disease is 3–4 per 1,000 in developed countries, but the incidence increases markedly after age 50 years and rises to 10 per 1,000 after age 75 years. Some studies suggest that lifetime incidence is 10–20% and may be as high as 50% among individuals older than 85 years (102). Estimates of the number of new HZ cases in the United States vary from 300,000 to 1,000,000 annually (102–104). Up to 10% of patients older than 65 years who develop HZ require hospitalization.

A common, debilitating complication of HZ is postherpetic neuralgia, which is pain along the affected cutaneous nerves that persists more than 90 days after the lesions have healed. Postherpetic neuralgia is more common with increasing age, occurring in 25–50% of HZ patients older than 50 years, and it may persist for months or years. Other severe complications include keratitis, uveitis, retinitis, and blindness from HZ in the ophthalmic nerve; motor paresis or paralysis; GBS; and skin complications, including bacterial skin infections, gangrene, and sepsis.

A live attenuated HZ vaccine, Zostavax (Merck), was developed to boost cell-mediated immunity against VZV in older individuals and was licensed by the FDA in 2006. Zostavax has 14 times the antigenicity of pediatric varicella vaccine. In a study involving 38,546 participants aged 60 years or older, the vaccine, compared to placebo, reduced the burden of illness caused by HZ by 61.1%, the incidence of postherpetic neuralgia by 66.5%, and the incidence of HZ by 51.3%. Adverse events were similar in the vaccine and the placebo groups; injection-site reactions (erythema, pain, and tenderness) were more common among vaccine recipients but were generally mild (105). The cost effectiveness of the vaccine is uncertain, with estimates ranging from $2,000 to more than $100,000 per quality-adjusted life-year gained, depending on the method of calculation (106–108). However, using different assumptions, other estimates showed the cost to be similar to many other preventive measures used in elderly persons (109).

Indications

In 2006, the ACIP recommended the administration of Zostavax to all people age 60 years and older, whether or not they report a previous episode of shingles. Zostavax is not indicated for the treatment of HZ or postherpetic neuralgia.

Administration

The single-dose (0.65-mL) vaccine is intended for subcutaneous administration (preferably in the upper arm). It should be given immediately after reconstitution to minimize loss of potency. Unused reconstituted vaccine should be discarded after 30 minutes.

Adverse Effects

In the largest study of safety, rates of serious adverse events were similar (1.4%) in recipients of Zostavax and placebo. In a smaller study subset, serious adverse events were noted more frequently in those who received Zostavax (1.9%) than in those who received placebo (1.3%). The rates of deaths in each group were similar. Side effects reported more often in recipients of Zostavax (compared to placebo) include redness, pain, tenderness, and swelling at the injection site, and headache.

Because zoster vaccine, like varicella vaccine, is an attenuated live virus, transmission to other individuals is theoretically possible. Although further data will be needed to confirm this risk, it seems reasonable to follow the guidelines for varicella vaccine, in which viral transmission seems to occur only if the recipient develops a rash. If this occurs, it would be prudent for the patient to avoid contact with persons who do not have evidence of varicella immunity and who are at high risk of complications of varicella, such as immunocompromised persons, until the rash has resolved.

Precautions and Contraindications

Zostavax should not be administered to the following individuals: patients with a history of anaphylactic/anaphylactoid reaction to gelatin, neomycin, or any other component of the vaccine; those with a history of primary or acquired immunodeficiency states including leukemia, lymphomas of any type, or other malignant neoplasms affecting the bone marrow or lymphatic system; patients with AIDS or other clinical manifestations of HIV infection; patients on immunosuppressive therapy, including high-dose corticosteroids; patients with active untreated tuberculosis; and women who are or may be pregnant (110).

ROTAVIRUS VACCINE

Rotavirus affects virtually all children by age 5 years. Each year worldwide, rotavirus causes an estimated 111 million episodes of diarrhea, with 25 million clinic visits, 2 million hospitalizations, and a median of 440,000 deaths in children younger than 5, making it the principal cause of death from diarrheal disease in this age-group (111). In the United States it is responsible for approximately 500,000 office visits, 50,000 hospitalizations, and 20–60 deaths per year. The financial burden of rotavirus infections in the United States is estimated at more than 1 billion dollars annually. Therapies such as oral rehydration have had a minimal impact on the disease burden. Therefore, vaccination appears to be the predominant way to reduce its severity.

In 1998, the first rotavirus vaccine was licensed in the United States, and it appeared to offer excellent protection against this disease. However, the vaccine was withdrawn from the market in 1999 because it caused intussusception, at an estimated rate of one case per 10,000 vaccinated infants. In early 2006, placebo-controlled clinical trials for two new rotavirus vaccines showed excellent vaccine efficacy without an increased risk of intussusception and the ACIP approved a new pentavalent live attenuated oral rotavirus vaccine, RotaTeq (Merck), containing human serotypes G1, G2, G3, G4, and P[8]. In a study of 68,038 infants, the vaccine reduced hospitalizations and emergency department visits related to G1–G4 rotavirus gastroenteritis by 95%. Efficacy against any G1–G4 rotavirus gastroenteritis through the first full rotavirus season after vaccination was 74% and efficacy against severe gastroenteritis was 98%; the vaccine reduced clinic visits for G1–G4 rotavirus gastroenteritis by 86% and produced no increase in intussusception (112).

Also in 2006, a second rotavirus vaccine, Rotarix (GlaxoSmithKline), was approved and licensed in Europe by the European Medicines Agency. It has been licensed for use in more than 30 countries; as of 2007 it was not licensed for use in the United States. Rotarix is an attenuated monovalent vaccine derived from the most common human rotavirus strain, G1P[8]. It is administered in two oral doses 1–2 months apart. In a study of 63,225 infants in Finland and Latin America, two oral doses given at age 2 months and 4 months reduced severe rotavirus gastroenteritis and rotavirus-associated hospitalization by 85%, with no increase in the incidence of intussusception (113).

Indications
RotaTeq vaccine is indicated for all infants.

Administration

RotaTeq vaccine is given orally. The ACIP recommends that infants receive three doses of the oral vaccine at age 2, 4, and 6 months. Children should receive the first dose between age 6 and 12 weeks, with the subsequent doses administered at 4- to 10-week intervals. The third dose should be administered by age 32 weeks, and no doses of rotavirus vaccine should be given after this time. Although the ACIP recommends not initiating vaccination in infants older than 12 weeks (due to lack of safety and efficacy data), it is nonetheless recommended that if the first dose of rotavirus vaccine is inadvertently administered (off label) at age 13 weeks or older, the rest of the rotavirus vaccination series should be completed as per the schedule because the timing of the first dose should not affect the safety and efficacy of the second and third dose (114).

Adverse Effects

In more than 11,000 infants in 3 clinical trials, a vaccination report card was used to report the presence of adverse events for 42 days after each dose. Fever was observed at similar rates in vaccine and placebo recipients (43%). Adverse events that occurred at a statistically higher incidence within 42 days of any dose among recipients of RotaTeq as compared with placebo recipients were diarrhea (24 versus 21%), vomiting (15 versus 14%), otitis media (15 versus 13%), nasopharyngitis (7 versus 6%), and bronchospasm (1.1 versus 0.7%) (115).

Precautions and Contraindications

RotaTeq vaccine is contraindicated in infants with a history of hypersensitivity to any component of the vaccine. As of 2007 no safety or efficacy data were available to establish precautions for the administration of RotaTeq to infants who are potentially immunocompromised, including infants with blood dyscrasias, leukemia, or other lymphatic malignancies; infants who have an immunodeficiency disease; infants receiving immunosuppressive therapy; infants with HIV infection, cellular immune deficiencies, or hypogammaglobulinemic states; and infants who have received a blood transfusion or blood products within 42 days. Caution is advised when considering administration of RotaTeq to these infants. Caution is also advised for infants with a history of gastrointestinal disorders including infants with active acute gastrointestinal illness, chronic diarrhea and failure to thrive, and/or a history of congenital abdominal disorders, abdominal surgery, or intussusception. Viral shedding occurs in some vaccine recipients, primarily after the first dose (9%). Caution is advised when considering the administration of RotaTeq to individuals with immunodeficient close contacts such as individuals with malignancies or those who are receiving immunosuppressive therapy. Moderate or severe acute illness is a precaution for vaccination, but low-grade fever (less than 100.5°F) and mild upper respiratory infection do not preclude vaccination.

HUMAN PAPILLOMAVIRUS VACCINE

HPV is the most common sexually transmitted infection in the United States. An estimated 20 million Americans are currently infected with HPV, with an incidence of more than 6 million new cases per year. On the basis of present estimates, 75–80% of all sexually active people will become infected with HPV at some point during their lifetime.

Although the immune system eliminates the vast majority of HPV infections, in a minority of women persistent HPV infection may lead to the development of cervical cancer. As noted in Chapters 4 and 12, virtually all cervical cancer arises from high-risk types of HPV, particularly types 16, 18, 31, and 45. More than 99% of cervical cancers contain at least one high-risk HPV type, and approximately 70% contain HPV types 16 or 18. Worldwide, cervical cancer causes a significant disease burden, with approximately 270,000 deaths each year. An estimated 10,000 women in the United States develop cervical cancer each year, with approximately 3,700 deaths. Screening and treatment of cervical cancer are estimated to cost $6 billion annually in the United States. Prevention of HPV infection is difficult without changes in sexual behavior. Use of condoms has not been shown to be effective in eliminating transmission of the HPV virus (116). A vaccine against high-risk HPV types could significantly reduce not only cervical cancer but also HPV-related cancers of the vulva, penis, and anus.

Two HPV vaccines have been developed. Gardasil (Merck) was approved by the FDA in 2006 for use in females aged 9–26 years and is designed to prevent HPV types 16 and 18—the leading vectors of cervical cancers—as well as HPV types 6 and 11, which are linked to roughly 90% of genital warts. One study showed the vaccine to be 89% effective in preventing infection with these viral strains and 100% effective in preventing cervical cancer, precancerous lesions, or genital warts (117). However, the vaccine does not protect women against HPV strains with which they have already been infected before vaccination, nor is it designed to protect against less common HPV types. Therefore, routine Pap screening and counseling about protective sexual behaviors, as discussed in Chapters 4 and 11, respectively, will continue to remain an essential part of preventive care for women (118).

The second vaccine, Cervarix (GlaxoSmithKline), also protects against the two HPV strains that cause most cervical cancers. Cervarix has been shown to be 100% effective in preventing HPV strains 16 and 18; it is 100% effective for more than 4 years, according to data presented to the ACIP in 2006. The manufacturer applied for FDA approval in March 2007.

The vaccine has been licensed in more than 24 countries, and at this writing is pending licensing approval by the European Union.

The cost-effectiveness of HPV vaccine by routine vaccination of girls at age 12 years in several published studies ranged from $3,000 to $24,300 per quality-adjusted life year gained (118).

Indications

In March 2007, the ACIP published its recommendation for routine HPV vaccination for girls aged 11–12 years (118). The ACIP recommendation also allows for vaccination of girls beginning at age 9 years as well as catch-up vaccination of girls and women aged 13–26 years. The vaccine should be administered before onset of sexual activity (i.e., before females are exposed to HPV), but females who are sexually active (even if they have prior HPV exposure) should still be vaccinated, because they may still benefit from immunization against strains of HPV to which they have not yet been exposed. HPV vaccine is not licensed for females outside of the recommended 9- to 26-year age range, or for males. At the time of this publication, studies were ongoing among women older than 26 years and among men (no studies were under way among girls younger than 9 years) (118).

Administration

Quadrivalent HPV vaccine (Gardasil [Merck]) is available in single-dose vials (0.5 mL) and as single-dose, prefilled, Luer Lock syringes (0.5 mL). It is administered intramuscularly in a three-dose schedule. The second and third doses should be administered 2 and 6 months after the first dose. Quadrivalent HPV vaccine can be administered at the same visit when other age-appropriate vaccines are provided, such as Tdap and MCV4.

Adverse Effects

The most commonly reported side effects include pain, swelling, itching, and redness at the injection site. Fever, nausea, and dizziness have also been reported. Difficulty in breathing (bronchospasm) has been reported very rarely.

Precautions and Contraindications

See Tables in Appendix B for precautions and contraindications. Administration of HPV vaccine is not recommended during pregnancy but may be safely given to lactating mothers.

COMBINATION VACCINES

The Standards for Child and Adolescent Immunization Practices call for clinicians to administer simultaneously all vaccine doses for which a child is eligible at the time of each visit (19). However, most parents and clinicians are concerned about the administration of multiple injections at a single visit and hesitate to administer more than two or three simultaneous injections. These factors have created a demand for new combination vaccines that include multiple unrelated antigens. Combination vaccines have certain practical benefits: they reduce the psychological burden of the parents and office staff brought about by the concern that the infant experiences greater pain when receiving multiple injections; they lead to more efficiency in the office setting by decreasing shipping, handling, and vial storage needs; less time is needed to prepare vaccines and document their administration; handling fewer syringes reduces the potential for accidental needle sticks; administration costs are reduced; and the immunization schedule is simplified, which may lead to increased adherence and fewer missed opportunities for vaccination (20,21). For these reasons, the use of licensed combination vaccines is preferred over separate injection of their equivalent component vaccines (22).

Some parents, in part influenced by antivaccination activism in the media and on the Internet, express concerns about the use of multiple antigens in a single injection. There is no scientific evidence to support such concerns (119). Nonetheless, clinicians should be aware of these sentiments and should offer parents clear and concise information about the benefits of combination vaccines. Resources for counseling parents on certain myths about the dangers of vaccination are found on page 377.

Table 16.1 lists the currently available combination vaccines in the United States. Table 16.2 shows various strategies for using some combination vaccines. This can significantly reduce the number of shots given by age 2 years.

IMMUNIZATIONS FOR TRAVELERS

Patients traveling to other countries may require special immunizations against endemic diseases and/or chemoprophylaxis against malaria and other diseases. Some countries require an International Certificate of Vaccination against yellow fever. Vaccination against hepatitis A and hepatitis B, meningococcal disease, Japanese encephalitis, polio, plague, rabies, or typhoid fever may be indicated for travelers to certain countries. Depending on their destination, patients may also require counseling about measures to protect themselves against exposure to mosquitoes and arthropod vectors, risks from water and food, swimming and animal-related hazards, traveler's diarrhea, and motion sickness.

Clinicians who are unfamiliar with current recommendations for travel to specific countries can consult the CDC's *Traveler's Health* website at http://www.cdc.gov/travel/, which is updated continuously. Clinicians and patients can also obtain information from the CDC's automated traveler's hotline (877-FYI-TRIP), which is accessible 24 hours a day from a touch-tone telephone. *Health Information for International Travel*, known as the *Yellow Book*, is published by the CDC every 2 years as a reference for those who advise international travelers of health risks. The *Yellow Book* can be accessed online at http://wwwn.cdc.gov/travel/contentYellowBook.aspx or can be ordered by calling 800-545-2522.

Not all clinicians have access to all travel vaccines. For example, to administer yellow fever vaccine, clinics must be designated "yellow fever vaccination centers" by the WHO, and clinicians in the United States wishing to become "designated" must make arrangements with the CDC (120). Clinicians can refer patients to community referral resources, such as local public health departments, many of which operate travel medicine clinics, other health care facilities in the community offering immunization services for international travelers, and local infectious disease specialists with expertise in travel medicine.

OTHER IMMUNIZATIONS

Rabies infection is spread by contact with the saliva of infected animals. Worldwide, an estimated 35,000 to 50,000 human deaths from rabies occur every year (120). Before 1960 most of the U.S. cases occurred in domestic animals; at present, more than 90% of all animal cases reported annually occur in wildlife. Raccoons continue to be the most frequently reported rabid wildlife species (37.2% of all animal cases during 2001), followed by skunks (30.7%), bats (17.2%), foxes (5.9%), and other wild animals, including rodents and lagomorphs (0.7%) (121). The number of rabies-related human deaths in the United States has declined from more than 100 annually at the turn of the century to 1–2 per year in the 1990s. Modern day prophylaxis has proved approximately 100% successful (122). Rabies vaccination is indicated as preexposure prophylaxis for persons whose occupations, travel, or recreational activities expose them to potentially rabid animals, and (along with human rabies immune globulin) as postexposure prophylaxis following certain bite wounds.

Tetanus prophylaxis with tetanus immune globulin and/or toxoid is indicated in certain patients with wounds that are potentially contaminated with tetanus spores (see Table 16.3). Travelers to areas where postexposure tetanus immunization might be unavailable should consider receiving a booster dose of Td or Tdap before departure if 5 or more years have elapsed since their last vaccination. Measles, mumps, and rubella are still common throughout the world; travelers without evidence of adequate immunity should receive boosters (see "Suggested Readings" for guidance on MMR requirements for international travelers). Bacille Calmette–Guérin (BCG) vaccine is a live antituberculosis vaccine used in more than 100 countries throughout the world, primarily to prevent serious disease from *Mycobacterium tuberculosis*. It is more than 80% effective in protecting against meningeal and miliary tuberculosis in children. It is recommended in the United States only for certain children and health care workers in certain high-risk settings. It is not recommended for HIV patients (123).

OFFICE AND CLINIC ORGANIZATION

In spite of many advances in vaccine delivery, many national goals for universal immunization have not been reached. For clinicians, a number of organizational and logistical issues can interfere with adequate delivery of vaccination services (1,124). In response to this problem, Standards for Child and Adolescent Immunization Practices (SCAIP) (19) and objectives for adult immunization (125) have been issued by the National Vaccine Advisory Committee (see "Suggested Readings"). These standards suggest organizational practices to help clinicians ensure timely and comprehensive immunization of all appropriate patients. The SCAIP have been endorsed by the AAP, AAFP, American Medical Association, and 40 other health-related organizations. Although these recommendations were developed to improve the delivery of childhood and adolescent immunizations, the same office procedures can also enhance the delivery of adult immunizations. Many SCAIP recommendations are cited in the following discussion:

- **Vaccine product management** Office or clinic procedures for handling and storage of vaccines should be designed to comply with the recommendations in the manufacturer's package inserts. The SCAIP recommends daily monitoring of the temperature at which vaccines are stored and the expiration date of each vaccine. CDC-recommended storage and handling procedures are available at http://www.cdc.gov/vaccines/recs/storage/default.htm.
- **Use of appropriate contraindications.** Systems should be in place to ensure that parents are asked routinely about adverse events following prior immunizations and proper precautions or contraindications are considered before administering any vaccine (Tables in Appendix B). The SCAIP recommends posting up-to-date immunization protocols at all locations where vaccines are administered. Vaccines should only be administered by individuals with proper training and/or supervision.
- **Maintenance of vaccination records** SCAIP recommends that vaccination records be "accurate, complete, and easily accessible." Vaccination records should be recorded on a standard form or flow sheet in the medical record to help the clinician quickly determine whether the patient's immunizations

are up-to-date. Unfortunately, clinicians may be faced with incomplete or confusing immunization records because many patients change clinicians often as their health insurance coverage changes. Patient-held records, or shot cards, can be helpful, but these may be unavailable or incomplete.

A key plan to ensure the availability and completeness of the immunization record is the use of immunization registries. See Chapters 21 and 22 for general discussions of registries. Immunization registries are confidential, computerized information systems that collect vaccination data from multiple clinicians, generate reminder and recall notifications, and assess vaccination coverage within a defined geographic area (126). A registry with added capabilities, such as vaccine management, adverse event reporting, lifespan vaccination histories, and linkages with electronic data sources, is called an immunization information system (IIS). State registries receive funding under section 317b of the Public Health Service Act. Among the many benefits of such systems are consolidation of immunization records from many clinicians into one central location that can be accessed on demand by parents or clinicians; identification of due or overdue immunizations and generation of reminder notices; and the use of advanced centralized computer support to help clinicians determine needed immunizations at routine and catch-up visits, as well as to facilitate the integration of new vaccines into the recommended schedules (127).

The widespread use of electronic billing systems and electronic health records (EHRs) will not necessarily improve completeness of the vaccination record. A study of clinicians who submitted immunization data electronically from computerized billing records to an immunization registry in Philadelphia found that almost a fourth of the immunizations given were not submitted (128). At their present stage, EHRs do not use a standard format that allows communication with other EHR systems and do not uniformly offer immunization decision support. Furthermore, frequent updates in ACIP recommendations are unlikely to be distributed throughout the many proprietary EHR systems in a timely manner. An AAP task force recommended that "the ability [of EHRs] to flexibly format immunization data and support electronic data interchange with registries is vital." (129) Enhanced data exchange between EHRs and state registries would greatly increase the likelihood that immunization records would be accurate and available when needed. (See Chapter 22 for further discussion of data interface issues.)

SCAIP recommends that all administered vaccinations should be reported to state or local immunization registries, where available, to ensure that each patient's vaccination history remains accurate and complete. A CDC study showed that, in 2004, approximately 48% of U.S. children younger than 6 years participated in an IIS; furthermore, 76% of public vaccination provider sites and 39% of private vaccination provider sites submitted immunization data to an IIS during the last 6 months of 2004 (126). One of the national health objectives for 2010 is to increase to at least 95% the proportion of children younger than 6 years who participate in population-based immunization registries (130). More information about vaccine registries can be found at the National Immunization Program website at http://www.cdc.gov/vaccines/programs/iis/default.htm.

- **Reminder systems** Reminder systems can be helpful in ensuring that children return on time for their next immunization. Manual or automated systems can be used to trigger postcard, letter, or telephone reminders for parents to schedule their next vaccination appointment. Reminders, incorporated into EHRs, could also notify clinicians about overdue immunizations during acute care visits (129). See Chapters 21 and 22 for more details about reminder systems.

- **Medical record documentation** Physicians are required by statute to record the following information about childhood immunizations: name of vaccine, date of administration, manufacturer, lot number, signature and title of person administering the vaccine, and address where the vaccine was given. Adverse reactions to immunizations should be described in detail in the medical record. Vaccine refusal should also be documented.

    For vaccines requiring a VIS, the clinician should document which VIS was given, its date of publication, and the date the VIS was given. There is no federal requirement for written informed consent for vaccinations, and VISs are not informed consent documents, but some states do have such requirements. In such cases the clinician should have the recipients or their parents (or legal representatives) sign a separate "informed consent" form.

    According to SCAIP, clinicians should be aware of and report selected adverse events occurring after vaccination through the Vaccine Adverse Event Reporting System, a national vaccine safety surveillance program operated by the CDC and FDA. The National Childhood Vaccine Injury Act requires clinicians to report any event listed by the vaccine manufacturer as a contraindication to subsequent doses of the vaccine, and any event listed in the Reportable Events Table that occurs within a certain period after vaccination. Reportable events, which are specified, are generally those that require the patient to seek medical attention. Vaccines listed in the Reportable Events Table are tetanus in any combination; pertussis in any combination; measles, mumps, and rubella in any combination; rubella in any combination; measles in any combination; OPV; IPV; hepatitis A; hepatitis B; Hib conjugate; varicella; rotavirus; pneumococcal conjugate; and influenza vaccines. Report forms and assistance can be obtained by calling 800-822-7967. Report forms can be downloaded from http://vaers.hhs.gov/pubs.htm. The Reportable

Events Table can be viewed or downloaded from http://vaers.hhs .gov/reportable.htm.

SCAIP also recommends that clinicians should be familiar with the National Vaccine Injury Compensation Program. This is a no-fault, federally funded system designed to compensate persons who may have been injured by childhood vaccines. Any new vaccine recommended by the CDC for routine administration to children is covered. Vaccines currently covered under this program are DTP, DTaP, DT, tetanus toxoid (TT), Tdap, Td, MMR or its components, OPV, IPV, hepatitis A, hepatitis B, Hib, varicella, rotavirus, TIV, and LAIV, whether administered individually or in combination. Information about the Vaccine Injury Compensation Program can be obtained online at http://www.hrsa.gov/vaccinecompensation/or by calling 1-800-338-2382. It should be noted that this program is separate from the Vaccine Adverse Event Reporting System; a claim initiated in the former does not automatically generate an adverse event report, or vice versa.

• **Minimization of vaccine costs for children** Charges for vaccinations have become a major barrier to immunizations, especially among poor parents. The SCAIP recommends that patient costs should be kept as low as possible, and that "no child or adolescent should be denied vaccination because of inability to pay." One of the main publicly funded sources of low-cost vaccinations is the Vaccines for Children (VFC) Program. This is an entitlement program for children up to age 18 years, started in 1994 and paid for by federal funding, which supplies vaccines free of charge to participating clinicians. VFC is administered by the CDC, which contracts with vaccine manufacturers to buy vaccines at reduced rates and then distributes them to VFC providers. Children are eligible for VFC vaccines if they:

- Are 18 years or younger
- Are eligible for Medicaid
- Have no health insurance
- Are Native American or Alaskan Native
- Have health insurance that does not cover immunizations. In these cases, children must go to a federally qualified health center or rural health clinic for immunizations.

Further information about the VFC program can be obtained at http://www.cdc.gov/vaccines/programs/vfc/default.htm or by calling the CDC at 1-800-CDC-INFO (1-800-232-4636) [TTY (hearing impaired): 1-888-232-6348].

Some companies also offer patient assistance programs for certain individuals who cannot afford the vaccine and lack medical coverage

(Merck for all adult vaccines, e.g., HPV vaccine, Zostavax, Pneumovax 23; sanofi pasteur for rabies vaccine/immune globulin and meningococcal polysaccharide vaccine).

The SCAIP includes other recommendations that may help improve immunization practices but that, although often difficult, can be important for clinicians to implement. These include regular chart reviews to assess the effectiveness of vaccination coverage; working with other community organizations such as public health departments, health plans, and other clinicians to determine local needs and develop community vaccination programs; and allowing sufficient time during each visit to discuss with parents (or guardians) and adolescent patients the benefits and risks of vaccines in a culturally appropriate and easy-to-understand manner.

ELECTRONIC RESOURCES FOR POINT-OF-CARE IMMUNIZATION INFORMATION

With the constantly evolving complexity of recommended vaccinations, it becomes progressively more difficult for clinicians to remain up-to-date with current recommendations. For example, a study of pediatricians and family physicians found serious deficiencies in their ability to correctly choose appropriate catch-up regimens for children with immunization delay. For six questionnaire scenarios sent to clinicians, the median score was 1.83 correct out of a possible score of 6.0. The study also documented substantive knowledge gaps regarding immunization contraindications (14).

A number of regularly updated web-based resources provide the relevant information. One of the best point-of-care resources for immunization information is the "SHOTS" software program, developed by the Society of Teachers of Family Medicine with support from the CDC. The SHOTS program runs on a handheld digital device using either the Palm or Pocket PC operating system, or it can be used online (http://www.immunizationed.org/ShotsOnline.asp). It contains the complete immunization schedules for children, adults, and persons with special medical conditions. In addition, information can be quickly viewed for each individual vaccine regarding immunization basics, high-risk indications, adverse reactions, contraindications, and administration. There is also information on how to catch up on each vaccine if behind, as well as a section on how to discuss common vaccine misconceptions. The program also has photographs of common vaccine-preventable diseases. The SHOTS program is updated regularly, and users can request email notification of new releases and updates.

ACKNOWLEDGMENT

The author wishes to thank Donald B. Middleton, MD, Professor of Family Medicine at the University of Pittsburgh School of Medicine, and Chairman of the Group on Immunization Education of the Society of Teachers of Family Medicine, for invaluable help in reviewing this chapter.

RESOURCES — PATIENT EDUCATION MATERIALS

Vaccine Information Statements are available online at:
http://www.cdc.gov/nip/publications/VIS/default.htm and
Immunization Action Coalition web site at:
http://www.immunize.org/vis/

National Immunization Program Publications: Immunization Educational and Training Materials.
http://www.cdc.gov/nip/publications/default.htm

Immunization Action Coalition has a collection of free print materials.
http://www.immunize.org/catg.d/free.htm

SUGGESTED READINGS

Atkinson WHJ, McIntyre L, Wolfe S, eds. Centers for Disease Control and Prevention. *Epidemiology and prevention of vaccine-preventable diseases*, 10th ed. Washington, DC: Public Health Foundation, 2007. "*The Pink Book*." Available online at: http://www.cdc .gov/nip/publications/pink/.

Centers for Disease Control and Prevention. Recommended immunization schedules for persons aged 0–18 years—United States, 2007. *MMWR Morb Mortal Wkly Rep* 2007;55(51):Q1–Q4 Available online at: http://www.cdc.gov/mmwr/preview/ mmwrhtml/mm5551a7.htm.

Centers for Disease Control and Prevention. Recommended adult immunization schedule—United States, October 2006–September 2007. *MMWR Morb Mortal Wkly Rep* 2006;55(40):Q1–Q4. Available online at: http://www.cdc.gov/mmwr/preview/ mmwrhtml/mm5540a10.htm.

Centers for Disease Control and Prevention. Updated U.S. Public Health Service guidelines for the management of occupational exposures to HBV, HCV, and HIV and recommendations for postexposure prophylaxis. *MMWR Recomm Rep* 2001;50(RR-11):22. Available at: http://www.cdc.gov/mmwr/PDF/rr/rr5011.pdf.

Dosages for influenza vaccine: See http://www.cdc.gov/flu/professionals/vaccination/. Accessed June 7, 2007.

Middleton DB, Zimmerman RK, Mitchell KB. Dosages for Hepatitis B vaccine: vaccine schedules and procedures, 2007. *J Fam Pract* 2007;56(2):S47–S60. Available online at: http://www.jfponline.com/uploadedFiles/Journal_Site_Files/Journal_of_Family _Practice/supplement_archive/JFPSupp_Vaccines07_0207.pdf (p. 58 of pdf document).

National Vaccine Advisory Committee. Standards for child and adolescent immunization practices. *Pediatrics* 2003;112(4):958–963.

Pickering LK, Baker CJ, Long SS, eds. American Academy of Pediatrics. *Red book: 2006 Report of the committee on infectious diseases*, 27 ed. Elk Grove Village: American Academy of Pediatrics, 2006.

Zimmerman RK, Middleton DB. Vaccines for persons at high risk, 2007. *J Fam Pract* 2007;56(2):S38–S46. Available online at: http://www.jfponline.com/uploadedFiles/ Journal_Site_Files/Journal_of_Family_Practice/supplement_archive/JFPSupp _Vaccines07_0207.pdf. (pp. 48–56 of pdf document).

References

1. Kimmel SR, Burns IT, Wolfe RM, et al. Addressing immunization barriers, benefits, and risks. *J Fam Pract* 2007;56(Suppl 2):S61–S69.
2. Kroger AT, Atkinson WL, Marcuse EK, et al. General recommendations on immunization: recommendations of the Advisory Committee on Immunization Practices (ACIP). *MMWR Recomm Rep* 2006;55(RR-15):1–48.
3. Centers for Disease Control and Prevention. Recommendations of the Advisory Committee on Immunization Practices (ACIP): use of vaccines and immune globulins for persons with altered immunocompetence. *MMWR Recomm Rep* 1993; 42(RR-4):1–18.
4. Williams BC, Miller CA. American Academy of Pediatrics. Preventive health care for young children: findings from a 10-country study and directions for United States policy. *Pediatrics* 1992;89(5 Pt 2):981–998.
5. Zimmerman RK, Giebink GS. Childhood immunizations: a practical approach for clinicians. *Am Fam Physician* 1992;45(4):1759–1772.
6. Centers for Disease Control and Prevention. Retrospective assessment of vaccination coverage among school-aged children–selected U.S. cities, 1991. *MMWR Morb Mortal Wkly Rep* 1992;41(6):103–107.
7. Centers for Disease Control and Prevention. *Childhood immunization rates surpass healthy people 2010 goal.* http://www.CDC.gov/od/oc/media/pressrel/r050726.htm. Accessed February 4, 2006.
8. World Health Organization. *Immunization surveillance, assessment and monitoring.* http://www.who.int/immunization_monitoring/routine/immunization_coverage/ en/index.html. Accessed February 4, 2006.
9. Luman ET, Barker LE, Shaw KM, et al. Timeliness of childhood vaccinations in the United States: days undervaccinated and number of vaccines delayed. *JAMA* 2005;293(10):1204–1211.
10. Sloan FA, Berman S, Rosenbaum S, et al. The fragility of the U.S. vaccine supply. *N Engl J Med* 2004;351(23):2443–2447.
11. Goldfarb NI, Patel NM, Clarke JL. Improving quality by encouraging providers to use pediatric combination vaccines. *Manag Care* 2005;14(Suppl 6):3–12.
12. Zimmerman RK, Schlesselman JJ, Baird AL, et al. A national survey to understand why physicians defer childhood immunizations. *Arch Pediatr Adolesc Med* 1997;151(7):657–664.
13. Prislin R, Sawyer MH, Nader PR, et al. Provider-staff discrepancies in reported immunization knowledge and practices. *Prev Med* 2002;34(5):554–561.
14. Cohen NJ, Lauderdale DS, Shete PB, et al. Physician knowledge of catch-up regimens and contraindications for childhood immunizations. *Pediatrics* 2003; 111(5):925–932.

15. Schaffer SJ, Humiston SG, Shone LP, et al. Adolescent immunization practices: a national survey of U.S. physicians. *Arch Pediatr Adolesc Med* 2001;155(5):566–571.

16. Szilagyi PG, Roghmann KJ, Campbell JR, et al. Immunization practices of primary care practitioners and their relation to immunization levels. *Arch Pediatr Adolesc Med* 1994;148(2):158–166.

17. Taylor JA, Darden PM, Brooks DA, et al. Practitioner policies and beliefs and practice immunization rates: a study from pediatric research in office settings and the National Medical Association. *Pediatrics* 2002;109(2):294–300.

18. King GE, Hadler SC. Simultaneous administration of childhood vaccines: an important public health policy that is safe and efficacious. *Pediatr Infect Dis J* 1994;13(5): 394–407.

19. National Vaccine Advisory Committee. Standards for child and adolescent immunization practices. *Pediatrics* 2003;112(4):958–963.

20. Dodd D. Benefits of combination vaccines: effective vaccination on a simplified schedule. *Am J Manag Care* 2003;9(Suppl 1):S6–12.

21. Decker MD. Principles of pediatric combination vaccines and practical issues related to use in clinical practice. *Pediatr Infect Dis J* 2001;20(Suppl 11):S10–S18.

22. Centers for Disease Control and Prevention. Combination vaccines for childhood immunization. Recommendations of the Advisory Committee on Immunization Practices (ACIP), the American Academy of Pediatrics (AAP), and the American Academy of Family Physicians (AAFP). *Am Fam Physician* 1999;59(9):2565–2574.

23. Zimmerman R. Principles for using combination vaccines. *Am Fam Physician* 1999; 59(9):2422, 2424, 2427.

24. Centers for Disease Control and Prevention. General recommendations on immunization. In: Atkinson WHJ, McIntyre L, Wolfe S, eds. *Epidemiology and prevention of vaccine-preventable diseases*, 10th ed. Washington, DC: Public Health Foundation, 2007:9–30.

25. Bohlke K, Davis RL, Marcy SM, et al. Risk of anaphylaxis after vaccination of children and adolescents. *Pediatrics* 2003;112(4):815–820.

26. Murphy KR, Strunk RC. Safe administration of influenza vaccine in asthmatic children hypersensitive to egg proteins. *J Pediatr* 1985;106(6):931–933.

27. Watson JC, Hadler SC, Dykewicz CA, et al. Measles, mumps, and rubella–vaccine use and strategies for elimination of measles, rubella, and congenital rubella syndrome and control of mumps: recommendations of the Advisory Committee on Immunization Practices (ACIP). *MMWR Recomm Rep* 1998;47(RR-8):1–57.

28. Centers for Disease Control and Prevention. Thimerosal in vaccines: a joint statement of the American Academy of Pediatrics and the Public Health Service. *MMWR Morb Mortal Wkly Rep* 1999;48(26):563–565.

29. Centers for Disease Control and Prevention. Summary of the joint statement on thimerosal in vaccines. American Academy of Family Physicians, American Academy of Pediatrics, Advisory Committee on Immunization Practices, Public Health Service. *MMWR Morb Mortal Wkly Rep* 2000;49(27):622, 631.

30. U.S. Food and Drug Administration—Centers for Biologics Evaluation and Research. *Thimerosal in vaccines*. March 21, 2007; http://www.fda.gov/cber/vaccine/ thimerosal.htm. Accessed April 16, 2007.

31. Stratton K, Gable A, McCormick MC, et al. *Immunization safety review: thimerosal-containing vaccines and neuro-developmental disorders*. Washington, DC: National Academy Press, 2001.

32. Heron J, Golding J. The ALSPAC Study Team. Thimerosal exposure in infants and developmental disorders: a prospective cohort study in the united kingdom does not support a causal association. *Pediatrics* 2004;114(3):577–583.

33. Parker SK, Schwartz B, Todd J, et al. Thimerosal-containing vaccines and autistic spectrum disorder: a critical review of published original data. *Pediatrics* 2004;114(3): 793–804.

34. Hviid A, Stellfeld M, Wohlfahrt J, et al. Association between thimerosal-containing vaccine and autism. *JAMA* 2003;290(13):1763–1766.

35. Gellin BG, Maibach EW, Marcuse EK. Do parents understand immunizations? A national telephone survey. *Pediatrics* 2000;106(5):1097–1102.

36. AAFP. *Periodic survey of fellows no. 48: immunization administration practices.* Elk Grove Village:AAFP, 2001.

37. Flanagan-Klygis EA, Sharp L, Frader JE. Dismissing the family who refuses vaccines: a study of pediatrician attitudes. *Arch Pediatr Adolesc Med* 2005;159(10): 929–934.

38. Wolfe RM, Sharp LK. Vaccination or immunization? The impact of search terms on the internet. *J Health Commun* 2005;10(6):537–551.

39. Wolfe RM, Sharp LK, Lipsky MS. Content and design attributes of antivaccination websites [See Comment]. *JAMA* 2002;287(24):3245–3248.

40. Feikin DR, Lezotte DC, Hamman RF, et al. Individual and community risks of measles and pertussis associated with personal exemptions to immunization. *JAMA* 2000;284(24):3145–3150.

41. Diekema DS. The Committee on Bioethics. Responding to parental refusals of immunization of children. *Pediatrics* 2005;115(5):1428–1431.

42. Gust DA, Kennedy A, Shui I, et al. Parent attitudes toward immunizations and health care providers: the role of information. *Am J Prev Med* 2005;29(2):105–112.

43. Kimmel SR, Wolfe RM. Communicating the benefits and risks of vaccines. *J Fam Pract* 2005;54(Suppl 1):S51–S57.

44. Hopkins RS, Jajosky RA, Hall PA, et al. Summary of notifiable diseases–United States, 2003. *MMWR Morb Mortal Wkly Rep* 2005;52(54):1–85.

45. Jajosky RA, Hall PA, Adams DA, et al. Summary of notifiable diseases–United States, 2004. *MMWR Morb Mortal Wkly Rep* 2006;53(53): 1–79.

46. Cherry JD. The epidemiology of pertussis: a comparison of the epidemiology of the disease pertussis with the epidemiology of Bordetella pertussis infection. *Pediatrics* 2005;115(5):1422–1427.

47. Centers for Disease Control and Prevention. Pertussis. In: Atkinson WHJ, McIntyre L, Wolfe S, eds. *Epidemiology and prevention of vaccine-preventable diseases*, 10th ed. Washington, DC: Public Health Foundation, 2007:81–100.

48. Greenberg DP. Pertussis in adolescents: increasing incidence brings attention to the need for booster immunization of adolescents. *Pediatr Infect Dis J* 2005;24(8): 721–728.

49. Vitek CR, Pascual FB, Baughman AL, et al. Increase in deaths from pertussis among young infants in the United States in the 1990s. *Pediatr Infect Dis J* 2003;22(7): 628–634.

50. Centers for Disease Control and Prevention. Pertussis–United States, 1997–2000. *MMWR Morb Mortal Wkly Rep* 2002;51(4):73–76.

51. Ward JI, Cherry JD, Chang S-J, et al. Efficacy of an acellular pertussis vaccine among adolescents and adults. *N Engl J Med* 2005;353(15):1555–1563.

52. Centers for Disease Control and Prevention. Tetanus. In: Atkinson WHJ, McIntyre L, Wolfe S, eds. *Epidemiology and prevention of vaccine-preventable diseases*, 10th ed. Washington, DC: Public Health Foundation, 2007:71–80.

53. Kretsinger K, Broder KR, Cortese MM, et al. Preventing tetanus, diphtheria, and pertussis among adults: use of tetanus toxoid, reduced diphtheria toxoid and acellular pertussis vaccine recommendations of the Advisory Committee on Immunization Practices (ACIP) and recommendation of ACIP, supported by the Healthcare Infection Control Practices Advisory Committee (HICPAC), for use of Tdap among health care personnel. *MMWR Recomm Rep* 2006;55(RR-17): 1–37.

54. World Health Organization. *Measles: fact sheet No. 286.* January 2007; http://www .who.int/mediacentre/factsheets/fs286/en/index.html. Accessed April 22, 2007.

55. Mustin HD, Holt VL, Connell FA. Adequacy of well-child care and immunizations in U.S. infants born in 1988. *JAMA* 1994;272(14):1111–1115.

56. Centers for Disease Control and Prevention. Measles. In: Atkinson WHJ, McIntyre L, Wolfe S, eds. *Epidemiology and prevention of vaccine-preventable diseases*, 10th ed. Washington, DC: Public Health Foundation, 2007:129–148.

57. Centers for Disease Control and Prevention. Mumps epidemic–Iowa, 2006. *MMWR Morb Mortal Wkly Rep* 2006;55(13):366–368.

58. Centers for Disease Control and Prevention. Brief report: update: mumps activity–United States, January 1-October 7, 2006. *MMWR Morb Mortal Wkly Rep* 2006;55(42):1152–1153.

59. Centers for Disease Control and Prevention. Update: multistate outbreak of mumps–United States, January 1-May 2, 2006. *MMWR Morb Mortal Wkly Rep* 2006; 55(20):559–563.

60. Centers for Disease Control and Prevention. Notice to readers: updated recommendations of the Advisory Committee on Immunization Practices (ACIP) for the control and elimination of mumps. *MMWR Morb Mortal Wkly Rep* 2006; 55(22):629–630.

61. Reisinger KS, Brown ML, Xu J, et al. A combination measles, mumps, rubella, and varicella vaccine (ProQuad) given to 4–6-year-old healthy children vaccinated previously with M-M-RII and Varivax. *Pediatrics* 2006;117(2):265–272.

62. Lieberman JM, Williams WR, Miller JM, et al. The safety and immunogenicity of a quadrivalent measles, mumps, rubella and varicella vaccine in healthy children: a study of manufacturing consistency and persistence of antibody. *Pediatr Infect Dis J* 2006;25(7):615–622.

63. Shinefield H, Black S, Thear M, et al. Safety and immunogenicity of a measles, mumps, rubella and varicella vaccine given with combined haemophilus influenzae type b conjugate/hepatitis B vaccines and combined diphtheria-tetanus-acellular pertussis vaccines. *Pediatr Infect Dis J* 2006;25(4):287–292.

64. Offit PA, Jew RK. Addressing parents' concerns: do vaccines contain harmful preservatives, adjuvants, additives, or residuals? *Pediatrics* 2003;112(6):1394–1397.

65. American Academy of Pediatrics Summaries of Infectious Diseases: Haemophilus influenzae infections. In: Pickering LK, Baker CJ, Long SS, eds. *Red book: 2006 Report of the committee on infectious diseases*, Section 3. 27 ed. Elk Grove Village: American Academy of Pediatrics, 2006.

66. Zimmerman RK, Middleton DB, Burns IT, et al. Routine vaccines across the life span, 2007. *J Fam Pract* 2007;56(2):S18–S37.

67. Centers for Disease Control and Prevention. Prevention of pneumococcal disease: recommendations of the Advisory Committee on Immunization Practices (ACIP). *MMWR Recomm Rep* 1997;46(RR-8):1–24.

68. Centers for Disease Control and Prevention. Pneumococcal Disease. In: Atkinson WHJ, McIntyre L, Wolfe S, ed. *Epidemiology and prevention of vaccine-preventable diseases*, 10th ed. Washington, DC: Public Health Foundation, 2007: 257–270.

69. Centers for Disease Control and Prevention. Direct and indirect effects of routine vaccination of children with 7-valent pneumococcal conjugate vaccine on incidence of invasive pneumococcal disease–United States, 1998–2003. *MMWR Morb Mortal Wkly Rep* 2005;54(36):893–897.

70. Kellner JD, Church DL, MacDonald J, et al. Progress in the prevention of pneumococcal infection. *CMAJ* 2005;173(10):1149–1151.

71. Jackson LA, Neuzil KM, Yu O, et al. Effectiveness of pneumococcal polysaccharide vaccine in older adults. *N Engl J Med* 2003;348(18):1747–1755.

72. Dear K, Holden J, Andrews R, et al. Vaccines for preventing pneumococcal infection in adults. *Cochrane Database Syst Rev* 2003(4):CD000422.

73. Christenson B, Hedlund J, Lundbergh P, et al. Additive preventive effect of influenza and pneumococcal vaccines in elderly persons. *Eur Respir J* 2004;23(3):363–368.

74. Fisman DN, Abrutyn E, Spaude KA, et al. Prior pneumococcal vaccination is associated with reduced death, complications, and length of stay among hospitalized adults with community-acquired pneumonia. *Clin Infect Dis* 2006;42(8):1093–1101.

75. Vila-Corcoles A, Ochoa-Gondar O, Hospital I, et al. Protective effects of the 23-valent pneumococcal polysaccharide vaccine in the elderly population: the EVAN-65 study. *Clin Infect Dis* 2006;43(7):860–868.

76. Gluck T. Vaccinate your immunocompromised patients! 10.1093/rheumatology/kei237. *Rheumatology (Oxford)* 2006;45(1):9–10.

77. Centers for Disease Control and Prevention. Outbreak of invasive pneumococcal disease–Alaska, 2003–2004. *MMWR Morb Mortal Wkly Rep* 2005;54(3):72–75.

78. Pollard AJ. Global epidemiology of meningococcal disease and vaccine efficacy. *Pediatr Infect Dis J* 2004;23(Suppl 12):S274–S279.

79. Bilukha OO, Rosenstein N. Prevention and control of meningococcal disease. Recommendations of the Advisory Committee on Immunization Practices (ACIP). *MMWR Recomm Rep* 2005;54(RR-7):1–21.

80. Centers for Disease Control and Prevention. Update: Guillain-Barre syndrome among recipients of Menactra meningococcal conjugate vaccine–United States, June 2005-September 2006. *MMWR Morb Mortal Wkly Rep* 2006;55(41):1120–1124.

81. Gardner P. Clinical practice. Prevention of meningococcal disease. *N Engl J Med* 2006;355(14):1466–1473.

82. Centers for Disease Control and Prevention. Hepatitis B. In: Atkinson WHJ, McIntyre L, Wolfe S, ed. *Epidemiology and prevention of vaccine-preventable diseases*, 10th ed. Washington, DC: Public Health Foundation, 2007:211–234.

83. Mast EE, Margolis HS, Fiore AE, et al. A comprehensive immunization strategy to eliminate transmission of hepatitis B virus infection in the United States: recommendations of the Advisory Committee on Immunization Practices (ACIP) part 1: immunization of infants, children, and adolescents. *MMWR Recomm Rep* 2005; 54(RR-16):1–31.

84. Mast EE, Weinbaum CM, Fiore AE, et al. A comprehensive immunization strategy to eliminate transmission of hepatitis B virus infection in the United States: recommendations of the Advisory Committee on Immunization Practices (ACIP) part II: immunization of adults. *MMWR Recomm Rep* 2006;55(RR-16):1–33. [Quiz CE31-34.]

85. Fiore AE, Wasley A, Bell BP. Prevention of hepatitis A through active or passive immunization: recommendations of the Advisory Committee on Immunization Practices (ACIP). *MMWR Recomm Rep* 2006;55(RR-7):1–23.

86. Centers for Disease Control and Prevention. Hepatitis A. In: Atkinson WHJ, McIntyre L, Wolfe S, eds. *Epidemiology and prevention of vaccine-preventable diseases*, 10th ed. Washington, DC: Public Health Foundation, 2007:197–210.

87. Tellier R. Review of aerosol transmission of influenza A virus. *Emerg Infect Dis* 2006;12:1657–1662.

88. Thompson WW, Shay DK, Weintraub E, et al. Mortality associated with influenza and respiratory syncytial virus in the United States. *JAMA* 2003;289(2):179–186.

89. Smith NM, Bresee JS, Shay DK, et al. Prevention and control of influenza: recommendations of the Advisory Committee on Immunization Practices (ACIP). *MMWR Recomm Rep* 2006;55(RR-10):1–42.

90. Jefferson T. Influenza vaccination: policy versus evidence. *BMJ* 2006;333(7574):912–915.

91. Zimmerman RK. Recent changes in influenza vaccination recommendations, 2007. *J Fam Pract* 2007;56(2):S12–S17.

92. Juckett G. Avian influenza: preparing for a pandemic. *Am Fam Physician* 2006;74(5):783–790.

93. Centers for Disease Control and Prevention. *Avian influenza infection in humans.* October 25, 2006; http://www.CDC.gov/flu/avian/gen-info/avian-flu-humans.htm. Accessed April 16, 2007.

94. U.S. Food and Drug Administration. *FDA approves first U.S. Vaccine for humans against the avian influenza virus H5N1.* April 19, 2007; http://www.fda.gov/cber/vaccine/thimerosal.htm. Accessed April 26, 2007.

95. Jefferson T, Demicheli V, Rivetti D, et al. Antivirals for influenza in healthy adults: systematic review. *Lancet* 367(9507):303–313.

96. Centers for Disease Control and Prevention. Influenza. In: Atkinson WHJ, McIntyre L, Wolfe S, eds. *Epidemiology and prevention of vaccine-preventable diseases*, 10th ed. Washington, DC: Public Health Foundation, 2007:235–256.

97. Heininger U, Seward JF. Varicella. *Lancet* 2006;368(9544):1365–1376.

98. Centers for Disease Control and Prevention. Varicella. In: Atkinson WHJ, McIntyre L, Wolfe S, eds. *Epidemiology and prevention of vaccine-preventable diseases*, 10th ed. Washington, DC: Public Health Foundation, 2007.

99. Centers for Disease Control and Prevention. Prevention of varicella. Update recommendations of the Advisory Committee on Immunization Practices (ACIP). *MMWR Recomm Rep* 1999;48(RR-6):1–5.

100. Jumaan AO, Yu O, Jackson LA, et al. Incidence of herpes zoster, before and after varicella-vaccination-associated decreases in the incidence of varicella, 1992–2002. *J Infect Dis* 2005;191(12):2002–2007.

101. Centers for Disease Control and Prevention. A new product (VariZIG) for postexposure prophylaxis of varicella available under an investigational new drug

application expanded access protocol. *MMWR Morb Mortal Wkly Rep* 2006;55(8): 209–210.

102. Schmader K. Herpes zoster in older adults. *Clin Infect Dis* 2001;32(10):1481–1486.

103. Gilden DH, Kleinschmidt-DeMasters BK, LaGuardia JJ, et al. Neurologic complications of the reactivation of varicella-zoster virus. *N Engl J Med* 2000;342(9): 635–645.

104. Insinga RP, Itzler RF, Pellissier JM, et al. The incidence of herpes zoster in a United States administrative database. *J Gen Intern Med* 2005;20(8):748–753.

105. Oxman MN, Levin MJ, Johnson GR, et al. A vaccine to prevent herpes zoster and postherpetic neuralgia in older adults. *N Engl J Med* 2005;352(22):2271–2284.

106. Gilden DH. Varicella-zoster virus vaccine–grown-ups need it, too. *N Engl J Med* 2005;352(22):2344–2346.

107. Hornberger J, Robertus K. Cost-effectiveness of a vaccine to prevent herpes zoster and postherpetic neuralgia in older adults. *Ann Intern Med* 2006;145(5):317–325.

108. Rothberg MB, Virapongse A, Smith KJ. Cost-effectiveness of a vaccine to prevent herpes zoster and postherpetic neuralgia in older adults. *Clin Infect Dis* 2007; 44(10):1280–1288.

109. Levin MJ. Herpes zoster vaccine: update (January 2007). In: Plotkin SA, Orenstein WA, eds. *Vaccines*, 4th ed. Philadelphia: Elsevier Science, 2004.

110. *Zostavax* Whitehouse Station: Merck & Co, June 2006 [Package insert].

111. Parashar UD, Hummelman EG, Bresee JS, et al. Global illness and deaths caused by rotavirus disease in children. *Emerg Infect Dis* 2003;9(5):565–572.

112. Vesikari T, Matson DO, Dennehy P, et al. Safety and efficacy of a pentavalent human-bovine (WC3) reassortant rotavirus vaccine. *N Engl J Med* 2006;354(1): 23–33.

113. Ruiz-Palacios GM, Perez-Schael I, Velazquez FR, et al. Safety and efficacy of an attenuated vaccine against severe rotavirus gastroenteritis. *N Engl J Med* 2006;354(1): 11–22.

114. Parashar UD, Alexander JP, Glass RI. Prevention of rotavirus gastroenteritis among infants and children. Recommendations of the Advisory Committee on Immunization Practices (ACIP). *MMWR Recomm Rep* 2006;55(RR-12):1–13.

115. Centers for Disease Control and Prevention. Rotavirus. In: Atkinson WHJ, McIntyre L, Wolfe S, eds. *Epidemiology and prevention of vaccine-preventable diseases*, 10th ed. Washington, DC: Public Health Foundation, 2007:295–306.

116. Winer RL, Lee SK, Hughes JP, et al. Genital human papillomavirus infection: incidence and risk factors in a cohort of female university students. *Am J Epidemiol* 2003;157(3):218–226.

117. Villa LL, Costa RL, Petta CA, et al. Prophylactic quadrivalent human papillomavirus (types 6, 11, 16, and 18) L1 virus-like particle vaccine in young women: a randomised double-blind placebo-controlled multicentre phase II efficacy trial. *Lancet Oncol* 2005;6(5):271–278.

118. Markowitz LE, Dunne EF, Saraiya M, et al. Quadrivalent human papillomavirus vaccine: recommendations of the Advisory Committee on Immunization Practices (ACIP). *MMWR Recomm Rep* 2007;56(RR-2):1–24.

119. Halsey NA. Safety of combination vaccines: perception versus reality. *Pediatr Infect Dis J* 2001;20(Suppl 11):S40–S44.

120. Thompson MJ. Immunizations for international travel. *Prim Care* 2002;29(4): 787–814.

121. Centers for Disease Control and Prevention. *Rabies: epidemiology. November 6, 2006*; http://www.CDC.gov/ncidod/dvrd/rabies/Epidemiology/Epidemiology.htm. Accessed April 16, 2007.
122. Centers for Disease Control and Prevention. *Rabies: about rabies. December 1, 2003*; http://www.CDC.gov/ncidod/dvrd/rabies/introduction/intro.htm. Accessed April 16, 2007.
123. Centers for Disease Control and Prevention. The role of BCG vaccine in the prevention and control of tuberculosis in the United States. A joint statement by the Advisory Council for the Elimination of Tuberculosis and the Advisory Committee on Immunization Practices. *MMWR Recomm Rep* 1996;45(RR-4):1–18.
124. Randolph G, Fried B, Loeding L, et al. Organizational characteristics and preventive service delivery in private practices: a peek inside the "Black Box" of private practices caring for children. *Pediatrics* 2005;115(6):1704–1711.
125. Fedson DS. Adult immunization. Summary of the National Vaccine Advisory Committee report. *JAMA* 1994;272(14):1133–1137.
126. Centers for Disease Control and Prevention. Immunization information system progress–United States, 2004. *MMWR Morb Mortal Wkly Rep* 2005;54(45):1156–1157.
127. Linkins RW. Immunization registries: progress and challenges in reaching the 2010 national objective. *J Public Health Manag Pract* 2001;7(6):67–74.
128. Kolasa MS, Cherry JE, Chilkatowsky AP, et al. Practice-based electronic billing systems and their impact on immunization registries. *J Public Health Manag Pract* 2005;11(6):493–499.
129. American Academy of Pediatrics: Task Force on Medical Informatics. Special requirements for electronic medical record systems in pediatrics. *Pediatrics* 2001;108(2): 513–515.
130. U.S. Department of Health and Human Services. *Healthy people 2010: with understanding and improving health and objectives for improving health*, 2nd ed. Washington, DC: U.S. Department of Health and Human Services, 2000.

CHAPTER 17

Health Promotion and Disease Prevention for Children and Adolescents

Virginia A. Moyer and Laura E. Ferguson

INTRODUCTION

Being invited to take part in a child's upbringing is one of the greatest privileges of primary care. The joy of this opportunity is tempered by the recognition that there is never enough time to accomplish all that is desirable in these short visits. Given the limited time and other resources, how can a clinician best promote optimal growth and development of a child, and support the family and community that surround the child? This chapter briefly reviews health promotion and disease prevention in children, focusing on the ways it may differ from that in adults and on the specific interventions that are reasonably well supported by research evidence. In addition, the chapter offers a special focus on two special populations of children: newborns and adolescents.

Early in the 20th century well child care made its appearance in the form of public child health fairs (sometimes called milk fairs) and freestanding, publicly supported well baby clinics run mostly by women pediatricians and public health nurses. Starting in the 1920s, political action on the part of the American Medical Association to prevent what it viewed as a socialist scheme, as well as the recognition by academic pediatricians of the importance of care of the well child, resulted in the movement of well child care to private physicians (1). By the 1950s, well child care was firmly established as a part of primary care in the United States.

The content of well child visits has changed significantly since the days of clean milk and immunization fairs. Infectious diseases and premature birth are no longer the primary causes of morbidity and mortality in children; ill health related to environmental and social problems has become the "new morbidities" (2) of childhood and adolescence. Childhood obesity, diabetes, asthma, injuries, mental illness, and behavioral disorders may be devastating to children and have lifelong implications for children and their families, as affected children become adults whose potential contributions to society are impaired by chronic disease.

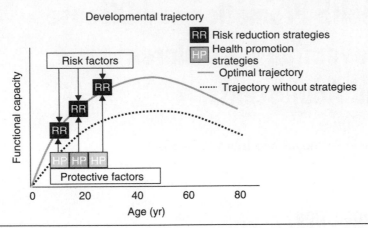

Figure 17.1 • Positive and negative influences on optimal human development. (From Halfon N, Hochstein M. Life course health development: an integrated framework for developing health, policy, and research. *Milbank Q* 2002;80(3):433–479, iii. Used with permission.)

Current notions about the important outcomes of child health care and supervision are evolving from the prevention of specific conditions to a broader view based on the concept of healthy developmental trajectories (3). This view holds that each child has an optimal developmental trajectory that is subject to both upward and downward pressure, so that small changes in the trajectory at an early age may result in very large differences in outcomes at a later age (see Fig. 17.1). What have traditionally been called risk factors *threaten* the child's health and development. Other factors can be identified that *promote* optimal health and development. The former should be identified and mitigated, and the latter should be identified and supported. Unfortunately, the preventive and protective factors that will turn out to be important for a specific child are often not known in advance.

Helping Families with Limited Resources

For disadvantaged families, paying for preventive health care may take a back seat to meeting other expenses. After early infancy, parents may dispense with preventive visits except to obtain required interventions such as the immunizations required for school attendance and mandatory sports or camp physicals. The negative effects of this situation can be mitigated if prevention is incorporated into every health care visit, no matter what the presenting complaint (see Chapter 20, page 527). These "opportunistic" discussions should focus on expressed parental concerns, issues noted on the physical examination, and the most common threats to the child's health at that age.

For exsample, a 3-year-old who is brought in for fever and rash but is noted to be very chubby will need to have the long-term problem of obesity addressed and may also benefit from brief discussion of prevention of the most common injuries in this age-group. Methods are being developed to help families keep up with well child care, such as patient-carried records, immunization registries, and automated reminders of services that are due (see Chapters 21 and 22). This chapter reviews the approach to the well child visit in children and adolescents in the order suggested by the "real-time" sequence of that visit: from taking the history through the physical examination and appropriate laboratory or other screening tests, to the provision of immunizations and the delivery of anticipatory guidance to the child and family. The end of the chapter gives special consideration to newborns and adolescent populations.

GENERAL CONSIDERATIONS

The optimal number and frequency of scheduled child health maintenance visits has not yet been fully determined. Many agencies, including state Medicaid programs and private insurance companies, mandate both the visit schedule and specific health interventions and screenings by age, and often link provider reimbursement to documentation of these services (see Chapter 23). More frequent visits are appropriate during periods of rapid growth and development, such as infancy and adolescence, than during the relative stability of middle childhood. However, it is important to carefully tailor both the schedule and the visit to the individual child and family and to avoid a one-size-fits-all approach. The evidence base is somewhat slim for much of what is routine in well child care. Discussion with families and patients regarding what we know and what we do not know about preventive health care in children, in the context of shared decision making, will be best when the balance of benefits and harms is either unknown or close (see discussion of "Shared Decision Making" in Chapter 4, pages 91–92).

CONTENT OF THE WELL CHILD VISIT

The well child visit is aimed at disease detection and prevention, along with health promotion and anticipatory guidance. The history and physical examination and selected screening tests are intended to detect existing conditions and risk factors for disease. Health promotion and anticipatory guidance are intended to prevent future illness and injury and to optimize development.

Pediatric History Taking

Every family arrives at the well child visit with an agenda—sometimes quite a long one. Determining what is on this agenda is essential to successfully engage both the patient and the family in the health supervision process. The concerns of the family can then be integrated with the clinician's agenda for health supervision so that a shared agenda guides the visit and so that both patient/family and clinician will be satisfied that the goals of the visit have been met.

Much like the taking of the history discussed in Chapter 2, the history taken during a well child visit is geared to discovering current problems and potential threats to the child's health, including inherited conditions, environmental risks, and psychosocial risks. As noted in Chapter 2, printed or online questionnaires, which can be completed before arriving for the visit or in the waiting room, are useful to obtain the new patient's medical history, family history, and social history as well as information about nutrition, diet, school performance, psychosocial adjustment, and health concerns. Examples of questionnaires designed for use with children are listed in the "Suggested Readings" at the end of this chapter.

A targeted pediatric history requires special attention to birth and perinatal history, childhood immunizations, developmental and school history, and a family history tailored to childhood-onset illnesses such as asthma, seizure disorders, learning disabilities, cardiovascular disease, hypertension, and diabetes. Clinicians using a "waiting room questionnaire" should be mindful of the literacy rates and relevant language or cultural barriers of their patient populations and should be prepared to review the questionnaire during the visit.

Some questionnaires (e.g., Vanderbilt Scale for attention deficit hyperactivity disorder; see "Suggested Readings" on page 459) have been developed to aid in screening for specific health risk behaviors, developmental status, and behavioral issues when they are identified as concerns during the course of the patient encounter. Others are considered a part of the standard assessment of a child and include lists of developmental "milestones" (such as the Modified Checklist for Autism in Toddlers [MCHAT] for autism screening, see page 458) and risk factors for tuberculosis (TB) exposure, environmental lead exposure, and the like. Alternatively, the interview with the family may be used by the clinician to evaluate these risks. The clinician should be alert for high-risk situations, such as the child's exposure to incarcerated persons (for which TB testing may be indicated), or substandard living conditions or diet, in which screening for lead toxicity or anemia, respectively, may be indicated.

The Physical Examination

The usefulness of a complete physical examination at each well child visit is not supported by evidence, but the examination may be expected by parents and can provide a good opportunity for discussion with parents about their child. Clinicians can reassure and teach the parents as they examine the child, generally assessing the overall state of the child's health and pace of development, and noting the interaction between the parent(s) and the child. For children beyond infancy, the physical examination can trigger a conversation about health issues with the child. Specific, formalized screening maneuvers as a part of the physical examination should be differentiated from surveillance. *Surveillance* is an ongoing process in which the clinician's conscientious, skilled observation permits detection of *obvious* abnormalities or concerns, whereas screening is a formal process applied to a patient in whom surveillance has not revealed a concern. Readers should consult a pediatric reference for detailed instructions on the nuances of physical examination in the infant and child; the discussion here focuses on only a few prevention-oriented aspects of the standard physical examination.

The focus of the routine physical examination in children varies with age, and it differs in important respects from the focus of the physical examination in adults. If the child presents with complaints, the examination should focus on these, but most infants and children have few or no physical complaints. Fair to good quality evidence is available for some aspects of the pediatric physical examination, which are discussed next. A comprehensive review of the evidence supporting these maneuvers, and the rationale for advising against other forms of screening, is beyond the scope of this chapter. The reader may consult the "Suggested Readings" for further discussion of the science supporting the physical examination.

GROWTH MEASUREMENTS

Growth is usually monitored at health maintenance visits. Weight, length, and head circumference (for children younger than 2 years and older children with developmental concerns) should be plotted on standardized gender-specific growth charts (http://www.cdc.gov/growthcharts). Growth since the last visit should be noted, and any deviations from expected growth investigated. It is well documented that measurements of height and weight are often inaccurate in office practice (4). If a clinician intends to monitor these parameters, they should be measured consistently in the following manner.

Before the second birthday, weight should be obtained with the child completely undressed, length should be measured with a reclining stadiometer, and head circumference should be measured with a nonelastic tape measure at the largest point. Taking three measurements and using the largest of the three is often advised. The toddler and older child should be weighed unclothed or in underwear only. Beginning at age 2 years, standing height rather than reclining length should be recorded, and it should be measured with the child standing firmly against a wall-mounted device that has a fixed right angle at the head. Special growth curves have been developed for children with common syndromes that affect growth, such as Down syndrome, achondroplasia and Turner syndrome, which are available from the American Academy of Pediatrics website (www.aap.org).

Body mass index (BMI) is calculated as (weight [in kilograms]) divided by (height [in meters]^2); measured in pounds and inches the formula is (weight [in pounds]) divided by (height [in inches]^2) multiplied by 703. An online calculator can be found at: http://www.cdc.gov/nccdphp/dnpa/bmi/calc-bmi.htm. Reference ranges for BMI change significantly as children grow; therefore obesity in children is defined by BMI percentile rather than by a single cutoff as it is in adults. Gender-specific BMI percentile growth charts are available for children starting at age 2 years, but the usefulness of this measure has not been confirmed in young children. BMI percentiles in young children are poor predictors of adult obesity, and data are lacking to demonstrate a benefit of monitoring BMI in young children. In children with obvious obesity, BMI percentile is a reasonable measure to follow the child's weight status. BMI percentile in adolescents is a better predictor of adult obesity, and BMI above the 85th percentile is also associated with insulin intolerance and other adverse health effects, making calculation and plotting of BMI in adolescents a more useful tool. A link from the calculator page provides the reference ranges for children: http://www.cdc.gov/nccdphp/dnpa/bmi/bmi-for-age.htm.

VITAL SIGNS

If vital signs are routinely obtained, age-based normal values such as those found in *The Harriet Lane Handbook* (see "Suggested Readings") should be used. Although evidence from trials is lacking, blood pressure screening has been recommended starting at age 3 years, as noted in Chapter 3. The clinician should measure blood pressure using a cuff of the appropriate size (see Chapter 3, Table 3.2), recalling that use of too small a cuff may result in a falsely elevated measurement. The clinician should also be careful to interpret blood pressure according to gender-, age-, and height-based norms (see Chapter 3, Table 3.3) (5).

OPHTHALMIC EXAMINATION

Funduscopy in children is difficult at best and rarely yields useful information in a child who has no visual complaints and normal visual acuity. In early infancy, the detection of symmetric red retinal reflexes may be useful in excluding retinoblastoma or congenital cataracts. To perform this test, the examiner should stand 2–3 ft from the patient and look through the direct ophthalmoscope with the largest white-light circle aimed at the face, then use the dial to focus on the face, illuminating both eyes simultaneously. With the infant looking at the light, the color of the red reflex (which may vary normally from yellow to orange or red) should be the same in both eyes. If the color is significantly different, or the reflex is absent in one eye, the infant should be referred to an ophthalmologist for further evaluation.

Young children should also be screened for amblyopia, strabismus, and defects in visual acuity. In infants and toddlers, the cover test and the Hirschberg light reflex test can be used to detect strabismus. To perform the cover test, the clinician should have the child look at an object 10 ft away (such as a colorful toy) and cover one of the child's eyes. Children may not cooperate with keeping one eye covered, in which case an eye patch can be taped over the eye. As the examiner covers the eye, he or she notes whether the uncovered eye moves in order to remain focused on the toy; this is repeated with the other eye. Movement of either eye suggests that the eyes are not aligned and requires referral. In the Hirschberg test, the examiner points a light source at the eyes and checks for an asymmetric light reflex. Convergent strabismus ("crossed eyes") may be seen in healthy infants until 6 months of age, but divergent strabismus is usually pathologic at any age.

Visual acuity screening in very young children typically requires specialized training and equipment. Visual acuity testing is often performed qualitatively during infancy by observing the patient's ability to fixate on a target and, by 3 months of age, to follow a moving object. By 6 months of age, the child should be able to grasp objects and recognize faces.

By age 3 years, most children can cooperate with office-based tests. Children who do not understand the instructions can sometimes participate if they are given a card with a large E and told to turn the card in the direction of the letter on the chart ("tumbling E" test). The "tumbling E" and similar tests, which are ideal for children aged 3–5 years, are performed with the child standing 10 ft from the chart and covering one eye. The child "reads" each line until reaching the line at which fewer than four of the symbols are identified correctly; the test is then repeated for the other eye. If the acuity is less than 20/40 in either eye *or* if there is a two-line difference between the eyes, the child should be referred for further evaluation

CARDIOVASCULAR EXAMINATION

Auscultation of the chest is often difficult in the child who is distressed by the examination and is crying. Therefore, it is useful to examine the chest when the child is quiet and to perform the chest examination before relatively more invasive examinations of the eyes, ears, and oropharynx. Familiarity with functional or innocent murmurs is important to avoid alarming the parents and to avoid an unnecessary workup for the child. Most children with significant congenital heart disease present with cyanosis or symptoms related to heart failure early in life. Identification of children with structural heart disease who are hemodynamically stable is still important from the standpoint of prophylaxis for endocarditis. Therefore, the clinician should be skilled in detecting valvular heart disease, including mitral valve prolapse, as well as septal defects.

GENITOURINARY EXAMINATION

Examination of the external genitalia is often omitted from well child visits due to concerns about invasion of privacy. This is a good example of an instance in which inclusion of the examination serves not only to detect abnormalities such as undescended testis or inguinal hernia, but also to offer an opportunity to discuss issues such as modesty, prevention of sexual molestation, and information about normal development. This discussion may be as important as the examination itself. It should be noted that most children who allege child sexual abuse have normal physical examinations without evidence of penetration.

SCOLIOSIS EXAMINATION

Screening for scoliosis (using a scoliometer or inclinometer, or using the forward bending test) by the clinician or in school-based screening is not recommended, as it results in overdetection of minor curvature or postural abnormalities. Most adolescents with mild scoliosis are not candidates for intervention as they approach the end of linear growth. An unclothed examination to rule out asymmetry (specifically of the scapulae or the iliac crests) is sufficient and is more important for the diagnosis of scoliosis in early to middle childhood. Plain spine films are not useful for the diagnosis of scoliosis.

Developmental And Behavioral Assessment

Developmental and behavioral assessment can begin in the waiting room with parent questionnaires, as discussed previously. Although developmental and language delay are important problems, and studies suggest that earlier intervention is likely to result in improved outcomes, formal screening has not been shown to result in improved outcomes. Clinicians are often not proficient in the use of formal instruments, and some commonly used screening tools, such as the Denver Developmental Screen II, have been shown to have very poor test performance (6). Validated tools include the Parents Evaluation of Developmental Status (PEDS) and Ages and Stages Questionnaire (ASQ) instruments (see "Suggested Readings"). Even under optimal circumstances, false-positive and false-negative results may occur. Parental concern is a sensitive indicator of developmental delay, so clinicians should be alert to issues raised by the parents, and their concerns should not be ignored or "brushed off" (7). Any concern about delay on the part of the parent or clinician should result in immediate referral for evaluation.

Speech delay is the single most common form of delay in children with otherwise normal development. In the past, some clinicians have falsely reassured parents who are concerned about delayed speech, calling such children "late bloomers." It is now clear that many children benefit from early referral for delayed speech milestones. Children with delayed language development may have either hearing loss or language delay, and both of these possible explanations should be investigated.

The apparent increase in the prevalence of autism concerns many parents and physicians. The two hallmarks of autism are impaired communication, for which speech delay may be the heralding sign, and impaired relationships, marked by a lack of "shared attention" with the parent or caretaker. If a child has deficiencies in speech acquisition or personal social skills, the primary care clinician may wish to use a screening instrument such as the MCHAT (see "Suggested Readings"), or may wish to immediately refer the child for further evaluation. Some experts recommend routine screening for autism, although the efficacy of this practice is not known.

Laboratory Screening

Laboratory screening tests that have been recommended during childhood include newborn metabolic screening and screening for anemia, lead poisoning, TB, lipid disorders, and urinary tract abnormalities. Newborn metabolic screening is discussed on page 450.

ANEMIA SCREENING

Screening during infancy for lead poisoning and anemia is mandated by many state Medicaid programs and is often recommended by other authorities. Although screening using venous blood samples is simple and straightforward for both conditions, what to do with the results is much less clear. The theoretic basis for screening for anemia or lead poisoning is the known adverse effects of elevated lead levels and of iron deficiency (even without anemia) on the developing brain. However, treatment of elevated lead levels (by abatement or chelation) has not been shown to improve developmental outcomes. Treatment of iron deficiency (the most common cause of anemia in childhood) improves hemoglobin levels but has not been shown to improve clinical outcomes. In both cases, it may be that treatment comes too late, and resources would be better spent on community-based efforts to prevent these conditions. All infants should receive an iron-rich diet, including iron fortified formula (if formula fed) and infant cereals. If screening for either lead poisoning or anemia is mandated, sampling by venipuncture is more accurate and less painful than sampling by fingerstick.

TUBERCULOSIS SCREENING

As noted in Chapter 4 (pages 117–118), TB skin testing is recommended only for children at high risk of exposure. Risk factors include recent immigration of the patient or household contacts from a country with a high prevalence of TB infection and exposure to a person with known infectious TB, to an adult with chronic cough and no other underlying diagnosis, to a person who has been incarcerated, to an injection drug user, or to a person with known immunosuppressive disease, especially human immunodeficiency virus (HIV) infection. Children with HIV infection must also be screened for TB. Testing should be performed using the Mantoux test, with interpretation of the skin test determined by local guidelines. See page 118 for further details on technique.

LIPID SCREENING

Cholesterol screening of the general pediatric population has been a subject of controversy, and recommendations vary widely. Currently the American Academy of Pediatrics, American Heart Association, and National Heart, Lung and Blood Institute do not recommend routine screening of well children without personal or family risk factors. Cholesterol screening (especially isolated cholesterol screening with no further lipid profile analysis) is sometimes done at health fairs. The discovery of elevated serum lipid levels is likely to result in anxiety for the parents, which is unnecessary unless there are comorbid disorders such as hypertension, obesity, or diabetes risk. In the context of the child's primary care setting, judicious evaluation may be warranted when children have a strong family history of cardiovascular disease, including cardiac death before age 55 years in first-degree relatives or relevant risk factors such as hypertension, obesity, or diabetes. There is little evidence that dietary change or the use of cholesterol-lowering drugs in childhood affect health outcomes during adulthood, or that these drugs are safe for long-term use in children. However, families with familial hyperlipidemia may represent a special case; hence the importance of an accurate family history. Normal lipid values for children differ from those for adults (see Table 17.1).

SCREENING URINALYSIS

Screening urinalysis has been recommended to detect asymptomatic bacteriuria, proteinuria, and glycosuria. However, there is little scientific rationale for screening for these conditions because their detection in the absence of symptoms may increase unnecessary investigation or therapy without evidence of improved outcomes.

TABLE 17.1 Classification of Serum Cholesterol Levels in High-Risk[a] Children and Adolescents

	Total Cholesterol (mg/dL)	LDL Cholesterol (mg/dL)
Acceptable	<170	<110
Borderline	170–199	110–129
High	≥200	≥130

Reproduced from the National Cholesterol Education Program. http://www.nhlbi.nih.gov/about/ncep/index.htm.
LDL = low-density lipoprotein.
[a]Children and adolescents from families with hypercholesterolemia or premature cardiovascular disease.

ANTICIPATORY GUIDANCE IN PEDIATRICS

Providing "anticipatory guidance" is a time-honored tradition in pediatric care. Many pediatric clinicians believe that their greatest contribution is in educating and guiding parents, especially first-time parents, with regard to their child's health. Rapid changes in a child's developmental status mean rapid changes in the most important threats to the child's health and safety. Therefore, specific counseling interventions change with the patient's age and individual circumstances. As the child gradually advances toward physical, cognitive, and emotional independence, the target of the counseling intervention will gradually shift from the parent(s) to the child and parent(s) together, and eventually to the patient alone in late adolescence.

For many specific counseling interventions, there is clear evidence that the recommended behavior change will lead to the desired outcome (e.g., wearing bicycle helmets decreases head injuries) but it is less clear that the clinician's advice has a causal role in changing the behavior. The clinician's advice is probably most effective when it is part of a multifaceted, community-based effort to change behavior.

Car Safety Seats

One of the most effective interventions in child safety has been the introduction and use of automobile safety seats. Until the infant is at least 1-year-old and weighs at least 20 lb, the car seat should face the back of the vehicle and preferably be placed in the back seat. It should never be placed on a seat within range of an airbag. Older children should wear seat belts in a booster seat, sized as appropriate, until they are approximately 8 years and 57 in. tall. Discussing child safety seats is a good opportunity to emphasize to parents the importance of wearing seat belts themselves, for their own benefit and to model good car safety behavior, to say nothing of complying with traffic safety laws. Table 17.2 provides one state's child car seat guidelines, but clinicians should familiarize themselves with applicable regulations in their state.

TABLE 17.2 General Guidelines for Child Car Seat Use

	Age/Weight	Seat Type/Seat Position	Usage Tips
Infants	Less than 1 yr and less than 20 lbs	Infant-only seat/rear-facing or (if child is at least 1 yr and at least 20 lbs) convertible seat/rear-facing *Seats should be secured to the vehicle by the safety belts or by the LATCH system*	a) Never use in a front seat where an air bag is present b) Tightly install child seat in rear seat, facing the rear c) Child seat should recline at approximately a 45 degree angle d) Harness straps/slots at or below shoulder level (lower set of slots for most convertible child safety seats) e) Harness straps snug on child; harness clip at armpit level
	Less than 1 yr/20–35 lbs	Convertible seat/rear-facing (select one recommended for heavier infants) *Seats should be secured to the vehicle by the safety belts or by the LATCH system*	1. Never use in a front seat where an air bag is present 2. Tightly install child seat in rear seat, facing the rear 3. Child seat should recline at approximately a 45 degree angle 4. Harness straps/slots at or below shoulder level (lower set of slots for most convertible child safety seats) 5. Harness straps snug on child; harness clip at armpit level

Preschoolers/ Toddler	1–4 yr/at least 20 lbs. to approximately 40 lbs.	Convertible seat/forward-facing **or** forward-facing only **or** high back booster/harness. **Seats should be secured to the vehicle by the safety belts or by the LATCH system.**	a. Tightly install child seat in rear seat, facing forward b. Harness straps/slots at or above child's shoulders (usually top set of slots for convertible child safety seats) c. Harness straps snug on child; harness clip at armpit level
Young Children	4 to at least 8 yr/unless they are 4'9" (57") tall.	Belt-positioning booster (no back) or high back belt-positioning booster. **NEVER use with lap-only belts—belt-positioning boosters are always used with lap AND shoulder belts.**	a. Booster used with adult lap and shoulder belt in rear seat. b. Shoulder belt should rest snugly across chest, rest on shoulder, and NEVER be placed under the arm or behind the back. c. Lap-belt should rest low, across the lap/upper thigh area—not across the stomach.

From the State of Indiana Government website http://www.in.gov/cji/traffic/occupant/images/CSSchart.pdf. Accessed 2007.

Injury Prevention

The leading fatal events in the home are poisonings, falls, fires and burns, and suffocation by an ingested object. Discussion by the clinician about the use of baby walkers, smoke alarms, safe water heater temperature, and the importance of keeping small objects away from young children who may choke on them may help reinforce what parents hear on such matters from public health campaigns. Parents who ride bicycles should be encouraged to use helmets for themselves (especially as it may be mandated by local law) and to insist that their children always wear helmets for activities such as bicycling, skateboarding, skating, and skiing. Use of helmets during these activities has been shown to reduce significant head injury by 88% (8).

Encouraging Literacy

Emerging evidence suggests that at the child health visit in late infancy through early childhood, physician-supported attention to early literacy through provision of books and encouragement of reading may be beneficial in achieving a measurable increase in vocabulary in early school years (9).

Dental Care

Every child should begin to receive oral health risk assessments by 6 months of age from a pediatrician or a qualified pediatric health care professional. Risk factors for caries include family history of caries (which may represent both genetic factors and the vertical transmission of cariogenic bacteria from caregivers), bottle-feeding, drinking juice, lack of an adequate fluoride source in the diet, and recent immigrant or low socioeconomic status. In general, clinicians should refer children for a "get acquainted visit" with a dental health professional at 1–2 years of age (usually a pediatric dentist, although some general dentists are comfortable with children older than 3 years).

Parents may clean the teeth of older infants and toddlers with a clean washcloth in plain water at the beginning of bath time. Adult toothpastes are not recommended for young children. Fluoride administration can help prevent caries but its risks include fluorosis or staining of the teeth from overzealous use of topical or dietary fluoride.

Exogenous fluoride supplementation should not be prescribed for infants younger than 6 months. Fluoride supplementation should be prescribed for older infants if the community water supply has inadequate fluoride content (10,11).

IMMUNIZATIONS

The eradication or near eradication of vaccine-preventable disease means that many 21st century clinicians will not see any cases of illnesses that were commonplace in the 20th century. Continued dedication to the provision of recommended immunizations is one of the hallmarks of primary care, not only for young children but also increasingly for adolescents and young adults. The recommended immunization schedule changes frequently as new immunizations and combination vaccines are developed. The reader is directed to Chapter 16 for a complete discussion of immunizations. "Best practice" for ensuring high vaccination rates entails review of the immunization record and a policy of "no missed vaccine opportunities" with regard to office visits for minor illness or injury (see page 360).

Some parents, not having seen firsthand the burden of illnesses such as polio, chickenpox, pertussis, and measles, may question the need or advisability of providing immunizations for their children. Of course, it is those very vaccines that have prevented the outbreaks that older clinicians can vividly remember. Helpful resources for patient and parent education about vaccines include websites such as that of the University of Pennsylvania Vaccine Education Center. This center provides vaccine information sheets that can be distributed in English and Spanish (see http://www.chop.edu/consumer/jsp/division/generic.jsp?id=75743). See also the resources and guidelines provided in Chapter 16.

SPECIAL POPULATIONS

Early infancy and adolescence are the times of greatest risk during childhood; perhaps this is why more evidence on evaluation and intervention has been developed for these age-groups than for the relatively quiet years in between.

The Newborn
HISTORY AND RISK ASSESSMENT

Evaluation of the newborn begins with a review of the child's prenatal course, including the mother's prenatal care, ultrasonography and laboratory screening results (if available), and perinatal events. Infants of adolescent mothers, mothers with a history of depression or substance abuse, and mothers with no prenatal care are at increased risk of neonatal problems and require closer follow-up.

PHYSICAL EXAMINATION

Two to 3% of children are born with congenital defects, some of which are not immediately obvious; furthermore, a newborn with one congenital abnormality is at increased risk of a second abnormality. The initial physical examination should be thorough, with particular attention to the most common and significant congenital abnormalities. A careful oral examination is required to detect submucous cleft palate, which may be associated with future respiratory and speech problems. A normal cardiac examination in the immediate newborn period does not rule out the presence of congenital heart disease, as the adaptation to extrauterine circulation continues for the first several weeks of life. An undescended testis increases the risk of both infertility and later testicular cancer. If the testis does not descend spontaneously in the first year of life, the infant should be referred for evaluation; bilateral undescended testes should be evaluated immediately.

Identification of developmental dysplasia of the hip (now known to not always be "congenital" but in some instances to first manifest itself in early infancy) remains important because this condition may result in lifelong difficulties with ambulation and in arthritis. However, the natural history of this disorder is poorly understood and evidence for the efficacy of screening examinations with the Ortolani or Barlow maneuvers or with ultrasonography is lacking. Spontaneous resolution occurs in the newborn period in most (60–80%) cases identified as abnormal or suspicious on physical examination and in greater than 90% of those cases so identified on ultrasonography. The common surgical and nonsurgical interventions are associated with a risk of avascular necrosis of the hip. Given the lack of evidence for routine screening, the best path may be attention to known risk factors for developmental dysplasia of the hip (such as female gender and breech positioning at birth) and careful follow-up of infants at risk (12).

Although extreme hyperbilirubinemia is very rare, and jaundice in the first 24 hours of life is always of concern, moderate jaundice is a common finding after the first 24 hours of life. Risk factors for extreme hyperbilirubinemia include gestational age below 37 weeks, blood group incompatibility, cephalohematoma, East Asian origins, a previous infant with severe hyperbilirubinemia, and exclusive breastfeeding, especially if breastfeeding has not gone well. Newborns should be assessed for jaundice and risk factors for developing jaundice before hospital discharge. If a serum bilirubin is obtained, a nomogram for interpreting the result based on age is available at: www.bilitool.org.

LABORATORY SCREENING

Newborn screening using dried blood spots on filter paper is mandated in all 50 states, and includes (at a minimum) screening for phenylketonuria and congenital hypothyroidism. Most states also require screening for sickle cell anemia and galactosemia. The evidence that screening for these conditions leads to improved outcomes is quite strong. The evidence in support of screening for cystic fibrosis or congenital adrenal hyperplasia is less strong, while the usefulness of dramatically expanded newborn screening panels made possible by tandem mass spectrometry has not yet been studied. Clinicians should have a thorough understanding of their state's screening policies and of systems for follow up of abnormal screens, and they should ensure that a normal screen has been reported within the first month.

Screening for congenital hearing loss is also mandated in most states and is provided in most hospitals before the newborn's discharge. The screening typically involves otoacoustic emission testing and/or auditory brainstem response. Such screening has led to earlier identification and intervention in children with congenital hearing loss, which is associated with improved language skills during childhood. The results of this test should be reviewed during the first month of life so that infants who are identified can be evaluated and intervention undertaken as early as possible.

ANTICIPATORY GUIDANCE

The initial in-hospital visit by the pediatric caregiver is a uniquely "teachable" moment for new parents. The clinician should be sure to admire the baby and help the parents understand the emotional roller coaster of new parenthood. The health benefits of breastfeeding, such as decreased rates of infant diarrhea and otitis media, are discussed in Chapter 7. As noted in that chapter, the clinician's support for breastfeeding, especially in concert with hospital programs, improves the rate and duration of breastfeeding.

The clinician should also emphasize the importance of supine sleep to decrease the risk of sudden infant death syndrome. Infants should be placed on their back for sleep in the first year of life. Parents should be warned that the side position is unstable and is therefore not recommended. Skull deformities resulting from prolonged supine positioning (positional plagiocephaly) are reported. However, this complication can be avoided by allowing the child plenty of "tummy time" when awake and by alternating to which side the child's head is positioned for sleep.

The clinician should discuss the importance of avoiding the child's exposure to cigarette smoke, which is associated with sudden infant death syndrome, otitis media, asthma, and other disorders. See Chapter 9 (page 248) for a further discussion of smoking by parents and passive exposure to "side-stream" environmental tobacco smoke. The clinician should also take the opportunity to begin counseling about the importance of using car safety seats for the first ride home from the hospital and every ride thereafter.

NEWBORN FOLLOW-UP

With the shortening of postpartum hospital stays, "early follow-up" visits are now routinely recommended to assess weight gain and breastfeeding and to detect neonatal jaundice and assess for physical signs suggestive of congenital cardiac or metabolic defects. It is recommended that these visits take place within 72 hours of discharge. The examination should include the following elements: infant weight, assessment of maternal/infant bonding, assessment of maternal lactation and infant feeding, and a targeted physical examination looking for ductal dependent congenital cardiac abnormalities, neonatal jaundice, evidence of normal hydration, and intact neuromuscular function. Newborns should be seen again at age 2 weeks to 1 month to assess weight gain, feeding, residual jaundice (which requires evaluation for cholestasis if it persists to the third week of age), the cardiac examination, and the general well-being of the infant and caretaker.

The Adolescent

Adolescent health maintenance deserves special discussion because risk reduction, health maintenance, and anticipatory guidance at this age are neither wholly in the domain of the child nor of the parent. Teenagers make the transition to adulthood at different rates, assuming increasing responsibility for their own health care but with their parents still involved to varying degrees. As teens mature, the encounter with the clinician (regardless of whether it was originally precipitated by an illness/injury or for health maintenance) must be structured to meet the needs of the patient primarily and the parent secondarily. This is a paradigm shift for many clinicians, and it can also be difficult for parents to accept. The issues most relevant to adolescent health maintenance revolve around physical and psychosocial maturation and health risk behaviors.

CONSENT AND CONFIDENTIALITY

For most health conditions, permission for treatment of an adolescent is given by the parent or legal guardian. However, with variations in minimum age, all states legally entitle adolescents to confidentiality and require their consent for treatment for "medically emancipated conditions" that may include contraception, pregnancy, diagnosis and treatment of sexually transmitted infections, HIV, or reportable diseases; substance abuse problems; and mental health issues. In addition, some adolescents may themselves be "emancipated" and therefore able to consent for most medical treatment: for example, when adolescents marry or join the armed forces before age 18 years (with parental consent and permission from the court), they become emancipated from their parents. In general, if adolescents can consent to treatment for a condition, they have a legal right to confidentiality about that treatment. The exception to these rules, in most states, is the matter of termination of pregnancy, which still requires parental notification or judicial permission for any minor, regardless of emancipated status. Chapter 12 (page 302) also discusses the potential for parents to learn inadvertently about visits through insurance billing.

Although parents must (legally) give permission for most treatments, adolescents who are capable of understanding can (and should) assent to any planned treatment. Certainly, coercing the adolescent to undergo testing (such as for drugs of abuse or pregnancy) or to accept treatment they object to is very likely to damage the relationship between the clinician and the patient. Clinicians should determine the limits of confidentiality based on the specific laws of their state and their own comfort level. State laws concerning confidentiality and consent may be found at: http://www.law.cornell.edu/topics/Table_Emancipation.htm.

As noted in Chapter 2, without the explicit reassurance of confidentiality, teens may not be willing to disclose important health concerns. Clinicians should reassure adolescent patients that what they tell the clinician will not be shared with anyone, including the patient's parents or guardians, without permission, with the sole exception being the determination of an immediate danger to someone's life. It may be helpful to parents to explain the need for confidentiality in terms of their child's appropriately increasing maturity and self-reliance.

THE ADOLESCENT HEALTH MAINTENANCE VISIT

Because adolescents often know little about their family's medical history and the parent's concerns do need to be addressed, the visit may begin with the parent present in the examination room. A family history of obesity, hypertension, diabetes, or cardiovascular disease may indicate a need to screen and then counsel the adolescent. The family's social situation and the current health status of siblings, parents, and grandparents will alert the clinician to concerns the adolescent may have but be unable to voice on his or her own. Once the family history has been obtained and the parents' concerns are heard, the remainder of the adolescent examination should be conducted without the parents in the examination room.

It bears repeating that the one-on-one interview should begin with an explicit assurance to the adolescent patient that the rest of the conversation is confidential. Taking a psychosocial history is facilitated by using the mnemonic "HEEADSSS," which stands for **H**ome, **E**ducation/employment, **E**ating, **A**ctivities, **D**rugs, **S**exuality, **S**uicide/depression, and **S**afety. Designed for both genders, it allows a clinician to rapidly assess a teen's psychosocial development and behavior, moving from less-sensitive areas, such as home environment, to more sensitive topics, such as suicidal feelings. Although this chapter discusses anticipatory guidance after the physical examination and laboratory screening, counseling can be woven into the visit by allowing the history and physical examination to provide an opening for discussion of particular issues. For example, questions about activities provide an opportunity to promote physical activity, and questions about sexual activity provide an opportunity to discuss the prevention of sexually transmitted infections.

Targeted screening for depression, cardiovascular risk, and sexually transmitted infections will be guided by the information gathered in the history. No one specific method of screening for depression has been proved to benefit adolescent mental health, but the clinician should be alert for signs of depression and for behavioral problems and drug use, which may be manifestations of adolescent depression. See Chapters 10 and 13 for further details about screening for substance abuse and depression, respectively.

PHYSICAL EXAMINATION

Few specific aspects of the adolescent physical examination have been empirically evaluated. However, simply performing a physical examination and being alert to the adolescent's demeanor during the examination may give the clinician insight into the patient's concerns and offer clues as to what areas to explore further. Adolescents are often anxious about whether their bodies are normal and about the pace of their development. The examination gives both the patient and the clinician an opening to discuss these sensitive topics. All adolescents should have growth parameters and blood pressure measured and compared to age-based norms at each visit (see Table 3.3 on page 55). Areas that may be particularly fruitful for discussion will include the mouth, the skin (even one pimple can make a teenager anxious), and the breasts, and genitalia. Formal screening by the clinician for scoliosis, breast cancer, or testicular cancer is not useful. As discussed in Chapter 14, there is also little evidence to support teaching breast or testicular self-examination.

THE "SPORTS PHYSICAL" AND OTHER PREPARTICIPATION EVALUATIONS

Adolescents may visit the clinician for preparticipation "physicals" for sports, camp, employment, or school (13). Although the usefulness of the "sports physical" has been debated, three purposes can be defined: identifying conditions that would make participation unsafe, screening for underlying illness, and identifying and ameliorating existing patterns of injury in the young athlete. The family history should include evaluation for premature cardiac death and inherited cardiac conditions such as prolonged QT or Marfan's syndrome. The patient should be asked about symptoms associated with exertion, including excessive breathlessness, fatigue, chest pain, lightheadedness, or syncope, and should be asked about prior injuries, particularly musculoskeletal injuries and concussion (whether from sports or other causes).

The physical examination should focus on the cardiovascular and musculoskeletal systems, and include documentation of blood pressure, cardiac examination (both supine and upright), inspection for stigmata of Marfan's syndrome, and examination of bones and joints for prior injury. The clinician should be alert for nutritional issues, including the use of supplements and the appearance of eating disorders, which are associated with weight-class sports (e.g., wrestling) and aesthetic sports (e.g., gymnastics). Highly conditioned female athletes may develop amenorrhea, especially if they have markedly decreased body fat. Although the young athlete may not be seeing the clinician for general health maintenance, the sports physical is a good opportunity to ask about and discuss smoking and drug use, because they relate directly to sports performance. As with adults (see Chapter 19), screening electrocardiograms or echocardiograms have not been shown to be useful in adolescent preparticipation evaluations, nor have any screening laboratory tests.

The so-called station examination is often hosted by a school or other party with a vested interest in obtaining a normal examination result. Parents should be advised to avoid having their children go through such events. The venue generally does not allow for confidential clinician–patient interaction or for a comprehensive, meaningful physical examination. Indeed, the sports physical may be the only reason that some adolescents ever visit the clinician. Although time may not permit a truly comprehensive patient evaluation during such a visit, the opportunity to build rapport and encourage the teen to return for regular care is valuable.

LABORATORY SCREENING

Diabetes Screening

As with adults, universal screening of children and adolescents for diabetes is not recommended (see page 94 and Chapter 19). However, children with *both* a family history of insulin resistance *and* physical evidence of obesity, acanthosis nigricans, or other risk factors may benefit from early screening by glucose tolerance testing. Simple random blood glucose measurement is not helpful.

Screening for Sexually Transmitted Infections

As discussed in Chapters 4 and 12, screening for sexually transmitted infections is recommended for all sexually active adolescents. In the past, complete pelvic examinations and cultures were recommended for the detection of disease, but now less invasive screening of asymptomatic young women may be accomplished with urine probes for chlamydia and gonococcal disease (see pages 108–109). The potential benefit of a pelvic examination and Pap smear in later adolescence and young adulthood may rest more in the teaching of good health habits and conveying the risk of unprotected intercourse as a precursor to cervical cancer, infections, and unwanted pregnancy. As noted in Chapter 4, the first Pap smear should take place within 3 years of sexual debut (see pages 104).

Human Immunodeficiency Virus Screening

Adolescents of both genders may benefit from HIV screening. See pages 98–99 in Chapter 4 for further details regarding the risk groups most likely to benefit. A decision to perform HIV screening should include a discussion with the teen that addresses the consequences of that diagnosis and a plan for follow-up medical care.

COUNSELING AND ANTICIPATORY GUIDANCE

Sexual Behavior

Although sexual abstinence and condom use decrease the risk of unwanted pregnancy and sexually transmitted infections (see Chapters 11 and 12), it is not clear whether clinician counseling is effective in helping to establish those habits and life skills. This counseling may be more important, more consistent, and more effective when provided in conjunction with messages delivered by school programs or by other community groups. Specific counseling to achieve sexual abstinence in adolescents has not been proved to prevent adolescent pregnancy. See Chapter 11 for details on how to counsel patients about contraceptive choices, such as Depo-Provera injections, use of emergency contraception, and sustained oral contraceptives.

Alcohol and Tobacco Screening

As discussed in Chapters 9 and 10, avoiding tobacco use and ethanol abuse early in life will reduce the risk of a wide host of diseases in later years. Physician counseling of young people appears to have a modest effect on tobacco cessation (14). Direct evidence of its effect on substance use is lacking. See Chapters 9 and 10, respectively, for detailed guidance on how to counsel patients about smoking and about alcohol and drug abuse.

Injury Prevention

Wearing safety belts has been clearly shown to reduce injury and death in motor vehicle accidents but it is not clear whether guidance from clinicians regarding this intervention helps promote this practice. Law enforcement and school and community efforts may be chiefly responsible for compliance when it occurs. Similarly, use of safety gear (e.g., helmets) when riding bicycles or motorcycles, skateboarding, and skiing reduces injury during accidents involving rapid deceleration. Clinician counseling for injury prevention is probably most effective when offered in combination with reinforcing messages from community and school-based health promotion programs.

Lastly, the absence (or locked storage) of firearms in the home prevents access to both guns and ammunition and is associated with lower risk of youth suicide, homicide, and unintentional shootings. It is not known whether brief counseling by clinicians is likely to influence handgun safety practices. Unless evidence emerges that doing so is counterproductive, it seems prudent for clinicians to continue to address gun safety in discussions with young people and their parents.

OFFICE AND CLINIC ORGANIZATION

The organization of the office in which children are seen should be somewhat different from that of the office where adults are seen exclusively. Separate waiting areas for sick children or even areas or procedures for caring for patients with known infections (chickenpox, etc.) may be useful in some practices. Age-appropriate reading material is important and conducive to literacy development in young children (9). Toys provided for a waiting area or examination room should be child safe and diminish hazardous play. Adolescents are most comfortable when either a section of the waiting room relates to their interests or they are promptly moved to an area not decorated and equipped for young children.

Some practices use the waiting room time and experience to foster anticipatory guidance, to deliver other useful health information with proprietary video or television programming for patients and parents, and to display health information and periodicals relevant to the patient population. For example, the pediatric waiting room might have brochure racks with information about newborn care, adolescent health concerns, immunizations, safety, and the like. As previously discussed, much information can be elicited before the initial child health maintenance visit through questionnaires that address both the general patient history and information targeted to the purpose of the visit if indicated.

Examination room furnishings should be equally safe and comfortable for children and should minimize potential for falls (e.g., rolling stools may be a hazard). Private areas to discuss such issues as adolescent sexuality, perinatal infections, and child abuse allegations are frequently needed. A separate supervised area for children to play while parents discuss issues with the clinician may be useful. The use of an office without an examination table or other medical equipment may be useful for the follow-up of children with behavioral or other concerns and may be less threatening once the medical examination has finished.

CONCLUSION

The "mantra" of caring for the pediatric population has always been that "the child is not a little adult." As well child health care continues to progress toward evidence-based interventions, the pediatric health care provider will remain pivotal as an advocate and participant, along with schools and community organizations, in improving the health of children. The clinician also plays a role in working with the community to develop those resources, advocating for change when evidence suggests it will better children's environment, and encouraging early childhood education for young children and support for their parents. Policy initiatives to promote health and prevent disease, combined with efforts by clinicians in their individual relationships with patients and their parents, offer the best opportunity for advancing the health of today's children and enhancing their well-being as tomorrow's adults.

RESOURCES—PATIENT EDUCATION MATERIALS

American Academy of Family Physicians
Health information for the whole family
http://familydoctor.org/online/famdocen/home/children.html. Accessed 2007.

American Academy of Pediatrics
Parenting corner
http://www.aap.org/parents.html. Accessed 2007.

Children's Physicians Network
Pediatric advisor (English and Spanish)
http://www.cpnonline.org/CRS/CRS/pa_index.htm. Accessed 2007.

Schmitt B. *Instructions for pediatrics patients*, 2nd ed. University of Colorado, Denver: WB
Saunders, 1998, English and Spanish.

SUGGESTED READINGS

Ages and Stages Questionnaire. One of several evidence-based developmental assessment
questionnaires available in English and Spanish in hard copy or on CD-ROM.
http://www.brookespublishing.com/store/books/bricker-asq/index.htm

Bright Futures Guidelines for Health Supervision for Infants, Children and Adolescents,
American Academy of Pediatrics in conjunction with the Maternal and Child Health
Bureau, 2002 (revision pending). A collection of materials (manuals and pocket guides)
including guidelines for health supervision visits for children of all ages and materials
regarding nutrition, physical activity and other patient and family instructional
material in English and Spanish.
http://brightfutures.aap.org/web/

Modified Checklist for Autism in Toddlers (MCHAT). Available at several websites
including: http://www.ddhealthinfo.org/documents/ASD_Best_Practice.pdf

Neinstein LS. *Adolescent health curriculum. Includes discussion of the HEEADSSS exam.*
http://www.usc.edu/student-affairs/Health_Center/adolhealth/info/intro.html

Parents Evaluation of Developmental Status. A computer-based or hard copy
questionnaire to evaluate parental concern about children's development.
http://www.pedstest.com/

Pediatric Symptom Checklist (PSQ). This waiting room questionnaire may be used as
an initial instrument for detecting problems outside the realm of normal childhood
behavioral and emotional disturbances, although care must be taken with any "broad"
screening tool to use it only as a screen prior to using other instruments such as depression inventories or prior to treatment or referral for depression. Available in the public domain at http://www.mgh.harvard.edu/allpsych/PediatricSymptomChecklist/
psc_home.htm. See Chapter 13 for further details about screening for depression.

Robertson J, Shilkofski N, eds. *The Harriet Lane handbook*, 17th ed. The Johns Hopkins
Hospital: Elsevier Science, 2005. Available for PDA as well as soft cover book.

U.S. Preventive Services Task Force. *Counseling About Proper Use of Motor Vehicle
Occupant Restraints and Avoidance of Alcohol Use While Driving: U.S. Preventive Services
Task Force Recommendation Statement.* August 2007. First published in *Ann Intern*

Med 2007;147:187–93. Agency for Healthcare Research and Quality, Rockville, MD. http://www.ahrq.gov/clinic/uspstf07/mvoi/mvoirs.htm.

Vanderbilt scale for ADHD. This questionnaire also includes subtests for screening for anxiety and oppositional behavior comorbid with ADHD. Available at the National Institute for Child Health Quality website: http://www.nichq.org/NICHQ/Topics/ChronicConditions/ADHD/Tools/screening.

References

1. Baker J. Women and the invention of well child care. *Pediatrics* 1994;94(4):527–531.
2. American Academy of Pediatrics Committee on Psychosocial Aspects of Child and Family Health. The pediatrician and the "new morbidity." *Pediatrics* 1993;92(5): 731–733.
3. Halfon N, Inkelas M, Hochstein M. The health development organization: an organizational approach to achieving child health development. *Milbank Q* 2000; 78(3):447–497.
4. Lipman TH, Hench KD, Benyi T, et al. A multicentre randomized controlled trial of an intervention to improve the accuracy of linear growth measurement. *Arch Dis Child* 2004;89(4):342–346.
5. National High Blood Pressure Education Program Working Group on Hypertension Control in Children and Adolescents. The fourth report on the diagnosis, evaluation, and treatment of high blood pressure in children and adolescents. *Pediatrics* 2004; 114(2 Suppl 4th Report):555–576.
6. Glascoe FP, Byrne K, Ashford LG, et al. Accuracy of the Denver-II in developmental screening. *Pediatrics* 1992;89(6 Pt 2):1221–1225.
7. Committee on Children with Disabilities, American Academy of Pediatrics. Developmental surveillance and screening of infants and young children. *Pediatrics* 2001;108(1):192–196.
8. American Academy of Pediatrics. Committee on Injury and Poison Prevention. Bicycle helmets. *Pediatrics* 2001;108(4):1030–1032.
9. Needlman R, Silverstein M. Pediatric interventions to support reading aloud: how good is the evidence? *J Dev Behav Pediatr* 2004;25(5):352–363.
10. American Academy of Pediatrics. Policy statement: oral health risk assessment timing and establishment of the dental home section on pediatric dentistry. *Pediatrics* 2003;111(5):1113–1116.
11. Lewis CW, Milgrom P. Fluoride. *Pediatr Rev* 2003;24:327–336.
12. Shipman SA, Helfand M, Moyer VA, et al. Screening for developmental dysplasia of the hip: a systematic literature review for the U.S. Preventive Services Task Force. *Pediatrics* 2006;117:e557–e576.
13. Smith DM, Kovan JR, Rich BSE, et al. *Preparticipation physical evaluation*, 2nd ed. Minneapolis: McGraw-Hill, 1997. Available from the AAP.
14. Grimshaw GM, Stanton A. Tobacco cessation interventions for young people. *Cochrane Database Syst Rev* 2006(4):CD003289.

CHAPTER 18

What to Do with Abnormal Screening Test Results

Alex H. Krist and Terence McCormally

INTRODUCTION

This chapter examines what clinicians should do when they find abnormal results arising from screening tests, as recorded in the history, physical examination, and laboratory procedures (see Chapters 2–4). The tests specifically considered in this chapter are those that identify lipid disorders, hypertension, abdominal aortic aneurysm, asymptomatic coronary artery disease, certain cancers (breast, colorectal, cervical, prostate, oral, testicular, and skin), diabetes, abnormal hearing, impaired vision, and latent tuberculosis (TB). Approaches to abnormal results for screening for sexually transmitted infections and for neonatal screening are discussed in Chapters 12 and Chapter 17, respectively. Topics not addressed in this book are the evaluation of abnormalities found through prenatal screening, nonrecommended screening interventions, tests used to evaluate specific patient complaints (e.g., thyroid-function studies to evaluate fatigue), and chronic disease monitoring.

This chapter presents the recommended steps for initiating appropriate management. The reader should consult the references and "Suggested Readings" at the end of this chapter for more detailed information. For the most part, the "Suggested Readings" contain or reflect formal guidelines produced by relevant national medical organizations. With medical advances over time, recommended workups will change and guidelines will be updated. By performing literature and Internet searches using the "Suggested Readings" as a starting point, the reader should be able to easily update outdated references (e.g., searching for a new hypertension guideline using "Joint National Committee AND hypertension").

A general limitation of recommendations concerning the evaluation and management of abnormalities detected by screening tests is that the supporting evidence for intervention may be less rigorous than the evidence justifying screening itself. Management recommendations often rely on expert opinion or only apply to select patient populations rather than being totally evidence based. This chapter compiles and combines recommendations from many sources. Diagnostic and evaluation algorithms presented here have been derived from key national guidelines and are accompanied by supporting references. The reader should consult the "Suggested Readings" to examine the supporting evidence and obtain a broader understanding of the nuances of the issues involved.

Screening tests do not necessarily lead directly to the alleviation of symptoms but instead are focused on the immediate goal of identifying patients at increased risk of disease, either for further testing to clarify the diagnosis or for identifying a modifiable risk factor that affects the probability of developing disease. For example, blood pressure screening is meant to identify hypertension, a risk factor for cardiovascular disease. Patients may not necessarily derive an immediate benefit from treating hypertension; they may not feel better with a lower blood pressure. For benefits to occur (i.e., a reduction in cardiovascular risks), treatments must be maintained and monitored for long periods. Most often, patient education and a long-term relationship centered on patient–clinician collaboration are essential to ensure that management of the condition identified by the screening test results in an improved health outcome.

Additionally, risk factors are interdependent. Interpretation of one test result and appropriate next steps may be influenced by the awareness of other coexisting risk factors (e.g., the appropriate goal for lipid lowering therapy depends on the patient's overall cardiovascular risk profile). Often, management must extend beyond dealing with the identified condition (e.g., in a hypertensive patient the priority is not only blood pressure control but also the control of other cardiovascular disease risk factors such as smoking, diet, physical inactivity, and serum lipid levels).

Although the results of some screening tests are binary—"positive" or "negative"—they do not necessarily determine whether the patient has or does not have the target condition. False positives often occur more frequently than true positives, for two reasons: First, screening tests are designed to "cast a wide net" to ensure that patients with the target condition are not missed (i.e., some tests have relatively high sensitivity, but low specificity). Second, the disease prevalence in asymptomatic populations is often low. For example, the positive predictive value of a positive fecal occult blood test (FOBT)—the chance that a patient with a positive test has colorectal cancer or a polyp—is only 10% (1) (90% of positive results are falsely positive). The intent of the FOBT is not to diagnose disease but rather to identify patients most likely to benefit from the more definitive but invasive test, colonoscopy. Likewise, a negative bimodal screening test rarely rules out the target condition; the FOBT test detects only about one-third of colorectal cancers or abnormal polyps.

Other types of screening tests measure continuous variables (e.g., blood pressure or prostate-specific antigen [PSA] concentration). For these conditions, the risk increases as the abnormal value changes, but not necessarily in a linear manner. A threshold or "cutoff" value is used to define "normal" and "abnormal." The cutoff value at which intervention is recommended is often selected arbitrarily, depending on epidemiologic information, the morbidity of the disease, the risks of further intervention, and the efficacy of the interventions contemplated. For example, a common definition of an abnormal PSA test is a value greater than 4 ng/mL. Patients with lower PSA values can also have prostate cancer, but the risk that they do is lower. The likelihood that a patient will have a positive biopsy for prostate cancer is 15% with a PSA value less than 4 ng/mL whereas the likelihood is 25% for values equal to or greater than 4 ng/mL (2). A slight change in a result that carries little biological significance may cross the threshold and make the difference in labeling the patient as having the target condition. For example, a blood pressure of 138/88 is normal but a slightly higher reading (e.g., 142/92) classifies the patient as being hypertensive.

Steps in Responding to an Abnormal Screening Result

Responses to an abnormal screening test result should include the following:

1. Verifying the accuracy of the result
2. Interpreting the result's significance in the context of the individual patient
3. Applying the result to the diagnostic criteria for the target condition
4. Developing a plan for assessment of other risk factors for the target condition
5. Setting treatment goals
6. Recommending a treatment plan
7. Implementing longitudinal follow-up and monitoring

Steps 1 and 2 may include repeating the test or looking for clinical factors that may influence the significance of the result. It may include verifying that the patient was fasting when the blood was drawn, had been following proper dietary restrictions, or had not been taking medications that might interfere with the test result. Step 3 emphasizes that an abnormality on screening is not tantamount to a diagnosis. Step 4 places the findings in the broader context of the patient's overall risks and other priorities. Steps 5 and 6 apply only if the results represent true disease or indicate that the patient is at greater risk of developing disease, and if there is evidence that treatment is beneficial. They also present an opportunity for patient education about risk reduction. Step 7 is often necessary regardless of whether the results are abnormal, although the frequency and method of follow-up depend on prior test findings. There are many barriers to reaching appropriate closure on normal and abnormal test results (see Table 18.1). The ability of screening to achieve its proven health benefits

TABLE 18.1 Barriers to Closure in Appropriately Responding to Screening Test Results

Results of Test Not Reviewed by Clinician
- Test recommended by clinician but not obtained by patient because of disinterest, resistance, or financial barriers
- Test obtained in another setting but results not forwarded to clinician
- Results filed in patient's chart without review by clinician

Knowledge Deficit
- Clinician unaware of guidelines, recommendations, or current literature
- Clinician unaware of other patient factors that influence patient's risk profile

Resistance to Diagnosis by Patient or Clinician (Clinical Inertia)

may ultimately be lost if these barriers are inadequately addressed and managed.

General Patient Education

Since an abnormal result on a screening test may for the first time label a previously well individual as ill, the clinician should address the patient's readiness to accept the label or recommended interventions. Ideally, much of the groundwork required to help patients understand abnormal screening test results should be accomplished before the performance of the test (pages 91–92). Ideally, patients should not be asked to undergo a test without understanding the implications of an abnormal result. In practice, however, it is quite common for patients to be subjected to testing without a full understanding of the downstream consequences. It is therefore necessary to educate the patient about the chances that an abnormal result is falsely positive, the diagnostic steps that will follow, initial treatments if the diagnosis is confirmed, and any prognostic implications. Even when clinicians attempt to provide this information before performing tests, patients may only partially grasp or retain the details. To assist patients and clinicians in managing these considerations, high quality, accessible patient education and motivation tools are essential. Recommended resources are listed at the end of this chapter (see "Resources—Patient Education Materials").

SCREENING TESTS FOR CARDIOVASCULAR RISK FACTORS

General Information

The modifiable risk factors for coronary artery disease—hypertension, hyperlipidemia, smoking, diabetes, and obesity—are both continuous and additive.

Identification of any risk factor for cardiovascular disease should prompt a search for the presence of other risk factors. This will allow for a more accurate estimation of the patient's total cardiovascular risk, the adoption of appropriate therapeutic targets, and a determination of the proper intensity of therapy for risk factor modification. The principal cardiovascular abnormalities considered here involve blood pressure, serum lipids, and metabolic syndrome. Screening for diabetes is covered on page 482. Chapters that discuss counseling about other cardiovascular risk factors include those on exercise, nutrition, obesity, and smoking (see Chapters 6–9).

An increased risk of cardiovascular disease is associated with other biochemical markers, including elevated C reactive protein, homocysteine, and uric acid levels. Using them as first-line tests for risk stratification is not very beneficial. However, these tests may have a role in determining therapeutic options for patients with borderline lipid values or for those with early cardiovascular disease but no identifiable risk factors (3).

Hypertension
ABNORMAL SCREENING TESTS

The seventh report of the Joint National Committee on Prevention, Detection, Evaluation, and Treatment of High Blood Pressure (JNC-VII) provides a succinct and authoritative guideline for clinicians managing hypertension. It classifies patients into four blood pressure categories: normal, prehypertension, stage I hypertension, and stage II hypertension (see Table 18.2). A patient's blood pressure reading is defined as the mean of two or more properly obtained seated blood pressure measurements obtained during a single office visit. Before a patient is categorized as having prehypertension or hypertension, the blood pressure should be measured during at least two office visits. See Chapter 3 (pages 53–57) for further details on measurement technique.

TABLE 18.2 Classification of Blood Pressure (JNC VII)

	Systolic BP (mm Hg)	Diastolic BP (mm Hg)
Normal	<120	<80
Prehypertension	120–139	80–89
Stage I hypertension	140–159	90–99
Stage II hypertension	>160	>100

BP = blood pressure.
(Adapted from Chobanian AV, Bakris GL, Black HR, et al. The seventh report of the Joint National Committee on Prevention, Detection, Evaluation, and Treatment of High Blood Pressure: the JNC 7 report. *JAMA* 2003;289:2560–2572.)

INITIAL DIAGNOSTIC STRATEGY

There are three components to the initial diagnostic evaluation of patients with elevated blood pressure:

1. Assessment for the presence of other cardiovascular risk factors
2. Screening for end-organ damage
3. Assessment of possible causes of secondary hypertension

As noted in the preceding text, all patients with elevated blood pressure should have an assessment for the presence of other cardiovascular risk factors. This includes asking the patient about diabetes, tobacco use, whether they have been told that they have an elevated serum cholesterol level, and whether a family history of premature heart disease (defined as onset before 45 years for male relatives or 55 years for female relatives) applies to any first-degree relative. The clinician should also measure the patient's body mass index (BMI), waist circumference, lipid profile, and fasting blood sugar. The JNC-VII guidelines recommend that all patients with stage I or II hypertension should have a basic assessment for end-organ damage before initiating therapy. This includes performing a12-lead electrocardiogram, a urinalysis, and determination of the creatinine level. For patients with protracted exposure to more severely elevated blood pressure, clinicians should consider performing other tests for assessing the presence of end-organ damage to the optic nerve, heart, lungs, kidneys, and carotid arteries.

All patients with stage I or II hypertension should have several additional tests that may prompt an evaluation for secondary hypertension or that may be important for monitoring adverse medication effects. These include measuring the serum potassium and calcium levels, and the hematocrit. A more extensive evaluation for secondary hypertension is unnecessary in most patients. However, it may be considered for patients with sudden onset of hypertension, an elevation of blood pressure with no apparent cause after being well controlled, or failure to achieve target blood pressures despite appropriate medication management. A secondary cause may also be suspected based on the patient's age, pertinent findings on the history or physical examination, the severity of hypertension, or initial laboratory findings. Table 18.3 outlines the causes of secondary hypertension and their potential diagnostic evaluations.

TREATMENT OPTIONS

The optimal management for patients with hypertension is outlined in Figure 18.1. The first step is to agree with the patient on a therapeutic blood pressure goal. Since most patients will achieve the target range for diastolic pressure when the systolic pressure is under control, the systolic blood pressure can serve as the primary target for control. An in-office blood pressure measurement of less than 140/90 is an appropriate goal

TABLE 18.3 Evaluation for Secondary Causes of Hypertension

Cause	Suggestive Findings	Evaluation
Renovascular disease	Onset before age 30 yrs or after age 55 yrs; abdominal bruit	Doppler flow study; magnetic resonance angiography
Chronic kidney disease	Risk factors for renal disease	Estimated glomerular filtration rate
Pheochromocytoma	Abrupt onset, episodic, episodes of flushing and headache	24-hr urinary metanephrine and normetanephrine concentration
Coarctation of aorta	Early onset, characteristic murmur	Computerized tomographic angiography
Sleep apnea	Obesity, history from sleep partner	Sleep study with monitoring of oxygen saturation
Cushing's syndrome	Obesity, striae, glucose intolerance	History, dexamethasone suppression test
Primary aldosteronism	Hypokalemia	24-hr aldosterone level
Drug or substance induced[a]	History of use	History, observation when not using substance
Thyroid or parathyroid disease	Tachycardia; skin, hair, or nail changes; anxiety; tremor	Thyroid stimulating hormone and serum parathyroid hormone levels

[a]Examples of suspect drugs include sympathomimetics (e.g., cocaine, amphetamines, ephedra), steroids, overuse of alcohol, licorice, tobacco, oral contraceptives, nonsteroidal anti-inflammatory drugs, erythropoetin, tacrolimus, and cyclosporine.
(Adapted from National Heart, Lung, and Blood Institute. *Complete report: the seventh report of the Joint National Committee of Prevention, Detection, Evaluation, and Treatment of High Blood Pressure.* National Heart, Lung, and Blood Institute. Available at: http://www.nhlbi .nih.gov/guidelines/hypertension/. Accessed February 2007.)

for most patients. For patients with diabetes or chronic kidney disease the target should be 130/80. Although self-measurement and automated 24-hour readings can provide valuable information regarding blood pressure control, ambulatory blood pressure readings tend to be lower than office measurements. Therefore, when relying on ambulatory readings, an average below 135/85 is an indicator of satisfactory control.

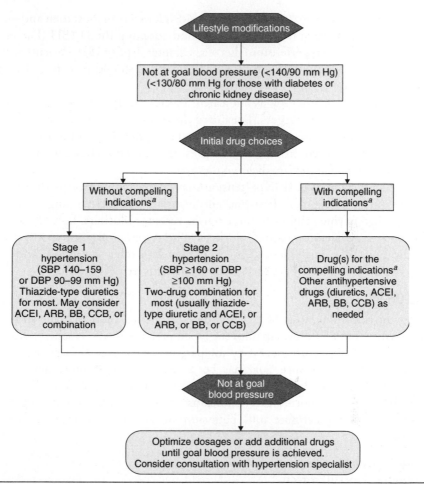

Figure 18.1 • Treatment algorithm for hypertension. ACEI, angiotensin converting enzyme inhibitor; ARB, angiotensin receptor blocker; BB, beta blocker; CCB, calcium channel blocker; DBP, diastolic blood pressure; SBP, systolic blood pressure.
[a]Compelling indications include heart failure, post-myocardial infarction, high risk of coronary artery disease, diabetes, chronic kidney disease, and recurrent stroke prevention. See Table 12 in the JNC-VII guidelines for further details.
(Reproduced with permission from National Heart, Lung, and Blood Institute. *Complete Report: the seventh report of the Joint National Committee of Prevention, Detection, Evaluation, and Treatment of High Blood Pressure*. National Heart, Lung, and Blood Institute. Available at: http://www.nhlbi.nih.gov/guidelines/hypertension/. Accessed February 2007.)

All patients with either prehypertension or hypertension should be counseled about hypertension-ameliorating lifestyle modifications, which include smoking cessation (see Chapter 9); normalizing weight to a BMI less than 25 kg/m^2 (see Chapter 8); increasing physical activity to 30 minutes a day of moderate exercise most days of the week (see Chapter 6); limiting alcohol consumption to a maximum of two drinks a day in most men and one drink a day in women (see Chapter 10); and adopting the DASH (Dietary Approach to Stop Hypertension) diet (see Chapter 7, page 182). Patients who have difficulty adopting dietary recommendations should be referred to a dietitian for medical nutrition therapy.

Pharmacologic therapy is indicated if lifestyle modifications do not achieve blood pressure targets. The initial therapy of choice for most patients is a thiazide diuretic. Many patients will need more than one antihypertensive agent to adequately control their blood pressure and should be advised of this possibility at the onset of medication therapy.

Patients with stage II hypertension may be started on two medications at the outset. Acceptable first-line antihypertensives include angiotensin-converting enzyme inhibitors, angiotensin-receptor blockers, beta blockers, diuretics, and calcium channel blockers. The selection of antihypertensive medications may be influenced by the presence of other conditions and by the medication side effects experienced by patients (see Figure 18.1).

FOLLOW-UP

After an initial diagnosis of elevated blood pressure, most patients should return for monthly follow-up until the blood pressure goal is reached. Often, more frequent visits are necessary for patients with stage II hypertension. After the blood pressure goal has been reached and stability achieved, follow-up visits should be provided on a 3- to 6-month schedule dictated by complicating comorbidities. Clinicians should consider monitoring the patient's serum creatinine and potassium levels at least once or twice per year.

Lipid Disorders
ABNORMAL SCREENING TESTS

The National Cholesterol Education Program-Adult Treatment Panel III (NCEP-ATPIII) established an evidence-based guideline for the detection, evaluation, and treatment of high blood cholesterol. For the purposes of the program, hypercholesterolemia is considered an elevated serum low-density lipoprotein (LDL) as defined in Table 18.4. A high-density lipoprotein (HDL) serum level of 35 mg/dL or less is a cardiovascular risk factor. An elevated serum triglyceride level (equal to or greater than 200 mg/dL) is a secondary risk factor. A total serum cholesterol level equal to or greater than 200 mg/dL is abnormal and, by itself, warrants follow-up measurements of the LDL, HDL, and triglyceride levels.

INITIAL DIAGNOSTIC STRATEGY

Risk of cardiovascular disease in the population appears to rise steadily with increasing cholesterol levels. Because the benefits of lipid management depend on a patient's overall risk for cardiovascular disease, no single "abnormal" lipid level applies to all patients. Instead, the threshold for initiating therapy depends on the presence or absence of other risk factors (see Table 18.4). For patients with intermediate serum lipid levels, it is recommended that the patient's 10-year risk of coronary artery disease be calculated, using an instrument that is based on data from the Framingham study. A point system and automated tools for making this calculation are described in Chapter 1 (pages 19–20).

A diagnostic evaluation for secondary dyslipidemia may be warranted for patients with hyperlipidemia at an early age, poorly controlled lipid levels despite proper medical management, or unexplained worsening of serum lipid levels after being well controlled for some period of time. Renal disease, diabetes, hypothyroidism, obstructive liver disease, or drug use (progestins, corticosteroids, or anabolic steroids) cause secondary dyslipidemia.

INITIAL MANAGEMENT STRATEGY

Management options for hyperlipidemia include therapeutic lifestyle modifications (diet and exercise) and medications. Few patients can achieve a LDL of less than 100 mg/dL without drug therapy. Therefore, simultaneous initiation of lifestyle modification and drug therapy is appropriate for patients at high risk. For other patients, a 6-month trial of lifestyle changes alone, including dietary counseling, may be warranted. Medical nutrition counseling provided by a dietitian or nutritionist may be more effective than written patient education materials or physician counseling. For most patients, drug therapy is initiated with a single statin. Combination therapy with a second lipid-lowering agent may be necessary for some patients.

FOLLOW-UP

For patients attempting lifestyle modification for hyperlipidemia, serum lipid levels should be rechecked in 3 to 6 months. A shorter interval to assess success with lifestyle modifications may assist some patients with improving their diet and exercise habits. Once a patient starts using a lipid-lowering agent, serum cholesterol should be rechecked in 4 to 6 weeks, allowing the regimen time to achieve its full effect. Once the serum cholesterol target level has been reached, it is reasonable to monitor lipid levels and liver function every 6 months.

Metabolic Syndrome
DIAGNOSTIC STRATEGY

A constellation of cardiovascular risk factors, none of which independently meets the criteria for a specific diagnosis, is termed *metabolic syndrome*. The presence of at least three of the risk factors listed in Table 18.5 qualifies for the diagnosis of metabolic syndrome.

TABLE 18.4 Treatment Targets for Low-Density Lipoprotein (LDL) Level

Risk Category	LDL Goal (mg/dL)	LDL Level to Initiate Lifestyle Modifications[d]	LDL Level to Initiate Drug Therapy
CHD; CHD equivalent;[a] 10 yr Framingham risk[b] ≥20%	<100 (for high-risk patients, optional[e] goal of LDL <70)	100	130 (optional[e] for 100–129)
2+ risk factors[c] and Framingham risk <20%	<130	130	130 if 10-yr risk >10% 160 if 10-yr risk <10%
0–1 risk factor	<160	160	190 (optional[e] for 160–189)

CHD = Coronary heart disease.

[a]CHD equivalents include diabetes and other vascular diseases.

[b]See pages 19–20 for details on calculating Framingham risk.

[c]Risk factors include smoking, hypertension, HDL cholesterol less than 40 mg/dL, older than 45 years for men or 55 years for women, a family history of heart disease in a first degree relative with onset earlier than 55 years in a man or 65 years in a woman. An HDL cholesterol greater than 60 mg/dL is a "negative risk factor": 1 point should be subtracted from the risk factor count.

[d]Therapeutic lifestyle changes include smoking cessation, weight reduction, a low-fat, low cholesterol diet, increased physical exercise and inclusion of plant stanols and viscous fiber in the diet (see Chapters 6–8 for further details about exercise, diet, and weight management).

[e]The designation of "optional" targets allows for the inclusion of patient values in goal setting.

(As recommended by: National Cholesterol Education Program. *Detection, evaluation, and treatment of high blood cholesterol in adults [Adult Treatment Panel III].* Adapted from: http://www.nhlbi.nih.gov/guidelines/cholesterol/atp3_rpt.htm. Last reviewed January 2006.)

TABLE 18.5 Diagnostic Criteria for Metabolic Syndrome[a]

Waist circumference	>102 cm in men; >88 cm in women
Fasting triglyceride	>150 mg/dL
HDL cholesterol	<40 mg/dL in men; <50 mg/dL in women
Fasting blood sugar	>100 mg/dL
Blood pressure	>130/85 mm Hg

[a]Having any three criteria is diagnostic for metabolic syndrome.
(As recommended by: National Cholesterol Education Program. *Detection, evaluation, and treatment of high blood cholesterol in adults [Adult Treatment Panel III].* Adapted from: http://www.nhlbi.nih.gov/guidelines/cholesterol/atp3_rpt.htm. Last reviewed January 2006.)

MANAGEMENT STRATEGY

Whether metabolic syndrome qualifies as a distinct clinical entity is currently in dispute. Therefore, therapy for metabolic syndrome is directed at the individual risk factors and begins with therapeutic lifestyle changes.

Abdominal Aortic Aneurysm
ABNORMAL SCREENING TESTS

Follow-up is indicated if an ultrasound measurement of the abdominal aorta reveals a diameter of greater than 3 cm.

DIAGNOSTIC STRATEGY

Aneurysms between 3 and 4.5 cm do not require immediate intervention but do require repeated measurement at defined intervals (see Table 18.6). Depending on a patient's overall health status, an aneurysm equal to or greater than 4.5 cm warrants referral to a vascular specialist for a likely aortogram and consideration of surgical options. Decisions regarding further imaging and endovascular versus open repair depend on clinical circumstances and on local resources and expertise.

INITIAL MANAGEMENT RECOMMENDATIONS

Cessation of smoking and control of blood pressure are important to prevent progression of an aortic aneurysm. Beta-blocker therapy may be particularly useful in this regard. If follow-up screening demonstrates rapid dilatation (e.g., greater than 0.5 cm within 6 months) referral to a vascular specialist is warranted even if the aneurysm has not reached 4.5 cm in diameter. Aortic aneurysms identified in women and nonsmokers require similar management, although, as noted on page 119, screening is not routinely recommended in these populations.

TABLE 18.6 Approach to Results of Aortic Aneurysm Screening

Size	Recommended Follow-up
<3 cm	No further testing
3–4 cm	Annual ultrasonography
4–4.5 cm	Ultrasonography every 6 mo
>4.5 cm or rapid dilation[a]	Referral to vascular specialist

[a]Dilatation of more than 0.5 cm within 6 months or 1.0 cm in 1 year.
(Adapted from Kent KC, Zwolak RM, Jaff MR, et al. Screening for abdominal aortic aneurysm: a consensus statement. *J Vasc Surg* 2004;39(1):267–269.)

FOLLOW-UP

See Table 18.6

Tests for Asymptomatic Coronary Artery Disease

Tests to detect asymptomatic coronary artery disease—for example, resting electrocardiography, exercise stress testing, and electron beam coronary artery calcium scoring—are available but are not recommended for asymptomatic average risk populations (see Chapter 19). Nonetheless, the clinician will frequently encounter patients who present with abnormalities found on one or more of these tests, and further follow-up with more invasive testing may be necessary. Exercise stress testing, stress echocardiography, myocardial perfusion scintigraphy, or cardiac catheterization can clarify the presence of significant disease. Treatment and follow-up should be dictated by the presence of significant clinical findings. Consultation with a cardiologist is frequently necessary.

SCREENING SUGGESTIVE OF NEOPLASIA

General Information

Clinicians can encounter a range of findings from cancer screening tests that include negative results, the presence of an abnormal finding that *suggests* the possibility of malignancy (e.g., positive FOBT), or a result that is diagnostic of cancer (e.g., a biopsy report indicating invasive carcinoma). In a patient diagnosed with cancer, coordination among numerous health professionals may be necessary in both the evaluation of abnormal cancer screening test results and the delivery of the indicated medical care. The potential team includes medical specialists (e.g., surgeons, pulmonologists, gynecologists, gastroenterologists, urologists, medical oncologists, and radiation oncologists), pain specialists, dieticians, home care staff, social service workers, and counseling and support groups. The patient struggling with cancer evaluation or treatment may be overwhelmed by and tends to focus solely on that problem. The primary care clinician should also address the other aspects of primary care, including other preventive services, and is responsible for the long-term care of cancer survivors (4).

Breast Cancer
ABNORMAL SCREENING TESTS

On the clinical breast examination, abnormal findings that could indicate the presence of breast cancer include palpable masses, lymphadenopathy, skin dimpling, nipple retraction or discharge, or rashes such as *peau d'orange* (see Figure 3.2 on page 71). Potential abnormal findings on a mammogram include calcification, cystic masses, and solid masses.

DIAGNOSTIC STRATEGY

The evaluation of a palpable breast mass depends upon the patient's age, the history of the lesion, and characteristics of the lesion on examination. Further diagnostic tests that can be undertaken include imaging (ultrasonography or mammography) and obtaining a tissue sample (fine needle aspiration, core needle biopsy, or incisional or excisional surgical biopsy). Figure 18.2 depicts one useful diagnostic algorithm. Since mammography fails to detect 10% of breast cancers, tissue diagnosis of a palpable mass should be pursued even if a mammogram is normal.

Abnormalities detected on screening mammography may warrant additional mammographic images, ultrasonographic examination, or magnetic resonance imaging. Some abnormal findings require tissue diagnosis, as outlined in the preceding text for palpable masses. Interpreting the radiographic criteria that define abnormalities on a mammogram is beyond the purview of primary care clinicians and is not discussed here. Since mammograms have a poor positive predictive value, patients should be counseled that an abnormal mammogram usually does not mean that breast cancer is present. In community settings, only 4–20% of abnormal mammograms are indicative of breast cancer.

Women who are identified as having breast cancer on the basis of tissue diagnosis will need a staging evaluation to determine the next appropriate treatment steps. This evaluation includes a comprehensive history and physical examination, chest radiography, liver function tests, and the measurement of serum tumor markers.

TREATMENT OPTIONS

Noncancerous breast lesions may not require further treatment. Treatment for localized lobular and ductal breast carcinomas entails some combination of surgical excision, lymph node dissection, radiation, and hormonal therapy

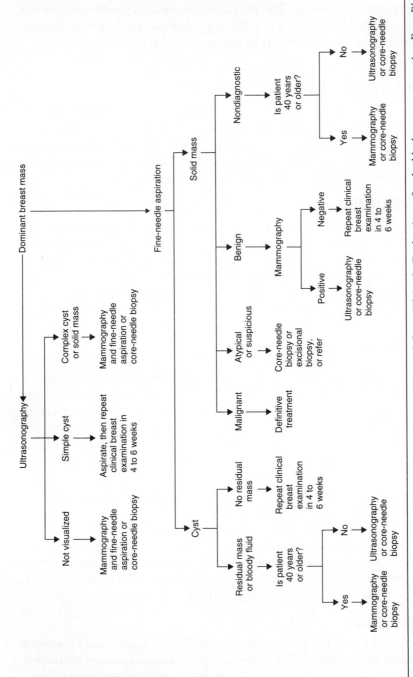

Figure 18.2 • Evaluation of a palpable breast mass. (Adapted from Klein S. Evaluation of palpable breast masses. *Am Fam Physician* 2005;71:1731–1738.)

(e.g., tamoxifen). Radiation therapy and chemotherapy may also be beneficial for women with more extensive breast cancers. For many women, either breast conserving therapy (lumpectomy and radiation therapy) or a modified radical mastectomy may be equally appropriate. Less aggressive therapy may be warranted for *in situ* breast disease but this is an area of ongoing controversy.

FOLLOW-UP
See Figure 18.2

Colorectal Cancer
ABNORMAL SCREENING TESTS
A range of potential abnormal findings from colorectal cancer screening includes a positive FOBT, a radiographic abnormality on barium enema, a polyp (hyperplastic, adenomatous, or villous) detected by endoscopy, or cancer detected by endoscopy.

DIAGNOSTIC STRATEGY
Positive Fecal Occult Blood Test
All patients who have a positive screening FOBT should have a colonoscopy to rule out a malignancy (see also Chapter 4). Repeating the FOBT or performing sigmoidoscopy or barium enema are inappropriate responses to a positive FOBT.

Abnormal Radiographic Finding on Double Contrast Barium Enema
The presence of a suspicious radiographic abnormality usually indicates that direct visualization by colonosocopy is necessary.

Polyp Detection
All colonic polyps detected by endoscopy should be completely removed and sent for pathologic evaluation. Individuals with an adenomatous or villous polyp that is taken on sigmoidoscopic biopsy should have a subsequent colonoscopy to rule out the presence of proximal lesions.

Mass Detection
Individuals with colorectal masses should have a partial or complete surgical biopsy for pathologic evaluation to rule out malignancy. Patients diagnosed with a malignancy will need a further evaluation for staging. This evaluation may include surgical resection for determination of the depth and extent of lesion penetration, blood work (complete blood count, liver function tests, and carcinoembryonic antigen), and imaging studies (abdominal/pelvic computerized tomography and chest radiography).

TREATMENT OPTIONS

Central to the treatment and diagnosis of colorectal lesions is their complete removal when possible. Polyps can be removed at the time of endoscopy through resection and fulguration. Masses and larger polyps may require *en bloc* surgical resection. Malignancies, depending on their stage, may also be treated with radiation or adjuvant chemotherapy.

FOLLOW-UP

Although 80% of colorectal cancers arise from adenomatous polyps, an adenomatous polyp of less than 1 cm in diameter has less than 1% chance of progressing to cancer in 10 years. An adenomatous polyp greater than 1 cm has a 10% chance of becoming malignant in the same period. Hyperplastic polyps, which are normal variants, are not precancerous, nor do they portend an increased risk for precancerous polyps or cancer elsewhere in the colon. On the basis of the principles outlined in the preceding text, the American Cancer Society and a consortium of gastroenterological organizations have issued recommendations on when to repeat a colonoscopy following abnormal endoscopy findings (Table 18.7) (5,6). Individuals with normal screening tests or hyperplastic polyps can be retested using any of the recommended colorectal cancer screening tests at the same intervals recommended for low-risk individuals (see Chapter 4, pages 110–115).

TABLE 18.7 Recommended Follow-up Intervals After Colonoscopy

Colonoscopy Findings	Repeat Screening Interval
Normal colonoscopy	10 yr
Hyperplastic polyps	10 yr
1–2 small (<1 cm) tubular adenoma(s)	5–10 yr
3–10 adenomas, any adenoma >1 cm, or high grade dysplasia	3 yr
>10 adenomas on one examination	<3 yr
Adenomas that are removed piecemeal	2–6 mo
Family history of colon cancer[a]	5 yr

[a]Defined as a first degree relative diagnosed before the age of 60 years or two first degree relatives diagnosed at any age.
(Adapted from: Winawer SJ, Zauber AG, Fletcher RH, et al. Guidelines for colonoscopy surveillance after polypectomy: a consensus update by the US Multi-Society Task Force on Colorectal Cancer and the American Cancer Society. *CA Cancer J Clin* 2006;56:143–159. [Quiz 184–185.])

It is common to find polyps during an endoscopy; they are present in 25% of persons by age 50 years and in 50% by age 75 years. Accordingly, an essential role of the primary care clinician is to ensure that patients receive the appropriate follow-up after abnormal findings. Repeating colonoscopy too infrequently may create an opportunity for invasive cancer to progress, but repeating the colonoscopy too frequently may subject patients to unnecessary risks.

Cervical Cancer
ABNORMAL SCREENING TESTS

Red or white lesions found on cervical inspection raise concerns about the presence of either cervical atypia or cancer. Pap smear abnormalities include reactive and inflammatory changes (variants of normal); squamous cell abnormalities such as atypical cells of unknown significance (ASCUS); low-grade squamous intraepithelial lesions (LGSIL); high-grade squamous intraepithelial lesions (HGSIL); and glandular abnormalities such as atypical glandular cells of unknown significance (AGCUS).

DIAGNOSTIC STRATEGY

Cervical lesions seen on inspection should be biopsied, even if the Pap smear is normal. Screening for human papilloma virus (HPV) infection is not recommended as an initial screening test for cervical cancer as HPV may be transiently present in the absence of current or even future cervical pathology, particularly in younger women. However, in patients with ASCUS or LGSIL, HPV status may help determine whether a patient should undergo colposcopy or early repeat Pap testing. Diagnostic steps for evaluating squamous abnormalities (ASCUS, LGSIL, and HGSIL) found by a Pap smear heighten in Figure 18.3. Glandular abnormalities (e.g., ASCUS) found on Pap smear heighten concern for malignancy and require endometrial sampling, colposcopy, and endocervical sampling.

TREATMENT OPTIONS

Treatment of cervical cancer and precancerous lesions varies depending on the patient's risk of progression. The considerations vary, for example, for patients with human immunodeficiency virus (HIV) infection or immunosuppression, for adolescents or postmenopausal women, and for women who are currently pregnant or interested in becoming pregnant in the future. Treatment options for low-risk individuals are presented in Figure 18.3. High-risk individuals require more aggressive treatments.

FOLLOW UP

See Figure 18.3.

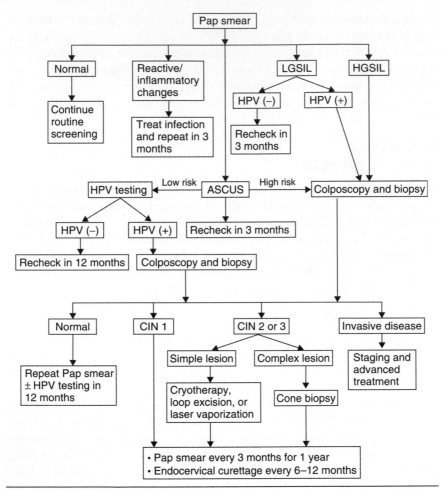

Figure 18.3 • Evaluation of an abnormal Pap smear. HPV, human papilloma virus; LGSIL, low grade squamous intraepithelial lesion; HGSIL, high grade squamous intraepithelial lesion; ASCUS, atypical squamous cells of unknown significance; CIN, cervical intraepithelial neoplasia. (Adapted from Wright TC Jr, Cox JT, Massad LS, et al. 2001 consensus guidelines for the management of women with cervical intraepithelial neoplasia. *Am J Obstet Gynecol* 2003;189:295–304 and Saslow D, Runowicz CD, Solomon D, et al. American Cancer Society guideline for the early detection of cervical neoplasia and cancer. *CA Cancer J Clin* 2002;52(6):342–362.)

Prostate Cancer
ABNORMAL SCREENING TESTS

A prostate nodule palpable on digital rectal examination and a PSA value of 4 ng/mL or greater are considered abnormal. A PSA velocity, or rate of increase, greater than 0.7–1.0 ng/mL/year is also considered abnormal.

DIAGNOSTIC STRATEGY

The evaluation of a prostate mass includes measuring the PSA level and considering a prostate biopsy. The evaluation of an abnormal PSA value can include (a) observation (doing nothing immediately), (b) measuring the free-to-total PSA ratio, (c) rechecking the PSA in 3–6 months, or (d) performing a prostate biopsy. The most appropriate diagnostic step should be determined jointly between a patient and clinician. The clinician should use a shared or informed decision-making process (see pages 91–92) to review the false-positive rate of PSA screening and the downstream implications of the workup, and to gauge how aggressively the patient wishes to evaluate the abnormal results.

Considerations influencing next steps include, but are not limited to, patient preferences and beliefs (e.g., beliefs about the benefits of early treatment, beliefs about the harms of treatment, and comfort with uncertainty), the likelihood that the elevated value could represent another condition (e.g., benign prostatic hypertrophy), and the patient's overall health and life expectancy. More aggressive diagnostic steps (such as prostate biopsy) may be warranted for patients who are at increased risk of prostate cancer (e.g., marked elevation in PSA concentration, suspicious symptoms, a family history of prostate cancer, or African American race), men with a relatively long life expectancy (and therefore at greater risk of developing complications from prostate cancer) and patients who are particularly concerned that they might have prostate cancer (and are willing to tolerate the risks associated with diagnosis and treatment of prostate cancer).

For patients at lower risk of experiencing complications from prostate cancer, or for those with greater apprehensions about unnecessary diagnostic or therapeutic procedures, a more cautious approach is indicated. For example, the clinician might initially measure the free-to-total PSA ratio and, if it is normal, recheck the PSA level in 3 to 6 months. This less aggressive approach is supported by evidence that men with prostate cancer who defer treatment demonstrate no increase in mortality from prostate cancer for 8–15 years (7). A 6- to 12-month observation period to assess the persistence of a PSA elevation over time appears reasonable.

TREATMENT OPTIONS

Treatments for prostate cancer are dictated by the Gleason score assigned to the biopsy specimen (the score is a rating of cell pathology based on histologic characteristics, ranging from 2–10, with higher scores assigned to more aggressive cancers), whether the cancer has expanded beyond the prostatic capsule, the age of the patient, and the patient's personal preferences. For cancers confined to the prostate, treatment options include watchful waiting, implantation of radioactive seeds, external beam radiation, or prostatectomy. More aggressive treatments have greater risks of side effects such as incontinence or impotence. Radiation, chemotherapy, and/or antitestosterone therapy may be indicated for cancers that have extended beyond the prostatic capsule.

FOLLOW-UP

Men with PSA abnormalities should have their PSA rechecked every 3–6 months until the value has normalized, an alternative diagnosis is established (e.g., benign prostate hypertrophy), or a determination is made to proceed further with diagnostic evaluation(s). Similarly, men treated for prostate cancer should have their PSA rechecked every 3–6 months for 1–2 years. Beyond that time, it is sufficient to recheck the PSA annually.

Oral Cancer
ABNORMAL SCREENING TESTS

Abnormal findings indicating concern for oral cancer include suspicious visible lesions on physical examination, a palpable oral mass, or head and neck lymphadenopathy.

DIAGNOSTIC STRATEGY

Diagnostic evaluations include oral exfoliative cytology, toluidine blue/ tolonium chloride mucosal staining, fine needle aspiration, or biopsy.

TREATMENT OPTIONS

If cancer is detected, treatment options include surgical resection, potentially accompanied by neck dissection, radiation therapy, or chemotherapy. The specifics of treatment vary depending on the extent and location of involvement as well as the specific type of cancer.

FOLLOW-UP

Clinical monitoring through reexamination and imaging studies are potentially indicated on a periodic basis after treatment.

Testicular Cancer
ABNORMAL SCREENING TESTS

Palpable scrotal masses are all potentially abnormal.

DIAGNOSTIC STRATEGY

A thorough history and physical examination should be performed to rule out common benign scrotal masses including varicoceles, spermatoceles, hydroceles, and hernias. Masses that are irregular, nontender, and fixed to the testes and that do not transilluminate are more suggestive of testicular cancer. An ultrasonographic examination should be performed on suspicious lesions followed by tissue sampling for cytopathology (through fine needle aspiration or incisional/excisional biopsy). Imaging (chest radiography and chest/abdominal/pelvic computed tomography) and measurement of serum tumor markers (β-human chorionic gonadotropin and α-fetoprotein) can be performed for further diagnostic clarification and staging.

TREATMENT OPTIONS

Treatment options include radical or partial orchiectomy, retroperitoneal lymph node resection, radiation, and chemotherapy.

FOLLOW-UP

Follow-up tests include monitoring the concentration of serum tumor markers and chest, abdominal, and pelvic computed tomography.

Skin Cancer
ABNORMAL SCREENING TESTS

Skin lesions that change in size, shape, or color as well as lesions that hurt, itch, or bleed for protracted periods are possibly indicative of skin cancer. Characteristics of pigmented lesions that are worrisome for melanoma can be recalled using the "A-B-C-D-E" mnemonic: (A) asymmetry, (B) (irregular) borders, (C) (irregular or multiple) colors, (D) diameter (equal to or greater than 6 mm), or (E) (recent) elevation (of a flat mole) (see Figure 3.7).

DIAGNOSTIC STRATEGY

Expert clinicians can frequently establish the diagnosis of basal or squamous cell skin cancer by examination alone. If the diagnosis is uncertain, a biopsy is indicated. Any lesion that raises even a slight suspicion of melanoma requires a full thickness biopsy. Shave biopsy or procedures that result in tissue destruction such as cryotherapy are contraindicated for lesions that are suspicious for melanoma. Full thickness skin biopsy is essential to ascertain the depth of penetration, which in turn determines both the correct treatment regimen and the prognosis.

TREATMENT OPTIONS

Nonmelanomatous skin cancers can be treated by excision, cryotherapy, topical chemotherapy, curettage and electrodesiccation, or laser vaporization. Melanomatous skin cancers require a 1–5 cm wide re-excision, sentinel node biopsy (or lymph node dissection), and potentially chemotherapy.

FOLLOW-UP

The American Cancer Society recommends that patients with a history of melanoma perform weekly skin self-examinations, undergo total skin examinations by a clinician every 3–6 months, and obtain a yearly chest radiograph. Liver enzymes, chemistry panels, and chest/abdominal/pelvic computed tomography may also be indicated for some patients.

SCREENING RESULTS SUGGESTIVE OF ENDOCRINE AND METABOLIC DISORDERS

Diabetes

ABNORMAL SCREENING TEST

A fasting blood glucose level of 100 mg/dL or greater, or a random plasma glucose level of 200 mg/dL or greater are considered abnormal.

DIAGNOSTIC STRATEGY

In the symptomatic patient, in the absence of factors causing transient hyperglycemia (such as use of steroids or the presence of a critical illness), a single random plasma glucose level of 200 mg/dL or more is diagnostic for diabetes. For such patients, no further workup is required to establish the diagnosis. Asymptomatic patients with an elevated fasting blood glucose level should have a second fasting measurement before a diagnosis is made. Fasting glucose measurements of 100–125 mg/dL are consistent with *prediabetes* whereas a fasting glucose level of 126 mg/dL or more is consistent with *diabetes*. Clinicians should review the patient's history and age as well as consider evaluating for ketosis and measuring the C-peptide and insulin levels to differentiate type 1 from type 2 diabetes. Typically type 1 can be differentiated from type 2 diabetes based on age and history alone. Further tests are necessary to evaluate the severity of hyperglycemia (e.g., glycosylated hemoglobin) and to assess the possible presence of comorbid conditions (e.g., hypercholesterolemia, hypertension).

TREATMENT OPTIONS

Long-term management of diabetes requires a package of interventions. The cornerstone is lifestyle modification: the adoption of a "diabetic diet" and engaging in a program of regular exercise (see Chapters 6 and 7). Medications such as oral hypoglycemic agents and insulin can assist with maintaining glucose within the target range (fasting glucose level of 130 mg/dL or less and glycosylated hemoglobin level of 7% or less). The pneumococcal and influenza vaccine should also be administered (see pages 393 and 405). Most importantly, comorbid cardiovascular disorders should be aggressively controlled. Tight control of blood pressure (less than 135/85 mm Hg) and lipids (LDL less than 100 mg/dL) produces even greater reductions in overall mortality than does optimal glycemic control (8).

FOLLOW-UP

Diabetes is a chronic condition that requires careful longitudinal follow-up to help patients minimize both macrovascular and microvascular complications. Long-term management is complex and difficult for patients (Table 18.8). It

TABLE 18.8   Follow-up of Patients with Diabetes

Follow-up Test	Monitoring Frequency	Goal
A. Monitoring Glucose Control		
Review glucometer readings	Every 3 mo	Fasting glucose <130 mg/dL
Check for hypoglycemia	Every 3 mo	No hypoglycemic episodes
Glycosylated hemoglobin	Every 3–6 mo	Glycosylated hemoglobin <7%
Medication review	Every 3 mo	Taking medications as prescribed
B. Monitoring Lifestyle Behaviors		
Weight measurement	Every 3 mo	Body mass index <25 lb/in^2
Review food plan	Every 3 mo	• Five servings vegetables and fruits per day • Limiting simple sugars and fats
Review exercise regimen	Every 3 mo	Aerobic activity most days of the week
Re-evaluate smoking status	Every 3 mo	Not smoking
C. Monitoring for Diabetic Complications		
Review history	Every 3 mo	No complaints
General examination, including neurological evaluation	Every 12 mo	No macrovascular or microvascular disease, including neuropathy
Measure microalbumen	Every 12 mo	Normal renal function
Dilated funduscopic eye examination	Every 12 mo	No diabetic retinopathy
Complete foot examination	Every 12 mo	Normal sensation with no skin breakdown or infection
D. Monitoring Cardiovascular Comorbidities		
Blood pressure measurement	Every 3 mo	<135/85 mm Hg
Lipid measurement	Every 12 mo	LDL <100 mg/dL and HDL >35 mg/dL

(Adapted from: American Diabetes Association. Standards of medical care in diabetes—2006. *Diabetes Care* 2006;29(Suppl 1):S4–S42.)

extends beyond glycemic control and includes management of cardiovascular comorbid disorders, lifestyle reassessment and counseling, and monitoring for diabetic complications. A team-based approach utilizing dieticians, exercise physiologists, and nurse educators can provide patients with the necessary tools to control their diabetes. Ophthalmologists, neurologists, nephrologists, cardiologists, podiatrists, and endocrinologists often play important roles in monitoring and managing the potential complications of the disease.

Osteoporosis
ABNORMAL SCREENING TESTS

Decreased bone mineral density noted on radiographs taken for other reasons is an insensitive but specific predictor for osteoporosis and likewise deserves further evaluation. Decreased bone mineral density as measured by dual-energy x-ray absorptiometry (DEXA) scans or ultrasonography is also considered abnormal and can be diagnostic for osteoporosis. Patients who sustain a "fragility fracture," defined as a fracture occurring with less intense trauma than the equivalent of falling from a standing position (e.g., a spontaneous vertebral fracture) also deserve evaluation for osteoporosis.

DIAGNOSTIC STRATEGY

Osteoporosis can be diagnosed with the DEXA scan's T-score, a measure of the standard deviation of a patient's bone mineral density compared to the peak bone density of a gender and ethnically matched young adult. A T-score between −2.5 and −1.0 standard deviations is diagnostic for *osteopenia*, whereas a T-score less than −2.5 standard deviations is diagnostic for *osteoporosis*. A T-score decrease of 1.0 standard deviation correlates with a decrease in bone mineral density of 10–12% and an increased fracture risk of 1.5. Further laboratory evaluation may be necessary for patients younger than 60 years found to have low bone mineral density after a fragility fracture and to rule out conditions other than postmenopausal or senile osteoporosis. These tests may include parathyroid hormone, thyroid-stimulating hormone, cortisol level, serum calcium, and phosphorous levels.

TREATMENT OPTIONS

Treatment for osteopenia includes supplementation with vitamin D (400–800 IU daily) and calcium (1,500 mg/daily) and weight-bearing activity. Treatment for osteoporosis includes these measures but can also include pharmacotherapy with bisphosphonates, calcitonin, selective estrogen receptor binders, or bone metabolism modulators. While these medications have demonstrated benefit for some women, they can also incur significant risks and costs. Clinicians should engage patients in a shared decision-making process (see pages 91–92) to select the most appropriate treatment regimen.

The patient's overall risk for an osteoporotic fracture and the potential risks from the medication as well as the patient's values and beliefs should all be taken into consideration.

FOLLOW-UP

Follow-up should include periodic reassessment of the bone mineral density. Because bone turnover and new deposition are slow processes and the precision of the DEXA scan is relatively low, there is no benefit to measuring bone density more frequently than every 3 years.

SCREENING RESULTS SUGGESTIVE OF HEARING AND VISION DISORDERS

Impaired Hearing
ABNORMAL SCREENING TESTS

The clinician should initiate an evaluation when a patient or family member of a patient reports any concerns with the patient's hearing. An evaluation could also be considered if a patient fails a whispered voice test. Follow-up is also required when newborns fail hearing screening tests such as otoacoustic emissions testing.

DIAGNOSTIC STRATEGY

Clinicians should perform a physical examination to rule out reversible causes of hearing loss such as middle ear effusion or cerumen impaction. Comprehensive audiometry can ascertain if a hearing loss is conductive or sensorineural and can test for acoustic reflexes and speech discrimination. For a progressive sensorineural hearing loss with no obvious cause, investigation for diabetes, thyroid disease, or other metabolic problems may be in order. Imaging of the posterior fossa and internal auditory canal may also be warranted. The severity of hearing loss can be categorized as in Table 18.9.

TREATMENT OPTIONS

Correction of underlying metabolic problems is essential, as is treatment of conditions such as otosclerosis, Meniere's disease, or acoustic neuroma. Neurosurgical or otolaryngological consultation is often needed. For patients with stable deficits, amplification with hearing aids is often useful.

FOLLOW-UP

Because hearing loss tends to increase with age, the clinician should be attentive to signs of social withdrawal or other signs that may be indicative of increased hearing difficulty.

TABLE 18.9 Categorization of Hearing Loss

Hearing Threshold	Category	Implications
0–20 db	Normal hearing	
20–40 db	Mild hearing loss	Trouble hearing soft speech or filtering out background noise; increased work of listening
40–60 db	Moderate hearing loss	Difficulty hearing conversational speech
60–80 db	Severe hearing loss	Marked difficulty with conversational speech
>80 db	Profound hearing loss	Clinically deaf

(Adapted from: American Speech, Language, Hearing Association. *Type, Degree, and Configuration of Hearing Loss*. Website available at: http://www.asha.org/public/hearing/disorders/types.htm. Accessed 2007.)

Impaired Visual Acuity
ABNORMAL SCREENING TESTS

Chapter 17 discusses vision disorders that affect children, such as amblyopia and strabismus. Visual difficulties at any age, particularly those impacting daily activities and quality of life, may warrant further evaluation. Symptoms can include decreased reported visual acuity, limitations in central or peripheral vision, and diminished contrast sensitivity (the visual ability to see objects that may not be outlined clearly or that do not stand out from their background). Individuals with diminished visual acuity detected on a Snellen eye chart examination warrant further evaluation.

Visual acuity is categorized as follows:

- Normal vision: 20/10 to 20/25
- Near normal vision: 20/25 to 20/60
- Moderate visual impairment: 20/70 to 20/160
- Severe visual impairment: 20/200 to 20/400

The U.S. Social Security Administration defines legal blindness as remaining vision of 20/200 or worse in the better eye after best correction OR contraction of the peripheral visual field in the better eye to 10 degrees or less (9).

DIAGNOSTC STRATEGY

The diagnostic evaluation of visual impairment in the elderly can be complicated. Multiple conditions affect vision, including refractive errors, cataracts, glaucoma, macular degeneration, and diabetic retinopathy, and these conditions may coexist simultaneously. When patients are identified with visual difficulties in the primary care setting, the most effective next step for most patients is referral to an eye care specialist (optometrist or ophthalmologist). Diagnostic evaluation generally includes a vision-specific history and physical examination (including external examination and central and peripheral fundus examination), visual acuity testing (distance and near), refraction, ocular motility and binocular vision assessment, visual field evaluation, tonometry, and evaluation of contrast sensitivity.

TREATMENT OPTIONS

The diagnosis dictates the treatment. Treatments include the following:

- Correction of refractive errors using glasses or contact lenses
- Use of magnifiers for decreased near visual acuity
- Medications to reduce ocular hypertension
- Surgical treatments for glaucoma, macular degeneration, and cataracts

Patients with decreased nighttime vision may need to be advised to alter their driving patterns; those with severe visual deficits may need to discontinue driving. Counseling patients and their family members to maintain well-lit and uncluttered living areas may prevent falls and subsequent injuries.

FOLLOW-UP

The underlying diagnosis determines the appropriate follow-up interval.

Tuberculosis
ABNORMAL SCREENING TESTS

Test results that prompt concern for TB include an abnormal tuberculosis skin test (TST) or an abnormal chest radiograph suggesting active or latent TB infection. Another potential finding is a positive score on a questionnaire, such as that developed by the Centers for Disease Control and Prevention for identifying high-risk children (see Table 18.10) (10). If a positive score is found, the next step is application of a TST.

DIAGNOSTIC STRATEGY

A TST should be ordered if the questionnaire result is positive, or if a chest radiograph presents suspicious findings. The TST is read by determining the number of millimeters of induration (not erythema) in the transverse diameter perpendicular to the long axis of the arm at the site of application. Whether the diameter is abnormal depends on the risk category of the person being tested (see Table 18.11). Although prior immunization with Bacillus Calmette-Guérin (BCG) can cause a false-positive TST result, this effect wanes over a few years. For practical purposes, BCG administration more

TABLE 18.10 New York City Department of Health Tuberculosis Screening Questionnaire (adapted)

1. Has the child been in contact with a person with known tuberculosis?
2. Does the child have HIV infection?
3. Was the child born in or has the child traveled to areas where tuberculosis is endemic in Latin America, the Caribbean, Africa, or Asia?
4. Does the child have regular contact with an adult at high risk for tuberculosis such as a HIV infected person, an incarcerated person, a homeless person, or a user of illicit drugs?

If any of the above is true, a tuberculosis skin test should be administered.

HIV = human immunodeficiency virus.
The questionnaire has a sensitivity of 85.2% and a specificity of 86%, with a positive predictive value of 32.5% and a negative predictive value of 99.8%.

than 1 year before the TST has no bearing on the interpretation of the TST result.

As noted in Chapter 4 (page 118), individuals subjected to serial TSTs (e.g., health care workers, long-term care facility residents) are at risk of a "booster phenomenon," which could falsely suggest a recent conversion. A booster phenomenon occurs when the first TST result is negative in an individual with latent tuberculosis infection, but the TST itself stimulates immunologic memory cells. When the TST is next administered, it appears positive. As a result, all individuals undergoing serial TSTs should have an initial two-step TST. If the initial TST result is negative, the test should be repeated in 1–2 weeks. If the test is still negative, the person can be considered truly negative. If this second-step test is positive, the positive TST result represents remote infection and not a new conversion.

TREATMENT OPTIONS

If an asymptomatic patient has a positive TST result, including a positive test in the second step of a two-step TST, an evaluation to determine appropriateness for drug therapy should begin with a chest radiograph. If the chest radiograph is suggestive of TB, or if the patient has symptoms consistent with TB, the clinician should consider further evaluation with sputum cultures and possibly consultation with an infectious disease or pulmonary specialist for consideration of bronchoscopy.

Asymptomatic patients who have a normal chest radiograph but a positive TST result are candidates for therapy with isoniazid (INH) to decrease the risk of progression to active TB. While in the past INH therapy was withheld from those older than 35 years because of concerns about

TABLE 18.11   Threshold for Positive Tuberculosis Screening Test Given the Patient's Risk Status

Risk Status	Criteria for Abnormal Tuberculosis Skin Test
Household or close contact of an active case, HIV infection, or clinical suspicion of tuberculosis including abnormal chest radiography	>5 mm induration
Foreign born persons from high prevalence countries; medically undeserved, low income populations including high risk ethnic minorities; injection drug users; the homeless; residents and employees of nursing homes, group homes or correctional institutions; persons with medical conditions associated with a higher risk of tuberculosis, such as long term use of steroids or immunosupressants	>10 mm induration
All others	>15 mm induration

HIV = human immunodeficiency virus.
(Adapted from: Centers for Disease Control and Prevention. *Tuberculin skin testing*. *National Center for HIV, STD, and TB Prevention*. Available at: http://www.cdc.gov/nchstp/tb/pubs/tbfactsheets/250140.htm. Accessed February 2007.)

hepatotoxicity, the 2003 management guidelines recommend treatment of any patient with a documented positive TST result regardless of age (11). INH should be administered at a dose of 300 mg/day for adults and 10–15 mg/kg/day for children (not to exceed 300 mg a day) for 9 months, along with pyridoxine 10–50 mg/day to prevent neuropathy. Patients should be advised to avoid regular alcohol consumption. They should be assessed monthly for symptoms and signs of hepatotoxicity and for medication adherence. Routine laboratory monitoring is not recommended, except in patients at increased risk of hepatitis. Special considerations apply to pregnant or recently pregnant women, persons whose exposure was from a patient with INH-resistant TB, or patients at risk of poor medication adherence. Consideration should be given to twice weekly, directly observed therapy, supervised by the local health department, for patients who are at high risk to progress to active TB or who are unlikely to adhere to therapy without direct observation.

FOLLOW-UP

Once a person has had a positive TST result, there is little to gain from a repeated TST and there is a potential risk of skin necrosis. Patients who successfully complete a course of INH therapy still face some, albeit reduced, risk of progression to active TB and should therefore contact the clinician if they develop prolonged cough, fever, night sweats, or weight loss. Interpretation of TST results may be difficult in patients who require serial testing either because of their living situation, employment, or travel history.

OFFICE AND CLINIC ORGANIZATION

As noted in Chapter 4, practices should establish reminder and referral systems to identify patients overdue for follow-up tests and to ensure that the clinician receives test results, that patients return for repeat visits and testing at recommended intervals, and that patients with positive results receive appropriate follow-up and treatment. For patients screened for infectious diseases, reminder systems should also ensure that infected patients receive appropriate antibiotic therapy; that potential contacts of infected patients are notified, tested, and treated according to guidelines; and that the public health department is notified of reportable cases. Patient education materials, such as those listed in the subsequent text, should be available to help patients learn more about these disorders and related diagnostic tests and treatments and to facilitate shared decision making.

CONCLUSION

The clinician's ability to respond appropriately to the results of abnormal screening tests ultimately determines the value of a screening program. Clinicians who deliver preventive care must understand not only the evaluation of abnormal results but also the range of therapeutic options. By definition, the process of screening involves an asymptomatic patient. Any potential future health benefit must be weighed against the assured expense, inconvenience, anxiety, and risk of the workup prompted by an abnormal screening test. Particularly when the potential benefits are small or unproven, it is essential to elicit and include the patient's values in making both screening and evaluation recommendations.

Clinicians should expect that the guidelines for appropriate evaluation of an abnormal screening test will continually evolve as diagnostic tests improve and treatment options expand. Clinicians delivering preventive care must remain vigilant for changes in screening, evaluation, and treatment recommendations for a broad range of clinical topics.

RESOURCES—PATIENT EDUCATION MATERIALS

Hypertension

American Academy of Family Physicians
High blood pressure: things you can do to help lower yours
http://familydoctor.org/092.xml

American Heart Association
High blood pressure
http://www.americanheart.org/presenter.jhtml?identifier=2114

National Heart, Lung, and Blood Institute
High blood pressure
http://www.nhlbi.nih.gov/health/dci/Diseases/Hbp/HBP_WhatIs.html

Lipids

American Academy of Family Physicians
Cholesterol: what your levels mean
http://familydoctor.org/029.xml

American Academy of Family Physicians
Cholesterol lowering medications
http://familydoctor.org/801.xml

American Heart Association
Cholesterol
http://www.americanheart.org/presenter.jhtml?identifier=1516

National Heart, Lung, and Blood Institute
High blood cholesterol
http://www.nhlbi.nih.gov/health/dci/Diseases/Hbc/HBC_WhatIs.html

Metabolic Syndrome

American Academy of Family Physicians
Metabolic syndrome
http://familydoctor.org/826.xml

Abdominal Aortic Aneurysm

American Heart Association
Aneurysm, aortic
http://www.americanheart.org/presenter.jhtml?identifier=4455

Coronary Artery Disease

American Heart Association
Atherosclerosis
http://www.americanheart.org/presenter.jhtml?identifier=4440

National Heart, Lung, and Blood Institute
Coronary artery disease
http://www.nhlbi.nih.gov/health/dci/Diseases/Cad/CAD_WhatIs.html

Breast Cancer

American Cancer Society
Learn about breast cancer
http://www.cancer.org/docroot/lrn/lrn_0.asp

National Cancer Institute
What you need to know about breast cancer
http://www.cancer.gov/cancertopics/wyntk/breast

Colorectal Cancer

American Cancer Society
Learn about colon and rectum cancer
http://www.cancer.org/docroot/lrn/lrn_0.asp

National Cancer Institute
What you need to know about cancer of the colon and rectum
http://www.cancer.gov/cancertopics/wyntk/colon-and-rectum

Cervical Cancer

American Cancer Society
Learn about cervical cancer
http://www.cancer.org/docroot/lrn/lrn_0.asp

National Cancer Institute
What you need to know about cancer of the cervix
http://www.cancer.gov/cancertopics/wyntk/cervix

Prostate Cancer

American Cancer Society
Learn about prostate cancer
http://www.cancer.org/docroot/lrn/lrn_0.asp

National Cancer Institute
What you need to know about prostate cancer
http://www.cancer.gov/cancertopics/wyntk/prostate

Oral Cancer

American Cancer Society
Learn abut oral cavity and oropharyngeal cancer
http://www.cancer.org/docroot/lrn/lrn_0.asp

National Cancer Institute
What you need to know about oral cancer
http://www.cancer.gov/cancertopics/wyntk/oral

Testicular Cancer

American Cancer Society
Learn about testicular cancer
http://www.cancer.org/docroot/lrn/lrn_0.asp

National Cancer Institute
Testicular cancer: questions and answers
http://www.cancer.gov/cancertopics/factsheet/Sites-Types/testicular

Skin Cancer

National Cancer Institute
What you need to know about skin cancer
http://www.cancer.gov/cancertopics/wyntk/skin

Diabetes Mellitus

American Academy of Family Physicians
Diabetes
http://familydoctor.org/x3092.xml

American Diabetes Association
All about diabetes
http://www.diabetes.org/about-diabetes.jsp

Osteoporosis

American Academy of Family Physicians
Osteoporosis in women: keeping your bones healthy and strong
http://familydoctor.org/136.xml

National Osteoporosis Foundation
Medications to prevent and treat osteoporosis
http://www.nof.org/patientinfo/medications.htm

Impaired Hearing

American Speech-Language-Hearing Association
Hearing loss
http://www.asha.org/public/hearing/disorders/default.htm

NIH Senior Health
Hearing loss
http://nihseniorhealth.gov/hearingloss/toc.html

Impaired Visual Acuity

American Optometric Association
Eye Health Topics
http://www.aoa.org/

NIH Senior Health
Low vision
http://nihseniorhealth.gov/lowvision/toc.html

Tuberculosis

American Academy of Family Physicians
Tuberculosis: treatment of tuberculosis infection
http://familydoctor.org/120.xml

SUGGESTED READINGS

Hypertension

Chobanian AV, Bakris GL, Black HR, et al. The seventh report of the Joint National Committee on Prevention, Detection, Evaluation, and Treatment of High Blood Pressure: the JNC 7 report. *JAMA* 2003;289:2560–2572. Available at: http://www.nhlbi.nih.gov/guidelines/hypertension/jnc7full.htm.

Lipids

Grundy SM, Cleeman JI, Merz CN, et al. Implications of recent clinical trials for the National Cholesterol Education Program Adult Treatment Panel III guidelines. *Circulation* 2004;110:227–239.

National Cholesterol Education Program. *Detection, evaluation, and treatment of high blood cholesterol in adults (Adult Treatment Panel III)*. Available at: http://www.nhlbi.nih.gov/guidelines/cholesterol/atp3_rpt.htm. Last reviewed January 2006.

Metabolic Syndrome

National Cholesterol Education Program. *Detection, evaluation, and treatment of high blood cholesterol in adults (Adult Treatment Panel III)*. Available at: http://www .nhlbi.nih.gov/guidelines/cholesterol/atp3_rpt.htm. Last reviewed January, 2006.

Abdominal Aortic Aneurysm

Kent KC, Zwolak RM, Jaff MR, et al. Screening for abdominal aortic aneurysm: a consensus statement. *J Vasc Surg* 2004;39(1):267–269.

Coronary Artery Disease

American College of Cardiology Foundation and the American Heart Association. *ACC/AHA 2002 guideline update for exercise testing—full text*. Available at: http://www.acc.org/qualityandscience/clinical/guidelines/exercise/exercise_clean.pdf. Accessed 2007.

American College of Cardiology Foundation and the American Heart Association. *ACC/AHA/ASNC guidelines for the clinical use of cardiac radionuclide imaging*. Available at: http://www.acc.org/qualityandscience/clinical/guidelines/radio/index.pdf. Accessed 2007.

Breast Cancer

Evans WP III, Mendelson E, Bassett L, et al. Appropriate imaging work-up of palpable breast masses. American College of Radiology. ACR Appropriateness criteria. *Radiology* 2000;215(Suppl):961–964.

Klein S. Evaluation of palpable breast masses. *Am Fam Physician* 2005;71:1731–1738.

Colorectal Cancer

Smith RA, Cokkinides V, Eyre HJ. American Cancer Society guidelines for the early detection of cancer, 2006. *CA Cancer J Clin* 2006;56:11–25.

Winawer SJ, Zauber AG, Fletcher RH, et al. Guidelines for colonoscopy surveillance after polypectomy: a consensus update by the US Multi-Society Task Force on Colorectal Cancer and the American Cancer Society. *CA Cancer J Clin* 2006;56:143–159. [Quiz 184–5].

Cervical Cancer

Wright TC Jr, Cox JT, Massad LS, et al. 2001 consensus guidelines for the management of women with cervical intraepithelial neoplasia. *Am J Obstet Gynecol* 2003;189: 295–304.

Prostate Cancer/Oral Cancer/Testicular Cancer/Skin Cancer

Abeloff MD, Armitage JO, Niederhuber JE, et al. *Clinical oncology*, 3rd ed. Philadelphia: Churchill Livingstone, 2004.

Rakel RE. *Textbook of family practice*, 6th ed. Philadelphia: WB Saunders, 2002.

Diabetes Mellitus

American Diabetes Association. Standards of medical care in diabetes–2006. *Diabetes Care* 2006;29 (Suppl 1):S4–S42.

Osteoporosis

National Osteoporosis Foundation. *Osteoporosis clinical practice guidelines*. Available at: http://www.nof.org/professionals/clinical.htm.

Impaired Visual Acuity

American Optometric Association. *Clinical practice guidelines.* Available at: http://www.aoa.org/x4813.xml. Accessed 2007.

American Optometric Association. *Care of the patient with low vision.* Available at: http://www.aoa.org/documents/CPG-14.pdf. Accessed 2007.

Tuberculosis

American Thoracic Society, CDC and Infectious Diseases Society of America. Treatment of tuberculosis. *MMWR Recomm Rep* 2003;52:1–77.

References

1. U.S. Preventive Services Task Force. *Screening for Colorectal Cancer: Recommendations and Rationale.* July 2002. Agency for Healthcare Research and Quality, Rockville, MD. http://www.ahrq.gov/clinic/3rduspstf/colorectal/colorr.htm. Accessed 2007.
2. Thompson IM, Pauler DK, Goodman PJ, et al. Prevalence of prostate cancer among men with a prostate-specific antigen level < or =4.0 ng per milliliter. *N Engl J Med* 2004;350:2239–2246.
3. Pearson TA, Mensah GA, Alexander RW, et al Markers of inflammation and cardiovascular disease: application to clinical and public health practice: a statement for health care professionals from the Centers for Disease Control and Prevention and the American Heart Association. *Circulation* 2003;107:499–511.
4. Sunga AY, Eberl MM, Oeffinger KC, et al. Care of cancer survivors. *Am Fam Physician* 2005;71:699–706.
5. Winawer SJ, Zauber AG, Fletcher RH, et al. Guidelines for colonoscopy surveillance after polypectomy: a consensus update by the US Multi-Society Task Force on Colorectal Cancer and the American Cancer Society. *CA Cancer J Clin* 2006;56: 143–159. [Quiz 184–5.]
6. Smith RA, Cokkinides V, Eyre HJ. American Cancer Society guidelines for the early detection of cancer, 2006. *CA Cancer J Clin* 2006;56:11–25.
7. Johansson JE, Andren O, Andersson SO, et al. Natural history of early, localized prostate cancer. *JAMA* 2004;291:2713–2719.
8. Adler AI, Stratton IM, Neil HA, et al. Association of systolic blood pressure with macrovascular and microvascular complications of type 2 diabetes (UKPDS 36): prospective observational study. *Br Med J* 2000;321:412–419.
9. United States Department of Commerce, Economics and Statistics Administration, Bureau of the Census. *Statistical brief: sixty-five plus in the United States.* Washington, DC: United States Department of Commerce, 1992.
10. Ozuah PO, Ozuah TP, Stein RE, et al. Evaluation of a risk assessment questionnaire used to target tuberculin skin testing in children. *JAMA* 2001;285:451–453.
11. American Thoracic Society, CDC and Infectious Diseases Society of America. Treatment of tuberculosis. *MMWR Recomm Rep* 2003;52:1–77.

CHAPTER 19

What Not to Do and Why: The Arguments against Some Forms of Screening and Chemoprevention

Janelle Guirguis-Blake and Russell Harris

As well as deciding which preventive services to routinely offer to patients, clinicians must also decide which services not to offer. Ardent advocates of preventive services argue that any potential for preventing disease is worthwhile and that it would be unethical to not offer patients all preventive services because it may deprive them of a possible benefit. In the face of what appears to be a "simple blood test" or noninvasive x-ray or ultrasonography, many clinicians and patients alike wonder, "why not order the test?"

Attempts to prioritize preventive services may strike some as a means of rationing or cost control in order to protect payers. This is not necessarily the case. In fact, as has been observed throughout this book, the wellbeing of patients is often protected by the clinician who prioritizes preventive services and is selective in offering patients targeted, effective preventive services that are evidence-based. The purpose of preventive services is not just to detect "abnormalities" or to prescribe medications, but to help people live longer, better lives. Examples throughout this book demonstrate that indiscriminate delivery of preventive services can actually cause more harm than good. Therefore, the burden of proof in favor of provision of a given preventive service lies with its advocates to demonstrate how a specific screening test or chemopreventive medication will improve health outcomes before the service comes to be routinely recommended.

CRITERIA FOR AVOIDING SOME PREVENTIVE SERVICES

Not all preventive services result in improved health. In fact, the provision of a given preventive service can be inappropriate if it is harmful, has little or no effectiveness, or has an uncertain balance of benefits and harms. Preventive services that are not recommended can fall into one or more of these categories. For example, screening for a condition with low prevalence in the target population may have limited effectiveness because few people have the condition. At the same time, its routine usage may cause harm by generating a large number of false-positive results. Examples are presented in the subsequent text. Each example may highlight only one of the arguments against

---

Rationale for Not Offering Preventive Services

1. The service causes net harm in the target population.
2. The service benefits few or no people in the target population.
3. The balance between benefits and harms is uncertain.

---

routinely providing the service, but often there are multiple reasons for discouraging use of the service (see Table 19.2).

The Preventive Service Produces Net Harm in the Target Population

Certain previously popular preventive services have proved harmful for patients. For example, for many years asymptomatic postmenopausal women were advised to take hormone replacement therapy. Such therapy was thought to prevent a number of chronic diseases as well as to improve the quality of life. As detailed in Chapter 15, evidence from the Women's Health Initiative, a large randomized controlled trial (1), has since shown that for most women combined hormone replacement therapy actually *increases* the risk of the very diseases that were once thought to be prevented by hormone therapy, such as cardiovascular disease and dementia.

Harm from screening tests may result directly from the use of the test itself, from the downstream diagnostic workup, or from overtreatment. Although most screening tests seem innocuous, some (e.g., colonoscopy) can cause direct harm (e.g., perforation of the colon). Although such complications occur to a small percentage of patients, given the large number of persons screened in a population, the absolute number injured may be significant. The use of screening tests can also cause considerable indirect harm by producing far more false-positive than true-positive results, leading to added anxiety for both patients and their families.

The "downstream" consequences of screening tests may also be harmful. Patients with positive screening test results must undergo further diagnostic testing in order to determine whether they truly have the target condition. If these diagnostic tests are invasive, the resulting harms can outweigh the benefits, especially when the target condition has a relatively low prevalence. For example, screening for ovarian cancer (with CA-125 and/or ultrasonography) leads to invasive laparoscopies with associated harms (bleeding, pain, and infection) (see Figure 19.1). Modeling shows that screening 10,000 women aged 50–64 years for ovarian cancer would result in 300 women who do not have ovarian cancer being recalled each year for a diagnostic workup, resulting in potential distress and anxiety in otherwise healthy women. Of these, 20–65 women without ovarian cancer would undergo unnecessary surgery each year (2). Similarly, screening average-risk people for carotid artery stenosis may cause more strokes than it prevents, due to complications from screening angiography and carotid endarterectomy.

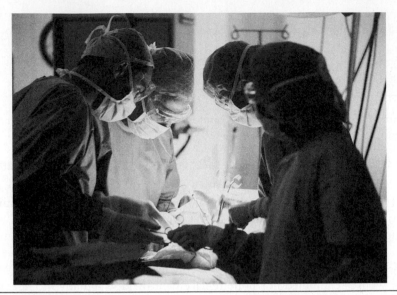

Figure 19.1 • Unnecessary surgery is among the potential complications of false-positive results from seemingly innocuous screening tests.

Screening can also cause harm by precipitating overtreatment (3,4). *Overtreatment* refers to the treatment of conditions that would never have become clinically important (e.g., radical prostatectomy or radiation therapy for prostate cancers that would never have progressed). The risk of overtreatment is greatest in situations where there are "borderline" conditions that are neither completely normal nor completely pathologic (e.g., small colonic polyps, ductal carcinoma *in situ* of the breast, and cervical intraepithelial neoplasia I and II), or where there is great heterogeneity in the natural history of conditions that appear to be pathologic (e.g., breast cancer, prostate cancer, and bladder cancer). As it is impossible to know which persons with these conditions will experience clinically meaningful progression, all are usually treated.

Preventive services may result in *net* harms, although they offer some health benefits. Chapter 15 provides specific examples of these tradeoffs, such as the use of tamoxifen, which reduces the risk of developing breast cancer in women but also increases the risk of thromboembolic events. Although aspirin chemoprevention may prevent myocardial infarction, it can also cause gastrointestinal bleeding and hemorrhagic strokes. In certain subgroups, the harmful effects of aspirin may outweigh its benefits (see pages 350–351).

For some preventive services, net population harm can be minimized by offering the service selectively to subgroups of patients. The tradeoff between benefits and harms is usually most favorable among people who are at increased risk for the target condition. For example, aspirin prophylaxis will prevent 1–4 myocardial infarctions in low-risk men (those with a 5-year coronary heart disease [CHD] risk of 1%) and 6–20 myocardial infarctions in higher-risk men (those with a 5-year CHD risk of 5%) for every 2–4 major gastrointestinal bleeds it causes (5).

When screening is offered to a population subset with a higher prevalence of the condition, more patients will benefit, with fewer false-positive results generated. For example, the U.S. Preventive Services Task Force (USPSTF) reports that screening for osteoporosis (a condition that becomes more prevalent with age) would prevent 14 hip fractures per 10,000 women screened over a 5-year period among women aged 65–69 years but would prevent only 1 hip fracture over the same time period among women aged 50–54 years.

The Service Benefits Few or No People

There are at least three reasons why a screening or chemoprevention program might benefit few or no people:

- The service has little or no effectiveness in the target population.
- The target condition has low prevalence in the target population.
- The screening or chemoprevention is unfocused.

PREVENTIVE SERVICES OF LITTLE OR NO EFFECTIVENESS

A preventive service is "ineffective" when it benefits few or none of those people who might be helped. Even relatively ineffective services may occasionally help someone. The "number needed to treat" (NNT) and "number needed to screen" (NNS) are metrics that estimate how many people would need to undergo a treatment (e.g., chemoprevention) or would need to be screened before a single individual would benefit from the service. The service is considered ineffective if the NNT or NNS is large relative to the benefit that results from the service.

There are two potential reasons why a service that is occasionally beneficial to patients may not be routinely offered to an entire population. First, routinely offering these services may result in *net harm*s. For example, only a small fraction of breast cancer cases is attributable to the *BRCA* genetic mutation. Screening of the general population would benefit very few women and create anxiety for many more. Moreover, because the *BRCA* gene is large, general screening would detect multiple mutations, most of which are not clinically important (6). The second reason for avoiding services of limited effectiveness, even when there is no net harm, is the *opportunity cost*. Opportunity costs are the services that will be crowded out and not performed because of the time and effort required to deliver the service in question.

Clinicians, patients, and society can experience opportunity costs. For clinicians, an unnecessary preventive service to discuss and monitor consumes time and effort that the clinician and the clinician's staff could use for more effective services. As discussed in Chapter 20, lack of time is a barrier to the delivery of preventive care. In today's world of limited time availability, in the course of a day it can prove impossible to provide even those services known to be effective (7). For every minute spent on ineffective prevention, 1 minute is lost from implementing effective prevention. Therefore, during a 15-minute office visit, the clinician has a choice: whether to offer a preventive service for which there is limited evidence of benefit (e.g., screening for thyroid disorders) or to discuss a service for which there is good evidence of a substantial benefit (e.g., colorectal cancer screening). It is important for clinicians to realize that prioritization of services based on available evidence is not a way to ration but rather a way to maximize the benefit to patients. Prioritization of preventive services is discussed further in Chapter 1 (see pages 16–18). Chapter 20 examines how practices can set their own priorities in identifying the preventive services to emphasize.

For patients, the opportunity costs of services with limited effectiveness include time, effort, and often financial cost. Given other demands, patients are able to attend to a limited number of health issues at any one time and often choose to focus on urgent symptomatic issues rather than prevention. Offering patients relatively ineffective services may result in an unfavorable "tradeoff," such as foregoing other, more effective services.

For society, using scarce resources such as medical personnel and dollars to deliver services that provide minimal return is a poor investment. Routinely providing ineffective services drives up the cost of health care without improving the health of the public. Providing relatively ineffective services reduces the time and effort devoted to services that are more effective, possibly resulting in a negative impact on the health of the population.

We refer here to services for which there is *evidence of ineffectiveness*, which is distinguished from *insufficient evidence of effectiveness*. The latter refers to a gap in the research whereas the former refers to good quality evidence that a service does not work (i.e., has little or no effectiveness). There are some preventive services for which science has shown no benefit in the general population. For example, studies find no benefit from routine screening for asymptomatic bacteriuria or pyuria in average or high-risk adults by urinalysis, urine microscopy, or urine culture (8).

Another category of ineffective prevention is screening or chemoprevention in patients with short life expectancy, such as the "frail" elderly or patients with severe comorbid disease. Since the benefit from screening or chemoprevention often occurs some years after starting the preventive service, many of these patients will not live long enough to benefit from the service. For example, screening for colorectal cancer in those older than 80 years, mammography in women older than 75 years, and cervical cancer screening of women older than 65 years are examples of services that are generally unlikely to be beneficial. As noted in Chapter 4, guidelines for many of these screening tests recommend discontinuation when the average life expectancy is less than 10 years.

Another common form of ineffective screening is so-called baseline screening. For example, baseline electrocardiograms are commonly ordered as a part of the periodic health examination with the rationale that they may be useful if the patient has chest pain in the future. The value of any test as a comparison for the future, however, rapidly decreases as the time from the provision of the "baseline" test increases. To maintain their usefulness, such "baseline" tests need to be repeated regularly. If there are benefits to such periodic screening, then the salient question is at what age such screening has been shown to yield benefits.

A final category of ineffective screening is increasing the frequency of a screening test for patients at higher risk of the target disease (e.g., more frequent Pap testing among women at increased risk of cervical cancer). For reasons explained in Chapter 20 (see page 525), the frequency of screening for a particular disease should be determined by the rate of progression of the disease rather than its incidence.

THE TARGET CONDITION HAS LOW PREVALENCE IN THE CHOSEN POPULATION

When screening or chemoprevention is applied to target groups in which the condition has low prevalence, many people must undergo the service and be exposed to risk to benefit a very few. Even relatively effective services may have a high NNT or NNS if used in a population where few have the potential to benefit. A preventive medication that must be taken by thousands to prevent one case of the target condition means that the vast majority of patients may unnecessarily suffer side effects of the medication with little potential benefit (e.g., as noted earlier, tamoxifen for those women at low risk for breast cancer). Also, as noted earlier, the harms from false-positive results are more likely to outweigh the benefits when screening is conducted in populations with a low prevalence of the target condition. Screening average-risk women in their 50s for osteoporosis benefits few women and is not recommended (9). For similar reasons, screening for gonorrhea is not recommended in low-risk groups (e.g., monogamous women older than 25 years) and screening for cancer is rarely advocated in young adults (see Chapter 4).

UNFOCUSED SCREENING AND CHEMOPREVENTION

Unfocused prevention—checking boxes on a laboratory requisition form—is easy to do. Why order a "chem 7" when one can order a "chem 21?" Certainly, "casting a wide net" will detect many abnormalities. The problem with unfocused prevention is that the conditions detected through the screening are often not clinically significant, nor is their detection beneficial to patients. When ordering a multicomponent blood chemistry panel, for example, it is important to be aware that an abnormal result is much more likely to be a false positive than a true positive. As noted in Chapter 4, an unfocused blood chemistry panel with 20 independent variables has a 64% probability of producing an "abnormal" result, even when no abnormality exists. The risk of false-positive results is especially high in a population of healthy individuals for which the suspicion and probability of disease are low.

Direct-to-consumer advertisements for whole body positron emission testing, spiral computed tomography, and other scans have become increasingly common. As a result, patients have come to believe that this new technology can detect any occult cancer and thereby allay any underlying fears of undetected disease. Such screening finds many conditions of uncertain significance and such detection is likely to be of little benefit. If there are benefits from such broad-based, nonfocused screening, they are likely to be outweighed by the harms of "downstream" testing and overtreatment of insignificant conditions, as discussed earlier. False-positive findings from whole body scans often precipitate anxiety as well. False negatives are also common, perhaps giving patients a false sense of security that everything is normal, with the risk of discouraging patients from undergoing specific screening tests that have been shown to be effective and help save lives (e.g., colonoscopy, mammography).

Likewise, patients often take multiple vitamins and herbal supplements to maintain their health. As opposed to targeted chemoprevention using supplements with known benefit (e.g., folic acid supplementation in pregnant women), such unfocused use of multivitamins likely has little or no benefit to individuals (see Chapter 7, page 190) (10).

Uncertain Balance of Benefits and Harms

Some preventive services should be avoided because there is uncertainty about the balance between their benefits and harms. This occurs because there is insufficient or poor-quality evidence about the efficacy of the interventions. The potential upper and lower limits of benefit therefore cannot be estimated. Further research is often necessary to obtain the data to quantify the actual benefits and harms of routinely offering the preventive services that fall into this category.

For example, there is limited evidence concerning the benefits of diabetes screening in the general population. However, early detection of diabetes for those patients with hyperlipidemia or hypertension leads to tighter control of cholesterol and blood pressure with improved cardiovascular outcomes. Less clear is the extent to which early detection of diabetes in these patients prevents the microvascular disease outcomes that occur in people with diabetes, such as end-stage renal disease and blindness. Usually, microvascular complications become clinically apparent many years after the diagnosis of diabetes is established. Therefore, randomized controlled trials with more than 10 years of follow-up would be required to demonstrate improvements in these clinical outcomes as a result of screening (11). Similarly, uncertainty about the benefits of early detection of skin cancer and about the natural history of glaucoma makes the consequences of screening for these conditions difficult to predict.

In some cases, the probability of benefits and harms is clear but the relative significance of both harm and benefit depend on the patient's personal preferences. For example, approximately 50% of women regularly screened with mammography for breast cancer will have at least one false-positive screening test over a 10-year interval. Some women do not consider this to be harmful, but merely a minor inconvenience. For others, however, having to endure the anxiety of waiting for the results of further testing or even a biopsy to determine whether cancer is present would be considered a major harm. In these circumstances, placing a value on a particular potential harm often requires a discussion with the patient. Shared decision making, which is discussed further on pages 91–92, is often recommended to help patients make choices that reflect their personal preferences.

IMPLEMENTING EVIDENCE-BASED PREVENTION PROGRAMS IN CLINICAL PRACTICE

Clinicians face two opposing risks in deciding which preventive strategies to employ in clinical practice: adopting a service too early, before its effectiveness is established by properly conducted research, or adopting a service too late, after many missed opportunities for improving health. Clinicians are more vulnerable to the first risk if they immediately adopt new technologies before evidence of effectiveness is confirmed. Clinicians are more vulnerable to the second risk if they require direct evidence from randomized controlled trials for every intervention they implement.

Finding the middle ground between these two extremes is crucial. Clinicians must determine when the evidence is sufficient to justify action—whether positive (e.g., offering the intervention) or negative (e.g., not offering the intervention). The answer depends partly on the service and the condition. Services with little potential for harm and a large potential for benefit may be offered with less definitive evidence than services with a greater potential for harm. The opportunity costs discussed in the preceding text lead us to discourage the investment of time on services with uncertain benefits and harms.

As mentioned throughout this chapter, focusing limited time and resources on preventive services with a known benefit is more likely

TABLE 19.1 How to Appropriately Provide Preventive
Services

1. Routinely offer patients services with established effectiveness
2. Target prevention to those with a high chance of benefiting from
   intervention (e.g., high-risk groups)
3. Discourage patients from getting "parking lot van" or shopping
   mall testing (e.g., whole body scans)
4. Do not routinely offer preventive services for which there is
   insufficient evidence of effectiveness. If patients request such
   services, engage in shared decision making (see pages 91–92)
5. Do not offer preventive services for which there is evidence of
   ineffectiveness and harms. If patients request such services,
   discourage their use; be ready to negotiate
6. There are some screening tests that require up-front counseling
   with patients (e.g., colonoscopy, aspirin use for prevention of
   coronary heart disease, and screening for prostate cancer). Other
   screening services may require minimal discussion (e.g., screening
   for depression, alcohol misuse, and obesity). See related chapters in
   this book

to improve health outcomes for a clinician's panel of patients. Further suggestions are provided in Table 19.1. These strategies may not be immediately satisfactory to patients. It is always appropriate to discuss these issues with patients and families who request services of limited effectiveness. Clinicians should communicate to patients the uncertainty of the likely outcomes and help them to appreciate how they will benefit by focusing on a limited number of clearly effective preventive services. If feasible, it is best to deliver this important message in small doses, using multiple examples over a number of patient encounters. A clinician's willingness to discuss issues over time and negotiate mutually agreeable solutions to prevention is an attribute that most patients appreciate.

A clinician should not try to "talk the patient out of" an ineffective or potentially harmful preventive service; a single test usually carries with it little risk. Rather, clinicians should pursue continued efforts to provide accurate information to the patient. As discussed in Chapter 4, there are an increasing number of decision aids appropriate for primary care practices that facilitate this process, save time, and provide accurate information in an understandable format (see page 92) (12).

TABLE 19.2 Discouraged Preventive Services and the Target Groups to Which they Apply

Service	Population in Which Service Is Discouraged	Rationale for Discouraging Service[a]	Primary Exclusion Category[b]
		Endocrine	
Bone mineral density testing (e.g., DEXA scans)	Young women	Young women (<60 yr of age) have relatively low prevalence of osteoporosis. See http://www.ahrq.gov/clinic/3rduspstf/osteoporosis/osteowh.htm	2
Hormone therapy to prevent chronic disease	General population	Increased incidence of cardiovascular events, dementia, and breast cancer outweighs benefit of prevention of osteoporotic fractures. See Chapter 15 and http://www.ahrq.gov/clinic/uspstf/uspspmho.htm	1
Routine measurement of thyroid-stimulating hormone	General population	Clinical harm caused by overtreatment of subclinical disease and clinical improvement after treatment of subclinical disease are not known. See http://www.ahrq.gov/clinic/uspstf/uspsthyr.htm	3
Diabetes screening	General population (without hypertension or hyperlipidemia)	Unknown magnitude of incremental benefit from earlier detection and treatment in terms of patient-oriented outcomes due to microvascular disease. See Chapter 4 and http://www.ahrq.gov/clinic/uspstf/uspsdiab.htm	2, 3

(continued)

TABLE 19.2 (Continued)

Service	Population in Which Service Is Discouraged	Rationale for Discouraging Service[a]	Primary Exclusion Category[b]
		Hematology	
Screening for hemochromatosis	General population	Prevalence of clinical disease due to hemochromatosis in the general population is likely low; the natural history of people with increased iron stores is unknown; overtreatment is likely. See http://www.ahrq.gov/clinic/uspstf/uspshemoch.htm	1, 2, 3
		Cardiovascular and Pulmonary	
Beta-carotene supplements and vitamin E to prevent heart disease	General population	No health benefit; smokers harmed by beta-carotene. See http://www.ahrq.gov/clinic/uspstf/uspsvita.htm	1, 2
Routine chest radiography or computed tomography scans for lung cancer screening	General population	High false-positive rate; diagnostic workup (bronchoscopy, mediastinoscopy with biopsy) is invasive and potentially harmful. See http://www.ahrq.gov/clinic/uspstf/uspslung.htm	1

Routine electrocardiograms	General population	In average-risk population, no known benefit and minimal potential yield based on many false positives (nonspecific electrocardiographic findings have little clinical significance) and false negatives. See http://www.ahrq.gov/clinic/uspstf/uspsacad.htm	2
Routine pulmonary function testing	General population	Little or no potential benefit in asymptomatic individuals	2
Screening for abdominal aortic aneurysms	Women and nonsmoking men	Surgical repair has high morbidity/mortality; women have lower prevalence. See Chapter 4 and http://www.ahrq.gov/clinic/uspstf/uspsaneu.htm	1, 2
Routine aspirin chemoprophylaxis	Populations at low or intermediate risk of CHD	Net harms from increased gastrointestinal bleeding and hemorrhagic stroke. See Chapter 15 and http://www.ahrq.gov/clinic/uspstf/uspsasmi.htm	1
Tamoxifen in women	Women at low risk of breast cancer	Few women benefit; net harms from increased venous thromboembolic disease. See Chapter 15 and http://www.ahrq.gov/clinic/uspstf/uspsbrpv.htm	1, 2
Infectious Disease			
Screening for bacterial vaginosis	General population	No health benefit as few health consequences of asymptomatic condition. See http://www.ahrq.gov/clinic/uspstf/uspsbvag.htm	2

(continued)

TABLE 19.2 (Continued)

Service	Population in Which Service Is Discouraged	Rationale for Discouraging Service[a]	Primary Exclusion Category[b]
Screening for asymptomatic bacteriuria	Nonpregnant women	No health benefit as few health consequences of asymptomatic condition (in nonpregnant individuals). See http://www.ahrq.gov/clinic/uspstf/uspsbact.htm	2
Screening for syphilis	Low risk populations	Patients without risk factors have minimal potential benefit due to low prevalence and resulting false-positive results, which lead to unnecessary treatment. See Chapters 4 and 12, and http://www.ahrq.gov/clinic/uspstf/uspssyph.htm	2
Screening for gonorrhea or chlamydia	Low risk populations	Low-risk patients (>25 yr of age without risk factors) have minimal potential benefit due to low prevalence; false-positive results lead to unnecessary treatment. See Chapters 4 and 12, and http://www.ahrq.gov/clinic/uspstf/uspsgono.htm	2
Screening for hepatitis C	General population	General population has low prevalence and long-term benefits of treatment to improve health outcomes are not known. Treatment carries important harms. See http://www.ahrq.gov/clinic/uspstf/uspshepc.htm	1, 2, 3
Screening for genital herpes	General population	Detection does not alter care and confers little health benefit. See Chapter 12 and http://www.ahrq.gov/clinic/uspstf/uspsherp.htm	2

Screening for hepatitis B infection	General population	No treatment available to change health outcomes. See http://www.ahrq.gov/clinic/uspstf/uspshepb.htm	2
		Cancer	
Screening for pancreatic cancer	General population	No treatment has been shown to improve outcomes. See http://www.ahrq.gov/clinic/uspstf/uspspanc.htm	2
Screening for testicular cancer	General population	Treatment is effective even when condition is detected clinically so there is little incremental benefit from earlier detection through screening. See Chapter 14 and http://www.ahrq.gov/clinic/uspstf/uspstest.htm	2
Screening for *BRCA* mutations	General population	Minimal potential benefit in general population, as a minority of breast cancer cases is linked to this specific genetic mutation. See Chapter 4 and http://www.ahrq.gov/clinic/uspstf/uspsbrgen.htm	2
Screening for bladder cancer	General population	Minimal potential benefit, uncertain effectiveness of early detection, and harms due to overtreatment. See http://www.ahrq.gov/clinic/uspstf/uspsblad.htm	1, 2
Routine endometrial biopsy for endometrial cancer screening	General population	Minimal potential for benefit due to early clinical presentation of disease. Potential harms: pain, bleeding, uterine perforation, and infection	1, 2

(continued)

509

TABLE 19.2 (Continued)

Service	Population in Which Service Is Discouraged	Rationale for Discouraging Service[a]	Primary Exclusion Category[b]
Routine colposcopy for cervical cancer screening	General population	Minimal potential for incremental benefit over Pap screening. Potential harms: pain, bleeding, and infection	1, 2
Routine screening for prostate cancer (prostate-specific antigen, digital rectal examination)	General population	Important harms from overtreatment; uncertainty about benefits of earlier detection and treatment. See Chapter 4 and http://www.ahrq.gov/clinic/uspstf/uspsprca.htm	1, 3
Colonoscopy	Low risk populations younger than 50 yr	Net harms. See Chapter 4 and http://www.ahrq.gov/clinic/uspstf/uspscolo.htm	1
Mammography	Women younger than 40 yr	Minimal potential benefit as prevalence of invasive disease relatively low and false positive rate from mammography is high, leading to overdiagnosis and invasive workup; discuss appropriateness and balance of benefits and harms with women aged 40–50 yr. See Chapter 4 and http://www.ahrq.gov/clinic/uspstf/uspsbrca.htm	1, 2
Screening for ovarian cancer with ultrasonography or CA-125	General population	Screening inaccurate with high false-positive rate leading to invasive workup with laparoscopy. See http://www.ahrq.gov/clinic/uspstf/uspsovar.htm	1, 2

Screening for skin cancer	General population	Uncertain benefits; requires much time and effort. See Chapters 3 and 14, and http://www.ahrq.gov/clinic/uspstf/uspsskco.htm	3
Teaching breast self-examination	General population	Lack of evidence that teaching improves health outcomes; increases risk of diagnostic procedures. See Chapter 14.	1, 2
Vision			
Glaucoma screening	General population	Unknown balance of benefits and harms: earlier detection and treatment does improve vision-related function and quality of life but treatment involves some risks. See http://www.ahrq.gov/clinic/uspstf/uspsglau.htm	3
Mental Health			
Dementia screening	General population	Unknown balance of benefit and harms: current treatments have limited effectiveness in modifying instrumental activities of daily living. See Chapter 13 and http://www.ahrq.gov/clinic/uspstf/uspsdeme.htm	2, 3
Unfocused Screening			
Routine complete blood counts	General population	Identifies multiple hematologic abnormalities; detection of the most common disorders not associated with improved health outcomes in asymptomatic adults; false-positive results common.	1, 2

(continued)

TABLE 19.2 (Continued)

Service	Population in Which Service Is Discouraged	Rationale for Discouraging Service[a]	Primary Exclusion Category[b]
Routine chemistry panels	General population	Screens for dozens of abnormalities, many of which are rare; evidence of benefit scant, and false-positive results common. See Chapter 4.	1, 2
Routine liver function panel	General population	Screens for liver dysfunction but there is no effective treatment for isolated abnormalities in liver function tests in asymptomatic population; false-positive results common.	1, 2
Whole body scans	General population	Whole body ultrasonography, computed tomography, positron emission testing offered by mobile vans, senior centers, or shopping mall outlets do not provide targeted screening for those selected populations for which early detection improves outcomes (e.g., screening for abdominal aortic aneurysms in male smokers older than 65 yr); high rate of false-positive and false-negative results. See http://www.ahrq.gov/clinic/uspstf/uspslung.htm	1, 2
Routine urinalysis	General population	Detects asymptomatic bacteriuria, hematuria, and pyuria but these findings are nonspecific; bacteriuria not known to cause harms in asymptomatic adults; false-positive results common.	1, 2

DEXA = dual x-ray absorptiometry; ASA = acetylsalicylic; CHD = coronary heart disease.
[a]Space limitations preclude detailed explanations. In most cases the table provides the current website address for more detailed rationale statements from the U.S. Preventive Services Task Force.
[b]1 = The service benefits few or no people; 2 = The service causes important harms for a number of people; 3 = The balance between benefits and harms for the service is uncertain.

CONCLUSION

This chapter specifically focuses on those services that should not be routinely offered to the general population. Some of the services discussed in this chapter may have benefit in high-risk populations only (e.g., chlamydia/gonorrhea screening in high-risk populations, screening for abdominal aortic aneurysms in male smokers older than 65 years, and screening for the *BRCA* mutation in women with high-risk family histories). Differentiating those services that provide benefit to the general population, those that provide benefit in high-risk populations, and those that provide no benefit (or harm) in any population is critical to providing quality preventive care in clinical practice. Table 19.2 provides a selected list of preventive services and target groups that should not be routinely offered nor prioritized. The list is hardly exhaustive—for example, it does not include routine magnetic resonance imaging of the breasts, which is recommended only for high-risk women (see page 116). New preventive services that emerge after publication of this book and that also lack supporting evidence of net benefit should also join the list, whereas some services in Table 19.2 may become more important as supporting evidence accumulates.

RESOURCES—PATIENT EDUCATION MATERIALS

Welch HG. *Should I be tested for cancer? Maybe not and here's why.* Berkeley: University of California Press, 2004.

SUGGESTED READINGS

Agency for Healthcare Research and Quality. *Guide to clinical preventive services.* AHRQ Publication No. 06–0588, June 2005. Rockville: Agency for Healthcare Research and Quality, www.preventiveservices.ahrq.gov. 2006.

Jett JR. Limitations of screening for lung cancer with low-dose spiral computed tomography. *Clin Cancer Res* 2005;11(13 Pt 2):4988s–4992s.

Sirovich BE, Schwartz LM, Woloshin S. Screening men for prostate and colorectal cancer in the United States: does practice reflect the evidence? *JAMA.* 2003;289(11):1414–1420.

Sirovich BE, Welch HG. Cervical cancer screening among women without a cervix. *JAMA.* 2004;291(24):2990–2993.

Welch HG. Right and wrong reasons to be screened. *Ann Intern Med* 2004;140(9):754–755.

Woolf SH. The need for perspective in evidence-based medicine. *JAMA* 1999;282(24):2358–2365.

References

1. Anderson GL, Limacher M, Assaf AR, et al. Effects of conjugated equine estrogen in postmenopausal women with hysterectomy: the Women's Health Initiative randomized controlled trial. *JAMA* 2004;291(14):1701–1712.
2. U.S. Preventive Services Task Force. Screening for ovarian cancer: recommendation statement. *Ann Fam Med* 2004;2:260–262.

3. Kumar AS, Bhatia V, Henderson IC. Overdiagnosis and overtreatment of breast cancer: rates of ductal carcinoma *in situ*: a U.S. perspective. *Breast Cancer Res* 2005;7(6): 271–275.

4. Zackrisson S, Andersson I, Janzon L, et al. Rate of over-diagnosis of breast cancer 15 years after end of Malmö mammographic screening trial: follow-up study. *Br Med J* 2006;332:689–692.

5. U.S. Preventive Services Task Force. Aspirin for the primary prevention of cardiovascular events: summary of the evidence. *Ann Int Med* 2002;136(2):161–172.

6. U.S. Preventive Services Task Force. Genetic risk assessment and BRCA mutation testing for breast and ovarian cancer susceptibility: recommendation statement. *Ann Intern Med* 2005;143:355–361.

7. Yarnall KS, Pollak KI, Ostbye T, et al. Primary care: is there enough time for prevention? *Am J Public Health* 2003;93(4):635–641.

8. Harding GKM, Zhanel GG, Nicolle LE, et al. Antimicrobial treatment in diabetic women with asymptomatic bacteriuria. *N Engl J Med* 2002;347(20):1576–1583.

9. Nelson HD, Helfand M, Woolf SH, et al. Screening for postmenopausal osteoporosis: a review of the evidence for the U.S. Preventive Services Task Force. *Ann Intern Med* 2002;137:529–541.

10. Huang HY, Caballero B, Chang S, et al. *Multivitamin/mineral supplements and prevention of chronic disease.* Evidence Report/Technology Assessment No. 139. AHRQ Publication No. 06-E012. Rockville: Agency for Healthcare Research and Quality, 2006.

11. U.S. Preventive Services Task Force. Screening for type 2 diabetes mellitus in adults: recommendations and rationale. *Ann Intern Med* 2003;138(3):212–214.

12. Barry MJ. Health decision aids to facilitate shared decision making in office practice. *Ann Intern Med* 2002;136(2):127–135.

III

Putting Prevention Recommendations into Practice

CHAPTER 20

Developing a Health Maintenance Schedule

Paul S. Frame

Primary care clinicians are responsible for providing medical care to both sick and well patients. Their most challenging task may be the delivery of preventive services as recommended in current guidelines. Such guidelines are useless unless the services they advocate are routinely offered to eligible patients and are accepted by these patients. Clinicians encounter many barriers to implementation of preventive guidelines and often lack the motivation to incorporate preventive services into their practices due to the lack of direct incentives. The consequences of not treating an illness are more immediately apparent to the clinician than are the consequences of not offering recommended preventive services. For example, the failure to prescribe antibiotics for bacterial pneumonia creates immediate consequences, such as clinical deterioration or the need for referral to the emergency department. Forgetting to recommend health maintenance interventions, however, has deferred consequences, months or years in the future, and produces little effect in the near term to motivate clinicians to behave differently.

The proven benefits of preventive services cannot be fully realized unless practices develop systems to ensure their delivery. As shown in Figure 20.1, the organized delivery of preventive services in primary care settings requires a written health maintenance schedule—a protocol that describes the preventive services a practice intends to offer—and a system to ensure that the schedule is implemented. A health maintenance schedule defines the primary or secondary preventive services that should be offered to patients and their recommended periodicity. Interventions can include screening for disease, counseling patients about lifestyle changes, immunizations, and chemoprophylaxis. These services are indicated based on the patient's age, gender, and risk factors. The health maintenance schedule is a general guide for clinicians that can be modified based on the circumstances, characteristics, and needs of individual patients.

An explicit written health maintenance schedule is the foundation for developing an effective system of implementing prevention in patient care (see Chapter 21). It defines the goals of the practice for delivery of

```
┌─────────────────────────────┐
│  ┌───────────────────────┐  │
│  │ P Protocol            │  │
│  │ S System              │  │
│  │ A Audit               │  │
│  │ R Reinforcement       │  │
│  └───────────────────────┘  │
└─────────────────────────────┘
```

Figure 20.1 • Process for implementing prevention.

preventive services. The health maintenance schedule should be a written document so that there are no uncertainties about what the group is trying to achieve. Having a clearly stated standard for the practice does not mean, however, that individual clinicians cannot deviate from the basic protocol to accommodate their own preferences or the circumstances of individual patients. It does mean that the group's minimum standards are clearly stated. The health maintenance schedule is not a static document. It needs to be revised periodically based on changing evidence or group preference.

Carefully constructing a health maintenance schedule can be an intimidating task. For one thing, it takes time. It is an important task, though, because incorporating health promotion and disease prevention into the provision of acute medical care is a large part of what distinguishes primary care from specialty medicine. Designing the health maintenance schedule is also challenging because of conflicting expert recommendations, clinician preferences, expectations, time constraints, and costs that the clinician or group incurs in designing the schedule.

Chapters 21 and 22 describe systems and tools for implementing the health maintenance schedule. The system includes the following components: a plan for offering preventive services, a process for delivering the preventive services, a person responsible for making sure the goals of the practice are met, a clinician and patient reminder plan, and a plan for engaging patients in their own preventive care. Audits are necessary to monitor the progress of the practice in achieving its goals. Artificial reinforcements such as peer review and cajoling or more formal reinforcements such as monetary incentives (see Chapter 23) may also be needed, because the natural reinforcements that are found in acute care may not pertain to implementing a prevention program. Many tools can be helpful in implementing the preventive system—for example, flow charts, computer-based reminders, patient handouts, and web-based information resources—but tools alone do not ensure effective implementation of preventive medicine in practice. Tools should not be confused with a system.

Whereas the chapters that follow discuss systems and tools for implementation, this chapter focuses on the first step in adopting a system:

TABLE 20.1 Pearls for Developing a Health Maintenance Schedule

Get maximum clinician input in the developmental process

Develop a minimum, not a maximum, schedule

Allow individual clinician variation above the minimum

Make the schedule relevant to the local patient population and feasible to implement in the practice

Remember that the development of the schedule is an ongoing dynamic process

Remember that screening frequency is determined by the rate of progression of the disease and the sensitivity of the screening test

Remember that a person's risk status influences the cost-effectiveness of screening for a given disease, not screening frequency

reaching agreement on a health maintenance schedule. The discussion begins with an examination of barriers to the implementation of preventive services in practice. This is important primarily because the design of the health maintenance schedule must be sensitive to these barriers and deal with them constructively to be acceptable to clinicians and applicable to patient care. The chapter then discusses the three steps necessary to develop a health maintenance schedule: establishing a group process, determining which interventions to include in the schedule, and deciding on the recommended frequency for each of the interventions. Table 20.1 summarizes the important take-home points regarding this process.

BARRIERS TO PREVENTION

Barriers to implementing preventive services that affect the development of a health maintenance schedule include: lack of time, uncertainty about the value of preventive services, conflict among expert groups that issue recommendations, and lack of good systems to facilitate delivery of preventive services (1).

Lack of time is of paramount concern in primary care. A busy clinician sees 25–35 patients per day, and at each patient visit the question must be asked, "Is preventive care up-to-date?" Time does not permit clinicians to offer unlimited preventive services to all patients. Yarnall et al. estimated that a clinician would have to spend 7.4 hours of each work day in order to optimally implement all of the preventive services recommended by the U.S. Preventive Services Task Force (USPSTF) in 1996. Two hours each day would be required of an average primary care clinician to

TABLE 20.2 Criteria for Appropriate Screening Programs

The condition must have a significant effect on the quality or quantity of life

Acceptable methods of treatment must be available

The condition must have an asymptomatic period in which detection and treatment significantly reduce morbidity and/or mortality

Treatment in the asymptomatic phase must yield a superior result to that obtained by delaying treatment until symptoms appear

Tests that are acceptable to patients must be available at a reasonable cost to detect the condition in the asymptomatic period

The incidence of the condition must be sufficient to justify the cost of screening

Adapted from Frame PS, Carlson SJ. A critical review of periodic health screening using specific screening criteria: Part 1. Selected diseases of respiratory, cardiovascular, and central nervous systems. *J Fam Pract* 1975;2:29.

implement only the strongest ("A" grade) USPSTF recommendations (2). The health maintenance schedule must be sensitive to these time constraints by including only proven interventions that are feasible in the practice setting. In developing the schedule, the practice should prioritize interventions as essential or optional; it should include all the essential interventions and be selective about including the optional ones. In addition, the health maintenance schedule should be organized to enable clinicians to quickly determine which preventive services are indicated at any given patient visit.

Uncertainty about the value of preventive services is another barrier to effective implementation. For example, clinicians are unlikely to order a screening test if they do not believe it to be worthwhile. The practice should adopt and adhere to criteria of effectiveness that preventive interventions must meet to be considered worthwhile and appropriate for the health maintenance schedule. Clinicians and the practice must be comfortable with the criteria they adopt. An example of such criteria is provided in Table 20.2. Evidence-based guidelines explicitly state the evidence on which recommendations are based, allowing the group to discuss and debate the appropriateness of specific interventions.

Conflict among expert groups provides a further obstacle to preventive medicine. Although there is usually a core of agreement between the recommendations of different expert groups, there are often significant disagreements. For example, specialists often recommend intensive preventive efforts for conditions in their particular specialty, even when strong evidence of effectiveness is lacking. Primary care clinicians encounter a healthier population than do specialists, and they should not be reluctant to require evidence of benefit before adopting recommendations from

TABLE 20.3 Evidence-Based Preventive Medicine Guideline Resources

- **Agency for Healthcare Research and Quality**
  www.ahrq.gov
  Home of the U.S. Preventive Services Task Force (USPSTF) and the Put Prevention into Practice (PPIP) programs (see page 532); maintains a ListServ which sends e-mail notification of new USPSTF and PPIP recommendations
  - **U.S. Preventive Services Task Force:**
    http://www.ahrq.gov/clinic/uspstfix.htm
  - **Put Prevention into Practice** program materials:
    http://www.ahrq.gov/clinic/ppipix.htm
  - **Electronic Preventive Services Selector:**
    http://epss.ahrq.gov/PDA/index.jsp
- **National Guideline Clearinghouse**
  www.guideline.gov
  Single source for evidence-based guidelines on many topics including preventive services. Guidelines issued by specialty organizations can be accessed through this site.
- **Advisory Committee on Immunization Practices (ACIP)**
  www.cdc.gov/vaccines/pubs/acip-list.htm
  Authoritative source for immunization guidelines.
- **American Cancer Society Guidelines for the Early Detection of Cancer**
  http://Caonline.amcancersoc.org
  Recommendations are in the Jan-Feb issue yearly.

expert specialty sources. Resources for obtaining evidence-based preventive recommendations are described in Table 20.3.

Lack of good systems to facilitate delivery of preventive services is addressed by strategies discussed in Chapter 21. That chapter focuses on the importance of integrating the delivery of preventive services into the flow of patient care. Electronic tools to facilitate implementation of such a system, discussed in Chapter 22, are increasingly available.

Ultimately, clinicians must agree with the interventions contained in their practice's health maintenance schedule. After all, they are the ones who must implement the schedule, and they are the ones who will experience both the rewards and the frustrations that result from their efforts.

ESTABLISHING A GROUP PROCESS

Most clinicians practice in groups. Even clinicians in solo practice work closely with nurses and other health professionals. Therefore, a process is needed for the group to reach a consensus on the content of the health maintenance schedule. Although no single method for forging consensus is ideal for all groups, several common principles apply:

1. **Choose a leader.** In larger groups, there may be several clinicians with a particular interest in prevention. One of them is a logical choice to become the leader and should take charge of developing the health maintenance schedule. The leader should be respected by a majority of the group members. The leader should also be dedicated to the importance of disease prevention and be a good facilitator of group processes. It is helpful if the leader is knowledgeable about evidence-based preventive care recommendations. Such guidelines can be obtained from the resources listed in Table 20.3. Alternatively, an expert consultant can be retained to help the group understand the different prevention guidelines.

2. **Set a minimum standard.** The goal is not necessarily to develop full consensus, but to develop a protocol that establishes a minimum acceptable standard for the practice. The schedule should not list every preventive service recommended by an expert group. The USPSTF, one of the most conservative expert panels, has recommended approximately 20 services for low-risk adults and many more for patients with one or more known risk factors (see Appendix A). It is difficult and unnecessary for all the clinicians in a practice to reach a consensus on an identical schedule. What is necessary, however, is that the group agrees upon a *minimum* standard. Most of the proven benefits of early detection accrue from screening for a few conditions, namely risk factors for coronary artery disease, and cancer of the breast, cervix, colon and rectum. Clinicians who wish to add other procedures or adopt more frequent intervals may do so. In reality, most clinicians will find it challenging enough to comply with even the minimum standard for all patients. Screening is hard work.

3. **Group process.** The process should involve as many clinicians as possible. Ideally, unless the group is very large, all members should participate. Clinicians are unlikely to perform procedures on the health maintenance schedule that they do not believe are worthwhile. Clinicians' involvement in the development process is the best way to help them understand the rationale for each intervention. Depending on the size and dynamics of the group, it may also be desirable to involve nurses and nonmedical personnel when developing the health maintenance schedule. Clinician buy-in is essential to creating a health maintenance schedule that reflects the views of the group and will be used by the practice. If specific clinicians disagree with the schedule, they should be given the opportunity to suggest an alternate schedule and to discuss the merits of each option. An acceptable compromise is most easily reached by emphasizing the

concept that the group schedule is a minimum acceptable protocol, allowing clinicians the freedom to do more if they wish.

4. **Reevaluate.** The practice should not be reluctant to try an intervention for a specified time and to reevaluate its value at a later date. Developing a health maintenance schedule is a dynamic process that should result in changes to the document over time. If a major controversy over the schedule develops within the practice, the group should make a temporary decision about what to include, but should also commit itself to reevaluate the issue at a later date. The experience of either undertaking or not undertaking the intervention will, over time, help inform the clinicians' opinions about whether the schedule needs to be revised.

CHOOSING SPECIFIC INTERVENTIONS

Most practices will use a set of published guidelines as the starting point for deciding which interventions to include when developing a health maintenance schedule. Table 20.3 lists some of the major groups that issue evidence-based guidelines relating to prevention. The USPSTF, sponsored by the Agency for Healthcare Research and Quality (AHRQ), is considered the most comprehensive, authoritative, and unbiased source of clinical preventive recommendations. Appendix A to this book lists interventions recommended by the USPSTF for low-risk adults. The Advisory Committee on Immunization Practices, sponsored by the Centers for Disease Control and Prevention, is the leading source of recommendations relating to immunizations for vaccine-preventable disease (see Chapter 16). The American Cancer Society recommendations regarding cancer prevention are widely known and followed by many clinicians and the lay public. The National Guideline Clearinghouse is a website maintained by AHRQ, which catalogs evidence-based guidelines on a wide range of medical topics including preventive medicine. Most guidelines issued by specialty organizations can be accessed through this site. The Put Prevention into Practice (PPIP) initiative of AHRQ has produced an Electronic Preventive Services Selector that can be used online or can be downloaded to a personal digital assistant to provide ready access to the USPSTF recommendations.

Before a practice decides to include or exclude controversial interventions, the recommendations of several authoritative groups should be compared so that members understand the reasons that the experts disagree. The practice may find it useful to consider interventions for different age groups separately. Developing separate schedules for children (e.g., age 18 years and younger) young adults (e.g., ages 19–39 years), middle-aged adults (e.g., ages 40–64 years), and older adults (e.g., age 65 years and older) may be helpful.

The rationale for each potential recommendation should be understood. Clinicians should not hesitate to question or be critical of any recommendation, regardless of its acceptance in the medical community. Medicine has many examples of accepted screening interventions, such as pelvic examinations for the detection of ovarian cancer, for which there is little supporting scientific evidence. In addition to the scientific validity of the recommendation, the clinicians should consider the relevance of the recommendation to their patient population and the feasibility of implementing the recommendation under current practice conditions.

The definition of some preventive services in the health maintenance schedule may need special clarification. For example, whereas the meaning of blood pressure measurement is obvious, the exact operational meaning of more ambiguous services, such as "nutritional counseling," could have multiple interpretations. Is it, for example, a brief reminder to the patient to eat well or is it a lengthy dietary assessment? The practice should spell out in detail what is expected of the clinician to comply with the recommendation. If the practice cannot decide exactly what a recommendation means or how it should be implemented, then that one should probably be excluded from the schedule.

Keep the schedule simple. When developing health maintenance schedules, there is a strong tendency to become idealistic and include a variety of noble interventions with marginal evidence of benefit. As a general rule, if an adult or pediatric schedule cannot be clearly outlined in a flow sheet or table and limited to a single page, then it is too complex. A complex schedule will not be used routinely by clinicians because its implementation requires too much time and attention, and frustration can ensue. Clinicians will then likely ignore the schedule altogether, omitting worthwhile as well as marginal interventions.

The basic schedule should focus on interventions applicable to the general, low-risk population. Certain interventions are essential to include in the health maintenance schedule. An intervention is considered essential if its omission would be generally considered unacceptable medical care, would expose the clinician to high medicolegal risk, or is required by major payers, health plans, or statute. Examples of essential preventive interventions for adults include screening for tobacco use, obesity, hypertension, elevated serum lipids, colorectal cancer in patients age 50 years and older, and breast and cervical cancers in women. Given the caveats reviewed in Chapter 19 (see page 498), discussing the benefits and harms of prostate cancer screening with men older than 50 years and helping them decide if they wish to have screening is also an essential intervention (3).

Interventions that do not fulfill the above criteria should be considered optional. A practice can be more selective in deciding whether or not to include optional interventions in its health maintenance schedule. A few interventions relevant to large high-risk groups, such as influenza vaccination, might be included. Including services for all high-risk groups is unnecessary and should be avoided, however. Whatever the content of the practice's health maintenance schedule, most clinicians will individualize preventive care to the particular patient. This is partly because each patient has a unique set of risk factors and concurrent diagnoses, but it also reflects such factors as patient preferences. It is virtually impossible to account for all these factors in a preset schedule. Rather, the schedule should be seen as a basic guide to be modified, augmented, or pruned to reflect the needs of the individual patient.

FREQUENCY OF INTERVENTIONS

In addition to listing recommended interventions, the health maintenance schedule should specify the frequency for offering each intervention. For some recommendations, such as certain immunizations, the proper timing of the intervention is well established. For other preventive services, such as smoking cessation counseling, there are few scientific data to support a specific frequency. For most preventive interventions the evidence supports a range of frequencies (e.g., every 1–3 years for Pap smears).

The two most important determinants of screening frequency are the sensitivity of the screening test and the rate of progression of the disease. The risk of acquiring the disease (e.g., incidence rate) should not play a factor in determining screening frequency. For example, consider a cancer with a slow rate of progression of 10 years from dysplasia to an incurable stage. If a screening test with a sensitivity of 80% is performed every 3 years, the first screening will detect 80% of cases, the second will detect 80% of the remainder (96% of cases), and the third will detect 80% of the remainder (99% of cases). Unless the rate of progression of the disease or the sensitivity of the test changes (4), the same proportion of cases will be detected regardless of the patient's risk of acquiring the disease. Therefore, the health maintenance schedule should not recommend a shorter interval between screening tests for persons at high risk of disease simply because they are at higher risk. High-risk patients should receive more intensive outreach efforts to ensure their involvement in the health maintenance program of the practice, but they need not be screened more frequently. A patient's risk status does influence the cost-effectiveness of screening, however. Screening for tuberculosis, for example, will have a very low yield in an affluent suburban population but is very important in a correctional facility. Therefore, risk status influences the decision of whether or not to screen more than it affects the decision of how often to screen.

For many preventive interventions, a frequency cannot be specified based on scientific evidence and must be determined by the clinician. An excessively frequent interval will increase costs and take time away from other important tasks. In addition, more frequent testing increases the probability of generating false-positive results and unnecessary workups. Too long a screening interval will increase the risk of missing important disease. Because the practice will have to make an arbitrary decision about the recommended frequency that will appear in the schedule, the concept of a minimum schedule, with tolerance of individual variation, is again useful.

ANNUAL COMPLETE PHYSICAL EXAMINATIONS

The proper frequency of health maintenance *visits,* an issue separate from the frequency of doing specific *procedures*, is a subject of much controversy. The appropriateness of the "annual physical" has been debated since the 1940s, and the proper schedule for well child examinations has received greater attention in recent years. Several important questions underlie this controversy: What is the role of the annual complete physical examination (CPE)? How is the CPE different from the periodic health examination (PHE)? Should preventive interventions be delivered during acute-care visits or just during dedicated prevention visits?

The CPE was first popularized in the 1920s by the life insurance industry and became more entrenched after World War II. With increased acceptance of evidence-based preventive medicine in the 1970s and 1980s, however, major authoritative groups including the Canadian Task Force on the Periodic Health Examination, the American Medical Association, and the USPSTF recommended replacing the annual CPE with selective interventions tailored to the individual patient. Despite these recommendations, the annual CPE remains very popular with clinicians, patients, and the media. In a survey of primary care clinicians in Boston, San Diego, and Denver, 65% of respondents agreed that an annual CPE is necessary, 88% said they perform annual CPEs, and 63% said they believed the annual CPE was of proven value (5).

Several factors may explain the enduring appeal of the CPE. It is a simple concept that most health consumers have embraced, whereas the argument for a complex health maintenance schedule is less intuitive. This chapter has stressed the need for a system to deliver preventive care. The annual CPE is a system, albeit a crude and inefficient one. It may be better than no system, which may be the only alternative for practices that have not organized themselves to generate patient and clinician reminders. Finally, the CPE provides more time than an acute visit to focus on lifestyle issues and the delivery of preventive services.

There are disadvantages to the annual CPE, however. First, there is not enough time to perform a CPE on all patients. The average primary care clinician, with 2,000 patients in the practice and 200 workdays per year, would have to perform 10 CPEs every day and would have little time to do anything else. Therefore, clinicians who profess that the annual CPE is their system for delivering preventive care are probably offering it to selected patients.

Patients who elect to have annual CPEs and PHEs tend to be the affluent worried well with relatively healthy lifestyles. Therefore, in what has been called *reverse targeting*, patients who are in less need of preventive services may receive more preventive services than they need, whereas high-risk patients most in need of preventive services may receive little or no organized preventive care.

The annual CPE is also expensive and inefficient. "Complete" implies doing many tests, many of which offer no benefit to the asymptomatic patient but do generate false-positive results that must be evaluated, often at substantial costs (see Chapter 19). The word "complete" may also imply (falsely) to patients that everything possible has been done and that their good health can be assured for the next year. A final disadvantage of the annual CPE is that they are not covered by many third party payers including Medicare and Medicaid (see Chapter 23). New Medicare beneficiaries (within 6 months of enrollment) are eligible to receive a "Welcome to Medicare" visit in which some preventive services can be delivered (see page 576).

The concept of the PHE is distinct from the annual CPE in that its periodicity and content can be specified by the practice and tailored to individual patients. The PHE is dedicated to prevention and is less about the physical examination and laboratory testing—which are done for specific indications—and more about risk assessment and risk reduction (see Chapter 2). Evidence of the effectiveness of the PHE was reviewed by AHRQ in 2006 (see http://www.ahrq.gov/clinic/tp/phetp.htm). Practices may choose to include the PHE in their health maintenance schedule at specified intervals depending on age and gender. The schedule should specify the minimum content of those visits.

Clinicians can and do deliver preventive services during both acute and chronic care visits. Flocke et al., in a direct observation study of family physicians, reported that preventive services were delivered during 32% of illness visits (6). The limited time available to patients and clinicians during CPEs, PHEs, and illness visits can be put to best use by implementing reminder systems to help office staff quickly identify which preventive interventions are indicated when a patient checks in. Reminder systems enable the nurse to appropriately prepare the patient so that the clinician can more efficiently implement the scheduled preventive service. See Chapters 21 and 22 for a more detailed discussion about reminder systems. Chapters 2 and 21 also discuss the role of previsit procedures, reminders, prompts, and flow sheets to help clinicians rapidly identify preventive services needing attention.

Delivering preventive care during either acute or chronic illness visits captures the patient population that does not schedule CPEs or PHEs. Although lack of time is often considered the major disadvantage of implementing prevention during illness visits, most preventive interventions are brief and can be easily worked into the pace of acute care. This does not

ADULT HEALTH MAINTENANCE PROTOCOL

1. History of tobacco use: all adults, every 4 yr
2. History of alcohol use: all adults, every 4 yr
3. Blood pressure: all adults, every 2 yr
4. Weight: all adults, every 4 yr
5. Total and HDL cholesterol: all adults, every 4 years until age 70 yr
6. Fecal occult blood test: all adults, annually after age 50 yr
7. Tetanus-diphtheria booster: all adults, every 10 yr
8. Complete physical examination at age 50–55 yr: for midlife counseling (to establish data base and counsel about options for colorectal cancer screening and prostate cancer screening)
9. Screen for abdominal aortic aneurysm: ultrasound screen for men at age 65 yr
10. Pneumococcal vaccination: all adults, older than 65 yr
11. Pap smear: women, every 2 yr until age 70 yr
12. Clinical breast examination: women, every 2 yr, after age 40 yr
13. Mammogram: women, annually aged 40–49, every 2 yr beginning at age 50 yr
14. Assess osteoporosis risk: women, every 5 yr, after age 50 yr
15. Influenza vaccination: all adults, annually, after age 65 yr
16. Discuss prostate screening: men, every 5 yr, ages 50–70 yr

The following procedures will be available as options but are not part of the routine protocol

17. Sigmoidoscopy every 5 yr, OR
18. Colonoscopy every 10 yr

Figure 20.2 • Tri-County Family Medicine Preventive Protocol for Adult Health Maintenance, April 2005. HDL, high-density lipoprotein; AAA, abdominal aortic aneurysm. The protocol assumes the patient is asymptomatic. A complete physical examination is indicated when the patient is first seen to establish a database.

apply when patients are new to the practice, have multiple issues to address, or require a comprehensive health risk appraisal. The most effective strategy to maximize the delivery of preventive care to as many patients as possible is for the clinician to try to address preventive health needs during all illness visits and to recommend PHEs as needed for those patients who require a more complete health risk appraisal and prevention plan. As discussed in Chapter 2, continuity (longitudinal) relationships also enable primary care clinicians to initiate preventive services at a given visit and to return to the topic, or address other needed services, at future appointments.

Figure 20.2, the adult health maintenance schedule currently used at the author's practice, is presented only as an example of a feasible health maintenance schedule. Its inclusion by no means implies that it is ideal. Each group should develop a customized schedule that is appropriate for the practice.

SUMMARY AND CONCLUSION

Developing a health maintenance schedule requires an upfront effort to create the health maintenance protocol, an ongoing practice commitment, and cooperation. The group should select a designated leader to champion the effort. Participation and support should be sought from as many clinicians as possible. The schedule should include essential preventive interventions and optional services of proven effectiveness. It should provide a minimum standard for the group, with the understanding that it will be individually tailored to the particular patient and clinician. The frequency of specific screening interventions is not determined by the patient's risk, but by the sensitivity of the screening test and rate of progression of the disease. A structured approach should be developed to ensure that the health maintenance schedule is offered to all patients. A system for delivering preventive services, which is discussed in the following chapter, rests upon the foundation of a well-defined health maintenance schedule.

References

1. Frame PS. Health maintenance in clinical practice: strategies and barriers. *Am Fam Physician* 1992;45:1192–1200.
2. Yarnall KS, Pollak KI, Ostbye T, et al. Primary care: is there enough time for prevention? *Am J Pub Health* 2003;93:635–641.
3. Woolf SH. Screening for prostate cancer with prostate-specific antigen. *N Eng J Med* 1995;333:1401–1405.
4. Frame PS, Frame JS. Determinants of cancer screening frequency: the example of screening for cervical cancer. *J Am Board Fam Pract* 1998;11:87–95.

5. Prochazka AV, Lundahl K, Pearson W, et al. Support of evidence-based guidelines for the annual physical examination: a survey of primary care providers. *Arch Intern Med* 2005;165:1347–1352.
6. Flocke SA, Stange KC, Goodwin MA. Patient and visit characteristics associated with opportunistic preventive services delivery. *J Fam Pract* 1998;47:202–208.

CHAPTER 21

How to Organize the Practice for Improved Delivery of Clinical Preventive Services

John M. Hickner and Leif I. Solberg

> *To think is easy. To act is hard.*
> *But the hardest thing in the world is to act in accordance with your thinking.*
>
> —Johann Wolfgang von Goethe

Primary care practices that perform at a high level of effectiveness and efficiency strive to provide the right care for the right person at the right time. This dictum applies to preventive care as well as to the care of acute and chronic problems. Two hundred years ago, Goethe anticipated the challenge primary care clinicians and their office staffs would face in living up to this ideal for preventive care. Although most primary care clinicians know most of the right things to do for prevention and do the right thing some of the time, it is very difficult to do the right thing consistently for every patient. This variability has been demonstrated in many studies (1–3). It occurs despite the best intentions of primary care clinicians, most of whom are strong advocates for smoking cessation, healthy eating, optimal physical activity, moderation in use of alcohol, immunizations, and appropriate cancer screening. Chapter 20 describes the barriers that result in this apparent disconnect between clinicians' intentions and actions. In addition to those barriers, most primary care offices lack office systems designed for prevention; they use the same procedures and practices that evolved years ago to efficiently take care of patients' acute illnesses and exacerbations of chronic diseases. The problem is that those approaches simply do not work for preventive services, or for routine chronic disease care. The target conditions for preventive care are usually asymptomatic, so patients do not come in seeking care for them. That means that the practice must have ways to identify, monitor, and proactively manage problems that the patient does not recognize and may not even care much about.

How can clinicians overcome this gap between the ideal and the current practice of preventive medicine? Over the last 20 years, there has been sufficient credible research to show that continuing medical education, a "change of attitude," or trying harder are insufficient for making preventive

531

services a routine part of patient care (4). What *does* work is permanent office systems changes. However, making this happen requires clinicians to do something they were not trained to do: build office practice systems with procedures and processes for both staff and clinicians that will provide the proper preventive services as automatically as possible. In other words, the "default" mode becomes providing the right preventive service to the right patient at the right time. It must become easier to provide the preventive service than not to do so.

This chapter describes how to approach prevention systematically in primary care practice. Whereas Chapter 20 describes how to develop the prevention protocols of a practice, this chapter describes how to implement and sustain prevention protocols. We show how to develop and implement office systems with automatic procedures and processes, auditing of results, and reinforcement of clinician and staff behavior. We base our advice on techniques that have been shown to be effective in the authors' own practices and by many recent research studies. In this chapter, we discuss the general principles for providing high quality preventive care.

In building successful office systems for preventive care, the KISS principle applies: "**K**eep **I**t **S**imple and **S**ystematic" (5). For the details of implementation, we highly recommend the resources available on the Agency for Healthcare Research and Quality (AHRQ) website, notably *Put Prevention into Practice (PPIP). A Step by Step Guide to Delivering Clinical Preventive Services: A Systems Approach*, available at http://www.ahrq .gov/ppip/manual/. The "PPIP" Guidebook is a 176-page manual that is also available as a downloadable PDF file. For those serious about systems change, this guide provides detailed instructions and many useful tools for implementing and sustaining preventive services.

PREPARING THE PRACTICE FOR PREVENTION SYSTEMS

Before embarking on office systems changes, it is essential that there be agreement among the clinicians *and* staff that prevention is a high priority of the practice mission. Further, the clinicians must agree on specific prevention practice guidelines that they all will follow (see Chapter 20). If there is substantial disagreement about these ideas, the disagreement must be resolved before proceeding further because a lack of cohesion will make it impossible to develop or implement common care processes. Twenty years ago, one of the authors was an early adopter of the health risk appraisal concept and introduced a health risk questionnaire for adults into his practice. It never caught on because the nursing staff did not see its value. About the same time, the other author decided that smoking cessation would be a top priority in his practice. He developed consensus among the partners and staff, developed an office-wide system, and achieved a 12-month smoking cessation rate of 25% for all smoking patients in the practice.

Agreement on the priority and guidelines for preventive services, however, is not sufficient for success. The practice *culture* also must support the methods that are necessary for the mission of prevention. Culture in the business world has been studied thoroughly by Edward Schein, who defines business culture as "the way we get things done around here" (6). Research shows that, in order for preventive services to be delivered consistently in a primary care practice, the practice culture must value teamwork, appropriate task delegation, standardization, and standing orders. Teamwork and task delegation are essential because primary care clinicians do not have sufficient time in their day to do an adequate job of caring for all of the acute problems, chronic illnesses, and preventive needs of each of their patients (7). Standardization and standing orders facilitate the consistent delivery of preventive care. Teamwork and task delegation do not come naturally to many clinicians. Medical training puts high value on clinicians' individual accountability for diagnosis and treatment. "If I want to be sure it is done right, I must do it myself" is a commonly held work ethic. Furthermore, clinicians are trained to be diagnosticians and problem solvers and are not necessarily good at routine prevention tasks. Only when nurses, medical assistants, and receptionists have active and well-defined roles is it likely that appropriate preventive services will be offered to all patients on a routine basis. Clinicians who have learned this lesson usually find their own work more satisfying, with less hassle and better results.

Clinicians are ready for the next steps only after they discuss and agree with this systems approach in both its theoretical and practical implications. If there is disagreement, clinicians need to approach system implementation differently, or not at all. The key is to understand the inefficiency of building different systems for each clinician rather than one system for all that allows some room for individual clinician style and patient differences. If some clinicians are unsure about the value of whole practice systems, it may be possible to change this perception by demonstrating the value of a systems approach for one preventive service (e.g., immunizations) with one clinician-medical assistant team that is willing to try it. After showing how a system improves their success rates (assuming this is measured) and work lives, it may be easier to expand to other teams and other preventive services in the practice.

KEY BASIC PRACTICE SYSTEMS FOR PROVIDING PREVENTIVE SERVICES TO PATIENTS AS THEY PRESENT FOR CARE

Where should a practice begin in its efforts to create office systems for improved preventive care? After the clinicians have reached agreement on their guidelines for the preventive services they will deliver consistently to their patients, we recommend focusing efforts first on patients who present to the office for care. Approximately 80% of adult patients are seen in the office by their primary care clinician at least once every 2 years, so this approach will address preventive care for the great majority of patients. Furthermore, because there is such a large gap between recommended and received preventive services in most practices and because there is so much preventive work to do, it will be most efficient to start with the patients with whom a practice has the greatest chance of achieving success: the ones right in the office. Therefore, the first system to put in place is one that seeks to identify the prevention needs for each patient at each visit and to document adherence to the prevention guidelines upon which the group has agreed. In many offices, this identification and monitoring function can be delegated to front office staff and medical assistants. An integral step in designing an office prevention program is to assign appropriate roles for *all* staff and clinicians for delivering and monitoring preventive care. The PPIP Guidebook provides a worksheet to assist practices in doing this. Some examples of staff roles are given in Table 21.1.

Once preventive service needs have been identified for individual patients, the medical assistant or nurse who rooms patients can have a central role in assuring that needed preventive services are delivered. If the clinicians have agreed to routine standing orders, the assistant can prepare referrals for needed routine preventive services such as mammograms and deliver some

---

TABLE 21.1 Roles of Office Staff in Identifying Patients' Prevention Needs

Receptionists can

Ask patients to complete a brief preventive services questionnaire as they check in

Encourage patients to ask the clinician about any preventive care questions they have

Place an age- and sex-appropriate preventive services flow sheet in each medical record

Medical assistants can

Review the preventive services flow sheet to determine what preventive services are due

Ask if the patient has received preventive services elsewhere and document these in the medical record

Document health habits: smoking status, alcohol use, physical activity, diet

Ensure that routine prevention screening instruments are completed

services such as immunizations. A clinician can be involved if the assistant is unsure of what to do or if the patient declines the recommended service. Some services, however, do require or benefit from the more routine involvement of a clinician. Clinician advice or counseling is especially powerful in helping to motivate patients to change health habits—e.g., smoking, risky alcohol use, poor diet, and physical inactivity—or where complex medical decisions are needed such as the evaluation of a positive depression screen. In these cases it is very helpful to provide reminders to the clinician that such advice or evaluation is needed, such as a red flag, post-it note, or screen prompt placed in a prominent spot so the clinician will not miss it.

Prevention and Visit Type

Many experts recommend that prevention be a part of every patient encounter, whether the patient is scheduled for a health maintenance examination, chronic illness visit, or acute problem visit. As noted in Chapter 20, it is not sufficient to address preventive needs only at "annual physicals" or other well-person checkups, because many of the patients most in need of preventive services do not come in for such checkups. On the other hand, clinicians may raise the reasonable objection that their first obligation is to tend to patients' current medical needs, leaving little time to address prevention issues. The answer to this is to use *standing orders* so that at least the services that can be routinely delegated will be included in the visit. In this section, we suggest ways to approach prevention at each type of visit without neglecting the competing demands of chronic disease follow-up and acute care. Prevention visits are the most straightforward, so we will address them first.

PREVENTION VISITS

Visits that traditionally include prevention activities are periodic health examinations ("physicals"), "Pap and pelvic" examinations, well-child examinations, sports preparticipation physicals, employment physicals, and preoperative examinations. As discussed in Chapter 20, a practice should have a written protocol and checklist to ensure that all of the preventive guidelines to which it has agreed are addressed at these visits. Although this could differ for each type of prevention visit, it is usually more efficient and effective to use a standardized approach tailored to age and gender rather than the reason for the prevention visit.

As recommended in Chapter 2, the patient, parent, or caretaker should complete a written or electronic health assessment form before the encounter to identify the patient's current preventive health needs. This need not be a separate form; it can be a section of a form that includes other necessary information such as the reason for the visit, past medical history, review of systems, current medications, and so on. When rooming the patient, the assistant can check the form for accuracy and completeness, review the patient's medical record for documentation of past preventive services, and probe further if needed. Using a checklist, flow sheet, or similar chart tool (see PPIP examples) that is based on the prevention protocol of the practice, the assistant can identify the preventive services that are due for this patient at this visit. The medical assistant can initiate as many preventive services as possible, leaving for the clinician only those requiring clinician expertise. In this manner, it is possible to identify and provide a wide array of preventive services efficiently at prevention visits without taking much clinician time. The patient, receptionist, medical assistant, and clinician all have critical roles, working as a team to identify and deliver the preventive services. The clinician's role is largely one of overseeing the visit, helping patients set prevention priorities, negotiating treatment plans, and helping patients in setting prevention goals that can be reviewed for progress at subsequent visits. Because staff are probably already busy, try to identify routine tasks that are not essential and reassign tasks when possible. For example, it may not be necessary to obtain certain vital signs routinely (e.g., respiration rate and pulse) and some types of information can be collected by receptionists or laboratory staff rather than the medical assistant. Chapters 9 (pages 238 and 248) and 10 (page 272) discuss procedures for systematically assessing tobacco and alcohol use when vital signs are taken.

CHRONIC ILLNESS VISITS

Many patients with chronic illnesses do not receive the preventive services that effective management requires. For example, patients with diabetes may not receive dietary and physical activity counseling and influenza immunization. Preventive services that reduce risk factors for a patient's existing chronic disease should take priority over less effective prevention activities. However, patients with chronic diseases are less likely than those without chronic disease to receive preventive services that are unrelated to their illness. For example, patients with chronic disease are less likely to receive some cancer screening tests than are those without those conditions (8). For patients with very short projected life spans, such "errors of omission" may not be errors at all but appropriate care. But for most people with chronic disease who live for many years, screening for other problems and providing appropriate preventive services may be especially important.

As with pure prevention visits, chronic disease visits provide an opportunity for the medical assistant or nurse to have a central role in prevention activities (e.g., determining which services are due and implementing standing orders).

ACUTE VISITS

Practices that are highly effective at delivering preventive services capitalize on visits for acute problems to address prevention issues. This may be the only time to address prevention with young men. Although prevention issues should not detract from addressing the patient's presenting complaint, there is often sufficient time to approach at least one prevention issue, especially if the receptionist, medical assistant, and clinician are all alert to prevention needs. If the medical record is well organized (preventive services tracked in one place) and the flow sheet is updated consistently, the preventive services for which a patient is due will be apparent at a glance. For example, consider a 65-year-old woman who presents with an upper respiratory infection that might take the clinician only 5 minutes to manage. A quick scan of her health maintenance flow sheet reveals that she is due for a mammogram and she has never had an influenza or pneumococcal immunization. The medical assistant notices these deficiencies and mentions them to the patient. The patient might agree to the mammogram and the flu shot because she has heard about their advantages but may hesitate to have the pneumococcal immunization.

The medical assistant orders the mammogram, gives a handout to the patient about pneumococcal immunization, and flags the chart for the clinician, noting that this patient wants the influenza vaccine but is unsure about pneumococcal immunization. After addressing the upper respiratory infection, if the clinician discusses the advantages of the pneumococcal immunization, the patient might agree to it. The small increase in clinician time can often be recompensed by a justifiably higher billing code (see Chapter 23, page 567). After the clinician departs, the nursing assistant returns and administers the immunizations. Perhaps this patient also screened positive today on the two-question depression screener. Because the clinician does not have time to address this issue today, she invites the patient to return later in the week for a 30-minute visit to follow up on this important problem.

PREVENTION TOOLS

The basic primary care office prevention tool kit requires screening forms, prevention flow sheets in each medical record, and some type of clinician reminders. The prevention tool kit can be paper, electronic, or a combination of paper and electronic. The practice will not be a high performer in preventive care unless its prevention tools are well designed and used regularly. (See Chapter 22 for guidance on electronic tools.) Practices that do not have electronic health records can make use of chart forms for preventive services that have been developed by a number of organizations. Although one may choose to use these forms as is, most practices will prefer to adapt forms to their own chart system. Off-the-shelf forms are typically too long and detailed to be practical or do not fit well with other chart forms used by the practice.

Screening Forms

Many prevention screening forms, also called *health risk profiles* or *health risk appraisal forms*, are available from vendors or are in the public domain. The PPIP Guidebook provides examples of detailed health risk profile forms for adults, children, and adolescents. Rather than using separate health risk profile forms, for efficiency and optimal use we recommend that health risk questions be a part of the practice's routine initial and periodic comprehensive patient health history forms. Figure 21.1 is a sample screening form. Patients

(This form is not meant to be used as is; it is an example of one possible format for a preventive screening questionnaire. You must decide on the content and format most appropriate for your practice.)

Name _____ Date _____ DOB _____

The following chart contains questions that ask you about certain tests and procedures that can help you and your doctor find potential health problems. The answers are important because they can help us prevent some illnesses such as the flu. The answers you give can also help to find problems such as breast or cervical cancer in their early stages.

PREVENTION QUESTION	YES	NO	NOT SURE	NURSE/DOCTOR COMMENTS
When was your last physical exam? (Please write the date in the Yes column)				
CHOLESTEROL				
Has your cholesterol been checked in the last 5 years?				
Do you have high cholesterol (hyperlipidemia)?				
TOBACCO USE				
Do you smoke or chew tobacco? If no, skip to the immunization question.				
Do you plan on quitting your use of tobacco soon, say in the next three months?				
IMMUNIZATIONS				
Have you had a tetanus shot in the last 10 years?				
Have you had a flu shot (influenza) in the last year?				
For those 65 and older:				
Have you had a pneumonia shot in your lifetime?				
COLON CANCER				
Have you had a test for colon cancer?				
WOMEN ONLY				
Do you perform self breast exams every month?				
Has a doctor examined your breasts in the last year?				
Have you had a Pap smear in the last 3 years?				
WOMEN 40-75				
Have you had a mammogram in the last year?				
MEN 50 AND OLDER				
Have you had a PSA test for prostate cancer in the past year?				
SAFETY				
Do you use a seat belt every time you ride in a car or truck?				

Figure 21.1 • Sample adult preventive services screening questionnaire.

can complete similar forms electronically using practice websites or software, and they can sometimes do so from the convenience of home before their appointments. See Chapter 2 (pages 45–46) for further details about the use and limitations of written and electronic screening questionnaires.

The health risk profile should be updated periodically because patient's health risks change with time. The PPIP Guidebook suggests that practices update a complete health risk profile for every patient every year. This may be impractical, but each practice should decide on the appropriate interval for its own patients, preferably applying different intervals for those in different age-groups.

Prevention Flow Sheets

Prevention flow sheets (or screen displays) are probably the most important prevention tool for a practice. There are certain principles for a good format: it should be simple, with a limited number of items, in a user-friendly layout, with an easily remembered periodicity. Similar types of prevention activities, such as cancer screening or health behaviors, can be grouped for quick reference. There are many possible designs for prevention flow sheets, and Figure 21.2 is an example. The PPIP Guidebook gives examples of

(This form is not meant to be used as is; it is an example of one possible format for a prevention flow sheet. You must decide on the content and format most appropriate for your practice.)

Name _____ DOB: _____

Procedure	Minimum Recommended Schedule	Dates of Procedures and Result Codes*		
Blood Pressure	Every 2 years			
Cholesterol	Every 5 years			
Risky Drinking Screen#	Yearly			
Pap Smear	Every 3 years after 3 consecutive yearly normals			
Breast Exam	Yearly (age >39)			
Mammogram	Every year (ages 50-74)			
Stool for Occult Blood	Yearly (age >49)			
Sigmoidoscopy, or	Every 5 years (age >49)			
Colonoscopy	Every 10 years (age >49)			
PSA	Offered yearly to men (age >49)			

#Greater than 14 drinks with alcohol a week for men and greater than 7 drinks a week for women

Immunizations	Minimal Recommended Schedule	Dates of Procedures and Result Codes*		
Influenza	Every year (age >64)			
Pneumococcal	Give once (age >64)			
Tetanus	Every 10 years			

*Suggested result codes: 0 = ordered, C = completed, R = refused, E = done

Figure 21.2 • Sample prevention flow sheet (gender neutral).

prevention flow sheets for adults, adolescents, and children. When flow sheets are updated and used diligently by staff and clinicians, they provide a current assessment of a patient's clinical preventive services needs at a glance. The problem is rarely with the forms themselves. Rather, without all the other steps—for example, clinician and patient reminders, audits, and reinforcements—the forms are unlikely to be used. The specific form is less important if it complies with the principles mentioned in the preceding text. The form is just a piece of paper or a display on a screen. Success is achieved not by any given form, but by using it as part of a system of care.

Reminders

The flow sheet is the ultimate "reminder" of what preventive services are due for which patients. Because clinicians and office staff are appropriately distracted at times because of more pressing patient needs, clever reminders can serve as double checks to ensure that intended services are provided. For example, receptionists can be delegated the task of scanning the prevention flow sheet to look for preventive services that are obviously due at the current visit. The receptionist then flags the chart for the medical assistant, perhaps by putting a check on the encounter form next to the needed service. The medical assistant notes the flag from the receptionist and double checks the prevention flow sheet as well. The medical assistant might provide a written and/or verbal reminder to the clinician about services to be addressed at this visit. Such "low-tech" reminder systems may eventually be replaced by electronic health records, which can automatically generate "pop-ups" and other screen prompts when preventive services are due (see Chapter 22). Computer-generated reminders, however, may not perform any better than an activated and aware office team that uses custom designed reminders for their office. The key is to tailor the reminder system to the desires, work flows, and record systems of each practice group. Whether reminders are low-tech or computerized, they will work much better if there is an activated and aware office team and if the reminders are tailored to the needs of the practice.

AUDITING DELIVERY OF PREVENTIVE CARE IN THE PRACTICE

Unless the practice systematically measures achievement of its preventive care goals, clinicians will not know how well they are doing and in what areas improvement is needed. Electronic health records, if properly configured, can make this task relatively painless (see Chapter 22). However, practices that do not have an electronic health record can use a combination of administrative data and chart audits. Many health plans and insurers, with their extensive billing and utilization data, provide summaries of performance on certain measures for which there is a specific billing code, such as a screening test (e.g., mammograms). But for other services, such as smoking cessation and physical activity counseling, a chart audit is often the only practical way to measure performance.

Chart audits are time consuming and therefore expensive, so sampling charts rather than auditing every one is the only feasible option. Although one needs a relatively large sample for statistical validity, 10 to 20 charts per measured subject are usually sufficient to obtain an adequate estimate of performance. The numbers get overwhelming, however, if a practice seeks to audit 20 charts per clinician on 20 different prevention activities, so consider whether the information needed about the system's function can be determined by just measuring performance at the whole practice level. The PPIP Guidebook provides guidance on chart audits. If a practice has not completed one before, the easiest way to start is to audit only at the practice level, not for each clinician. If there is a desire to obtain individual clinician data, it might be preferable to have the clinicians audit their own chart sample. It is more convincing when clinicians see their own care problems and experience how much time they waste by having to search a chart for information that could have been conveniently summarized on a single prevention flowsheet.

IMPROVING PERFORMANCE IN DELIVERING PREVENTIVE SERVICES

If a practice is serious about reaching a high level of performance in preventive care, there is a clear path to improvement that has been proved first in industry and subsequently in medicine (9). (a) Identify a small team of volunteers (including both staff and clinicians) to work on improving prevention for the whole practice. (b) Measure current performance against the guidelines the group has agreed upon. (c) Set feasible goals for improvement, but make them hard to reach so that system changes will be made. (d) Develop office systems for prevention, as described in the preceding text. (e) Measure performance periodically to identify areas where performance is not optimal. (f) Change systems in a way that will improve performance. (g) Measure again, and start the cycle of improvement over again. It may sound complicated, but as long as the practice keeps it as simple and systematic as possible, quality improvement should not be very difficult to accomplish.

ADVANCED OFFICE SYSTEMS FOR PREVENTION

So far, we have described office systems to support improved delivery of preventive services when patients are physically present in the office. Achieving an even higher level of performance may require developing outreach activities to engage patients who do not present to the office and enhancing prevention systems when patients are present. These activities require additional resources, so it is important to carefully prioritize these prevention enhancements.

Previsit Preparation

Reception staff can send patients a health history form that includes a health risk profile to complete at home before an office visit, or patients can be asked to complete the form online. Staff can also call a patient the day before the visit to remind them to bring the completed form to the visit. Staff can even review patients' records before health maintenance examinations and ask them to come in ahead of the visit for needed screening tests so that results can be available at the time of the visit. It may also be helpful to send the practice's recommendations for prevention and healthy living to patients (or post them on the practice website) to create an expectation that the clinician will be addressing these issues during the office visit.

During the Office Visit

Let patients know the philosophy of prevention by peppering the office with information about prevention and healthy living. Have easy-to-read health promotion materials available prominently in the waiting area and examination rooms, including a checklist of the screening and prevention guidelines for the practice. Consider displaying posters promoting healthy behaviors and screening throughout the office and playing health promotion videos in the waiting room. Use patient education handouts and websites liberally, offer decision aids when patients face complex choices about preventive services, and adopt systems to identify when the need for shared decision-making applies (see Chapter 4). Have hard copies and website addresses available in a convenient place where medical assistants and clinicians can quickly access the right ones for a given patient. For larger practices, consider hiring a health educator to assist patients with health behavior change for healthy eating, physical activity, weight loss, dealing with risky drinking, and smoking cessation. For smaller practices, medical assistants or nurses can be trained to perform these tasks. An alternative to in-office behavioral counseling is to refer patients to prevention resources available in the community (e.g., group classes, commercial weight loss programs) or elsewhere (e.g., tobacco quit lines, interactive websites). Practices should maintain an annually updated list of resources that they have evaluated and trust to share with patients. This is a task ideally assigned to an interested staff member who can develop special expertise about community resources. Finally, paper and electronic systems for determining body mass index and calculating an individual's risk of breast cancer (e.g., Gail model) or cardiovascular disease (e.g., Framingham model) can improve the accuracy of advice given to patients (see Chapters 1 and 15). Medical assistants can be trained to calculate the risk and record it prominently in patients' medical records, and electronic health records can display the indices as automatic prompts.

After the Visit

Staff can maintain a log of all screening tests ordered to ensure appropriate follow-up of results. When results are returned to the office, they can check off the test and send a copy of all test results to the patients after checking abnormal results with the clinician. Increasingly, patients will be able to obtain test results directly from password-secure websites, telephone recordings, or direct access to the electronic health record. (By law in many states mammogram results are mailed directly to patients by the testing facility.) Reception or laboratory staff can review the log monthly and contact those patients who have not yet had results returned. If the practice has the resources to determine who is overdue for preventive services, staff can mail reminders, call patients, or send reminder emails. The practice can maintain a registry of preventive visits by date of last visit and send reminders to patients who are overdue, as do many dentists. All of the enhancements we have listed are designed to optimize the reach and completeness of the practice's delivery of preventive services. It is unlikely that a practice can achieve the highest level of performance without some kind of outreach activities and enhancements of office prevention systems.

PATIENTS AS PREVENTION PARTNERS

Engaging patients as partners in prevention is essential. Patients who are educated about the importance of a healthy lifestyle and periodic screening, and who expect certain services from the practice, can serve as catalysts for improvement. The practice can activate patients in several ways that are complementary. For example, the prominent posting of prevention materials throughout the office can prompt patients to remind clinicians about their needed services. Staff can encourage patients to advocate for themselves, for example, to call if they do not receive test results within a reasonable time period.

CONCLUSION

If a medical practice or group really wants to survive and thrive in a world that is increasingly demanding and yet ready to pay more for consistently high quality medical services, it will have to invest in some of the systems described in this chapter. It will also have to learn how to manage change in an efficient and effective way. These are not skills taught in medical school, but many clinicians have learned them, often by trial and error. One common error is to simply try to implement a system from elsewhere without adapting it to the practice's individual situation and needs and to the needs of its patient population. Another is to skip the kind of thorough management of the process needed for effective change, including baseline and periodic simple measurement. Although it is important to Keep Improvement efforts both Simple and Systematic (KISS), it is as problematic to make it too simple by skipping essential steps, such as providing clear job responsibilities. Finally, no amount of practice redesign can solve problems that require system solutions beyond the practice. Health systems and health plans in which practices operate—not just the practices—bear some responsibility for system redesign to improve preventive care.

RESOURCES—PATIENT EDUCATION MATERIALS

Put Prevention Into Practice. *A Step by Step Guide to Delivering Clinical Preventive Services: A Systems Approach*. Agency for Healthcare Research and Quality. Accessible at: http://www.ahrq.gov/ppip/manual/

SUGGESTED READINGS

Dietrich AJ, Woodruff CB, Carney PA. Changing office routines to enhance preventive care: the preventive GAPS approach. *Arch Fam Med* 1994;3: 176–183.

Leininger Ls, Finn L, Dickey L, et al. An office system for organizing preventive services: a report by the American Cancer Society Advisory Group on preventive health care reminder systems. *Arch Fam Med* 1996;5: 108–115.

Pommerenke FA, Dietrich A. Improving and maintaining preventive services, Part 1: identifying barriers and opportunities by applying the patient path model. *J Fam Pract* 1992;34: 86–91.

Pommerenke FA, Dietrich A. Improving and maintaining preventive services, Part 2: practical principles for primary care. *J Fam Pract* 1992;34: 92–97.

Solberg LI, Brekke ML, Fazio CJ, et al. Lessons from experienced guideline implementers: attend to many factors and use multiple strategies. *Jt Comm J Qual Improv* 2000;26(4): 171–188.

Solberg LI, Kottke TE, Conn SA, et al.. Delivering clinical preventive services is a systems problem. *Ann Behav Med* 1997;19(3): 271–278.

Thompson RS, Taplin SH, McAfee TA, et al. Primary and secondary prevention services in clinical practice: twenty years' experience in development, implementation, and evaluation. *JAMA* 1995;273: 1130–1135.

References

1. Fisher ES, Wennberg DE, Stukel TA, et al. The implications of regional variations in Medicare spending. Part 1: the content, quality, and accessibility of care. *Ann Intern Med* 2003;138(4):273–287.
2. Solberg LI, Kottke TE, Brekke ML, et al. The case of the missing clinical preventive services systems. *Eff Clin Pract* 1998;1(1):33–38.

3. Wennberg JE, Freeman JL, Culp WJ. Are hospital services rationed in New Haven or over-utilised in Boston? *Lancet* 1987;1(8543):1185–1189.
4. Solberg LI, Brekke ML, Kottke TE. How important are clinician and nurse attitudes to the delivery of clinical preventive services? *J Fam Pract* 1997;44(5):451–461.
5. Solberg LI. The KISS principle in family practice: keep it simple and systematic. *Fam Pract Manag* 2003;10(7):63–66.
6. Schein E. *The corporate culture survival guide*. San Francisco: Jossey-Bass, 1999.
7. Yarnall KS, Pollak KI, Ostbye T, et al. Primary care: is there enough time for prevention? *Am J Public Health* 2003;93(4):635–641.
8. Fontana SA, Baumann LC, Helberg C, et al. The delivery of preventive services in primary care practices according to chronic disease status. *Am J Public Health* 1997;87(7):1190–1196.
9. Langley GJ, Nolan KM, Norman CL, et al. *The improvement guide: a practical approach to enhancing organizational performance*. San Francisco: Jossey-Bass, 1996.

CHAPTER 22

Improving Preventive Care Using Automated Tools

J. Marc Overhage

INTRODUCTION

Information technology that is based evermore on the digital media has evolved rapidly in recent years. It now plays a significant role in the everyday lives of many people. The public makes regular use of e-mail, digital photography, cellular telephones, personal digital assistants (PDAs), and their progeny (e.g., Blackberry-type devices) to manage many aspects of their daily routines. Modern information technology has also transformed many industries in the United States. However, health care lags behind in this transformation. Although some venues in health care, such as the laboratory and the pharmacy, have adopted modern information technology, direct patient care processes have made less use of this resource. In fact, most physician practices in the United States continue to rely on paper-based medical records and likely will for some time to come (1). Clinicians in such practices can find suggestions in Chapter 21 on how to improve preventive care with manual systems. This chapter focuses on the role of automated tools. Even clinicians who have not yet adopted computerized information technology may nonetheless find in this chapter useful ideas about the directions their practices could take in the future.

Those practices that have adopted electronic systems to improve preventive care have taken a number of different approaches. Some have implemented a computerized *registry* for diseases or risk factors. This is a system by which a practice maintains a list of patients with specific risk factors (e.g., elevated serum lipids) or diseases/conditions (e.g., diabetes) along with selected data that are critical to monitoring their condition (e.g., glycosylated hemoglobin levels). As noted in Chapter 21, these systems can be used, for example, to generate lists of patients who need specific screening tests or treatments at given times. Chapter 16 notes the value of immunization registries. Such lists can facilitate the sending of reminder letters to these patients in order to facilitate their monitoring and management over time.

However, although these systems can be quite effective, they often require the practice staff to perform a great deal of data entry. Therefore, they may be less practical for preventive care because almost every patient in the practice must be entered into the registry. Despite the effort involved, some practices have effectively utilized registry systems to improve their preventive care. In recent years, large practices and a few communities (2) have begun to implement registries using data from sources such as radiology centers, laboratories, and public health departments combined with practice management or claims data. These systems reduce the time and effort required to maintain the data and may offer economies including avoiding capital expenses for the individual practice.

Electronic Record Keeping and Management

One way to overcome the challenges of implementing a registry—at the expense of meeting other challenges—is to implement an *electronic medical record* (EMR). As defined by the American Health Information Management Association, an EMR consists of electronic versions of the data and documents found in a paper-based legal medical record, such as structured data, diagnostic images, wave forms, scanned images of paper documents, and other types of documentation.

Some experts view the term "electronic medical record" as too narrow and too steeped in the traditional medical model of care. They prefer the term *electronic health record* (EHR). The EHR is far more than simply an electronic version of the traditional paper record. According to the Health Information Management Systems Society, EHRs aid clinicians by providing access to health information from patients, when needed, and guidance to help clinicians make evidence-based decisions. EHRs automate and streamline clinician workflow, ensuring that clinical information is effectively communicated, thereby decreasing the potential for delays or gaps in care. Some systems also support the collection of data for uses other than clinical care, such as billing, quality management, outcomes reporting, and public health disease surveillance and reporting. This chapter focuses on the evidence-based decision and clinical decision support capability of EHRs.

Patient-centered information technology can be used to empower the consumer with important tools. In recent years, the concept of a *personal health record* (PHR) has emerged. According to the Markle Foundation (www.markle.org), a PHR is a digital health record that is owned, updated, and controlled by the consumer. It contains a summary of health information gathered throughout an individual's entire lifetime. In addition to immunizations, a personal and family health history, medication lists, and other medical information, the PHR may contain information such as certain symptoms, home health monitoring results (e.g., capillary blood glucose measurements), and exercise patterns that are typically not recorded in the clinician's record. Some PHRs even provide simple clinical decision support. A number of large employers and payers, including the Medicare program, provide patients with access to PHRs that generate reminders to carry out preventive services such as mammograms or colonoscopies based on diagnoses or procedures included in claims.

In reference to the issue of self-management of chronic illnesses, Bodenheimer et al. concluded that "Patients with chronic conditions self-manage their illness. This fact is inescapable. Each day, patients decide what they are going to eat, whether they will exercise, and to what extent they will consume prescribed medications" (3). Although their comments were directed at patients with chronic illnesses, they apply equally to preventive behaviors as well. Information technology is introducing tools to help patients manage their health and adopt healthy behaviors (4). Most of these tools are available through the Internet. Some are included in PHRs and cellular telephones, and PDAs are increasingly being discussed as a delivery device. These tools can help patients track their behaviors, participate in online support groups, provide information and, in a few cases, provide rewards for behavior change.

THE RATIONALE FOR USING AUTOMATED SYSTEMS IN PRACTICE

There are four reasons why a practice might want to utilize a clinical decision support system (CDSS) to reliably deliver preventive care:

1. **Too many data.** There is an ever increasing number of preventive services recommended for patients and an expanding amount of clinical data that must be reviewed by clinicians in order to assess the appropriateness of preventive interventions. Without electronic aids, it becomes impossible for even the best clinician to synthesize and act upon this information in the time available during a typical visit.

2. **The decision space has become too complicated.** The correct implementation of recommendations such as those from the *Expert Panel on Detection, Evaluation, and Treatment of High Blood Cholesterol in Adults* depend on appropriate assessments of the patient's risk of a cardiovascular event (5). Even the much-simplified classifications developed by this panel to assist clinicians in managing such patients are too complicated to readily remember, much less calculate. As discussed in Chapter 1 (page 19), automated systems can easily perform these computations and provide precise estimates of risk based on the formal risk models developed for the guidelines (e.g., Framingham and Gail models).

3. **Too little time.** As discussed in Chapter 20, the number of psychosocial, medical, and remunerative tasks that occupy the typical patient encounter leave little time to address preventive care.

4. **Cognitive limitations.** As Clement McDonald wrote as far back as 1976 (6), man is a fallible data processor. The human brain is not

designed to reliably, reproducibly, and repetitively complete such tasks—computers are.

As Chapters 20 and 21 have already emphasized, the key to high quality health care can be summed up in the popular phrase "Do it right, the first time, every time" The frequency and importance of preventive services requires clinicians to create and adopt systems and processes of care to ensure that they are addressed with each patient, as early as appropriate, each and every time they are indicated.

Systematic reviews have documented that automated tools, especially reminder and clinical decision support functions, are among the most effective methods to help clinicians achieve high levels of performance and improve adherence to clinical care protocols. These studies have demonstrated, for example, that rates of influenza vaccination, pneumococcal vaccination, and fecal occult blood testing increased from 12% to 33% when such tools were used (7–9). Because most of this evidence comes from a few "benchmark" institutions and there are few studies of commercial systems, these findings may not generalize to an individual practice (10).

Implementing an automated disease registry or an EHR is a challenge for most practices, but even more work is required to use that system to improve preventive care. This chapter will now focus on four of those issues: (a) the importance of the knowledge base or rules that define what the EHR will do, (b) the need for the computer system to have access to the data that guidelines demand for decision making in a format that the computer system can interpret, (c) the five criteria required for reminders or feedback delivered by the computer system to be effective, and (d) how to integrate the reminders that a computer system generates into the clinical workflow of a practice. Specialty societies, government agencies, and others are creating practice guidelines. However, these guidelines are intended for a clinician—not a computer system—to interpret. In order to involve the computer as an effective aid for the clinician, these guidelines have to be translated into a format that a computer can understand and use—a knowledge base.

Telling the System What it Needs to Do

Computers are powerful tools but they can only do what they are told to do. In order to have automated systems support preventive care delivery, the practice must define the tasks they want the system to perform. Fortunately, most systems do not require the user to write computer programs to accomplish these goals. However, the tasks defined for the system must be stated in terms that a computer can understand, which many describe as a *knowledge base*. A "knowledge base" contains information about care policies, whereas the *database* stores data about the patient. The programming combines information in the knowledge base with the clinical data for each patient to determine which care the patient should receive. Compared with disease management guidelines, preventive care guidelines are relatively simple. This makes them ideally suited for having automated systems produce reliable clinical recommendations.

The research discussed in the preceding text, which demonstrates the effectiveness of automated systems for improving adherence to guidelines, was performed largely by organizations that developed their own systems and knowledge bases. Most practices, however, will purchase commercial products that may provide limited knowledge bases or lack processes to import further knowledge developed by the particular user. Many of these products do advertise the ability of practices to create their own knowledge base for the system. In reality, however, few clinicians have the energy, expertise, or time to create their own knowledge bases. They will need to understand the knowledge base that is available from the vendor. Fortunately, preventive care is probably the most common area covered by knowledge bases offered in commercial products.

If a practice is forced to create its own knowledge base, it should first define the "knowledge" to include. That is, the practice should determine which preventive guidelines or protocols it wishes to adopt. Chapter 20 discusses this process in detail. Although some guidelines are readily accessible electronically, clinical guidelines often lack explicit criteria and often use vague terms (11). Because automated systems require explicit definitions, creating a functional knowledge base may require the practice to conduct painstaking research and make difficult decisions about how to define these ambiguities in terms of fields of data (12). As guideline developers have become more aware of these translational challenges, they have begun to provide more explicit criteria and produce simpler guidelines (13).

Not all decisions surrounding preventive care are simple, however. As society enters an age of "personalized medicine," in which screening and treatment are tailored to an individual's genomic, proteomic, and pharmacodynamic characteristics, automated systems will become essential tools for performing the complicated computations required. Already, the scope of the data and the complexity of the models far outstrip the clinician's capacity to properly perform these computations. However, although automated systems can readily perform the complex computations, if their products are to be useful it is vital that they deliver the results of these computations to clinicians in forms that they can understand and communicate to their patients.

Making Sure the System Has the Data It Requires

An automated system requires access to appropriate data to create reminders. These data are likely to come from a variety of different sources, inside or outside the practice. But they always have to be captured and stored in a way that the system can interpret.

DATA FROM INSIDE THE PRACTICE

Some of the most important data to capture from inside the practice include patient demographics (e.g., date of birth which is needed to compute age, gender), vital signs (e.g., height, weight), blood pressures, operational and functional components (OFCs), and in-office laboratory test results. Many of these data are recorded by hand, typically on paper. Some of them are generated by simple instruments such as automated blood pressure measurement devices, electrocardiographs, or table-top laboratory instruments. Recovering data from these two types of sources—manual and automated—pose different challenges. Information recorded by hand must be entered into a computer system to be of use to automated CDSSs. Arranging for such data entry may well require a change in practice workflow. When data such as a glycosylated hemoglobin result is created by a table-top instrument, it can often be captured from a printer port or another connection on the instrument for storage in the computer system. However, although such data are now available from these instruments in a format the computer can understand, they are rarely linked to patient identifiers. In many cases, the practice staff must add this information into the system in order to match the laboratory data to the corresponding patient.

DATA COLLECTED DIRECTLY FROM PATIENTS

As noted in Chapters 1 and 2, patient questionnaires and health-risk appraisals help patients identify risks and make positive behavior choices particularly when employers or health plans offer financial incentives for program participation. Such instruments can be administered through automated health risk appraisal systems, PHRs (14), or in-office systems (15). In addition to their role in assisting patients directly, these automated tools can also provide patient-entered data that are useful to the clinician in providing preventive care. For example, patients may report health behaviors (e.g., smoking) that might otherwise escape the attention of the clinician.

Because health information standards and uniform policies for such systems are not yet widely adopted, few practices are currently able to incorporate data from health risk appraisal systems or PHRs except by entering results that patients bring to the practice on paper. Even if the technical challenges of transferring data from patient sources to EHRs can be overcome, policy and practice challenges require resolution before practices can confidentially incorporate these data directly into an EHR. Privacy concerns must be addressed so that patients are aware that their answers will enter the medical record. Moreover, it is unclear whether a clinician can rely fully on a patient's description of the name and date of preventive services they have received or of the medications they are taking. Patients are certainly the best source for reporting health habits (e.g., diet) and whether they are taking medications, but they may confuse the name of tests or immunizations they have received, the names of drugs they have taken, or the correct date on which tests or immunizations were administered.

DATA FROM OUTSIDE HEALTH SYSTEMS

Data that come from outside the practice often start life in a computer system. For example, laboratory test results are usually stored in a commercial laboratory information system, the record of dispensed drugs is usually stored in a pharmacy information system, and images and interpretations reside in a radiology information system. These systems typically have the capability to send results to practice computer systems using standard message formats that can be interpreted and linked with the correct patient. Unfortunately, because a practice typically receives these data from a wide variety of laboratories and other sources, creating automated methods to capture them can be a daunting task. Some practices are able to identify and work with a limited number of key sources that provide significant amounts of data. It is feasible for current technology to interface electronically with a limited number of outside data sources.

MESSAGE FORMATS FOR EXCHANGED DATA

In order to receive data from outside systems such as laboratories, the automated system of a practice should only use standard message formats. "Message formats" are agreed upon conventions about where and how different types of information will be transmitted. Just as envelopes could not be used for mailing if return and recipient addresses appeared in inconsistent locations and formats, data transferred to practice computer systems cannot be interpreted without a standard format. HL/7 (Health Level 7; see www.hl7.org) is the most common.

CODING SYSTEMS FOR REPRESENTING DATA

As mentioned earlier, in order to provide highly specific, clinically appropriate reminders, automated systems require access to patient data in a form that the systems can use. The data must be identified using terminologies or codes that the system can understand. The associated value must be clearly interpretable. For example, in order to calculate a patient's body mass index, the system must have access to the patient's weight and height and must know the units in which they are measured so that it can make the appropriate calculation.

All practices share a need to represent these types of data in an understandable way. In particular, using a consistent set of terms or codes to identify data greatly simplifies the interpretation of information (e.g., laboratory results) that the automated system receives from either other outside sources or automated devices in the office. Just as International Classification of Diseases (ICD-9) and Current Procedural Terminology

(CPT) codes are used across health systems as a common language for identifying diseases and procedures (see Chapter 23), automated systems use generally accepted coding systems or vocabularies for most important clinical content. These include RxNORM (http://www.nlm.nih.gov) for medications, LOINC (http://www.loinc.org) for laboratory results, and SNOMED (http://www.snomed.org) codes for other clinical findings. A clinician does not need great familiarity with these coding systems but should recognize their importance and insist that their vendor use them whenever possible.

Effective Reminders

Chapter 21 discusses the importance of reminder systems to improve preventive care. If a practice uses an EHR or other software with which the clinician interacts during a patient encounter, reminders can be delivered at the point of care. These reminders can potentially incorporate data such as vital signs or relevant risk factors entered earlier during the encounter. The most sophisticated systems can even generate "orders" for preventive services that the clinician can review and approve (Fig. 22.1).

Automated systems are well suited to generate such reminders, but they must adhere to five important principles to be effective. They must be:

1. Available at the time of care
2. Specifically actionable
3. Concise
4. Specific to the patient and appropriate to the setting
5. Correct at least 75% of the time

When evaluating a given vendor's knowledge base, the practice should keep these principles in mind and look at practical examples of the reminders that the product will generate. When practices must create their own knowledge base, they will want to apply these principles in designing the prompts the system will generate.

1. **Available at the time of care.** Reminders are most effective when they are delivered at the point of care ("just in time"). They stand in contrast with periodic reminders delivered intermittently in batches (e.g., reminders generated at the start or end of the day or month) (16). Intermittent batches are superior to no reminders at all, but many actions are easier for the clinician to initiate if the patient is present. Reminders to obtain blood tests, collect information for and from the patient, start new therapies, or educate the patient are all more difficult to act upon when the patient must be contacted outside of an encounter. In addition, point-of-care prompts are more effective because the clinician is usually already thinking about the specific patient and because both the clinician and patient are more prepared to make decisions about their care. Finally, point-of-care (just-in-time) reminders capture more

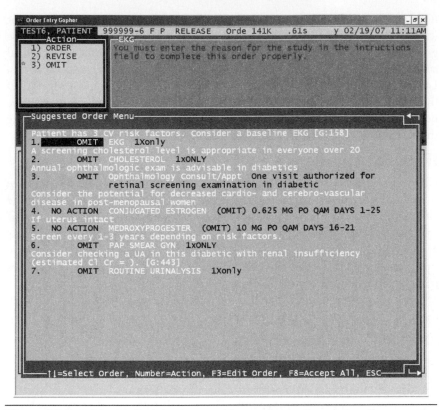

Figure 22.1 • The Medical Gopher provides sophisticated reminders for preventive care, diagnosis, and treatment.

current data, including information gathered during the course of the visit. However, they are more difficult to implement (9). Implementing point-of-care reminders is more difficult because they require identifying triggering events that the CDSS can utilize and creating a vehicle to deliver the reminders to the provider at precisely the moment that they are considering how to deal with that problem for that patient.

2. **Specifically actionable.** Actionable reminders are essential to changing clinician behavior. That is, the clinician must be able to respond to the reminder by taking some specific action. If the reminder provides some facts about the patient without a specific action to take or recommends interventions the clinician cannot implement for some reason, users will become frustrated and less likely to act on reminders in the future. Forcing clinicians to respond to reminders has been demonstrated to increase adherence by house staff physicians but not by experienced internists (17). Delivering reminders in the form of fully formed orders in an EHR is the ideal approach to making them actionable.

3. **Concise.** Concise, rather than verbose, reminders are preferred, although the verbose reminders may be informative. Reminders, just like commercial advertising, must catch the eye and convey a message in a very short time. The clinician should not have to work very hard to interpret the reminder. For example, a reminder to prescribe an angiotensin-converting enzyme (ACE) inhibitor might be "treat with ACE inhibitor because of diabetes and hypertension" followed by a suggested order for a specific ACE inhibitor at a standard dosage. The reminder conveys the underlying rationale but presumes that the clinician will recognize the connection. The practice might create a more detailed, explanatory version of the reminder for times when it is needed. This might be:

This 58-year-old diabetic patient (added to the problem list 12 years ago) has poorly controlled hypertension (mean of the last three systolic blood pressures was 158 and the mean of the last three diastolic blood pressures was 94). Because angiotensin-converting enzyme inhibitors have been demonstrated to slow the progression of renal disease and improve the quality of life in patients with diabetes, treatment with an ACE inhibitor appears warranted. R:14597; R:19390

This (relatively) verbose reminder provides links to supporting literature (the numbers preceded by R's) and to local guidelines that provide a detailed, authoritative explanation of the rationale. Providing links to supporting evidence improves the impact of reminders. However, the value of adding them is limited by the infrequency with which most clinicians will examine the references.

4. **Specific to the patient/appropriate to the setting.** The previous examples illustrate how reminders can be patient specific. General reminders to treat patients with diabetes and hypertension with ACE inhibitors will be less effective than the individualized prompt described in the preceding example. Nonspecific reminders force the clinician to first extract the facts (does the patient have hypertension or diabetes?), to determine whether the patient is already taking an ACE inhibitor, and, if not, to decide whether it should be prescribed. Making reminders specific to the patient also reduces the number of times clinicians are exposed to reminders and therefore enhances their impact when prompts do appear.

In addition to being specific to the patient, reminders that are specific to the setting are more effective in changing clinician behavior than those that lack such specificity. Clinicians are less likely to react to reminders that seem irrelevant to their domain of responsibility. For example, a reminder to administer an immunization, directed to the same clinician, is less likely to be acted upon when the patient is being seen at a Saturday morning "sick visit" than at a scheduled well child visit.

There is an evolving literature that advocates delivering preventive care at any opportunity (see page 527), including during visits to the emergency department or during hospital admissions. The clinician caring for the patient in these settings may not recognize that the patient is eligible for these interventions and may not feel it is their role to deal with these issues. Computer-generated reminders can directly address some of these issues by incorporating clinical data from a variety of sources, including evolving health information exchanges, and can use this information to generate reminders. In some cases these reminders may be delivered to someone other than the clinician in order to decrease the clinician's cognitive load and to increase the odds that the preventive service will be delivered.

The author's research team studied reminders for preventive care that were issued while patients were hospitalized, a strategy aimed at targeting a time when patients were available and when delivery of the preventive service would be easy. The study found that the reminder was ineffective when the clinician receiving it was not the patient's primary care clinician (18). When surveyed, the explanation given by the respondents was that physicians caring for hospitalized patients were not responsible for the preventive care of another physician's patients. A subsequent study of an intervention that dealt constructively with this issue achieved improved adherence to the reminders (19).

5. **Correct most of the time.** In order for clinicians to remain confident that the reminders are worth reading, in the clinicians view the reminders should be clinically appropriate approximately 75% of the time. In some cases, achieving this level of specificity may require trading off sensitivity. In other cases, it may require more elaborate logic (programming). Reminders are only as good as the data on which they are based. Clinicians should not use reminders unless the data they require are available and reliable. If a practice establishes a reminder for influenza vaccinations but lacks data about prior vaccinations or stores data only for influenza vaccinations for members of one health plan, then the system will generate a number of "false-positive" reminders. Clinician confidence in the system may then be jeopardized. Even small perturbations in their perceived validity can nullify the effect of reminders. For example, at a health system in which the reminders were appropriate for many years, a transient delay in capturing mammogram results severely eroded clinician confidence in mammography reminders. Clinicians' memory for mistakes or inconvenience is long.

In certain settings and for carefully selected preventive services, it may be possible and appropriate to put orders into effect as an automatic function (20). For example, the EHR can generate a referral for a screening mammogram when the system recognizes that more than 2 years have elapsed since the last screening. Before adopting this approach, the practice must decide who is qualified to authorize such decisions. For example, does the clinician have to be involved in the decision to administer a pneumococcal vaccination to a 68-year-old woman? Keeping the clinician on the critical path for reacting to every reminder can create an onerous burden; a clinician could easily be overwhelmed by the many preventive services that an automated system might flag. By creating "closed loop" control systems, a practice can focus a clinician's explicit decision making on the most critical issues rather than the routine, low risk issues.

INTEGRATING REMINDERS INTO THE WORKFLOW

As challenging as creating an automated clinical system can be, integrating the reminders into the workflow of a practice can be even harder. As already noted, it is ideal for reminders about preventive care to be delivered at the time the patient is on hand in the office. However, the system may also periodically generate a list of patients and the preventive care for which they are eligible. Clinicians may find this registry function useful for identifying patients for whom a preventive service is indicated but who have not presented for care, an example of the outreach discussed on pages 541–543 of Chapter 21.

Many preventive care guidelines include some temporal component (e.g., screening colonoscopy in average-risk patients is recommended beginning at age 50 years and every 10 years thereafter; see page 111). However, an otherwise healthy patient may not visit the clinician until after they turn 50 years of age, delaying the offer of screening for colorectal cancer. Automated systems can periodically query a database of patient information and identify all patients for whom a preventive service is indicated, or soon will be. In order to make the patient lists as specific as possible, such systems should take into account when the intervention was last completed, as well as other patient characteristics. Clinicians do not want the burden of reviewing the charts of all patients older than 50 years to determine whether they have been screened; that is what computers are good for.

Systems that generate point-of-care reminders can deliver these prompts on paper or on a computer display. As discussed in Chapter 21, reminders delivered on paper have been successfully used for many years. Paper does have its advantages. Printouts used as reminders were the only option in the early years of medical computing, before the existence of "personal computers" and when teleprinters were not amenable to use in clinical settings. Although as noted above society has many more technologic options now, including PDAs, cellular telephones, and wireless laptops and palmtops, paper can still be a viable and effective tool. Figure 22.2 illustrates early and

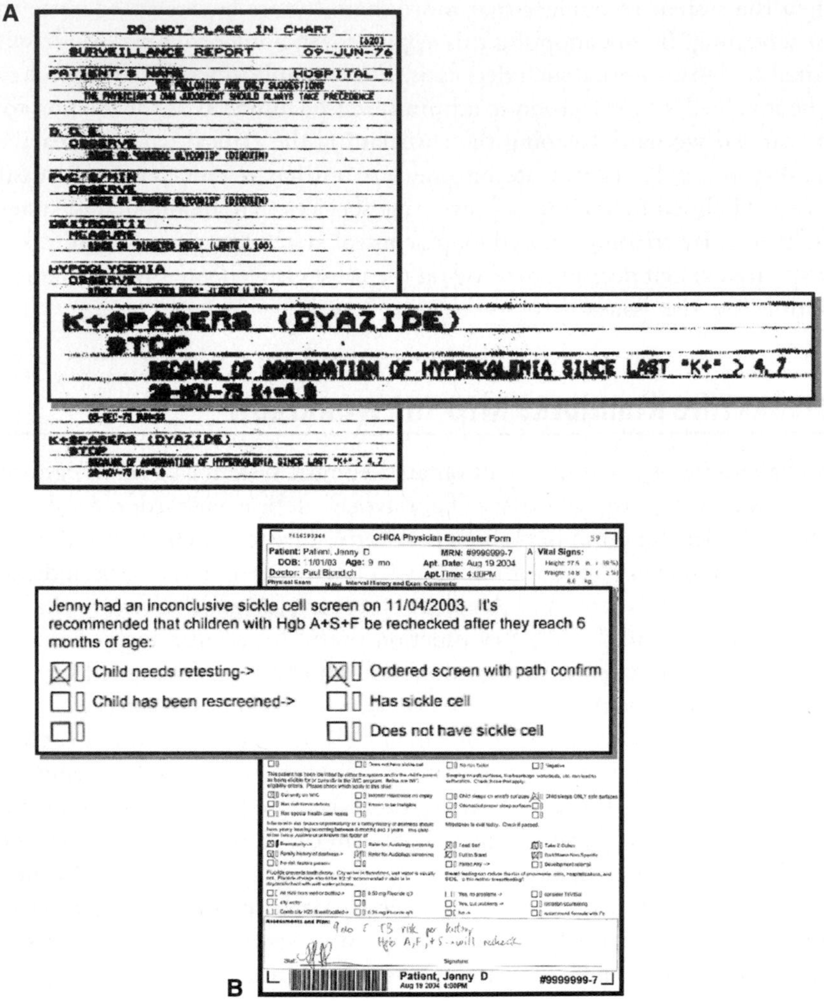

Figure 22.2 • Panel **A** illustrates a paper-based reminder from the 1970s and panel **B** illustrates a contemporary example.

contemporary examples of reminders delivered on paper. Advances in printer and computing technology, sophistication of software, and optical character recognition have combined to make paper a very attractive option in many settings. In addition to serving as a vehicle for reminding clinicians, the hard copy serves as a record for documenting actions taken. An advantage of paper reminders is that they can be more easily integrated into the existing workflow of some practices that cannot use screen displays. At practices that use paper charts, the staff can place paper reminders on the chart, either as they prepare charts the night before or when patients "check-in." The paper form is a convenient place to record information, make note of scheduling for tests, and list other follow-up tasks. Conversely, an advantage of paperless systems is that the reminding, documentation, and billing can all be done at once.

In the past, transferring information from hard copy to a computer system required manual data entry. However, contemporary technologies allow these data to be automatically imported into a database. One promising example of this technology is the Child Health Improvement through Computer Automation (CHICA) system (21), which is intended for practices that do not have an EHR or those that have an EHR but want to use simple paper-based interfaces to capture data from clinicians and patients. By using optical character recognition, "mark sense reading," and image capture, the CHICA system is designed to provide "just-in-time" clinical content to clinicians through a familiar, flexible paper interface. It uses patient-specific, computer-interpretable paper forms, known as *adaptive turnaround documents* (ATDs), to accurately capture handwritten data (15). The data captured on these forms allow CHICA to print clinical alerts and reminders on a clinician-directed ATD, along with relevant patient handouts. Interacting this way with clinicians allows CHICA to provide information in a manner that is exquisitely sensitive to work flow constraints.

PATIENT FOLLOW-UP

Whether the practice generates reminders as lists or when a patient presents for care, it must create a process for follow-up: determining whether the patient was offered the service, the decision, and the eventual result. For example, the practice might establish a routine to generate these lists, perhaps monthly, with clearly assigned responsibility for follow-up to ensure that the patient is contacted and offered the appropriate screening or other intervention. For an automated system to function correctly, the practice routine must include the steps of documenting these contacts, the patients' decisions to accept or decline the preventive care, and the date the preventive service was completed. Lacking this information, the system will endlessly issue reminders for preventive services that patients have already received. Entering these data will also provide a degree of medicolegal protection and can simplify a clinician's work by eliminating these patients from subsequent lists. The documentation may also provide opportunities for increased revenue as pay for performance programs proliferate (see page 579).

Over time many valuable and potentially interesting reminders could potentially be added to an established automated reminder system, but practices should think carefully about doing so. "Reminder overload" can be worse than no information, as clinicians are overwhelmed with dozens of reminders per patient and perhaps many hundreds of reminders in a single day. Aside from the difficulty of prioritizing so many reminders, clinicians who feel overwhelmed may be tempted to ignore them or to deactivate the prompts to eliminate the frustration.

In addition to reminding the clinician, automated systems can also be used to send reminders directly to patients. This approach has been shown to improve uptake of preventive services (22) and is discussed further in Chapter 21. Patient reminders can take the form of a personalized letter to the patient, often signed by the patient's clinician. The letter can inform patients that the practice wants to be sure that they receive the highest quality care possible and that current best practice is for them to receive a specific preventive service at a designated time (e.g., in the next 2 months). The letter can discuss the rationale for the service, what it entails, and how it can be obtained or scheduled; the clinician can offer to discuss the importance and implications by telephone or in person. Such correspondence, which can also take the form of postcards or e-mails, can as well be used to encourage patients to adopt healthy behaviors (e.g., exercise, smoking cessation) and to maintain healthy habits.

A practice that decides to incorporate direct-to-patient reminders as part of its preventive care strategy should create a regular process for generating, mailing, or otherwise delivering the reminders. The correspondence must be attentive to patient privacy concerns; patients may not wish information to be disclosed to spouses or other household members (see the next section).

PRIVACY AND CONFIDENTIALITY

Although patient privacy is always a paramount concern for clinicians, greater vigilance is required with an automated system. Automated systems can safeguard access to patient data by using security procedures for logging of all data accesses. However, many remain vulnerable to abuse—unauthorized access to personal data—if procedures are not followed conscientiously. As is well known, the Federal government passed the Health Insurance Portability and Accountability Act of 1996 (HIPAA), which defines a national "floor" for privacy and security of automated health information. Some states have enacted more stringent laws or regulations which supersede HIPAA. Under HIPAA, a practice may use a patient's personal health information for health care delivery or payment, as well as for public health or research purposes under certain circumstances. Practices must also enforce good physical, network, application, and procedural security. Given the complexity of the topic, practices should consider engaging consultation for assistance with creating and implementing their privacy and security practices. It is not an issue they can afford to ignore.

CONCLUSION

All clinicians want to deliver the best care possible for their patients. Doing so requires that they recognize their limitations in managing and delivering relevant information about, to, and for patients. Clinicians should consider the usefulness of automated systems and processes to compensate for these limitations and increase the odds for success. Automated systems can tirelessly execute logic; they can expand the amount of just-in-time data available to clinicians while also helping them focus on important preventive services to consider. They can provide automatic guardrails to enhance the safety and quality of the care that clinicians deliver. However, automated systems have their limitations. They do not necessarily take into account subtle aspects of the patient's social or medical situation. They cannot automate medicine nor can they replace the humans who deliver care or the human element they provide. Research has demonstrated, however, that automated reminder systems are effective in closing the gap between what is and what should be delivered. In the near future the use of automated systems will become the standard of care, and patients will expect nothing less.

SUGGESTED READINGS

American Academy of Family Physicians Center for Health Information Technology
EHR adoption
http://www.centerforhit.org/. Accessed 2007.

American College of Physicians
Medical computing
http://www.acponline.org/computer/. Accessed 2007.

American Medical Association
Health information technology
http://www.ama-assn.org/ama/pub/category/16195.html. Accessed 2007.

References

1. Ford EW, Menachemi N, Phllips T. Predicting the adoption of electronic health records by physiains: when will health care be paperless? *J Am Med Inform Assoc* 2006;13:106–112.
2. de Brantes F, Emery DW, Overhage JM, et al. The potential of HIEs as infomediaries. *J Healthc Inf Manag.* 2007;21(1):69–75.
3. Bodenheimer T, Lorig K, Holman H, et al. Patient self-management of chronic disease in primary care. *JAMA* 2002;288(19):2470.
4. Barrett MJ. *Patient Self Management Tool: an Overview*. Oakland, CA: California Healthcare Foundation, June 2005. http://www.chcf.org/topics/chronicdisease/index.cfm?itemID=111783. Accessed October 14, 2006.
5. National Heart Lung and Blood Institute. *Third Report of the Expert Panel on Detection, Evaluation and Treatment of High Cholesterol in Adults (Adult Treatment Panel III)*. Rockville, MD: National Institutes of Health, September

2002. http://www.nhlbi.nih.gov/guidelines/cholesterol/. Accessed October 12, 2006.

6. McDonald CJ. Computer reminders, the quality of care and the non-perfectibility of man. *N Engl J Med* 1976;295:1351–1355.

7. Dexter PR, Perkins SM, Maharry KS, et al. Inpatient computer-based standing orders vs physician reminders to increase influenza and pneumococcal vaccination rates: a randomized trial. *JAMA* 2004;292:2366–2371.

8. Litzelman DK, Dittus RS, Miller ME, et al. Requiring physicians to respond to computerized reminders improves their compliance with preventive care protocols. *J Gen Intern Med* 1993;8:311–317.

9. Tierney WM, Hui SL, McDonald CJ. Delayed feedback of physician performance versus immediate reminders to perform preventive care. Effects on physician compliance. *Med Care* 1986;24:659–666.

10. Chaudhry B, Wang J, Wu S, et al. Systematic review: impact of health information technology on quality, efficiency, and costs of medical care. *Ann Intern Med* 2006;144:E12–E22.

11. McDonald CJ, Overhage JM. Guidelines you can follow and can trust. An ideal and an example. *JAMA* 1994;271(11):872–873.

12. Tierney WM, Overhage JM, McDonald CJ. Computerizing guidelines: factors for success. *Proc AMIA Annu Fall Symp* 1996;459–462.

13. Shiffman RN, Shekell P, Overhage JM, et al. A proposal for standardized reporting of clinical practice guidelines: the COGS statement. *Ann Int Med* 2003;139:493–498.

14. Tang PC, Ash JS, Bates DW, et al. Personal health records: definitions, benefits, and strategies for overcoming barriers to adoption. *JAMA* 2006;13(2):121–126.

15. Biondich PG, Anand V, Downs SM, et al. Using adaptive turnaround documents to electronically acquire structured data in clinical settings. *AMIA Annu Symp Proc* 2003;86–90.

16. Tierney WM, Hui SL, McDonald CJ. Immediate vs. delayed feedback of performance: effect on physicians' preventive care behavior. *Clin Res* 1985;33:267A.

17. Litzelman DK, Dittus RS, Miller ME, et al. Requiring physicians to respond to computerized reminders improves their compliance with preventive care protocols. *J Gen Intern Med* 1993;8(6):311–317.

18. Overhage JM, Tierney WM, McDonald CJ. Computer reminders to implement preventive care guidelines for hospital inpatients. *Arch Intern Med* 1996;156:1551–1556.

19. Dexter PR, Perkins S, Overhage JM, et al. A computerized reminder system to increase the use of preventive care for hospitalized patients. *N Engl J Med* 2001;345(13):965–970.

20. Dexter PR, Perkins SM, Maharry KS, et al. Inpatient computer-based standing orders vs physician reminders to increase influenza and pneumococcal vaccination rates: a randomized trial. *JAMA* 2004;292:2366–2371.

21. Biondich PG, Overhage JM, Dexter PR, et al. A modern optical character recognition system in a real world clinical setting: some accuracy and feasibility observations. *Proc AMIA Symp* 2002;56–60.

22. Revere D, Dunbar PJ. Review of computer-generated outpatient health behavior interventions: clinical encounters "in absentia". *Am Med Inform Assoc* 2001;8:62–79.

CHAPTER 23

Reimbursement for Clinical Preventive Services

Betsy Nicoletti

This chapter is a resource to help clinicians understand coding and billing for preventive services provided in their office or clinic. The first section discusses the codes used to bill for preventive services, including screening tests and immunizations. The second section discusses coverage for preventive services under Medicaid, private health plans, and Medicare. The third section discusses the "pay-for-performance" initiative.

Although clinicians are admonished to "bill everyone the same," the challenge of obtaining reimbursement for preventive services reveals the difficulties to be encountered in attempting to follow this advice. Payers process claims using their own claims editing systems and in accordance with widely varying policies. This results in wide variations both in which claims receive reimbursement and in how much the plans pay, even when claims are billed "the same." This chapter addresses these variations in reimbursement practices and provides advice on effective billing in this complex subject area.

BILLING CODES

Periodic Health Examinations
CURRENT PROCEDURAL TERMINOLOGY CODES

Table 23.1 lists the *Current Procedural Terminology* (CPT) codes, developed by the American Medical Association (AMA), for the ambulatory care visit.

For the most commonly used codes for the office visit (99201–99215), documentation guidelines (developed jointly by the Centers for Medicare and Medicaid Services [CMS] and the AMA; see http://www.cms.hhs.gov/MLNEdWebGuide/25_EMDOC.asp) specify required elements that must be documented for reimbursement of *Evaluation and Management* (E/M) *services* (the standard codes for physician services in outpatient facilities). As most clinicians know, reimbursement of a "comprehensive" history requires documentation of four elements from the history of the present illness, the review of ten organ systems, and all of the past medical, family, and social history.

563

TABLE 23.1 Current Procedural Terminology (CPT) Codes for Office Visits

Office or Other Outpatient Services	
New patient[a]	99201–99205
Established patient	99211–99215
Preventive Medicine	
New patient[a]	99381–99387
Established patient	99391–99397

[a] A "new patient" is one who has not yet received a professional service from that particular physician, or from another physician of the same specialty in the same group, in the last 3 years.

These requirements do not apply to the history and physical examination conducted as part of periodic health examinations—what the documentation guidelines identify as "age- and gender-appropriate histories and examinations." For these visits, which can be billed under CPT codes 99381–99397, the clinician need only document those elements of the history and physical examination that are appropriate for the age and gender of the patient. The chief complaint and level of medical decision making, which must be documented for the reimbursement of other visits, need not be documented for the periodic health examination.

To determine which elements of the history and physical examination are age- and gender-appropriate for reimbursement under CPT codes 99381–99397, the *CPT Assistant* journal (see Suggested Readings on page 581) which provides coding guidance and additional details to providers, advises clinicians to consult guidelines from their specialty societies. Specifically, the *CPT Assistant* refers clinicians to the U.S. Preventive Services Task Force, the American Academy of Pediatrics, the American College of Physicians, and the Centers for Disease Control and Prevention, among other societies and organizations, for guidance on which services to provide. See Chapters 2–4 and Appendix A for more details about guidelines from these organizations, and see Chapter 20 for a discussion of how individual practices should decide which services they should provide.

Sports Physicals, College, and Camp Examinations

For children older than 2 years, most health plans will only pay for one preventive service examination yearly among those covered in the 99381–99397 series. When a child presents for an additional visit to have a form completed for playing sports or attending school or camp, the *CPT Assistant* advises billing these services with the office visit code (99201–99215) at the level of the history and examination that the clinician can document. The diagnosis code should indicate that the visit was for an examination, using the V20 or V70 series of codes. (As discussed in the subsequent text, *V codes* are used when a patient visits a clinician for reasons other than illness or injury.)

HEALTHCARE COMMON PROCEDURE CODING SYSTEM CODES

Medicare has its own set of codes for covered preventive and screening services. The Healthcare Common Procedure Coding System (HCPCS) definitions may be exactly the same as their CPT counterparts or may be slightly different. Using HCPCS codes allows Medicare to differentiate services delivered for diagnostic purposes from those done for screening. HCPCS codes are designated as "Level-2 CPT codes." These codes are described in the book, *Health Care Procedure Coding System National Level II Medicare Codes 2007*, which is published by AMA and Practice Management Information Corporation (PMIC). The book is reissued annually and is available for purchase from commercial vendors. The specific codes and their coverage are addressed in the section on Medicare coverage (see page 571).

INTERNATIONAL CLASSIFICATION OF DISEASES CODES

Medicare carriers and private plans pay claims based on procedure codes (e.g., CPT, HCPCS) but may deny claims based on diagnosis codes. Diagnosis codes indicate the reason for the visit and the patient's disease, illness, or injury, when known; they specify the patient's symptoms when the diagnosis is not known. As noted earlier, the series of "V diagnosis" codes designate the health status of the patient or may signify an office visit for screening or prophylactic care. As specified in the ICD-9-CM book, *International Classification of Diseases, Ninth Revision 2007* (published by the AMA and PMIC), many V codes are used as the primary diagnosis, but some may only be used for a secondary diagnosis. Many payers will reimburse for examination visits identified by a V code, but some payers will reimburse only those services that are billed for a diagnosis of an illness or injury.

Claims paying systems have "edits" that deny payment for screening services provided without mention of the corresponding diagnosis related to that service. For example, coverage of glaucoma screening under Medicare, using codes G0117 and G0118, requires the diagnosis code V80.1 ("special screening for neurologic, eye and ear diseases, glaucoma"). Coverage of pneumococcal vaccination under Medicare, using codes G0009 and 90732, requires the diagnosis code V03.82 ("need for prophylactic vaccination and inoculation against bacterial diseases, *streptococcus pneumoniae*").

Billing with a nonspecific examination-diagnosis code will usually result in denial. Some practices have incorporated these rules into their automated claims submission systems to alert them when claims are about to be submitted with the wrong diagnosis code. Practices that use a paper encounter form can avoid miscoding by printing the correct diagnosis code near the procedure code rather than listing them in separate sections.

Counseling and Risk Factor Reduction

Included in the services covered under the preventive medicine CPT codes 99381–99397 are counseling for risk factor reduction and anticipatory guidance related to health promotion and disease prevention. That these services were discussed with the patient should be documented in the note for the encounter. This includes, as appropriate to the patient, discussion of diet, exercise, smoking, car seat and seat belt use, alcohol and substance use, violent behavior, osteoporosis, depression, dementia, sexual activity, and infectious diseases.

Another series of preventive medicine CPT codes (see Table 23.2) are time based and intended to be used when counseling patients in a one-on-one discussion about disease prevention and risk factor reduction in the absence of disease or injury. As with all time-based codes, to enable billing under these codes, the time spent by the clinician must be documented in the medical record.

For patients with a medical illness, counseling regarding the history of their disease and the importance of adherence to treatment for that disease can be billed with a time-based E/M code. For example, if a clinician counsels an established patient with diabetes about the importance of adherence to diet and exercise recommendations, and more than half of the visit was spent in this discussion, the clinician could select an established patient visit code based on time (99211–99215). The clinician must document total time, the fact that more than 50% of the visit was devoted to this discussion, and the nature of the discussion. The codes in the 99401–99404 series are not used for advising patients with known disease but rather for services that are preventive in nature.

TABLE 23.2   Time-Based Current Procedural Terminology (CPT) Codes for Prevention-Focused Counseling Visits

	Preventive medicine counseling and/or risk factor reduction intervention(s) provided to an individual (separate procedure);
99401	~15 minutes
99402	~30 minutes
99403	~45 minutes
99404	~60 minutes

Two additional preventive medicine codes covering risk factor reduction services are the group counseling codes (99411 and 99412), which are also time-based codes (30 and 60 minutes, respectively). Typically, however, insurance plans do not currently pay for services billed under these codes. Most practices provide these services on a self-pay basis.

Immunizations

Practices bill separately for administration of the immunization and for the serum, if the latter is not provided by a state agency. If it purchased the serum, the practice should bill for both. Medicare and many insurers require practices to use vaccine-specific procedure and diagnostic codes, as are done in the HCPCS codes for Medicare (see pages 571–576). Use code 90471 for administration of a single vaccine (percutaneous, intradermal, subcutaneous, or intramuscular) and 90472 for each additional vaccine given. For example, if the practice administers three intramuscular immunizations to a patient, it should bill 90471 with one unit and 90472 with each of the other two units. In 2005, two new codes were added for circumstances when counseling regarding the risks and benefits of vaccinations accompanies the administration of immunizations to children younger than 8 years. These include code 90465 for counseling with administration of a single vaccine (percutaneous, intradermal, subcutaneous or intramuscular) and 90466 for counseling with additional vaccine administration. The clinician must personally document the discussion of the risks and benefits. Codes 90465 and 90466 should be used instead of 90471 and 90472, not in addition to them. Codes in the V03–V06 series are for encounters for inoculations or vaccinations.

Screening Tests

Advice about and referral for age- and gender-appropriate screening services are included in the definitions of the CPT preventive medicine codes. Recommended screening tests are discussed in Chapter 4. Coverage for these services varies by payer and by the patient's individual policy. Payment sometimes also depends on correct diagnostic coding, again varying by payer. Codes V70–V85 are used to report services delivered when patients lack a diagnosis and receive care related to a screening test or evaluation. Clinicians can choose from a series of V codes, including V28 and V73–V82, to report specific types of screening (e.g., screening for malignant neoplasms).

VISION SCREENING

Clinicians can use the 99173 CPT code to submit claims for screening for visual acuity that is quantitative and bilateral (e.g., using the Snellen chart, as described on pages 64 and 441). Although many private insurance companies bundle the payment for this service into the 99381–99397 series of codes and will not reimburse it separately, some Medicaid and private payers will pay for it as a separate service.

Medical Problems Addressed at a Prevention-Oriented Visit

In certain situations, clinicians may bill for an office visit made on the same day as a preventive service visit. If in the course of providing a preventive service, the clinician addresses a significant, separately identifiable medical problem of an acute or chronic nature that requires extra work, the clinician may bill for the office visit (99201–99215), adding a "-25 modifier" in addition to the preventive service (99381–99397). The AMA CPT manual defines -25 modifiers, which indicate that the same clinician provided a significant, separately identifiable E/M service on the same day as the examination. In general, this "extra work" should involve a change in the patient's medical condition as documented in the history of the present illness and treatment plan. In the assessment and plan, the clinician must document a significant change in treatment that qualifies as extra work. Renewing prescriptions, reviewing stable problems, or treating a minor, incidental problem found in the course of the examination (such as otitis media) is not considered significant enough to be separately payable.

Third-party payers rarely reimburse, on the *first* claims submission, an office visit with a -25 modifier that is performed on the same day as a preventive medicine service. Perhaps 10–20% of such claims will ultimately be paid on appeal with supporting documentation. If a patient has a policy requiring a copayment for each visit, some insurance companies require the clinician to collect two copayments if two E/M services are submitted. Some insurers will pay for both and some will pay the E/M service at 50% if the documentation supports both services. The clinician should document the sick-visit portion of the note separately from that for the preventive service. This shows the payer the additional work that was done, and will help the clinician see what level of additional service was really provided. When submitting claims for two E/M services, the clinician should check whether the payer processes the lower paid service and denies the other.

Billing for "split services" under Medicare is discussed later in this chapter (see "Split Visits" on page 577).

Clinicians can also submit claims for minor procedures, such as excising a lesion, which are performed on the same day as a preventive service. However, some insurers will not pay for both services in this circumstance, and therefore clinicians should clarify the carrier's policy beforehand.

Practices may prefer to bill for one or the other service because of the low payment when billing for both and the added work of appeals. If the patient has significant medical problems, it may be preferable to ask the patient to return for another visit devoted to those conditions or, if the medical problems are more urgent, it may be advisable to defer the preventive services to a future visit.

COMPLETION OF LIFE AND DISABILITY INSURANCE FORMS

Code 99450 can be used for the completion of a life and disability insurance form. This service includes measurement of height, weight, blood pressure, completion of a medical history form, collection of blood and/or urine samples (following the chain of custody for the sample), and completion of necessary certificates. This service is typically not covered by health insurance policies. If covered, it will be paid directly by the patient or the insurance company that is issuing the life or disability insurance. The specific diagnosis code for this service is V70.3 (other medical examination for administrative purposes).

WORK-RELATED OR MEDICAL DISABILITY EVALUATION

A history and physical examination that is required for work- or disability can be billed under one of two CPT codes: 99455, when provided by the treating physician, and 99456, when provided by a clinician other than the treating physician. Both require performance of the medical history and physical examination, forming an assessment and plan, and completion of necessary paperwork and reports.

HEALTH PLAN COVERAGE

The Uninsured, Medicaid, and Children's Health Insurance

According to the U.S. Census Bureau, 47 million Americans (15.8% of the population) lacked health insurance in 2006. Between 2005 and 2006 there was a decline in employment-based health insurance from 60.2 to 59.7% (1). For the uninsured, access to both preventive care and treatment of illness and injury is limited by ability to pay. Because of the availability of Medicaid coverage and the State Children's Health Insurance Program (SCHIP) (2), the percentage of children without insurance is lower than that of the general population, approximately 12%.

Medicaid pays for some preventive services through the Early Periodic Screening, Diagnostic, and Treatment (EPSDT) program. The two goals of this program are to assure the availability and accessibility of required health care for children and to help Medicaid recipients and their parents or guardians effectively use these resources. Although the individual features of state Medicaid programs vary considerably, these services are covered in all states. The screening services covered under EPSDT include a comprehensive health and developmental history, a comprehensive physical examination, immunizations, screening laboratory tests, and lead toxicity screening. The benefits include health education/anticipatory guidance as well as vision, dental, and hearing services. Access to practices that accept Medicaid varies widely. In particular, finding dentists who will accept Medicaid insurance can be difficult, leaving some patients without access to this mandated care.

In addition to the above, the federal government provides grants to states through SCHIP to provide health insurance to uninsured children at up to 200% of the federal poverty level. States may opt to cover all of the children in this group or to select a wider or narrower group of children to cover. The uninsured children must be younger than 19 years, ineligible for Medicaid, and be in families that meet the state's income eligibility requirements. The state selects a benefit package according to the terms of the law and may charge premiums, deductibles, and coinsurance to recipients. Coverage and eligibility vary by state, but covered children typically have access to preventive care. At this writing Congress is discussing potential expansions of the SCHIP program.

Private Health Coverage for Preventive Services

Many Americans have private health insurance coverage through their employers. Some can select from a menu of employee-sponsored plans and some must use a single plan offered by their employer. According to a Kaiser/Health Research and Educational Trust survey, 21% of enrollees in an employer-sponsored plan in 2005 had benefits in a health maintenance organization, which generally include complete coverage of preventive services, and 15% were enrolled in point-of-service plans, many of which also have prevention coverage.

According to the 2005 United Benefits Adviser/Ingenix Health Plan Survey, only 2.6% of employers offered their workers the option of enrolling in a consumer-directed health care plan. These are high-deductible plans with health savings accounts that can be used for preventive services (3). Healthy individuals who pay their own premiums may be more likely to select these types of policies. Patients with these types of coverage may be less willing to pay out of pocket for costly preventive services and other medical services than patients enrolled in traditional plans.

The claims processing systems for most insurers limit the frequency of the provision of preventive services. After infancy and early childhood, typically at age 2 years, preventive visits may be provided no more frequently than annually. Some plans will allow women one visit for primary care from either an internist/family physician or a gynecologist, but not both. In recent years, more plans have allowed a second preventive visit for women who want to see their gynecologist for their pelvic examination, Pap smear, or clinical breast examination. Coverage for bone densitometry varies by payer. Unfortunately, practices do not always know if an individual patient has coverage that allows more than one visit, nor can they always collect remuneration for the service upfront.

Medicare

Medicare provides health care coverage for Americans age 65 years and older and for those who are disabled. The original legislation that created the program in 1964 focused on diagnostic tests and treatment and included statutory prohibitions against coverage of either prevention or screening.

COVERAGE OF SPECIFIC CLINICAL PREVENTIVE SERVICES UNDER MEDICARE

Over the years, Congress has passed amendments that have markedly expanded coverage for specific preventive services in the Medicare benefit package. Table 23.3 lists the clinical preventive services covered under Medicare at this writing, along with their HCPCS codes, the time limits for periodicity, and the covered diagnosis codes. The services are covered within strict time limits and for only the diagnosis codes listed. Further details about specific coverage benefits follow:

Pelvic and Breast Examinations
As shown in Table 23.3, Medicare covers annual or biannual pelvic and breast examinations for women depending on their risk status (HCPCS code, G0101, "cervical or vaginal screening;" "pelvic and clinical breast examination"). Pelvic examinations, which have limited evidence of effectiveness, as discussed on page 75, are covered every 2 years for low-risk patients and every year for high-risk patients. The diagnosis code for the biannual screening is V76.2 ("special screening for malignant neoplasm, cervical"), and the code for the annual examination is V15.89 ("other specified personal history presenting hazards to health"). Diagnosis code V76.49 ("special screening for malignant neoplasms, other sites") should be used if the patient lacks a cervix.

G0101 can be used if the examination includes 7 of the following 11 elements:

- Inspection and palpation of the breasts for masses, lumps, tenderness, symmetry, or nipple discharge
- Digital rectal examination
- External genitalia (general appearance, hair distribution, or lesions)
- Bladder (fullness, masses, or tenderness)
- Urethral meatus (size, location, lesions, or prolapse)
- Urethra (masses, tenderness, or scarring)
- Vagina (general appearance, discharge, lesions, pelvic support, cystocele, or rectocele)
- Cervix (general appearance, lesions, or discharge)
- Uterus (size, position, mobility, tenderness, or support)
- Adnexa/parametria (masses, tenderness, nodularity, or organomegaly)
- Anus and perineum

TABLE 23.3 Clinical Preventive Services Covered Under Medicare

SERVICE	HCPCS/CPT CODES	ICD-9-CM CODES	WHO IS COVERED	FREQUENCY	BENEFICIARY PAYS
Initial preventive physical examination (IPPE) *Also known as the Welcome to Medicare Physical Exam*	G0344 – IPPE G0366 – EKG for IPPE G0367 – EKG tracing for IPPE G0368 – EKG interpret and report	No specific diagnosis code required for IPPE and corresponding EKG *Contact local Medicare Contractor for guidance*	All Medicare beneficiaries whose first Part B coverage began on or after January 1, 2005	Once in a lifetime benefit per beneficiary *Must be furnished no later than 6 mo after the effective date of the first Medicare Part B coverage begins*	Copayment/coinsurance Deductible
Ultrasound screening for abdominal aortic aneurysm (AAA)	G0389 – Ultrasound exam AAA screen	No specific code *Contact local Medicare Contractor for guidance*	Medicare beneficiaries with certain risk factors for abdominal aortic aneurysm *Important – Eligible beneficiaries must receive a referral for an ultrasound screening for AAA as a result of an IPPE*	Once in a lifetime benefit per eligible beneficiary, effective January 1, 2007	Copayment/coinsurance No deductible
Cardiovascular disease screenings	80061 – Lipid panel 82465 – Cholesterol 83718 – Lipoprotein 84478 – Triglycerides	Report one or more of the following codes: V81.0, V81.1, V81.2	All asymptomatic Medicare beneficiaries *12 hr fast is required before testing*	Every 5 yr	No copayment/coinsurance No deductible
Diabetes screening tests	82947 – Glucose; quantitative, blood (except reagent strip) 82950 – Glucose; post-glucose dose (includes glucose) 82951– Glucose tolerance test (GTT), three specimens (includes glucose)	V77.1 *Report modifier "TS" (follow-up service) for diabetes screening where the beneficiary meets the definition of pre diabetes*	Medicare beneficiaries with certain risk factors for diabetes or diagnosed with prediabetes *Beneficiaries previously diagnosed with diabetes are not eligible for this benefit*	• Two screening tests per year for beneficiaries diagnosed with prediabetes • One screening per year if previously tested but not diagnosed with prediabetes or if never tested	No copayment/coinsurance No deductible
Diabetes self-management training (DSMT)	G0108 – DSMT, individual session, per 30 min G0109 – DSMT, group session (2 or more), per 30 min	No specific code *Contact local Medicare Contractor for guidance*	Medicare beneficiaries at risk for complications from diabetes, recently diagnosed with diabetes, or previously diagnosed with diabetes *Physician must certify that DSMT is needed*	• Up to 10 hr of initial training within a continuous 12-mo period • Subsequent yr: Up to 2 hr of follow-up training each year	Copayment/coinsurance Deductible
Medical nutrition therapy (MNT)	97802, 97803, 97804, G0270, G0271 *Services must be provided by registered dietitian or nutrition professional*	*Contact local Medicare Contractor for guidance*	Medicare beneficiaries diagnosed with diabetes or a renal disease	• First yr: 3 hr of one-on-one counseling • Subsequent year: 2 hr	Copayment/coinsurance Deductible

Screening pap tests	G0123, G0124, G0141, G0143, G0144, G0145, G0147, G0148, P3000, P3001, Q0091	V76.2, V76.47, V76.49, V72.31	All female Medicare beneficiaries	• Annually if high-risk, or childbearing age with abnormal Pap test within past 3 yr • Every 24 mo for all other women	Copayment/coinsurance for Pap test collection *(No copayment/coinsurance for Pap lab test)* No deductible
Screening pelvic examination	G0101 – Cervical or vaginal cancer screening; pelvic and clinical breast examination	V76.2, V76.47, V76.49, V15.89, V72.31	All female Medicare beneficiaries	• Annually if high-risk, or childbearing age with abnormal Pap test within past 3 yr • Every 24 mo for all other women	Copayment/coinsurance No deductible
Screening mammography	77052, 77057, G0202	V76.11 or V76.12	All female Medicare beneficiaries age 40 or older Female Medicare beneficiaries ages 35–39	Annually One baseline	Copayment/coinsurance No deductible
Bone mass measurements	G0130, 77078, 77079, 77080, 77081, 77083, 76977	*Contact local Medicare Contractor for guidance*	Medicare beneficiaries at risk for developing osteoporosis	Every 24 mo *More frequently if medically necessary*	Copayment/coinsurance Deductible
Colorectal cancer screening	G0104 – Flexible sigmoidoscopy G0105 – Colonoscopy (high risk) G0106 – Barium enema *(alternative to G0104)* G0120 – Barium enema *(alternative to G0105)* G0121 – Colonoscopy (not high risk) G0122 – Barium enema (noncovered) G0328 – Fecal occult blood test *(alternative to 82270)* 82270 – Fecal occult blood test	Use appropriate code *Contact local Medicare Contractor for guidance*	• Medicare beneficiaries age 50 and older • Screening colonoscopy: individuals at high risk; no minimum age requirement • No minimum age for having a barium enema as an alternative to a high risk screening colonoscopy if the beneficiary is at high risk	• Fecal occult: Annually • Flexible sigmoidoscopy: Every 4 yr or once every 10 yr after having a screening colonoscopy • Screening colonoscopy: Every 24 mo at high risk; every 10 yr not at high risk • Barium Enema: Every 24 mo at high risk; every 4 yr not at high risk	No copayment/coinsurance or deductible for fecal occult blood tests For all other tests copayment/coinsurance apply No deductible
Prostate cancer screening	G0002 – Digital rectal exam (DRE)	V76.44	All male Medicare beneficiaries 50 or older (coverage begins the day after 50th birthday)	Annually	Copayment/coinsurance Deductible
	G0103 – Prostate specific antigen test (PSA)	V76.44	All male Medicare beneficiaries 50 or older (coverage begins the day after 50th birthday)	Annually	No copayment/coinsurance No deductible

(continued)

TABLE 23.3 (Continued)

SERVICE	HCPCS/CPT CODES	ICD-9-CM CODES	WHO IS COVERED	FREQUENCY	BENEFICIARY PAYS
Glaucoma screening	G0117 – By an optometrist or ophthalmologist G0118 – Under the direct supervision of an optometrist or ophthalmologist	V80.1	Medicare beneficiaries with diabetes mellitus, family history of glaucoma, African-Americans age 50 and older, or Hispanic-Americans age 65 and older	Annually for beneficiaries in one of the high risk groups	Copayment/coinsurance Deductible
Influenza (Flu)	90655, 90656, 90657, 90658, 90660 – Flu vaccine G0008 – Administration	V04.81 V06.6 – When purpose of visit was to receive both Flu and PPV vaccines	All Medicare beneficiaries	Once per flu season in the fall or winter Medicare may provide additional flu shots if medically necessary	No copayment/coinsurance No deductible
Pneumococcal	90732 – Pneumococcal polysaccharidevaccine (PPV) G0009 – Administration	V03.82 V06.6 –When purpose of visit was to receive both PPV and Flu vaccines	All Medicare beneficiaries	Once in a lifetime Medicare may provide additional vaccinations based on risk	No copayment/coinsurance No deductible
Hepatitis B (HBV)	90740, 90743, 90744, 90746, 90747– HBV vaccine G0010 – Administration 90471 or 90472– Administration (OPPS hospitals only)	V05.3	Medicare beneficiaries at medium to high risk	Scheduled dosages required	Copayment/coinsurance Deductible
Smoking and tobacco-use cessation counseling	G0375 – counseling visit, intermediate, greater than 3 min up to 10 min G0376 – counseling visit, intensive, greater than 10 min	Use appropriate code Contact local Medicare Contractor for guidance	Medicare beneficiaries who use tobacco and have a disease or adverse health effect linked to tobacco use or take certain therapeutic agents whose metabolism or dosage is affected by tobacco use	Two cessation attempts per year; each attempt includes maximum of four intermediate or intensive sessions, up to eight sessions in a 12-mo period	Copayment/coinsurance Deductible

This quick reference information chart was prepared as a service to the public and is not intended to grant rights or impose obligations. This chart may contain references or links to statutes, regulations, or other policy materials. The information provided is only intended to be a general summary. It is not intended to take the place of either the written law or regulations. We encourage Readers should review the specific statutes, regulations and other interpretive materials for a full and accurate statement of their contents.

Adapted from Centers for Medicare and Medicaid Services. *Quick reference information for Medicare preventive services.* http://www.cms.hhs.gov/MLNProducts/downloads/MPS_QuickReferenceChart.1.pdf. Accessed 2007.

Medicare also pays for the performance of a Pap smear at the same time under code Q0091 ("screening Pap smear; obtaining, preparing and conveyance of cervical or vaginal smear to laboratory"). This service is covered at the same frequency as the G0101 and is billable with the same diagnosis codes. The code is for use with screening, and not diagnostic, Pap smears.

If these services (G0101 and Q0091) are performed the same day as an office visit for another medical problem (for example, if the clinician also addressed the patient's hypertension on the same day), both can be billed, with a -25 modifier on the office visit as explained on page 568. If the pelvic examination is performed on the same day as a preventive service that Medicare does not cover, then the patient is responsible for the difference between the charges for the preventive medicine examination and the two HCPCS codes above, which are billed to Medicare.

Diabetes Screening

Testing of an individual at risk for diabetes can be billed using existing CPT codes, per the laboratory fee schedule: 82947 ("glucose; quantitative, blood, except reagent strip"); 82950 ("postglucose dose; includes glucose"); and 82951 ("glucose tolerance test [GTT] three specimens, includes glucose"). The clinician should designate ICD-9 code V77.1 ("special screening for diabetes mellitus"). Annual screening is covered for individuals with the following risk factors:

- Hypertension
- Dyslipidemia
- Obesity, defined as a body mass index greater than or equal to $30 \ kg/m^2$
- Previous identification of impaired fasting glucose
- Previous identification of impaired glucose tolerance
- A risk factor consisting of two of the following
  - Overweight, defined as a body mass index greater than $25 \ kg/m^2$, but less than $30 \ kg/m^2$
  - A family history of diabetes
  - A history of gestational diabetes or delivery of a baby weighing more than 9 lb.
  - Age 65 years or older

No screening coverage is provided for individuals with a previous diagnosis of diabetes; medically necessary laboratory services are covered under other Medicare benefits. Two screening tests per 12-month period are covered for patients with prediabetes, defined as a previous fasting glucose level of 100–125 mg/dL or a 2-hour postglucose challenge of 140–199 mg/dL (see page 482).

Cardiovascular Screening

Medicare covers screening blood tests for the early detection of cardiovascular disease or abnormalities associated with an elevated risk for that disease. These currently include measurement of total cholesterol (82465), high-density lipoprotein cholesterol (83178), and triglyceride (84478) levels. The tests can be billed every 5 years, as either a lipid panel (80061) or under the individual components. The appropriate diagnosis codes are V81.0 ("special screening for cardiovascular, respiratory, and genitourinary diseases, ischemic heart disease"), V81.1 ("special screening for cardiovascular, respiratory, and genitourinary diseases"), or V81.2 ("special screening for cardiovascular, respiratory, and genitourinary diseases; other and unspecified cardiovascular conditions").

Screening for Abdominal Aortic Aneurysms

In 2007, Medicare began paying for screening for abdominal aortic aneurysms when it is recommended as part of the Welcome to Medicare visit (see subsequent text) for men aged 65–75 years who have smoked 100 cigarettes in their lifetime and for individuals with a family history of such aneurysms.

COVERAGE OF PREVENTION-ORIENTED VISITS UNDER MEDICARE

Although Medicare does cover the specific preventive services listed in Table 23.3, it still does not cover periodic health examinations devoted to prevention. Therefore, patients covered by private insurance find that such visits are no longer covered when they become eligible for Medicare. Any claim billed with the 99381–99397 series of codes is denied as noncovered and is the patient's responsibility. As discussed in the subsequent text, the Medicare Modernization Act of 2004 added coverage for an initial "Welcome to Medicare" visit for new enrollees within the first 6 months as beneficiaries.

Except in this instance, Medicare patients who present for a periodic health examination should be told at the time of appointment booking that the service is noncovered. Some patients will have secondary coverage that will pay for the service, and the claims can be submitted to Medicare for processing by the secondary payer. The clinician can also bill Medicare for any covered services provided on that day, such as a pelvic or breast examination.

The "Welcome to Medicare" Visit

As noted, new Medicare beneficiaries are eligible for a "Welcome to Medicare" visit within the first 6 months of their enrollment. The Medicare deductible and coinsurance charges apply, so patients with no secondary coverage are responsible for the full amount. The visit may be performed by physicians, nurse practitioners, and physician assistants, but not by certified nurse midwives.

Seven components must be documented in the patient's medical record for such a visit to qualify for reimbursement. The seven elements include services that are covered under the statutory provisions of the legislation but that are not necessarily advocated elsewhere in this book. Routine electrocardiography, for example, is a covered benefit under the law but is among the proscribed practices discussed in Chapter 19 (see page 501). The seven elements include the following:

1. History
   - Past medical history, surgical history, including experience with illnesses, hospital stays, surgeries, injuries, allergies, and treatment
   - Current medications and supplements including calcium and vitamins
   - Family history, including a review of medical events in the patient's family and diseases that may be hereditary or place the individual at risk
   - Social history, including history of alcohol, tobacco, and illicit drug use; diet; and physical activities
2. Review of patient's potential for depression, using a screening tool recognized by national standards
3. Review of patient's functional ability, hearing, and level of safety using a screening tool recognized by national standards
4. Physical examination that includes height, weight, blood pressure, screening for visual acuity, and other examination components deemed appropriate by the clinician
5. Performance and interpretation of an electrocardiogram
6. Education, counseling, and referral, as appropriate, based on the results of the first five elements
7. Education, counseling, and referral, including a brief written plan given to the patient, such as a checklist for obtaining the appropriate screening and other preventive services covered by Medicare (Table 23.3). Table 23.4 lists the billing codes used for the "Welcome to Medicare" visit.

Split Visits

Medicare does allow physicians to bill Medicare for an illness-related visit provided on the same day as a noncovered, preventive medicine service, when both services are provided and documented. "Split visits" is the proper mechanism under Medicare to bill for visits for preventive medicine at which medical problems are addressed (see Table 23.5).

Under this provision, the practice should subtract the office visit portion of the fees from the preventive medicine portion and bill the patient for the difference. The practice's usual fee, not the Medicare-allowed amount, should be used in the calculation. For example, if the charge for the preventive medicine visit (99387) is $125 and the charge for the illness visit (99213) is $50,

TABLE 23.4 Billing Codes for "Welcome to Medicare" Visit

G0344: Initial preventive physical examination: face-to-face visit services, limited to new beneficiaries during their first 6 months of Medicare enrollment

G0366: Routine electrocardiogram with at least 12 leads, with interpretation and report, performed as a component of the initial preventive services examination

G0367: Electrocardiogram tracing only, without interpretation and report performed as a component of the initial preventive services examination

G0368: Electrocardiogram interpretation and report performed as a component of the initial preventive services examination

The diagnosis code is not specified in the final rule. Clinicians may wish to use V70.0 or specific medical diagnoses.

the patient would owe $75. The illness visit would be billed to Medicare and the patient would be responsible for the deductible and coinsurance amounts.

How should physicians select the level of service for which to bill Medicare when they perform an illness visit and a physical examination? Although the physical examination often entails a complete review of systems and a comprehensive examination, a high-level code is not always appropriate. The clinician should determine how much separate work was done during the visit that was not related to preventive care. The clinician should consider the history of the present illness and the medical decision making when selecting the proper level of the E/M code, remembering that the services are being carved out from one another and that the same service should not be reimbursed twice.

Split visits are inappropriate (the practice should bill for a preventive visit only) if the assessment focuses on preventive care and screening issues or even when it addresses other issues that are minor, such as refilling prescriptions. However, it may be appropriate to submit a claim for a split visit under one of the following circumstances:

- When the patient's underlying problems are deemed serious at the time of the visit.
- When the recorded history of the present illness documents the level of the complaint, such as multiple active symptoms or exacerbations of the patient's problems. (It is not appropriate when the clinician's note says "patient has no complaints.")
- When an unexpected, abnormal examination finding leads to further diagnostic tests, an indication that more than a preventive service was

TABLE 23.5   Billing for Medically Necessary Visit on the Same Occasion as a Preventive Medicine Service

"When a physician furnishes a Medicare beneficiary a covered visit at the same place and on the same occasion as a noncovered preventive medicine service (CPT codes 99381–99397), consider the covered visit to be provided in lieu of a part of the preventive medicine service of equal value to the visit. A preventive medicine service (CPT codes 99381–99397) is a noncovered service. The physician may charge the beneficiary, as a charge for the noncovered remainder of the service, the amount by which the physician's current established charge for the preventive medicine service exceeds his/her current established charge for the covered visit. Pay for the covered visit based on the lesser of the fee schedule amount or the physician's actual charge for the visit. The physician is not required to give the beneficiary written advance notice of noncoverage of the part of the visit that constitutes a routine preventive visit. However, the physician is responsible for notifying the patient in advance of his/her liability for the charges for services that are not medically necessary to treat the illness or injury.

There could be covered and noncovered procedures performed during this encounter (e.g., screening x-ray, ECG, lab tests). These are considered individually. Those procedures which are for screening for asymptomatic conditions are considered noncovered and, therefore, no payment is made. Those procedures ordered to diagnose or monitor a symptom, medical condition, or treatment are evaluated for medical necessity and, if covered, are paid."

Excerpt from: Publication 100-04, Medicare Claims Processing Manual, Chapter 12, Section 30.6.2http://www.cms.hhs.gov/Manuals/IOM/list.asp
CPT = Current Procedural Terminology; ECG = electrocardiogram.

performed. For example, the clinician may document a new heart murmur and order cardiac tests based on that finding.

- When the treatment plan includes changes to treatment of existing problems or an added treatment for a new problem.

When billing split visits, the clinician may find it helpful to write two notes, or a note within a note. Although not required by Medicare, having two notes helps the clinician separate the part of the visit that is billable to Medicare and provides more definitive documentation to support the split-visit claim.

PAY FOR PERFORMANCE

Pay for performance is a recent trend in reimbursement in which financial incentives are offered to clinicians who meet certain performance goals related to the quality of care. In some settings, the goals have been developed collaboratively by health plans and physicians. In some markets, health plans measure clinician performance without providing additional financial compensation. The indicators they monitor may include patient satisfaction, access to care, delivery rates for preventive services, and chronic care management.

In 2006, CMS launched the Physician's Voluntary Reporting Program, in which physicians voluntarily report their performance. At least initially, the program offered no additional reimbursement for reporting these services, but the move was part of the larger "pay-for-performance" initiative by private and public payers to offer greater reimbursement to clinicians who meet defined quality measures. The measures selected by CMS are reportedly evidence based, and physicians report their performance of these services by using a series of HCPCS codes and G-codes, developed for this purpose. The G-codes are submitted in addition to specific CPT and ICD-9-DM codes. Each G-code has specified CPT and ICD-9 codes for which the additional quality measure can be reported.

Performance indicators exist for both inpatient and outpatient services. Such indicators include osteoporosis assessment in elderly female patients and screening for hearing impairment and fall risk among elderly patients (75 years or older). Other indicators address mammography in women 40 years or older, influenza vaccination in patients 50 years or older, and pneumococcal vaccination in patients 65 years or older. The entire list of indicators and the G-codes that describe them can be found at http://www.cms.hhs.gov/PQRI/15_MeasuresCodes.asp#TopOfPage.

In legislation that updated the physician fee schedule for 2007, Congress added a provision to pay physicians for reporting on quality indicators and CMS published an expanded list of measures. Physicians who reported these measures in the latter half of 2007 were eligible for a 1.5% payment bonus. Further details about the program are available at http://www.cms.hhs.gov/PQRI/.

OFFICE AND CLINIC ORGANIZATION

Practices should include both the CPT and the HCPCS codes on their paper encounter forms, should clearly label the screening and diagnostic codes, and should place the correct diagnosis codes near the corresponding procedure codes. Electronic health records can employ prompts that remind clinicians to link diagnosis codes with the appropriate screening and immunization services and thereby reduce denials. Many practice management systems are able to track denials by reason code (the code representing the reason for denial). A practice can improve its billing and collecting for professional services if it knows why claims are denied. Standalone denial management systems are also available, but these must integrate with the practice management program to be useful.

In processing claims for preventive services, the practice's billing and coding staff should give feedback to clinicians about covered services, denials, and payer policy. If a practice disagrees with a payer policy, it may be worthwhile to discuss the issue with the payer representative or medical director. Having these discussions before contract renewal can be especially effective.

RESOURCES — PATIENT EDUCATION MATERIALS

Centers for Medicare and Medicaid Services
Preventive services: a healthier U.S. starts here. Website with resources about coverage benefits for preventive services under the Medicare program
http://www.medicare.gov/Health/Overview.asp. Accessed 2007.

SUGGESTED READINGS

Centers for Medicare and Medicaid Services
Website for health professionals regarding Medicare coverage of preventive services.
http://www.cms.hhs.gov/PrevntionGenInfo/. Accessed 2007.

Centers for Medicare and Medicaid Services
Medicare claims processing manual. Pub 100-04, Chapter 18. Baltimore, MD: Centers for Medicare and Medicaid Services, Accessed September 2007.
http://www.cms.hhs.gov/Manuals/IOM/

American Medical Association. *CPT Assistant* (monthly newsletter), *CPT Professional edition* (annual), and *CPT Changes: An Insider's View*. Chicago: American Medical Association.
These publications are updated regularly as serials and can be obtained online at the American Medical Association website (http://www.ama-assn.org/) by clicking on "CPT" under "Professional Resources." They can also be ordered by calling 800-621-8335.

References

1. DeNavas-Walt C, Proctor BD, Smith J. *Income, Poverty, and Health Insurance Coverage in the United States: 2006.* U.S. Census Bureau, Current Population Reports, P60-233. Washington, DC: U.S. Government Printing Office, 2007. Accessed September 4, 2007 at http://www.census.gov/prod/2007pubs/p60-233.pdf.
2. New York Times. *Health coverage of young widens with states' aid.* New York Times, December 4, 2005:1.
3. United Benefits Advisors. *2005 United Benefits Advisors/Ingenix Health Plan Survey.* Indianapolis: United Benefits Advisors, 2005. http://benefits.com/national _survey.htm.

CHAPTER 24

The Future of Health Promotion and Disease Prevention in Clinical Practice

Kevin Patrick

"The future is already here. It's just not very evenly distributed."

—William Gibson, Science fiction author

In the first edition of this book, Dr. Robert Lawrence began the final chapter with a sentiment that brought to mind William Gibson's observation: "The most reliable guide to predicting future developments in health promotion and disease prevention is a careful examination of current trends in society and progress in research" (1). This update, written a decade later, takes a similar approach. Because the health care system has emerged as one of the largest sectors of the economy, it is an inescapable reality that present-day social, technologic, and political forces shape what clinicians offer their patients and what patients expect of the health care system.

This chapter begins by "stepping back" and enumerating several of these changes, in particular those that by their magnitude or potentially disruptive nature seem most likely to affect such characteristics of the system as the accessibility, quality, cost, and impact of health promotion and disease prevention in clinical settings. Accompanying a brief description of each trend are a few comments on its potential impact on preventive care.

The chapter then moves on to consider how current conditions might lead to alternative futures, and how clinicians might work to increase the likelihood of a preferred future. This exercise is grounded in lessons this author has learned through participation in workshops led by Clem Bezold, Jonathan Peck, and others at the Institute for Alternative Futures in Alexandria, Virginia. Concluding this book with such speculation is offered in the spirit of optimism, anchored in the practical reality that society has at best only a modest ability to shape its destiny. However, those who spend most of their time promoting prevention are, in large measure, probably drawn to the field because of their inability to view things simply as they are. Perhaps more than others in medicine, they tend to wonder why things happen, what factors could have been changed to produce a different result, and how efforts can be refocused to improve conditions over time. Therefore, exercises in futurism fit well within the prevention paradigm.

TRENDS SHAPING PREVENTIVE CARE

A few observations help set the stage for this section. First, although the point of view in outlining these trends ranges from macro- to micro-level influences on health and disease, the artificiality of this approach is fully acknowledged. Many of these trends are strongly interrelated, for example, the globalization of the economy and technologic change. The former could not occur without the latter. A related corollary is that these trends interact with one another simultaneously at multiple levels. Population changes influence the allocation of economic resources; advancements in technology influence population dynamics as well as the cost of medical care. This reflects the richness of living systems and is what makes them so unpredictable. (It is also what provides the "Who knew it would happen?" exit strategy for all who are foolish enough to claim to be futurists.) Finally, although the focus of this book is primarily on clinical preventive care in the United States, because several trends that seem likely to influence health care in America are global in nature, worldwide trends are touched upon as well. Thus is the nature of the world in 2007, as this book appears.

Population Growth and Demographic Shifts

Demographic changes that can be predicted confidently at this writing include an aging population in the developed world and a burgeoning population in many parts of the less developed world. In 2005 the world's population reached 6.5 billion and was forecasted to grow to 9.1 billion by mid-century. Ninety-five percent of all new population growth is occurring in the developing rather than the developed world (2). The challenges that overcrowding and impoverishment will bring to the control of communicable diseases are likely to be compelling. On the other hand, for the United States, populated with its 300 millionth citizen at the time this chapter was written in 2006, and with its wave of post World War II baby boomers, demographic change will culminate in an unprecedented aging of the population with its attendant increase in the prevalence of chronic diseases.

This increase in longevity is mirrored in most other parts of the developed world. Combined with increases in obesity and the intractable nature of tobacco use in many populations, current trends promise a pipeline filled with health problems spilling out well into the middle of the 21st century and beyond. The effect of the demographic trends in the United States on preventive medicine depends on what resources are available for its provision, where and how it is being delivered, and what percentage of the population is at risk in any given health care setting. Tension is already apparent in policy discussions and decisions related to health care expenditures to control communicable versus chronic disease (3). The existence of an aging population will only exacerbate this tension, both within the developed world and between the developed and developing world.

Increased Diversity

In addition to the increase in the numbers of people, society is diversifying by culture and ethnicity at both the macro and micro level. Globally, this is resulting from a combination of high birth rates of selected subpopulations; migration, usually from less developed to developed areas; and differentials in death rates. In the United States, many groups (e.g., Hispanic Americans) once commonly settled in only a few regions are now more widely dispersed geographically because of such factors as local job and housing markets and family ties. In clinical settings these changes can influence the mix of patients in a given region, location, or practice; of presenting health problems; and of reimbursement patterns for health services delivery. Diversification and changes in the cultural background of patient populations also dictate changes in the required cultural competency of clinical staff. More so than for many medical services, cultural competency is needed for the optimal delivery of preventive services because they are so heavily dependent upon the quality of communication between clinicians and patients.

Rising Costs of Medical Care and Competition for Resources

Medical care costs as a share of overall gross domestic product vary from 7–8% in the United Kingdom and Japan to 15% in the United States (4); costs in the United States are expected to rise to 20% of the gross domestic product by 2015 (5). Owing to an aging population and higher costs of newer patented medications, expenditures on pharmaceuticals as a share of overall medical expenditures have been increasing annually at double-digit rates since 1995, faster than expenditures on hospital care or physician services (6). It remains to be seen whether the increase in the proportion of the economy devoted to health care will continue.

The greater the level of prosperity, the more willing is society to spend money on health care (7). However, even with this level of expenditure there is continued instability and variation in levels of medical care coverage and sources of funding for medical services. For example, in 2006 the National Center for Health Statistics estimated that 18.2% of the U.S. population spent at least part of the previous year without health insurance (8). The increase in medical spending is not limited to payments for expensive surgical procedures, hospitalization, and end of life care. Preventive services can also be costly, especially those that involve colonoscopy, imaging technologies, drugs, and expensive vaccines. How this will influence the share of the health care dollar devoted to prevention is uncertain. Continued growth in health care spending seems bound to force major policy discussions about who should pay for these increases and how. Sadly, this is a case where "what is old is new again," as these policy dilemmas were eloquently articulated in the early 1970s by the noted health policy scholar Victor Fuchs (9).

Although economic growth might be sufficient to supply the resources required for the anticipated increases in population and costs of medical services, there is also continued need for domestic investment in other important sectors such as education, transportation, housing, communications, defense, and basic public health. History suggests that the benefits of economic expansion are often unevenly distributed and that competition and tradeoffs for investment among these sectors are common, with "winners and losers" not always chosen rationally. In the face of this, it may be unclear what the optimal level of overall investment in health care should be, including that for prevention. Ideally, as the quantity and quality of the evidence supporting the cost-effectiveness of selected preventive services continue to improve, public and private decision makers will incorporate them into routine practice. But as is well known in health care, the lag time between knowledge and action can be substantial.

Advances in Science and Technology

The increasing pace of technologic change that began in the first half of the 20th century continues unabated. Some of the most profound changes seen in the present day, and likely to continue into the foreseeable future, are developments in three broad scientific domains: biology and the life sciences; computer, information, and telecommunications technology; and the social and behavioral sciences. In the biological sciences the fields of genomics and molecular biology, aided by the tools of bioinformatics, are yielding increasing knowledge about the fundamental building blocks of organisms and hold promise for the development of everything from new vaccines to precisely sensitive diagnostic technologies. Closely related to unfolding knowledge of the genome are advances in the chemical and pharmaceutical sciences that can enable a better understanding of how individuals with specific genetic profiles respond to specific drugs. This information holds considerable promise to help target and tailor the type and dose of medications used for individual preventive interventions.

Advances in computer, information, and telecommunications technologies continue to define much of contemporary society and transform most of its elements, including health care. From the increasingly ubiquitous silicon chips to advances in software and wireless devices, the options for storing, accessing, and communicating digitized information continue to expand in reach and impact. When the first edition of this book was written the Internet had only recently grown—through the invention of the http protocol and Mosaic—from a relatively obscure means of electronic messaging to a platform for easy transmission of multiple forms of text, graphic, and audio data. By 2005 the total number of extant web pages was estimated at 600 billion (10). At this writing, increases in available bandwidth and processing power are turning the Internet into a richly video-based medium.

One of the most important implications of these changes for health care is the ascendancy of the electronic health record. It is finally beginning to be adopted by sufficient numbers of clinicians so that it may eventually achieve the promise envisioned more than 40 years ago by experts in medical informatics. Concurrent developments in electronic personal health records, disease and vaccination registries, and systems that enable communication between and among clinicians, patients, and the public have the potential to greatly improve the delivery of preventive care. From identifying patients at risk through data mining to the application of fail-safe systems akin to those commonly used in fields such as aeronautics and manufacturing, much of the work of quality improvement in prevention can now be vested in automated rather than human-based systems. Chapter 22 discusses these themes in more detail.

Finally, the social and behavioral sciences, long the stepchildren of the "hard sciences," are benefiting from advances in everything from theory to measurement. At the pathophysiologic level, the use of functional magnetic resonance imaging and similar technologies is helping neuroscientists to better understand the biological basis of emotion, social interaction, learning, and cognition. These findings, combined with developments in genomics and bioinformatics, are engendering new transdisciplinary dialogue on the importance of social and behavioral influences on health risk and disease states. On a larger scale the application of technologies such as geographic information systems has helped to uncover previously obscure relationships between populations, the built and natural environment, health risk factors, and disease. Objective measurement strategies such as Systematic Social Observation (11) and the System for Observing Play and Leisure Activity in Youth (12) have supported advancements in both descriptive epidemiology and intervention research.

Because of the central role of behavioral and social factors as mediators, moderators, and correlators of health and disease risk, developments in these sciences hold great promise for health promotion and disease prevention (see Fig. 24.1). The benefits of much of this new knowledge may be most useful to inform population level interventions, such as the construction of more health-promoting neighborhoods and cities, schools, and workplaces. For example, improvements in understanding the impact of the built environment on opportunities for physical activity can inform policy in land use, zoning, transportation design, and building location (13). In addition, as detailed in Chapter 5, this new knowledge and skills have application in how

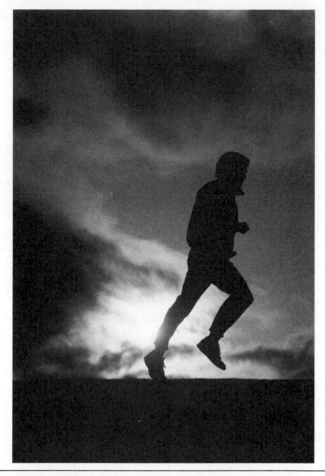

Figure 24.1 • The adoption of healthy lifestyles has the potential to alter substantially the trajectory of future disease trends.

clinicians care for patients. For example, increased knowledge in the social and behavioral sciences holds promise for helping to improve the content of messages delivered and reinforced in clinical settings.

Globalization of the Economy

Economies worldwide are experiencing major changes resulting from the increasing globalization of capital and labor markets and the development of an unprecedented and ever-expanding worldwide communication and transportation infrastructure. The socioeconomic rise of China, India, and to a lesser (but still important) extent other developing countries is projected to continue through the middle of this century. Relatively low costs of labor, and rapidly increasing industrialization through adoption of modern manufacturing methods, have moved many types of jobs from the developed world (including the United States) to the developing world.

This job shift is putting enormous stress on American companies and labor unions and on their traditional role in brokering relationships to assure health care coverage for employees. For example, some industries with current high-cost workforces and a significant number of retirees entitled to pensions with health benefits are reducing health care coverage for new employees. Reduced coverage for health care can restrict access and reduce opportunities for preventive care. On the other hand, some hold out hope that consumers, empowered with better information about how to manage their health—including the use of preventive services—might do a better job than the present "nonsystem" of health care. In response, some companies are changing the mix of health benefits they offer from cost-reimbursement models to "consumer-driven" health care (see page 570). These programs are beginning to demonstrate reduced costs in the near term, but the implications of this change for optimizing preventive care remain to be seen (14).

WITHER THE FUTURE?

How will these trends play out in the future, and how will they influence the provision of health care and preventive services? Along with Delphi surveys, statistical modeling, and simulation games, scenario development is used commonly by futurists to stimulate thinking and discussion about the world "to be" when all we know is "what is". These efforts often consider alternative scenarios, from the worst case to the best, which can be considered as "boundaries" of what the future might bring. Clearly these are exercises in fantasy. But in the often quoted words of Albert Einstein: "When I examine myself and my methods of thought, I come close to the conclusion that the gift of fantasy has meant more to me than my talent for absorbing positive knowledge" (15). With these thoughts in mind, the following three scenarios are representative of what this author can imagine.

Scenario 1: More of the Same

In this scenario, the health care system continues to consist of a Balkanized collection of payers, providers, and services. Most clinical care is episodic and provided in a reactive mode, reflecting the persistence of the disease orientation of American medicine. A few notable exceptions exist in some settings, such as forward-looking disease management programs for diabetes and cardiovascular disease that are based on the Chronic Care Model (16) (see page 322), or successful community approaches to achieve comprehensive levels of childhood vaccination supported through immunization registries that are open and accessible to all clinicians. Overall, however, the uneven adoption of preventive services continues to restrict their full potential. The health care system makes only marginal improvements in providing preventive services, only half of which are currently delivered as recommended.

Torpor in the system is also manifest in the failure to translate research-proven preventive strategies into practice. For example the Diabetes Prevention Program—which reported in early 2002 a 58% reduction in the risk of incident diabetes through the adoption of modest improvements in diet, improved physical activity, and weight loss (17)—continues to remain almost completely underimplemented in practice. Meanwhile, the cost of diabetes care in the United States, estimated at $92 billion in 2002 (18), increases each year at a double-digit rate along with the overall cost of medical care. Moreover, the responsibility for health promotion and preventive services in many health plans continues to fall more to the marketing department than to those managers who allocate resources for direct medical care. Research and development in preventive medicine, and its translation into practice, continue; the store of available evidence for its efficacy, effectiveness, and economic benefit increases. But with steady competition for the health care dollar from many sectors, and continued mixed messages about whether prevention is more a personal choice than a public good expected of the health care system, prevention languishes at the margins of the central efforts of the medical–industrial complex (19).

Scenario 2: The System Comes Apart at the Seams

The aging of the baby boomers continues to place pressure on the health care system to focus increasingly on medical services for chronic disease. An extended major economic recession results from increasing oil prices, accelerating job loss in both the traditional manufacturing and white collar service industries, and recurrent conflict in unstable parts of the world. The victims of chronic underinvestment in prior decades—sectors of society such as education, transportation, and the environment—become major competitors for new investments in public health and medicine. Consensus cannot be reached about how to address rising health care costs. Stakeholders are sharply divided along generational and socioeconomic lines over which are the correct solutions for the problems, and even over what the problems are.

Those with adequate financial resources increasingly opt out of pooled risk programs and purchase "boutique" health care, including certain preventive services that, at the "top end," benefit from innovative technologies, such as risk identification through genetic or other biomarker testing, imaging technologies, and pharmacologic interventions. Meanwhile, others with more modest financial resources find the costs for even basic medical care increasingly prohibitive. Rather than continuing the incremental gains in preventive care observed over the last decade, levels begin to decline for the provision of basic evidence-based preventive services such as smoking cessation counseling, established forms of cancer screening, and preventive pharmacotherapy. The "system" for providing these services begins to atrophy. To illustrate what might happen, this scenario envisions a particularly virulent strain of influenza virus emerging in Southeast Asia and sweeping across Europe and North America. Because of an essentially nonexistent system of quality control for even basic services such as immunizations, numbers of deaths mirror those seen in the 1918–1919 pandemic but are more heavily concentrated among the aging population as a result of demographic changes (20).

Scenario 3: Health Promotion and Disease Prevention Take Center Stage

As the resources spent in the U.S. economy that are apportioned to health care reach 20% of the gross domestic product, a sea change in thinking and action occurs. This comes about through a unique confluence of visionary leadership in both the administrative and legislative arms of the national government, reacting to trends in public opinion that reflect a sharply negative view of the costs, accessibility, and quality of health care. After extensive collaborative discussions among officials responsible for federal expenditures on programs such as Medicare and Medicaid and major groups representing employers and consumers, the importance of preventable causes of disease, disability, and reduced quality of life becomes fully acknowledged. This dialogue is partly informed by reviews of evidence by groups such as the U.S. Preventive Services Task Force, the Task Force on Community Preventive Services (see page xxxvi), and the Cochrane Collaboration. As with many things political, this recognition comes about because of a combination of crisis and common sense.

The need for investment in infrastructure in other areas of society is considered too great to allow health care costs to grow to 25%—or even more—of the gross domestic product. A reawakening of a sense of commonwealth prevails over arguments that prevention is a "personal responsibility," and support for collective investment in health promotion emerges. Surprisingly, there is also a renewed willingness to take the long-term view and recognize that preventable health problems that have taken generations to emerge—for example, obesity and its consequences such as diabetes and cardiovascular disease—will also take generations to reverse.

Prevention becomes the central organizing principle for health care services delivery. The curricula for health professional education at both the primary and continuing education levels change to reflect this emphasis, and new guidelines for medical care are adopted. Consensus emerges that it is essential to reduce the volume of chronic disease resulting from sedentary behavior, smoking, and other modifiable risk factors in the "pipeline." With the increasing burden of chronic disease that accompanies an aging population, a major social crisis is acknowledged. Similar to past national initiatives such as the development of the transcontinental highway system, the post–Sputnik era science education programs, and the effort to land a man on the moon, the political will is galvanized to make transformative changes to health care through new investments: for example, expansion of training programs for nurses, community health workers, and others capable of assuming the roles of health behavior coaches and disease case managers.

Systems engineers from other quality-dependent industries such as aircraft manufacturing and banking are recruited to help catalyze the adoption of methods of patient and population management to ensure 99.9% fidelity in the delivery of evidence-based primary, secondary, and tertiary prevention across the lifespan. Improvements in information technology such as the electronic health record, patient–clinician portals, data security systems, and consumer access to tailored health information help facilitate these efforts. Early in this process the pharmaceutical industry, sensing that its future is at stake, becomes a champion of this initiative and works with others to promote widespread use of current medications that can improve population health (e.g., aspirin, statins). Drug companies plan investments in new research and development with greater emphasis on the prevention paradigm than on the monetization of end-stage disease for which it was known in the past. Finally, the National Institutes of Health, a vital source of health science research, shifts its emphasis to public health, prevention, and translational sciences, including major new investments in behavioral, social, and environmental sciences. A particular emphasis is placed on addressing disparities in health and health care.

SEEKING THE PREFERRED FUTURE

Readers of this book, who presumably seek an improvement in the science and practice of preventive medicine, might reflect on the content of the preceding chapters and the potential scenarios presented here and ask themselves: What can be done to increase the likelihood of a *preferred* future for health promotion and disease prevention? Given the complex relationships involved in medical care and the impact of the trends outlined in the preceding text on the future of that care, strategies and solutions that involve actions outside of individual medical practices will almost certainly be necessary. There is no area of health care more dependent on social, cultural, and political determinants than health promotion. From the content and reach of marketing programs for cigarettes to whether the environment permits safe and affordable physical activity, policy matters. The good news is that clinicians can be highly influential voices in community-wide discussions of these issues. In addition to their scientific credibility, clinicians can contribute compelling stories based on the experiences of their patients, in particular those who either benefited greatly from preventive interventions or, on the other hand, suffered complications that optimal preventive care would have averted.

While advocacy for community-wide policy change will be important if a preferred future is to be reached, there is also considerable power in individual efforts at the local level. Through the professional and practice-level adoption of the evidence-based approaches discussed in this book, continued evaluation of their impact on outcomes, and implementation of improvements based on both experience and new knowledge, clinicians have the unequaled potential to make personal and meaningful differences in the lives of their patients and their families. With enough collective effort and in keeping with Mahatma Gandhi's well-known aphorism—"Be the change you want to see in the world"—the future may be favorable, indeed.

References

1. Lawrence RS. Future of health promotion and disease prevention in clinical practice and in the community. In: Woolf SH, Jonas S, Lawrence RS, eds. *Health promotion and disease prevention in clinical practice*, Philadelphia: Lippincott Williams & Wilkins, 1996:569.
2. The Department of Economic and Social Affairs, Population Division, United Nations. *World Population Prospects: The 2004 Revision*. New York: United Nations, 2005.
3. Yach D, Hawkes C Gould CL. The global burden of chronic diseases: overcoming impediments to prevention and control. *JAMA* 2004;291:2616–2622.
4. Organization for Economic Cooperation and Development (OECD). *Health data 2005: a comparative analysis of 30 countries*. Paris: Organization for Economic Cooperation and Development, 2005.
5. Borger C, Smith S, Truffer C, et al. Health spending projections through 2015: changes on the horizon. *Health Aff (Millwood)* 2006;25(2):w61–73.
6. Kaiser Family Foundation. *Prescription drug trends*. Menlo Park, CA: Kaiser Family Foundation, 2005. Accessed 2007 at www.kff.org/insurance/upload/3057-04.pdf.
7. Morris CR. *Too much of a good thing? Why health care spending won't make us sick*. New York: Century Foundation Press, 2000.
8. Cohen RA, Martinez M. *Health insurance coverage: early release of estimates from the National Health Interview Survey*. Hyattsville, MD: National Center for Health Statistics, 2006.
9. Fuchs V. *Who shall live?* New York: Basic Books, 1974.
10. Kelly K. *We are the web*. Wired, August, 2005.
11. Sampson RJ, Raudenbush SW. Systematic social observation of public spaces. A new look at disorder in urban neighborhoods. *Am J Sociol* 1999;(105):603–651.
12. McKenzie TL, Marshall SJ, Sallis JF, et al. Leisure-time physical activity in school environments: an observational study using SOPLAY. *Prev Med* 2000;30:70–77.

13. Handy SL, Boarnet MG, Ewing R, et al. How the built environment affects physical activity: views from urban planning. *Am J Prev Med* 2002;23(2S):64–73.
14. Buntin MB, Damberg C, Haviland A, et al. Consumer-directed health care: early evidence about effects on cost and quality. *Health Aff (Millwood)* 2006;25(6):w516–30.
15. Gardner H. *Creating minds: an anatomy of creativity seen through the lives of Freud, Einstein, Picasso, Stravinsky, Eliot, Graham and Ghandi.* New York. Basic Book. 1993; 105.
16. Wagner EH, Austin BT, Von Korff M, et al. Organizing care for patients with chronic illness. *Milbank Q* 1996;74(4):511–544.
17. Knowler WC, Barrett-Connor E, Fowler SE, et al. Diabetes Prevention Program Research Group. Reduction in the incidence of type 2 diabetes with lifestyle intervention or metformin. *N Engl J Med* 2002;346(6):393–403.
18. Hogan P, Dall T, Nikolov P. American Diabetes Association. Economic costs of diabetes in the US in 2002. *Diabetes Care* 2003;26(3):917–932.
19. Relman AS. The new medical-industrial complex. *N Engl J Med* 1980;303(17): 963–970.
20. Brundage JF. Cases and deaths during influenza pandemics in the United States. *Am J Prev Med* 2006;31(3):252–256.

Summary of Recommended Clinical Preventive Services

The proper clinical circumstances in which clinicians should routinely offer screening tests, immunizations, chemoprevention, and counseling regarding risk factors are discussed in the earlier chapters of this book and in greater detail in the source guidelines cited in those chapters. The following summary table is offered as a convenient reference for clinicians. However, it cannot substitute for the source guidelines, which provide details that a table cannot fully capture. Moreover, the table provides a snapshot of guidelines as of this printing; clinicians should consult current references to familiarize themselves with the latest recommendations and newer options for preventive care.

The following table draws heavily (although not exclusively) on the recommendations of the U.S. Preventive Services Task Force (USPSTF). The USPSTF, established by the U.S. Public Health Service in 1984, is an independent panel of nonfederal experts that uses a systematic methodology to review the evidence of effectiveness for clinical preventive services, assign ratings to the quality of the data, and issue clinical practice recommendations reflecting the strength of the supporting evidence. Preventive services are not recommended by the USPSTF unless there is compelling evidence that the service is effective and that the benefits outweigh the harms. The USPSTF works in close collaboration with primary care medical specialty societies (American Academy of Family Physicians, American Academy of Pediatrics, American College of Physicians, American College of Obstetricians and Gynecologists) and federal government health agencies (e.g., Centers for Disease Control and Prevention). Further details about the USPSTF and how its recommendations were developed are available in its publications, in reports posted on its website (http://www.ahrq.gov/), and in references listed at the end of the Introduction of this book (pages xliii–xlv).

The services listed in the table are not meant to exclude from consideration other preventive services that may also be effective and beneficial to patients. The list in the subsequent text is limited to clinical interventions that have been shown in well-designed studies to improve health outcomes when performed routinely and that have received "A" or "B" recommendations (see definitions in table) from the USPSTF, reflecting strong supporting evidence. Patients, especially those in special circumstances, may benefit from interventions that have not been the subject of such research. For example, although the USPSTF was unable to identify evidence that health outcomes are improved by routinely counseling all patients about diet or physical activity, clinicians or programs that are effective in helping patients to modify these behaviors and/or reduce weight are likely to be beneficial. Also, as is true for the book in general, the table does not include guidelines specific to pregnant women.

Owing to the considerations mentioned earlier, the preponderance of services listed in the table relate to adults; preventive services for infants, children, and adolescents are rarely the subject of well-designed intervention trials and therefore lack the scientific support necessary for endorsement by the USPSTF or other groups that adhere strictly to evidence-based analytic methods. The American Academy of Pediatrics and other groups provide useful tables that summarize the key elements of anticipatory guidance that clinicians should consider in caring for the pediatric population.

Target Condition	Preventive Service	Men	Women	Target Population	Periodicity	USPSTF Grade[a] (yr)	URL for Further Details on USPSTF Recommendation
Screening							
Abdominal aortic aneurysm	Abdominal ultrasonography	✓	—	Ever smokers, aged 65 years and older	Once	B (2005)	http://www.ahrq .gov/clinic/uspstf/ uspsaneu.htm
Alcohol misuse	Screening questionnaire; behavioral counseling	✓	✓	Adults	Not specified[b]	B (2004)	http://www.ahrq .gov/clinic/uspstf/ uspsdrin.htm
Amblyopia, strabismus, diminished visual acuity	Age-specific screening procedures to assess visual impairment	✓	✓	Children aged 5 years and younger	Not specified[c]	B (2004)	http://www.ahrq .gov/clinic/uspstf/ uspsvsch.htm
Breast cancer	Mammography with or without clinical breast examination	—	✓	Aged 40 years and older	1–2 years	B (2002)	http://www.ahrq .gov/clinic/uspstf/ uspsbrca.htm
	Genetic counseling and assessment for *BRCA* testing	—	✓	Women with family history consistent with *BRCA* gene mutation[d]	Not specified	B (2005)	http://www.ahrq .gov/clinic/uspstf/ uspsbrgen.htm

Cervical cancer	Pap smear	—	✓	Women who have been sexually active and have a cervix, from age 21 (or within 3 years of onset of sexual activity) to age 65 years	**High-risk:** 1 year; **low-risk:** 3 years	A (2003)	http://www.ahrq.gov/clinic/uspstf/uspscerv.htm
Chlamydial infection	Vaginal, urethral, or urine swab for nucleic acid amplification testing[e]	—	✓	Sexually active women aged 24 years and younger and other asymptomatic women at increased risk of infection	6–12 months[f]	A (2007)[g]	http://www.ahrq.gov/clinic/uspstf/uspschlm.htm
Colorectal cancer	FOBT[h] flexible sigmoidoscopy, barium enema, colonoscopy	✓	✓	**Average-risk:** aged 50 years and older	**FOBT:** 1 year; **sigmoidoscopy and barium enema:** 5 years; **colonoscopy:** 10 years	A (2002)	http://www.ahrq.gov/clinic/uspstf/uspscolo.htm

(continued)

Target Condition	Preventive Service	Men	Women	Target Population	Periodicity	USPSTF Grade[a] (yr)	URL for Further Details on USPSTF Recommendation
Depression	Screening questionnaire	√	√	Adults	Not specified[i]	B (2002)[j]	http://www.ahrq.gov/clinic/uspstf/uspsdepr.htm
Diabetes	Fasting plasma glucose	√	√	Adults with hypertension or hyperlipidemia[k]	Not specified[k]	B (2003)[j]	http://www.ahrq.gov/clinic/uspstf/uspsdiab.htm
Gonorrhea	Vaginal or urethral swab or urine specimen		√	Sexually active women aged 25 years and younger and other asymptomatic women at increased risk of infection.	Not specified	B (2005)[m]	http://www.ahrq.gov/clinic/uspstf/uspsgono.htm
Hypertension	Sphygmomanometry	√	√	Aged 18 years and older	Not specified[n]	A (2003)[j]	http://www.ahrq.gov/clinic/uspstf/uspshype.htm
Human immunodeficiency virus	Repeatedly reactive enzyme immunoassay	√	√	Adolescents and adults at risk of infection[o]	Not specified	A (2005)	http://www.ahrq.gov/clinic/uspstf/uspshivi.htm

Condition	Screening/Intervention			Population	Interval	Recommendation (Year)	Source
Lipid disorders (e.g., hyperlipidemia)	Total cholesterol, high-density lipoprotein	✓	✓	**Average-risk:** men aged 35 years and older, women aged 45 years and older[b]	Not specified[a]	A (2001)[c]	http://www.ahrq.gov/clinic/uspstf/uspschol.htm
Obesity	Measurement of body mass index; intensive counseling and behavioral interventions	✓	✓	Adults	Not specified	B (2003)	http://www.ahrq.gov/clinic/uspstf/uspsobes.htm
Osteoporosis in postmenopausal women	Bone density measurement		✓	Average-risk women aged 65 years and older and high-risk women aged 60 years and older	3 years	B (2002)	http://www.ahrq.gov/clinic/uspstf/uspsoste.htm
Ovarian cancer	Genetic counseling and assessment for BRCA testing		✓	Women with a family history associated with an increased risk of BRCA mutations[d]	Not specified	B (2005)	http://www.ahrq.gov/clinic/uspstf/uspsbrgen.htm

(continued)

599

Target Condition	Preventive Service	Men	Women	Target Population	Periodicity	USPSTF Grade[a] (yr)	URL for Further Details on USPSTF Recommendation
Syphilis infection	RPR or VDRL followed by confirmatory TP-PA or FTA-ABS	√	√	Persons at increased risk[r] and all pregnant women.	Not specified	A (2004)	http://www.ahrq .gov/clinic/uspstf/ uspssyph.htm
Chemoprophylaxis							
Cardiovascular disease	Discussion of aspirin chemoprophylaxis	√	√	Adults at increased risk of CHD (≥3% risk of CHD in 5 years)	Not specified[s]	A (2002)	http://www.ahrq .gov/clinic/uspstf/ uspsasmi.htm
Breast cancer	Discussion of tamoxifen		√	Women at high risk of breast cancer and at low risk of adverse effects of chemoprevention	Not specified	B (2002)	http://www.ahrq .gov/clinic/uspstf/ uspsbrpv.htm

| Dental caries | Fluoride supplementation | √ | √ | Preschool children (aged 6 months and older) whose primary water source is deficient in fluoride | Not specified | B (2004) | http://www.ahrq.gov/clinic/3rduspstf/dentalchild/dentchrs.htm |

Counseling

| Tobacco use | Identification of users and delivery of cessation interventions | √ | √ | Adults and pregnant women | Regular[t] | A (2003) | http://www.ahrq.gov/clinic/uspstf/uspstbac.htm |
| Diet | Intensive behavioral counseling | √ | √ | Adults with hyperlipidemia and other known risk factors for cardiovascular and diet-related chronic disease[a] | Not specified | B (2003) | http://www.ahrq.gov/clinic/uspstf/uspsdiet.htm |

Immunizations

See Chapter 16

(continued)

(Continued)

FOBT = fecal occult blood test; RPR = rapid plasma reagin; VDRL = Veneral Disease Research Laboratory test; TP-PA = *treponema pallidum* particle agglutination; FTA-ABS = fluorescent treponemal antibody absorbed; CHD = coronary heart disease.

Notes: The appropriate age to initiate and discontinue screening and the frequency of screening often vary with risk status and can be influenced by symptoms, comorbidities, family history, prior test abnormalities, or other factors that affect risk.

[a] The U.S. Preventive Services Task Force (USPSTF) grades its recommendations according to one of five classifications (A, B, C, D, I) reflecting the strength of evidence and magnitude of net benefit (benefits minus harms). **A:** The USPSTF strongly recommends that clinicians provide [the service] to eligible patients. The USPSTF found good evidence that [the service] improves important health outcomes and concludes that benefits substantially outweigh harms. **B:** The USPSTF recommends that clinicians provide [this service] to eligible patients. The USPSTF found at least fair evidence that [the service] improves important health outcomes and concludes that benefits outweigh harms. **C:** The USPSTF makes no recommendation for or against routine provision of [the service]. The USPSTF found at least fair evidence that [the service] can improve health outcomes but concludes that the balance of benefits and harms is too close to justify a general recommendation. **D:** The USPSTF recommends against routinely providing [the service] to asymptomatic patients. The USPSTF found at least fair evidence that [the service] is ineffective or that harms outweigh benefits. **I:** The USPSTF concludes that the evidence is insufficient to recommend for or against routinely providing [the service]. Evidence that the [service] is effective is lacking, of poor quality, or conflicting and the balance of benefits and harms cannot be determined.

[b] According to the USPSTF, "The optimal interval for screening and intervention is unknown. Patients with past alcohol problems, young adults, and other high-risk groups (e.g., smokers) may benefit most from frequent screening."

[c] Based on expert opinion, the American Academy of Pediatrics (AAP) recommends the following vision screening be performed at all well-child visits for children starting in the newborn period to age 3 years: ocular history, vision assessment, external inspection of the eyes and lids, ocular motility assessment, pupil examination, and red reflex examination. For children aged 3–5 years, the AAP recommends the aforementioned screening in addition to age-appropriate visual acuity measurement (using HOTV or tumbling E tests [see page 440] and ophthalmoscopy.

[d] For non–Ashkenazi Jewish women, relevant risk factors include two first-degree relatives with breast cancer, one of whom received the diagnosis at 50 years or younger; a combination of three or more first- or second-degree relatives with breast cancer regardless of age at diagnosis; a combination of both breast and ovarian cancer among first- and second-degree relatives; a first-degree relative with bilateral breast cancer; a combination of two or more first- or second-degree relatives with ovarian cancer regardless of age at diagnosis; a first- or second-degree relative with both breast and ovarian cancer at any age; and a history of breast cancer in a male relative. For women of Ashkenazi Jewish heritage, an increased-risk family history includes any first-degree relative (or two second-degree relatives on the same side of the family) with breast or ovarian cancer.

[e] Detailed guidance on available screening tests for chlamydia are provided at http://www.cdc.gov/STD/LabGuidelines/.

[f] The optimal screening interval is uncertain. For women with a previous negative screening test, the interval for rescreening should take into account changes in sexual partners. If there is evidence that a woman is at low risk of infection (e.g., in a mutually monogamous relationship with a previous history of negative screening tests for chlamydial infection), it may not be necessary to screen frequently. Rescreening at 6–12 months may be appropriate for previously infected women because of high rates of reinfection and for those at high risk. Pregnant women should be screened at the first prenatal visit and those at high risk should be retested in the third trimester.

[g] The USPSTF gave a B grade to screening pregnant women for chlamydial infection.

[h] FOBT = fecal occult blood test.

602

[i]The optimal interval for screening is unknown. Recurrent screening may be most productive in patients with a history of depression, unexplained somatic symptoms, comorbid psychological conditions (e.g., panic disorder or generalized anxiety), substance abuse, or chronic pain.

[j]The USPSTF recommends routine depression screening only at practices that have systems in place to assure accurate diagnosis, effective treatment and follow-up. At this writing the USPSTF is in the midst of updating this recommendation.

[k]The American Diabetic Association recommends initiating screening at age 45 years for average-risk individuals and earlier for high-risk individuals (those with an elevated body mass index [BMI], other cardiovascular risk factors, or a family history); if the value is normal, screening can be repeated every 3 years.

[l]At this writing the USPSTF is in the midst of updating this recommendation.

[m]The USPSTF also issued an A recommendation for the application of prophylactic ocular topical medication for all newborns against gonococcal ophthalmia neonatorum.

[n]The Joint National Committee on Hypertension VII recommends that adults undergo screening every 2 years if they have previously been normotensive and annually if they are prehypertensive (120–139/80–89 mm Hg).

[o]Those at increased risk (as determined by prevalence rates) include men who have had sex with men after 1975; men and women having unprotected sex with multiple partners; past or present injection drug users; men and women who exchange sex for money or drugs or have sex partners who do; individuals whose past or present sex partners were human immunodeficiency virus (HIV)-infected, bisexual, or injection drug users; persons being treated for sexually transmitted infections; and persons with a history of blood transfusion between 1978 and 1985. Persons who request an HIV test despite reporting no individual risk factors may also be considered at increased risk, since this group is likely to include individuals not willing to disclose high-risk behaviors. In September 2006, the Centers for Disease Control and Prevention (CDC) published revised guidelines recommending that all individuals age 13–64 years be screened for HIV regardless of recognized risk factors. In November 2006, the USPSTF reviewed the evidence considered by the CDC and reaffirmed its "C" recommendation for screening nonpregnant adolescents and adults who are not at increased risk of HIV infection.

[p]The 2001 USPSTF guidelines included a B recommendation for younger adults (men aged 20–35 years and women aged 20–45 years) if they have other risk factors for CHD, including: diabetes; a family history of cardiovascular disease before age 50 years in male relatives or age 60 years in female relatives; a family history suggestive of familial hyperlipidemia; or multiple CHD risk factors (e.g., tobacco use, hypertension). At this writing (2007) the USPSTF is preparing revised recommendations that, as discussed on page 97, recommend screening of average-risk men aged 35 years and older and high-risk men and women aged 20 years and older but do not recommend routine screening of average-risk women.

[q]The National Cholesterol Education Program recommends repeating the test in 5 years if previous results are normal.

[r]Men who have sex with men and engage in high-risk sexual behavior, commercial sex workers, persons who exchange sex for drugs, and those in adult correctional facilities.

[s]Although the optimal timing and frequency of discussions related to aspirin therapy are unknown, reasonable options include every 5 years in middle-aged and older people or when other cardiovascular risk factors are detected.

[t]The U.S. Department of Health and Human Services guideline on smoking cessation counseling recommends assessing tobacco use status at every clinical encounter.

[u]For patients without these risk factors (unselected patients), the USPSTF found evidence of limited quality that brief, low- to medium-intensity behavioral dietary counseling in the primary care setting can produce small-to-medium changes in average daily intake of core components of an overall healthy diet. Evidence that more intensive interventions are effective in unselected patients was not available at the time of the USPSTF review.

Immunization Guidelines

TABLE 1 Summary of Recommendations for Childhood and Adolescent Immunizations

Vaccine Name and Route	Schedule for Routine Vaccination[a]	Catch-Up Schedule and Related Issues	Contraindications and Precautions[b]
Hepatitis B *Give i.m.*	• Vaccinate all children aged 0 through 18 yr • Vaccinate all newborns with monovalent vaccine before hospital discharge. Give second dose at 1–2 mo and the final dose at 6–18 mo (the last dose in the infant series should not be given earlier than age 6 mo). After the birth dose, the series may be completed using two doses of single-antigen vaccine or up to three doses	• Do not restart series, no matter how long since previous dose • Three-dose series can be started at any age • Minimum spacing between doses: 4 wk between first and second, 8 wk between second and third, and at least 16 wk	**Contraindications** Previous anaphylaxis to this vaccine or to any of its components **Precautions** Moderate or severe acute illness

Hepatitis B (continued)	of Comvax (ages 2 mo, 4 mo, 12–15 mo) or Pediarix (ages 2 mo, 4 mo, 6 mo), which may result in giving a total of four doses of hepatitis B vaccine • **If mother is HBsAg-positive,** give the newborn HBIG + first dose within 12 h of birth; complete series at 6 mo of age or, if using Comvax, at 12–15 mo • **If mother's HBsAg status is unknown:** give the newborn first dose within 12 h of birth. If mother is subsequently found to be HBsAg positive, give infant HBIG within 7 d of birth and follow the schedule for infants born to HBsAg-positive mothers	between first and third (e.g., 0, 2, 4-mo; 0, 1-, 4-mo) ┌───┐ *Special Notes on Hepatitis B Vaccine (HepB)* ***Dosing of HepB:*** *Vaccine brands are interchangeable. For persons aged 0–19 yr, give 0.5 mL of either Engerix-B or Recombivax HB.* ***Alternative dosing schedule for unvaccinated adolescents aged 11–15 yr:*** *Give two doses Recombivax HB 1.0 mL (adult formulation) spaced 4–6 mo apart. (Engerix-B is not licensed for a two-dose schedule)* ***For preterm infants:*** *Consult ACIP hepatitis B recommendations (MMWR 2005; 54 [RR-16]).* └───┘
DTaP, DT (Diphtheria, tetanus, acellular pertussis) *Give i.m.*	• Give to children at ages 2 mo, 4 mo, 6 mo, 15–18 mo, 4–6 yr • May give first dose as early as age 6 wk • May give fourth dose as early as age 12 mo if 6 mo have elapsed since third and the child is unlikely to return at age 15–18 mo • Do not give DTaP/DT to children aged 7 yr and older • If possible, use the same DTaP product for all doses	• Second and third may be given 4 wk after previous dose • Fourth may be given 6 mo after third • If fourth is given before fourth birthday, wait at least 6 mo for fifth (age 4–6 yr) • If fourth is given after fourth birthday, fifth is not needed	**Contraindications** • Previous anaphylaxis to this vaccine or to any of its components • For DTaP/Tdap only: encephalopathy within 7 d after DTP/DTaP **Precautions** • Moderate or severe acute illness • Guillain-Barré syndrome within 6 wk of previous dose of tetanus toxoid–containing vaccine

(continued)

TABLE 1 (Continued)

Vaccine Name and Route	Schedule for Routine Vaccination[a]	Catch-Up Schedule and Related Issues	Contraindications and Precautions[b]

Td, Tdap (tetanus, diphtheria, acellular pertussis) *Give i.m.*	• Give Tdap booster dose to adolescents aged 11–12 yr if 5 yr have elapsed since last dose of DTaP/DTP; boost every 10 yr with Td
	• Give one-time Tdap to all adolescents who have not received previous Tdap. Special efforts should be made to give Tdap to persons aged 11 yr and older who are:
	   —in contact with infants younger than age 12 mo
	   —health care workers with direct patient contact
	• In pregnancy, when indicated, give Td or Tdap in second or third trimester. If not administered during pregnancy, give Tdap in immediate postpartum period
		• If never vaccinated with tetanus- and diphtheria-containing vaccine: give Td first dose now, second dose 4 wk later, and third dose 6 mo after second, and then give booster every 10 yr. A one-time Tdap may be substituted for any dose in the series
		• Intervals of 2 yr or less between Td and Tdap may be used if needed
			• For DTaP only: any of these occurrences following a previous dose of DTP/DTaP: (a) temperature of 105°F (40.5°C) or higher within 48 h; (b) continuous crying for 3 h or more within 48 h; (c) collapse or shock-like state within 48 h; (d) convulsion with or without fever within 3 d
			• For DTaP/Tdap only: unstable neurologic disorder
			Note: Use of Td or Tdap is not contraindicated in pregnancy. At the discretion of the clinician, either vaccine may be administered during the second or third trimester

Polio (IPV) *Give s.c. or i.m.*	• Give to children at ages 2 mo, 4 mo, 6–18 mo, 4–6 yr • May give first dose as early as age 6 wk • Not routinely recommended for those aged 18 yr and older (except certain travelers)	• All doses should be separated by at least 4 wk • If third dose is given after fourth birthday, fourth dose is not needed	**Contraindications** Previous anaphylaxis to this vaccine or to any of its components **Precautions** • Moderate or severe acute illness • Pregnancy

Human Papillomavirus (HPV) *Give i.m.*	• Give three-dose series to girls at ages 11–12 yr on a 0-, 2-, 6-mo schedule • May be given as early as age 9 yr • Vaccinate all older females (through age 26 yr) not previously vaccinated	• Second dose may be given 4 wk after first dose • Third dose may be given 12 wk after the second dose	**Contraindications** Previous anaphylaxis to this vaccine or to any of its components **Precautions** • Moderate or severe acute illness • Pregnancy
Varicella (Var) (Chickenpox) *Give s.c.*	• Give the first dose at age 12–15 mo • Give the second dose at age 4–6 yr. The second dose may be given earlier if at least 3 mo since the first dose • Give a routine second dose to all older children and adolescents with history of only one dose • MMRV may be used in children 12 mo through 12 yr	• If younger than age 13 yr, space the first and second dose at least 3 mo apart. If aged 13 yr or older, space 4–8 wk apart • May use as postexposure prophylaxis if given within 3–5 d • If Var and either MMR, LAIV, and/or yellow fever vaccine are not given on the same day, space them at least 28 d apart	**Contraindications** • Previous anaphylaxis to this vaccine or to any of its components • Pregnancy or possibility of pregnancy within 4 wk • Children immunocompromised because of high doses of systemic steroids, cancer, leukemia, lymphoma, or immunodeficiency **Note:** For patients with humoral immunodeficiency, HIV infection, or leukemia, or for patients on high doses of systemic steroids, see ACIP recommendations[c]

(continued)

TABLE 1 (Continued)

Vaccine Name and Route	Schedule for Routine Vaccination[a]	Catch-Up Schedule and Related Issues	Contraindications and Precautions[b]
Varicella (Var) (Chickenpox) (continued)			**Precautions** • Moderate or severe acute illness • If blood, plasma, and/or immune globulin (IG or VZIG) were given in the last 11 mo, see ACIP statement *General Recommendations on Immunization*[c] regarding time to wait before vaccinating
MMR (Measles, mumps, rubella) *Give s.c.*	• Give the first dose at age 12–15 mo • Give the second dose at age 4–6 yr. Second dose may be given earlier if at least 4 wk since the first dose • If a dose was given before 12 mo of age, it does not count as the first dose, so give the first dose at age 12–15 mo with a minimum interval of 4 wk between the invalid dose and first dose • MMRV may be used in children 12 mo through 12 yr	• If MMR and either Var, LAIV, and/or yellow fever vaccine are not given on the same day, space them at least 28 d apart • When using MMR (not MMRV) for both doses, minimum interval is 4 wk	**Contraindications** • Previous anaphylaxis to this vaccine or to any of its components • Pregnancy or possibility of pregnancy within 4 wk • Severe immunodeficiency (e.g., hematologic and solid tumors; congenital immunodeficiency; long-term immunosuppressive therapy; or severely symptomatic HIV) **Precautions** • Moderate or severe acute illness

MMR (continued)	• If blood, plasma, or immune globulin given in the last 11 mo or if on high-dose immunosuppressive therapy, see ACIP statement *General Recommendations on Immunization*[c] regarding delay time • History of thrombocytopenia or thrombocytopenic purpura **Note:** MMR is not contraindicated if a PPD (tuberculosis skin test) was recently applied. If PPD and MMR not given on same day, delay PPD for 4–6 wk after MMR
Trivalent inactivated influenza vaccine (TIV) *Give i.m.* Live attenuated influenza vaccine (LAIV) *Give intranasally*	• On an annual basis, vaccinate all children aged 6–59 mo, as well as all siblings and household contacts of children aged 0–59 mo • Vaccinate persons 5 yr and older who: —Have a risk factor (e.g., pregnancy, heart disease, lung disease, diabetes, renal dysfunction, hemoglobinopathy, immunosuppression, on long-term aspirin therapy, or have a condition that compromises respiratory function or the handling of respiratory secretions or that can increase the risk of aspiration) or live in a chronic-care facility —Live or work with at-risk people as listed above • Vaccinate any person wishing to reduce the likelihood of becoming ill with influenza	**Contraindications** • Previous anaphylaxis to this vaccine, to any of its components, or to eggs • For LAIV only: Pregnancy, asthma, reactive airway disease, or other chronic disorder of the pulmonary or cardiovascular systems; an underlying medical condition, including metabolic diseases such as diabetes, renal dysfunction, and

(continued)

TABLE 1 (Continued)

Vaccine Name and Route	Schedule for Routine Vaccination[a]	Catch-Up Schedule and Related Issues	Contraindications and Precautions[b]
Influenza (continued)	• LAIV may be given to healthy, nonpregnant persons aged 5–49 yr. For first-time vaccinees aged 6 mo through 8 yr. For TIV, space 4 wk apart; for LAIV, space 6 wk apart (no younger than 5 yr) • For TIV, give 0.25 mL dose to children aged 6–35 mo and 0.5 mL dose if aged 3 yr and older • If a child under age 9 yrs received the first influenza vaccination during a previous season and only received one dose, give two doses in the second season. If the child received only one dose for two previous seasons, only give one dose annually thereafter		hemoglobinopathies; a known or suspected immune deficiency disease or receiving immunosuppressive therapy; history of Guillain-Barré syndrome **Precautions** • Moderate or severe acute illness • For TIV only: History of Guillain-Barré syndrome within 6 wk of previous TIV
Rotavirus (Rota) *Give orally*	• Give a three-dose series at ages 2 mo, 4 mo, and 6 mo • May give the first dose as early as age 6 wk • Give the third dose no later than age 32 wk	• Do not begin series in infants older than 12 wk • Second and third dose may be given 4 wk after previous dose	**Contraindications** Previous anaphylaxis to this vaccine or to any of its components **Precautions** • Moderate or severe acute illness • Altered immunocompetence • Moderate to severe acute gastroenteritis or chronic gastrointestinal disease • History of intussusception

Vaccine	Schedule	Contraindications / Precautions
Hib (*Haemophilus influenzae* type b) *Give i.m.*	• HibTITER (HbOC) and ActHib (PRP-T): give at 2 mo, 4 mo, 6 mo, 12–15 mo (booster dose) • PedvaxHIB or Comvax (containing PRP-OMP): give at 2 mo, 4 mo, 12–15 mo • First dose of Hib vaccine may be given no earlier than age 6 wk • The last dose (booster dose) is given no earlier than age 12 mo and a minimum of 8 wk after the previous dose • Hib vaccines are interchangeable; however, if different brands of Hib vaccines are administered, a total of three doses are necessary to complete the primary series in infants • Any Hib vaccine may be used for the booster dose • Hib is not routinely given to children aged 5 yr and older	**All Hib vaccines:** • If first dose was given at 12–14 mo, give booster in 8 wk • Give only one dose to unvaccinated children from age 15 mo to 5 yr **HibTITER and ActHib:** • Second and third dose may be given 4 wk after previous dose • If first dose was given at 7–11 mo, only three doses are needed; second dose is given 4–8 wk after first dose, then booster at 12–15 mo (wait at least 8 wk after second dose) **PedvaxHIB and Comvax:** • second dose may be given 4 wk after first dose	**Contraindications** Previous anaphylaxis to this vaccine or to any of its components **Precautions** Moderate or severe acute illness
Pneumococcal conjugate (PCV) *Give i.m.*	• Give at ages 2-, 4-, 6-, and 12- to 15 mo • First dose may be given as early as age 6 wk • Give one dose to unvaccinated healthy children aged 24–59 mo • Give two doses at least 8 wk apart to unvaccinated high-risk[d] children aged 24–59 mo	• For ages 7–11 mo: If history of zero to two doses, give additional doses 4 wk apart with no more than three total doses by age 12 mo; then give booster 8 wk later	**Contraindications** Previous anaphylaxis to this vaccine or to any of its components **Precautions** Moderate or severe acute illness

(continued)

TABLE 1 *(Continued)*

Vaccine Name and Route	Schedule for Routine Vaccination[a]	Catch-Up Schedule and Related Issues	Contraindications and Precautions[b]
PCV (continued)	• PCV is not routinely given to children aged 5 yr and older	• For ages 12–23 mo: If zero to one dose before age 12 mo, give two doses at least 8 wk apart. If two to three doses before age 12 mo, give one dose at least 8 wk after previous dose • For ages 24–59 mo: If patient has had no previous doses, or has a history of 1–3 doses given before age 12 mo but no booster dose, or has a history of only one dose given at 12–23 mo, give one dose now	
Pneumococcal polysaccharide (PPV) *Give i.m. or s.c.*	• Give one dose at least 8 wk after final dose of PCV to high-risk[d] children aged 2 yr and older • For children who are immunocompromised or have sickle cell disease or functional or anatomic asplenia, give a second dose of PPV 3–5 yr after previous PPV (consult ACIP PPV	**Contraindications** Previous anaphylaxis to this vaccine or to any of its components **Precautions** Moderate or severe acute illness

recommendations in *MMWR* 1997;46 [RR-8] for details[c]

Hepatitis A *Give i.m.*	• Give two doses to all children at age 1 yr (12–23 mo) spaced 6 mo apart • Vaccinate all children and adolescents aged 2 years and older who: 　—Live in a state, county, or community with a routine vaccination program already in place for children aged 2 yr and older 　—Travel anywhere except United States, western Europe, New Zealand, Australia, Canada, or Japan 　—Wish to be protected from HAV infection 　—Have chronic liver disease, clotting factor disorder, or are MSM adolescents	• Minimum interval between doses is 6 mo • Consider routine vaccination of children aged 2 yr and older in areas with no existing program	**Contraindications** Previous anaphylaxis to this vaccine or to any of its components **Precautions** Moderate or severe acute illness
Meningococcal conjugate (MCV4) *Give i.m.*	• Give one-time dose of MCV4 to adolescents aged 11–12 yr, to adolescents at high school entry (approximately aged 15 yr), and to college freshmen living in dormitories	If previously vaccinated with MPSV4 and risk continues, give MCV4 5 yr after MPSV4	**Contraindications** Previous anaphylaxis to this vaccine or to any of its components, including diphtheria toxoid (for MCV4)

(continued)

TABLE 1 (Continued)

Vaccine Name and Route	Schedule for Routine Vaccination[a]	Catch-Up Schedule and Related Issues	Contraindications and Precautions[b]
Meningococcal vaccine (continued) Polysaccharide (MPSV4) *Give s.c.*	• Vaccinate all children aged 2 yr and older who have any of the following risk factors (use MPSV4 if younger than 11 yr and MCV4 if 11 yr and older): —Anatomic or functional asplenia, or terminal complement component deficiencies —Travel to or reside in countries in which meningococcal disease is hyperendemic or epidemic (e.g., the "meningitis belt'" of sub-Saharan Africa) **Note:** Other adolescents who wish to decrease their risk of meningococcal disease may be vaccinated with MCV4		**Precautions** Moderate or severe acute illness. For MCV4 only: history of Guillain-Barré syndrome **Note:** MCV4 is not licensed for use in children younger than 11 yr

Adapted with permission from *Summary of Recommendations for Child and Adolescent Immunization,* Immunization Action Coalition, St. Paul, MN 2007; available online at: http://www.immunize .org/catg.d/p2010.pdf. Accessed September 2007.

HBsAg = hepatitis B surface antigen marker; HBIG = hepatitis B immune globulin; DTaP = diphtheria-tetanus-acellular pertussis; DT = diphtheria-tetanus; DTP = diphtheria-tetanus-pertussis; Td = diphtheria toxoid; IPV = inactivated poliovirus vaccine; MMRV = measles-mumps-rubella-varicella; VZIG = varicella zoster immunoglobulin; HIV = human immunodeficiency virus; PPD = purified protein derivative.

[a] Any vaccine can be given with another.

[b] Mild illness is not a contraindication.

[c] For specific ACIP recommendations, refer to the official ACIP statements published in *MMWR.* To obtain copies of these statements, call the CDC-INFO Contact Center at (800) 232–4636; visit CDC's website at www.cdc.gov/nip/publications/ACIP-list.htm; or visit the Immunization Action Coalition (IAC) website at www.immunize.org/acip.

[d] High-risk: Those with sickle cell disease; anatomic/functional asplenia; chronic cardiac, pulmonary, or renal disease; diabetes; cerebrospinal fluid leaks; HIV infection; immunosuppression; or who have or will have a cochlear implant.

TABLE 2 Summary of Recommendations for Adult Immunizations

Vaccine Name and Route	Population For Whom Vaccination Is Recommended	Schedule for Vaccine Administration[a]	Contraindications and Precautions[b]
Trivalent inactivated influenza vaccine (TIV) *Give i.m.*	• Persons aged 50 yr and older • Persons with medical problems (e.g., heart disease, lung disease, diabetes, renal dysfunction, hemoglobinopathy, immunosuppression) and/or people living in chronic-care facilities • Persons with any condition that compromises respiratory function or the handling of respiratory secretions or that can increase the risk of aspiration (e.g., cognitive dysfunction, spinal cord injury, seizure disorder, or other neuromuscular disorder) • Persons working or living with at-risk people • Women who will be pregnant during the influenza season (December–March) • All health care workers and other persons who provide direct care to at-risk people • Household contacts and out-of-home caregivers of children aged 0–59 mo	• Given every year in the fall or winter • October and November are the ideal months to give TIV • LAIV may be given as early as August • Continue to give TIV and LAIV through the influenza season from December through March (including when influenza activity is present in the community) and at other times when the risk of influenza exists	**Contraindications** Previous anaphylactic reaction to this vaccine, to any of its components, or to eggs **Precautions** • Moderate or severe acute illness • History of Guillain-Barré syndrome within 6 wk of previous TIV

(continued)

TABLE 2 *(Continued)*

Vaccine Name and Route	Population For Whom Vaccination Is Recommended	Schedule for Vaccine Administration[a]	Contraindications and Precautions[b]
TIV (continued)	• Travelers at risk for complications of influenza who visit areas where influenza activity exists or who may be among people from areas of the world where there is current influenza activity (e.g., on organized tours) • Persons who provide essential community services • Students or other persons in institutional settings (e.g., dormitory residents) • Anyone wishing to reduce the likelihood of becoming ill with influenza		
Live attenuated influenza vaccine (LAIV) *Give intranasally*	• Healthy, nonpregnant persons 49 yr and younger who meet any of the conditions listed below: —Working or living with at-risk people as listed in the section above —Health care workers or other persons who provide direct care to at-risk people (except persons in close contact with severely immunosuppressed persons) —Household contacts and out-of-home caregivers of children ages 0–59 mo		**Contraindications** • Previous anaphylactic reaction to this vaccine, to any of its components, or to eggs • Pregnancy, asthma, reactive airway disease, or other chronic disorder of the pulmonary or cardiovascular system; an underlying medical condition, including metabolic disease such as diabetes, renal dysfunction, and hemoglobinopathy; a known or

LAIV (continued)	—Travelers who may be among people from areas of the world where there is current influenza activity (e.g., on organized tours) —Persons who provide essential community services —Students or other persons in institutional settings (e.g., dormitory residents) —Anyone wishing to reduce the likelihood of becoming ill with influenza	suspected immune deficiency disease or receiving immunosuppressive therapy; history of Guillain-Barré syndrome **Precautions** Moderate or severe acute illness
Pneumococcal polysaccharide vaccine (PPV) *Give i.m. or s.c.*	• Persons 65 yrs and older • Persons who have chronic illness or other risk factors, including chronic cardiac or pulmonary disease, chronic liver disease, alcoholism, diabetes, CSF leak, as well as people living in special environments or social settings (including Alaska Natives and certain American Indian populations). Those at highest risk of fatal pneumococcal infection are persons with anatomic asplenia, functional asplenia, or sickle cell disease; immunocompromised	• Routinely given as a one-time dose; administer if previous vaccination history is unknown • One-time revaccination is recommended 5 yr later for persons at highest risk of fatal pneumococcal infection or rapid antibody loss (e.g., renal disease) and	**Contraindications** Previous anaphylactic reaction to this vaccine or to any of its components **Precautions** Moderate or severe acute illness

(continued)

TABLE 2 *(Continued)*

Vaccine Name and Route	Population For Whom Vaccination Is Recommended	Schedule for Vaccine Administration^a	Contraindications and Precautions^b
PPV *(continued)*	persons including those with HIV infection, leukemia, lymphoma, Hodgkin's disease, multiple myeloma, generalized malignancy, chronic renal failure, or nephrotic syndrome; persons receiving immunosuppressive chemotherapy (including corticosteroids); those who received an organ or bone marrow transplant; and candidates for or recipients of cochlear implants	for persons 65 yr and older if the first dose was given before age 65 and 5 yr or more have elapsed since the previous dose	
Hepatitis B (Hep B) *Give i.m.* Brands may be used interchangeably	• All adolescents; any adult wishing to obtain immunity • High-risk persons, including household contacts and sex partners of HBsAg-positive persons; injection drug users; heterosexuals with more than one sex partner in 6 mo; men who have sex with men; persons with recently diagnosed STIs; patients receiving hemodialysis and patients with renal disease that may result in dialysis; recipients of certain blood products; health care workers and public safety workers who are exposed to blood; clients	• Three doses are needed on a 0-, 1-, 6-mo schedule • Alternative timing options for vaccination include 0, 2, 4 mo and 0, 1, 4 mo • There must be 4 wk between the first and the second dose, and 8 wk between the second and third dose. Overall, there must be at least 16 wk between the first and third dose	**Contraindications** Previous anaphylactic reaction to this vaccine or to any of its components **Precautions** Moderate or severe acute illness

Hepatitis B (continued)	and staff of institutions for the developmentally disabled; inmates of long-term correctional facilities; and certain international travelers • Persons with chronic liver disease **Note:** Provide serologic screening for immigrants from endemic areas. When HBsAg-positive persons are identified, offer appropriate disease management. In addition, screen their sex partners and household members, and give the first dose of vaccine at the same visit. If found susceptible, complete the vaccine series	• Schedule for those who have fallen behind: If the series is delayed between doses, DO NOT start the series over. Continue from where you left off • For Twinrix (hepatitis A and B combination vaccine [GSK]), three doses are needed on a 0-, 1-, 6-mo schedule. Recipients must be aged 18 yr or older	
Hepatitis A (Hep A) *Give i.m.* Brands may be used interchangeably	• Persons who travel or work anywhere except the United States, western Europe, New Zealand, Australia, Canada, and Japan • Persons with chronic liver disease, including persons with hepatitis B and C; injection and noninjection drug users; men who have sex with men; people with clotting-factor disorders; persons who work with hepatitis A virus in experimental laboratory settings (not routine medical laboratories); and food	• Two doses are needed • The minimum interval between the first and second dose is 6 mo • If the second dose is delayed, do not repeat the first dose. Just give the second dose	**Contraindications** Previous anaphylactic reaction to this vaccine or to any of its components **Precautions** • Moderate or severe acute illness • Safety during pregnancy has not been determined, so benefits must be weighed against potential risk

(continued)

TABLE 2 (Continued)

Vaccine Name and Route	Population For Whom Vaccination Is Recommended	Schedule for Vaccine Administration[a]	Contraindications and Precautions[b]
Hepatitis A (continued)	handlers when health authorities or private employers determine vaccination to be cost effective • Anyone wishing to obtain immunity to hepatitis A **Note:** Prevaccination testing is likely to be cost effective for persons older than 40 yr, as well as for younger persons in certain groups with a high prevalence of hepatitis A virus infection		
Td, Tdap (tetanus, diphtheria, pertussis) *Give i.m.*	• All adults who lack a history of a primary series consisting of at least three doses of tetanus- and diphtheria-containing vaccine • A booster dose of tetanus- and diphtheria-containing toxoid may be needed for wound management as early as 5 yr after receiving a previous dose, so consult ACIP recommendations[c] • Using tetanus toxoid (TT) instead of Td or Tdap is *not* recommended • In pregnancy, when indicated, give Td or Tdap in second or third trimester. If not administered during pregnancy, give Tdap in immediate postpartum period	• For persons who are unvaccinated or behind, complete the primary series with Td (spaced at 0, 1–2-mo, 6–12-mo intervals). One dose of Tdap may be used for any dose if aged 19–64 yr • Give Td booster every 10 yr after the primary series has been completed. For adults aged 19–64 yr, a one-time dose of Tdap is recommended to replace the next Td	**Contraindications** • Previous anaphylactic reaction to this vaccine or to any of its components • For Tdap only, history of encephalopathy within 7 days following DTP/DTaP **Precautions** • Moderate or severe acute illness • Guillain-Barré syndrome within 6 wk of receiving a previous dose of tetanus toxoid–containing vaccine • Unstable neurologic condition

| Td, Tdap (continued) | For Tdap (tetanus- and diphtheria-toxoids with acellular pertussis vaccine) only:
• All adults younger than age 65 yr who have not received Tdap
• Health care workers who work in hospitals or ambulatory care settings and have direct patient contact and who have not received Tdap
• Adults in contact with infants younger than age 12 mo (e.g., parents, grandparents younger than 65 yr, child care providers, health care workers) who have not received a dose of Tdap | • Intervals of 2 yr or less between Td and Tdap may be used if needed
Note: The two Tdap products are licensed for different age groups: Adacel (sanofi) for use in persons aged 11–64 yr and Boostrix (GSK) for use in persons aged 10–18 yr | **Note:** Use of Td or Tdap is not contraindicated in pregnancy. At the discretion of the clinician, either vaccine may be administered during the second or third trimester |
| Polio (IPV)
Give i.m. or s.c. | Not routinely recommended for persons aged 18 yr and older
Note: Adults living in the United States who never received or completed a primary series of polio vaccine need not be vaccinated unless they intend to travel to areas where exposure to wild-type virus is likely (i.e., India, Pakistan, Afghanistan, and certain countries in Africa). Previously vaccinated adults can receive one booster dose if traveling to polio endemic areas | • Refer to ACIP recommendations[c] regarding unique situations, schedules, and dosing information | **Contraindications**
Previous anaphylactic or neurologic reaction to this vaccine or to any of its components
Precautions
• Moderate or severe acute illness
• Pregnancy |

(continued)

TABLE 2 (Continued)

Vaccine Name and Route	Population For Whom Vaccination Is Recommended	Schedule for Vaccine Administration[a]	Contraindications and Precautions[b]
Varicella (Var) (Chickenpox) *Give SC*	All adults without evidence of immunity. Immunity is defined as any one of the following: • A history of two doses of Var • Born in the United States before 1980 • History of varicella disease or herpes zoster based on health care provider diagnosis • Laboratory evidence of immunity or laboratory confirmation of disease	• Two doses are needed • Second dose is given 4–8 wk after the first dose • If Var and either MMR, LAIV, and/or yellow fever vaccine are not given on the same day, space them at least 28 d apart • If the second dose is delayed, do not repeat the first dose. Just give the second dose	**Contraindications** • Previous anaphylactic reaction to this vaccine or to any of its components • Pregnancy or possibility of pregnancy within 4 wk • Persons immunocompromised because of malignancies and primary or acquired cellular immunodeficiency including HIV/AIDS. (See *MMWR* 1999, Vol. 48, No. RR-6.) **Note:** For those on high-dose immunosuppressive therapy, consult ACIP recommendations regarding delay time.[c] **Precautions** • If blood, plasma, and/or immune globulin (IG or VZIG) were given in the last 11 mo, see ACIP statement *General Recommendations on Immunization*[c] regarding time to wait before vaccinating • Moderate or severe acute illness

Vaccine		
Meningococcal conjugate vaccine (MCV4) *Give i.m* Polysaccharide vaccine (MPSV4) *Give s.c.*	• College freshmen living in dormitories • Adolescents and adults with anatomic or functional asplenia or with terminal complement component deficiencies • Persons who travel to or reside in countries in which meningococcal disease is hyperendemic or epidemic (e.g., the "meningitis belt" of sub-Saharan Africa) • Microbiologists who are routinely exposed to isolates of *Neisseria meningitidis*	• One dose is needed • If previous vaccine was MPSV4, revaccinate after 5 yr if risk continues • Revaccination after MCV4 is not recommended • MCV4 is preferred over MPSV4 for persons 55 yr and younger, although MPSV4 is an acceptable alternative	**Contraindications** • Previous anaphylactic or neurologic reaction to this vaccine or to any of its components, including diphtheria toxoid (for MCV4) **Precautions** • Moderate or severe acute illness • For MCV4 only, history of Guillain-Barré syndrome
MMR (measles, mumps, rubella) *Give s.c.*	• Persons born in 1957 or later (especially those born outside the United States) should receive at least one dose of MMR if there is no serologic proof of immunity or documentation of a dose given on or after the first birthday • Persons in high-risk groups, such as health care workers, students entering college and other post–high school educational institutions, and international travelers, should receive a total of two doses	• One or two doses are needed • If second dose is recommended, give it no sooner than 4 wk after first dose • If MMR and either Var, LAIV, and/or yellow fever vaccine are not given on the same day, space them at least 28 d apart	**Contraindications** • Previous anaphylactic reaction to this vaccine or to any of its components • Pregnancy or possibility of pregnancy within 4 wk • Persons immunocompromised because of cancer, leukemia, lymphoma, immunosuppressive drug therapy, including high-dose steroids or radiation therapy

(continued)

TABLE 2 (Continued)

Vaccine Name and Route	Population For Whom Vaccination Is Recommended	Schedule for Vaccine Administration[a]	Contraindications and Precautions[b]
MMR (continued)	• Persons born before 1957 are usually considered immune, but proof of immunity (serology or vaccination) may be desirable for health care workers • Women of childbearing age who do not have acceptable evidence of rubella immunity or vaccination	• If a pregnant woman is found to be rubella susceptible, administer MMR postpartum	**Note:** HIV positivity is NOT a contraindication to MMR except for those who are severely immunocompromised **Precautions** • If blood, plasma, and/or immune globulin were given in the last 11 mo, see ACIP statement *General Recommendations on Immunization*[c] regarding time to wait before vaccinating • Moderate or severe acute illness • History of thrombocytopenia or thrombocytopenic purpura **Note:** MMR is not contraindicated if a PPD (tuberculosis skin test) was recently applied. If PPD and MMR are both needed but not given on same day, delay PPD for 4–6 wk after MMR

Human-papillomavirus (HPV) *Give i.m.*	All previously unvaccinated women through age 26 yr	• Three doses are needed • Second dose is given 4–8 wk after first dose, and third dose is given 6 mo after first dose (at least 12 wk after second dose)	**Contraindications** Previous anaphylactic reaction to this vaccine or to any of its components **Precautions** Data on vaccination in pregnancy are limited; therefore, vaccination during pregnancy should be delayed until after completion of the pregnancy
Zoster (shingles)[d] (Zos) *Give s.c.*	All persons aged 60 yr and older, including those who have had a previous episode of shingles	• One dose is needed	**Contraindications** • History of anaphylactic reaction to gelatin, neomycin, or any other component of the vaccine • History of primary or acquired immunodeficiency states including leukemia; lymphomas of any type, or other malignant neoplasms affecting the bone marrow or lymphatic system; or AIDS/HIV

(continued)

TABLE 2 *(Continued)*

Vaccine Name and Route	Population For Whom Vaccination Is Recommended	Schedule for Vaccine Administration[a]	Contraindications and Precautions[b]
Zoster (continued)			• On immunosuppressive therapy, including high-dose corticosteroids (defined on page 387) • Active untreated tuberculosis • Pregnancy **Precautions** • Moderate or severe acute illness

Adapted with permission from *Summary of Recommendations for Adult Immunization*, Immunization Action Coalition, St. Paul, MN 2007; available online at: http://www.immunize.org/catg.d/p2011.pdf. Accessed September 2007.

CSF = cerebrospinal fluid; STI = sexually transmitted infection; Td = diphtheria toxoid; IPV = inactivated poliovirus vaccine; VZIG = varicella zoster immunoglobulin; PPD = purified protein derivative.

[a] Any vaccine can be given with another.

[b] Mild illness is not a contraindication.

[c] For specific ACIP recommendations, refer to the official ACIP statements published in *MMWR*. To obtain copies of these statements, call the CDC-INFO Contact Center at (800) 232–4636; visit CDC's website at www.cdc.gov/nip/publications/ACIP-list.htm; or visit the Immunization Action Coalition (IAC) website at www.immunize.org/acip.

[d] Based on the ACIP provisional recommendations of 10-25-06, and the vaccine package insert.

INDEX

Note: Page numbers followed by *f* indicate figures; those followed by *t* indicate tables.